Critical Thinking Study Guide to Accompany

MEDICAL-SURGICAL NURSING
Critical Thinking for Collaborative Care

Fifth Edition

Donna D. Ignatavicius, MS, RN, C
Presenter and Consultant for Nursing Programs
President, DI Associates, Inc.
Placitas, New Mexico

M. Linda Workman, PhD, RN, FAAN
Gertrude Perkins Oliva Professor of Oncology
Frances Payne Bolton School of Nursing
Case Western Reserve University
Cleveland, Ohio

Critical Thinking Study Guide prepared by

Julie S. Snyder, MSN, RN, BC
Adjunct Faculty
School of Nursing
Old Dominion University
Norfolk, Virginia

Linda L. Kerby, RNC, BSN, MA, BA
Educational Consultant
Mastery Educational Consultations
Leawood, Kansas

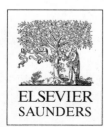

ELSEVIER
SAUNDERS

ELSEVIER
SAUNDERS

11830 Westline Industrial Drive
St. Louis, MO 63146

Notice

Nursing is an ever-changing field. Standard safety precautions must be followed, but as new research and clinical experience broaden our knowledge, changes in treatment and drug therapy may become necessary or appropriate. Readers are advised to check the most current product information provided by the manufacturer of each drug to be administered to verify the recommended dose, the method and duration of administration, and contraindications. It is the responsibility of the licensed health care provider, relying on experience and knowledge of the patient, to determine dosages and the best treatment for each individual patient. Neither the publisher nor the editor assumes any liability for any injury and/or damage to persons or property arising from this publication.

Critical Thinking Study Guide to Accompany *Medical-Surgical Nursing: Critical Thinking for Collaborative Care*, 5th edition

ISBN-13: 978-0-7216-0614-9
ISBN-10: 0-7216-0614-8

Printed in the United States of America

Last digit is the print number: 9 8 7 6 5 4 3

Contents

Preface vii

Tips for Student Success ix
   Diane Herrera Shepard

UNIT I   **HEALTH PROMOTION AND ILLNESS**
Chapter 1   Critical Thinking in the Role of the Medical-Surgical Nurse 1
Chapter 2   Community-Based Care 7
Chapter 3   Introduction to Managed Care and Case Management 11
Chapter 4   Introduction to Complementary and Alternative Therapies in Nursing..................... 15
Chapter 5   Health Care of Older Adults 19

UNIT II   **BIOPSYCHOSOCIAL CONCEPTS RELATED TO HEALTH CARE**
Chapter 6   Cultural Aspects of Health.. 25
Chapter 7   Pain: The Fifth Vital Sign 29
Chapter 8   Substance Abuse 41
Chapter 9   End-of-Life Care 49
Chapter 10   Rehabilitation Concepts for Acute and Chronic Problems...................................... 55
Chapter 11   Genetic Concepts for Medical-Surgical Nursing 63

UNIT III   **CONCEPTS OF EMERGENCY NURSING**
Chapter 12   Emergency and Mass Casualty Nursing.. 69
Chapter 13   Interventions for Clients with Common Environmental Emergencies 75

UNIT IV   **MANAGEMENT OF CLIENTS WITH FLUID, ELECTROLYTE, AND ACID-BASE IMBALANCES**
Chapter 14   Fluid and Electrolyte Balance 85
Chapter 15   Interventions for Clients with Fluid Imbalances.. 93
Chapter 16   Interventions for Clients with Electrolyte Imbalances... 99
Chapter 17   Infusion Therapy 113
Chapter 18   Acid-Base Balance 121
Chapter 19   Interventions for Clients with Acid-Base Imbalances.. 127

UNIT V   **MANAGEMENT OF PERIOPERATIVE CLIENTS**
Chapter 20   Interventions for Preoperative Clients 135
Chapter 21   Interventions for Intraoperative Clients 141
Chapter 22   Interventions for Postoperative Clients... 149

UNIT VI   **PROBLEMS OF PROTECTION: MANAGEMENT OF CLIENTS WITH PROBLEMS OF THE IMMUNE RESPONSE**
Chapter 23   Concepts of Inflammation and the Immune Response.. 155
Chapter 24   Interventions for Clients with Connective Tissue Disease and Other Types of Arthritis.............. 163
Chapter 25   Interventions for Clients with HIV/AIDS and Other Immunodeficiencies 177
Chapter 26   Interventions for Clients with Immune Function Excess: Hypersensitivity (Allergy) and Autoimmunity... 185
Chapter 27   Altered Cell Growth and Cancer Development 193
Chapter 28   General Interventions for Clients with Cancer 199
Chapter 29   Interventions for Clients with Infection 209

UNIT VII **PROBLEMS OF OXYGENATION: MANAGEMENT OF CLIENTS WITH PROBLEMS OF THE RESPIRATORY TRACT**

Chapter 30 Assessment of the Respiratory System 217
Chapter 31 Interventions for Clients Requiring Oxygen Therapy or Tracheostomy 231
Chapter 32 Interventions for Clients with Noninfectious Problems of the Upper Respiratory Tract 245
Chapter 33 Interventions for Clients with Noninfectious Problems of the Lower Respiratory Tract 257
Chapter 34 Interventions for Clients with Infectious Problems of the Respiratory Tract 275
Chapter 35 Interventions for Critically Ill Clients with Respiratory Problems 291

UNIT VIII **PROBLEMS OF CARDIAC OUTPUT AND TISSUE PERFUSION: MANAGEMENT OF CLIENTS WITH PROBLEMS OF THE CARDIOVASCULAR SYSTEM**

Chapter 36 Assessment of the Cardiovascular System 303
Chapter 37 Interventions for Clients with Dysrhythmias 317
Chapter 38 Interventions for Clients with Cardiac Problems 335
Chapter 39 Interventions for Clients with Vascular Problems 349
Chapter 40 Interventions for Clients with Shock 363
Chapter 41 Interventions for Critically Ill Clients with Acute Coronary Syndromes 373

UNIT IX **PROBLEMS OF TISSUE PERFUSION: MANAGEMENT OF CLIENTS WITH PROBLEMS OF THE HEMATOLOGIC SYSTEM**

Chapter 42 Assessment of the Hematologic System 385
Chapter 43 Interventions for Clients with Hematologic Problems 393

UNIT X **PROBLEMS OF MOBILITY, SENSATION, AND COGNITION: MANAGEMENT OF CLIENTS WITH PROBLEMS OF THE NERVOUS SYSTEM**

Chapter 44 Assessment of the Nervous System 405
Chapter 45 Interventions for Clients with Problems of the Central Nervous System: The Brain 413
Chapter 46 Interventions for Clients with Problems of the Central Nervous System: The Spinal Cord 419
Chapter 47 Interventions for Clients with Problems of the Peripheral Nervous System 423
Chapter 48 Interventions for Critically Ill Clients with Neurologic Problems 427

UNIT XI **PROBLEMS OF SENSATION: MANAGEMENT OF CLIENTS WITH PROBLEMS OF THE SENSORY SYSTEM**

Chapter 49 Assessment of the Eye and Vision 437
Chapter 50 Interventions for Clients with Eye and Vision Problems 443
Chapter 51 Assessment of the Ear and Hearing 451
Chapter 52 Interventions for Clients with Ear and Hearing Problems 455

UNIT XII **PROBLEMS OF MOBILITY: MANAGEMENT OF CLIENTS WITH PROBLEMS OF THE MUSCULOSKELETAL SYSTEM**

Chapter 53 Assessment of the Musculoskeletal System 463
Chapter 54 Interventions for Clients with Musculoskeletal Problems 471
Chapter 55 Interventions for Clients with Musculoskeletal Trauma 481

UNIT XIII **PROBLEMS OF DIGESTION, NUTRITION, AND ELIMINATION: MANAGEMENT OF CLIENTS WITH PROBLEMS OF THE GASTROINTESTINAL SYSTEM**

Chapter 56 Assessment of the Gastrointestinal System 491
Chapter 57 Interventions for Clients with Oral Cavity Problems 497
Chapter 58 Interventions for Clients with Esophageal Problems 503
Chapter 59 Interventions for Clients with Stomach Disorders 511
Chapter 60 Interventions for Clients with Noninflammatory Intestinal Disorders 519
Chapter 61 Interventions for Clients with Inflammatory Intestinal Disorders 529
Chapter 62 Interventions for Clients with Liver Problems 539
Chapter 63 Interventions for Clients with Problems of the Biliary System and Pancreas 549
Chapter 64 Interventions for Clients with Malnutrition and Obesity 557

UNIT XIV   **PROBLEMS OF REGULATION AND METABOLISM: MANAGEMENT OF CLIENTS WITH PROBLEMS OF THE ENDOCRINE SYSTEM**

Chapter 65   Assessment of the Endocrine System 565
Chapter 66   Interventions for Clients with Pituitary and Adrenal Gland Problems 575
Chapter 67   Interventions for Clients with Problems of the Thyroid and Parathyroid Glands 587
Chapter 68   Interventions for Clients with Diabetes Mellitus 599

UNIT XV   **PROBLEMS OF PROTECTION: MANAGEMENT OF CLIENTS WITH PROBLEMS OF THE SKIN, HAIR, AND NAILS**

Chapter 69   Assessment of the Skin, Hair, and Nails 613
Chapter 70   Interventions for Clients with Skin Problems 617
Chapter 71   Interventions for Clients with Burns 623

UNIT XVI   **PROBLEMS OF EXCRETION: MANAGEMENT OF CLIENTS WITH PROBLEMS OF THE RENAL/URINARY SYSTEM**

Chapter 72   Assessment of the Renal/Urinary System 633
Chapter 73   Interventions for Clients with Urinary Problems 641
Chapter 74   Interventions for Clients with Renal Disorders 649
Chapter 75   Interventions for Clients with Acute and Chronic Renal Failure 657

UNIT XVII   **PROBLEMS OF REPRODUCTION: MANAGEMENT OF CLIENTS WITH PROBLEMS OF THE REPRODUCTIVE SYSTEM**

Chapter 76   Assessment of the Reproductive System 669
Chapter 77   Interventions for Clients with Breast Disorders 675
Chapter 78   Interventions for Clients with Gynecologic Problems 681
Chapter 79   Interventions for Male Clients with Reproductive Problems 687
Chapter 80   Interventions for Clients with Sexually Transmitted Diseases 693

Preface

The *Critical Thinking Study Guide* is a companion publication for Ignatavicius & Workman's *Medical-Surgical Nursing: Critical Thinking for Collaborative Care*, 5th Edition. This study guide, written by experts in the fields of adult medical-surgical nursing and nursing education, will help to ensure mastery of the textbook content and help you learn about collaborative practice in the care of the adult medical-surgical client.

This revised edition has been redesigned in a more user-friendly, linear format. Additional blank space has been provided so that you can write notes and answers directly on the study guide rather than on a separate sheet of paper.

The overall organization of the *Critical Thinking Study Guide* directly corresponds to the unit/chapter name and number in the textbook so that you or your instructor can readily select the corresponding learning exercises in the study guide. Chapters are organized by the following sections:

- **Learning Outcomes** correspond directly to the Learning Outcomes listed in the textbook. They represent the essential learning outcomes that you should achieve for each chapter.
- **Learning Activities** provide a step-by-step approach for mastering the material. First, key prerequisites are provided for review as needed. Next, you will have the opportunity to review critical terms and their definitions that are highlighted in each chapter. These steps maximize the impact and benefit of the Study/Review Questions that are provided for each chapter.
- **Study/Review Questions** are designed to encourage prioritizing, critical thinking, and application of the steps of the nursing process. They are much more varied in this edition and include cutting-edge information, as well as fun learning activities such as crossword puzzles. Multiple-choice questions are written in NCLEX® Examination style and emphasize delegation, management of care, and pharmacology.
- In addition, more real-world **Case Studies** are presented in this edition, allowing you to further develop your critical thinking abilities in a variety of clinical situations. Also new to the fifth edition is an introductory "pre-chapter" that includes concrete study tips to help you make the most of your individual learning style.

Answers to the Study/Review Questions and Answer Guidelines to the Case Studies, with some rationales and references to the text, are provided on the companion EVOLVE Web site at *http://evolve.elsevier.com/Iggy/*.

The *Critical Thinking Study Guide* is a practical tool to help you prepare for classroom examinations and standardized tests, as well as a review for clinical practice. This improved format will help you obtain a greater understanding of medical-surgical content.

Tips for Student Success

Diane Herrera Shepard, BS, MA
College Instructor
TVI Albuquerque Community College
Albuquerque, New Mexico

INTRODUCTION

Have you ever been in a class, looked around and thought that most of the students in the class were learning more, knew more, or were more effective students than you were? Did you think that they had skills that enabled them to study more easily, remember more, and do better on tests? Well, look no longer. It's time for you to start thinking about yourself as a successful and high achieving student! This Student Success Study Guide, accompanying the text, *Medical-Surgical Nursing: Critical Thinking for Collaborative Care* by Ignatavicius and Workman, will provide you with strategies, tips, and techniques for helping you become an even more successful nursing student. You can further develop or learn to observe, read, write, critically think, and apply your understanding of adult nursing topics to numerous classroom, laboratory, clinical, and professional settings. Becoming an effective student in a nursing program is hard work, but that hard work can be made easier if you can learn to use or continue to develop specific learning and study techniques. You've already proven that you are a capable learner in being admitted to the nursing program. You'll need to apply those skills as well as develop new ones in order to excel in your demanding nursing and clinical classes.

Nursing programs will ask more of you than just refining or learning new study techniques; you'll also be asked to critically think and work with a diverse group of nursing students, instructors, and patients in both academic and clinical settings. Becoming successful in the nursing program is not just important, it is critical to your success in your profession. Consider developing, practicing, and using some of the following student success topics to achieve success in your nursing program:

- Use an "academic tool kit."
- Be an active listener.
- Take effective notes.
- Learn to mark and take notes in your textbooks.
- Read your textbook—and remember what you've read.
- Learn about your learning preferences.
- Improve your memory.
- Be healthy.

YOUR STUDENT SUCCESS "TOOL KIT"

Develop and use an affordable and effective student "tool kit" as you "go to work" in your classes, laboratories, and clinical settings. *Being organized* and having essential study tools will help you succeed in your nursing program. Basic, essential materials needed to manage the vast amounts of information you will encounter in your nursing courses might include the following supplies:

- Three-ring dedicated notebook for each course
- Subject dividers (Always label them.)
  - Syllabus
  - Class notes
  - Text notes
  - Extra paper
- Loose-leaf paper (three-hole punched)
- Index cards (Colored cards are also available.)

- Mini stapler
- Pencils, pens
- Mini, three-hole paper punch that fits in your binder
- Two contrasting color highlighter pens
- Liquid paper
- Zippered, pencil/pen pouch
- Dictionary—minimum 50,000 entries
- Clear, plastic paper protectors
- Removable (or "sticky") notes and/or page flags
- Adhesive hole reinforcers

Many students create personal study systems that work for them in their home study area, library, or classes. You might consider a way to make your tools portable for use in any study area. Some students carry basic items in a pocket in their backpack; others place everything in a three-ring, zippered pouch inside their notebook. Develop a system for yourself that includes easy access and use of your "student success tools."

An important aspect of using your tool kit successfully is to go through it daily, adding or deleting pages, updating projects, restocking supplies, and organizing it so it's ready for the next day. Your tool kit may be your most important organizational tool. It keeps your materials and supplies at hand so you can use it "at work." Creating and using your binder effectively can help improve grades, increase participation, and build confidence. Here are some notebook essentials:

Use one binder for each course. You will be taking extensive notes and receiving many handouts for each course. Carrying a semester's worth of notes, handouts, and old quizzes or exams can get heavy.

Identify your binder. Keep your name and phone number on the inside front cover for easy identification in case it gets lost or left behind in class.

Use a calendar. Keep a month-at-a-glance calendar in the front of your binder or in your backpack and refer to it several times a day. Write all assignments on the date they're due. To create more writing space, use removable notes. One problem is that many students keep several calendars. Some have a calendar at home for personal appointments and events, a calendar in their backpack, calendars for separate courses, and some keep a family calendar on the refrigerator. All these calendars can cause confusion. Try to consolidate all your calendars into *one master* calendar and carry it with you at all times. Refer to that calendar for *all* events, appointments, class assignments, exams, and personal needs. If necessary, create other calendars for home or work by copying information from your master calendar. Keep your master calendar current keep it with you at all times, and refer to it several times a day.

Section your binder by using color-tabbed subject dividers. Colored subject dividers help keep your binder and class requirements organized and easily accessible. Label each section. Common section dividers include the following: Course Syllabus, Notes, Homework, Study Group Information, New Paper, and Special Projects.

Use clear vinyl sheet protectors. Protect, organize, and use important course handouts by keeping them in sheet protectors. They won't fall out of your binder or get lost. Frequently referenced handouts stand out and can be used over and over without destroying the page.

Carry a three-hole punch. Place a small notebook-style three-hole punch in the front of your binder. When receiving a course handout, immediately three-hole punch it, *date it*, and place it in the appropriate section.

Use a zippered plastic pouch or bag. Keep a small zippered bag to store pencils, pens, mini stapler, paperclips, removable notes, index cards, and other organizational tools.

Use loose-leaf paper. With the number of handouts you'll receive in your nursing classes, keeping them organized can be a major task. Use loose-leaf paper in a binder to store notes, handouts, and course materials. Many students choose to use spiral-bound notebooks. Unfortunately, these do not allow for the addition or deletion of notes, handouts, tests, or other class materials. As a result, important course materials can get lost. With a portable three-hole punch and a three-ring binder, you can organize your course paper-work so you can locate essential information and use it when necessary. For example, instructor-prepared handouts can help you understand key concepts and old exams can become important tools when studying for finals.

Carry a dictionary. New, lightweight, binder-sized dictionaries are now available. You can purchase three-hole punched dictionaries for placement in a notebook binder. Make sure it has enough entries for your skill level. In the nursing program, you'll need a dictionary that has more than 50,000 entries. Improve your vocabulary and writing skills!

Locate new paper easily. Dedicate one section of the notebook for new paper. It's easier to go to one section than thumb through several sections to find a new sheet of paper.

Use colored, ruled paper. Some students choose to use colored paper to reduce light glare or to organize different topics or subjects. You might find it easier to locate a specific subject or topic by color. Pastel-colored paper is available at stationery stores.

Keep quizzes and tests in the same section as the subject. Don't lump all quizzes into one "test" section. Old tests can be helpful for review for a future test or final exam. Keeping them in the same section as the topic helps you locate them more easily

File your old notes. When a particular unit or topic is completed, staple together all notes, including tests, and file in a file cabinet or plastic storage box. Don't throw away old course mate-rials. They can be used for future reference and study.

Organize and work on your binder daily. Check your paper supply. Plan ahead for tomor-row's activities. Keep your notebook up to date.

Put it where you can find it. Put your binder in the same place daily after completion of homework or study. Having everything in place before you go to bed makes it easier in the morn-ing to grab your materials and go, knowing that you have everything you'll need for classes.

Becoming more organized is a key skill that will help you make sense of all the materials and tools you will be using in a nursing program. Re-search tells us that students who are organized tend to get higher grades. So take some time *before* the start of the term to get organized. Avoid the crowds, reduce your "beginning-of-the-term" stress by being ready with the tools that will serve you best. Buy the supplies you need and personalize your binder for immediate use the first day of the term. Being organized also impresses your instructors, so impress yourself and your teachers by being ready to take in, use, and remember essential information. Now that you're organized, you'll need to use those tools to actively listen to and record class, lab, and clinical notes.

ACTIVE LISTENING AND NOTE TAKING

Actively listening and taking effective class notes are two of the most effective keys to academic success. Your notes not only contain lecture content, but may also include course informa-tion, text notes, lab notes, diagrams, mind maps, assignments, and review information to prepare for quizzes and exams. Based on the style you use to take notes, the information you write down and remember will largely be the questions you'll face on quizzes and exams. If you have difficulty taking notes or if you don't think that your notes are effective, show your notes to your instructor or an academic advisor. Ask him or her if you're capturing essential lecture information. There are different note taking styles to help you record and remember critical course information. If your note taking is not as effective as it should be, try a different method and explore styles that you may enjoy using and that will serve you better.

Active listening and note taking are not just han-dy tools for remembering important information, they are essential job skills. Note taking itself fa-cilitates learning and recall of lecture material.

Dale's Cone of Learning (see figure) is often used to show how students can retain more informa-tion when they become active learners. *Active learners* are those who get involved in gathering, participating, and remembering essential information. The more you physically do, say, and hear (or mentally rehearse) while learning new information, the more you will remember. We sometimes call this *multisensory learning*. Examples include speaking while reading, explain-

ing while looking at a diagram or picture, or critically thinking while looking at a slide or visual presentation. Each of these processes helps us connect new information in our brain by stimulating more than one sense. **The more you participate, the more you will remember.**

Dale's Cone of Experience and Learning

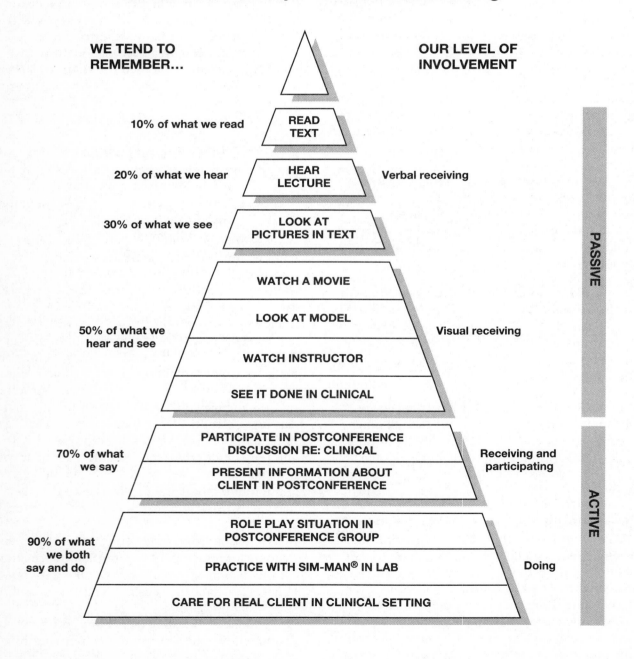

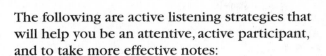

The following are active listening strategies that will help you be an attentive, active participant, and to take more effective notes:

Plan to be an active listener. You must *want* to be a better listener and view listening as a participative rather than a passive process. Sit up straight, lean forward, have your essential materials with you, and plan to listen for key or main ideas. Then, if you have enough time, try to add some details or an explanation to the main idea.

Keep an open mind about the course content. Students sometimes make up their mind about an idea, procedure, or information being presented before listening to a lecture. You may or may not agree with an idea or you may possibly know something about the topic, but you need to be able to give it your full attention and take notes that will help you understand the concept more fully. Be open to new information, new points of view, different styles of lecturing, and new ideas. Research tells us that if a student believes that he or she already knows the material, then the student will likely divert his or her attention elsewhere. Such students will stop listening, reading, working, or participating because they believe they already "know the answer" and they stop paying attention. This can happen in lectures or while reading a textbook. Keep your mind open and actively listen for key points.

Observe and pay attention to details. As you listen and take notes, observe your instructor and watch for obvious verbal and nonverbal clues as to what information may be important. If your instructor spends a lot of time talking about a concept, it's obviously important. If your instructor writes information on the board, uses overhead transparencies, or pays special attention to a diagram, list, or idea, be sure to write down that information. Instructors often raise the level of their voice, smile, move, or get excited when they explain a key concept. Watch them! If it's important to them, it should be important for you to write down.

Arrive to class a little early. Instructors often talk about the class plans, answer questions, and provide extra information before class. You can also ask questions and prepare yourself for the lecture. Take out your materials, review your notes, open your textbook, if appropriate, and be ready when the lecture starts. Your instructor will notice your efforts!

Determine where and how you learn best. Even before the class starts, you have probably made some subconscious decisions about where and how you take in and learn new information. Become conscious of these decisions and begin to ask yourself a few questions about your study location preferences:

- Where do you usually like to sit in a lecture or lab? Do you tend to sit near the front or back, near a window, near a door, or near friends?
- Where can you best see the instructor and hear the lecture?
- What about lighting? Do you prefer sitting under a light, a dim area, or in the bright light near a window?
- How do you control your temperature? Bring a sweater if it's cold or sit by an open window if it's warm.
- Are you hydrated? Bring bottled water with you and sip throughout the lecture, if allowed. Always ask your instructor about bringing water, snacks, or beverages into the classroom or lab.
- What kind of chair do you prefer? Although not always available, some newer classrooms offer adjustable chairs. Feel free to adjust yours to a height and angle that is comfortable.
- Are you able to reduce distractions and noise? For example, even though cell phones are not allowed in clinical settings, students do carry them to class. They have become major distractions for instructors as well as students. As a courtesy to others, turn off your cell phone during class. If necessary, check for phone messages before or after class.

By answering these questions, you will start to consciously make decisions about where and how you like to work in a classroom. We know that students who are actively involved—those who sit near the front of the class, actively make eye contact with the instructor, ask questions, participate in group work, or volunteer to comment—tend to be more successful in classes compared to students who do not actively participate. Be involved, active, and alert! Research shows that students who sit in the front of the class are able to listen more effectively, take better notes, be more involved, and, as a result, receive higher grades.

Participate! More and more, instructors are using critical thinking, collaborative, and problem-solving activities in classes. Groups are often formed to discuss and consider possible solutions to a problem, condition, or nursing situation. Participate in these groups with enthusiasm. You will find that sharing ideas and solving problems in small groups will enhance your learning and create opportunities to discuss nursing practices. It will also help you learn to make clinical decisions that may require critical thinking.

As you learn to actively listen and participate in your classes you will need to pair those skills with actually recording information from lectures, labs, individual study, and study groups. Being able to take effective notes is based on active listening, maintaining a positive and active attitude, and knowing how to use specific note taking strategies for different types of subjects, topics, and settings. To enhance your ability to take effective notes, consider using some of the popular styles used in adult classrooms today.

STRATEGIES FOR TAKING EFFECTIVE NOTES

Why take notes? Some students believe they can remember important information presented in classes by simply listening and occasionally jotting down a word or two. Learning how to take effective notes is one of the most powerful memory tools we can acquire and use. As a student, you can learn effective strategies that can improve your ability to "pull out" essential information from a lecture or text, remember more, and help you perform better on quizzes and exams.

You can take notes in a variety of ways. The important thing is to take notes! Students who are actively trying to identify key points or main ideas while listening to a lecture are more successful in recording that information on paper than those who sit back and assume that they will remember everything they heard. We now know that we remember more when we're actively involved.

To record and use your notes for effective study, consider the following:

- Arrive at your class early. Take out your materials. Get ready to take notes.
- Sit where you can see and hear the instructor. Watch the instructor for note taking clues. For example, if the instructor writes something on the board, write it down. If the instructor presents information on an overhead projector or computerized projector, write it down. If the instructor repeats a concept or point, write it down. If the instructor spends a lot of time explaining a concept, write it down. The key is to recognize that your instructors spend a great deal of time preparing lectures. If they're working hard to present those concepts to you, write them down!
- Use a three-ring binder.
- Label, date, and number each page.
- Use an established system or develop your own.

There are many systems for taking notes. However, no single method is best. Some students make lists, write outlines, draw mind maps, develop concept maps, create diagrams, or tape record their lectures. Some use more formal systems including the SQ3R System (Survey, Question, Read, Recite, Review) and the Cornell System of Note Taking. Experiment with a variety of systems to find one or more that work well for you. One of the most popular and effective ways to take notes is to use the Cornell System of Note Taking. This system is widely used in schools and colleges. Created by Walter Pauk of Cornell University, it was originally developed for soldiers returning to college after World War II. It has become one of the most used and successful systems developed. It is important to try not only this system, but also other popularly used systems to familiarize yourself with a variety of ways to record and remember information. The following description demonstrates the Cornell System of Note Taking format.

When using the Cornell System, use any standard sheet of paper (see diagram) and re-draw your left margin line about an inch to the right of the original red line. You can carefully draw it using a ruler or simply draw a quick freehand line down the paper. This expands the left side of the paper to allow you to write down key words, main points, definitions, mind maps, and important concepts. Use the entire right margin to write details. Summarize notes in one or two sentences at the bottom of the sheet. Develop questions from your main points. *These are your exam questions.*

Subject: <u>Cornell Note Taking Example</u>   Date _____

Main Ideas	Details
——— 2 1/2 inch column ———	————————— 6 inch column —————————
Cornell Notes	• Organized by main ideas and details • Helps you listen for and record main ideas • Easy to use • Diagrams and mind maps easy to include • Write only on one side • Leave lots of white space on page • When ready to study, remove selected pages and lay them on a table—exposing only the left column. These are your test questions!
In this column, write main ideas, key words, important points, definitions, or diagrams.	
Create a Mind Map or Concept Map 	• Can be used to provide a "big picture" of a chapter, lecture, or lab procedure • Organized by main ideas and subtopics • Very visual • Provides a quick overview • Promotes clinical correlation mapping
Summary:	Write one or two sentences here to summarize the page.

Other important points to remember about taking effective notes follow. Work to develop these skills and you will become more successful in recording and using your notes to study for tests, review important concepts, and create notes for future study and reference.

- Develop a positive attitude.
- Decide which supplies work best for you. Do you prefer pencils, pens, mechanical pens, color highlighters, or specialized paper? Use color, if helpful, but don't create a "coloring book" look to your notes.
- Plan to be active! Look for opportunities to write down a main idea or key points.
- Examine your pencil grip. Do you write with ease? If necessary, learn to adjust your grip to prevent pain and write more effectively. Many of us have forgotten what we learned about handwriting in grade school. Using a three-finger, gentle hold will allow you to take notes without the "pain." You can write more effectively if you're writing with a relaxed, comfortable style.
- Write quickly.
- Write as neatly as possible.
- Use good posture. Try to sit up and lean forward. Keep your feet on the floor.
- Always keep a pen or pencil in your hand. Be ready.
- Listen for and write down key points or ideas.
- Summarize key points.
- Use mind maps. Using pictures and diagrams in your notes helps you remember information as you organize your ideas.
- Draw diagrams or pictures.
- Use arrows to join ideas.
- Write down notes from the board or from charts.
- Use standard abbreviations. Abbreviations can be helpful when your instructor is talking rapidly. Use standard scientific symbols in math and science lectures. Leave out short words such as "a," "the," and "and," or leave out adjectives and word endings.

- Try not to tape record your lectures or use shorthand unless necessary. Transcribing your notes and listening to tapes takes too long. Generally you won't have the time. If you have trouble keeping up with the speed of the lecture, talk with your instructor or academic advisor for some suggestions. Also consider asking fellow study group members or other classmates to share a copy of their notes with you.
- Keep your calendar nearby. You will often be asked to write down important dates for tests, important reviews, study group sessions, and the like.

REVIEW, REVIEW, REVIEW

We tend to forget much of what we've heard almost immediately. You will remember more if you review several times a day for short periods of time. Develop a system of frequent review. Start to review immediately after class. Actively listening and taking notes in your lectures and labs will help you organize, retrieve, and remember more information. But classtime is not the only time to take notes. Consider marking in and taking notes from your textbooks.

EFFECTIVELY MARKING AND TAKING NOTES FROM YOUR TEXTBOOKS

Effectively marking and taking notes from your textbooks can help you more easily read and remember important information as well as to locate key words, important ideas, and concepts. It can also help you save time. You'll enjoy taking, organizing, and reviewing your text notes when you know they contain essential text information that you can quickly access for test preparation or future reference. Using them for individual, group study, or major reviews, your notes will reinforce major concepts and help you remember key information. Marking your textbooks helps you concentrate and be purposeful in your efforts to learn new information. Because you will read vast amounts of information from a variety of nursing and medical texts, it is important to develop and use a system that helps you organize and access specific information from your texts and from your class and lab notes. Marking your textbooks can be important in helping you identify key ideas and improve your retention of a variety of course reading material. Thinking critically as you read is an essential nursing skill. Critically thinking is also important as you read your textbook. You must decide and judge what to highlight, underline, or add in the margins of your textbook.

Marking your text as you read is a multilevel approach to learning. You are using your vision to identify key text, selecting color to stimulate retention, and feeling your muscles move as you write or mark. You might also be verbalizing important information as you mark text. This combined effect can strengthen the retention of important information.

Your job is to be an active and critically thinking learner. That is, you need to use clinical thinking or judgment in a variety of academic and practical settings. Taking effective notes from your textbook is a critical nursing skill that will enable you to more easily locate and retain essential clinical information.

Almost exclusively, nursing students use the popular technique of highlighting to mark their texts. In addition to highlighting your text, there are other strategies you can use to identify and locate key information. Here are some tips to consider when marking and taking notes from your texts:

- **Select just one highlighter pen for highlighting.** You can also use a pen or pencil for underlining, if you choose. Yellow is often best for highlighting. Darker colored highlighters are often too dark for ease of reading. Frequently they bleed through the page and make the other side of the page difficult to read. Some students are afraid of marking their textbooks because they plan to sell them back to the bookstore at the end of the term. You paid a lot of money for your nursing textbooks. Keep them as valuable

investments and part of your professional nursing library. You'll use them over and over for future study and reference. *Mark your texts—make them yours!*

- **Highlight or underline to identify a key word, main idea, passage, or important point that you may want to remember or read again.**
- **If necessary, use a second, contrasting highlighter color for cross-referencing information.** To cross-reference, use a second highlighter color that will allow you to "connect" a similar concept or idea presented in one text to another text. Use a specific-colored highlighter to indicate the importance of a passage. Then use that same colored highlighter in another text passage to indicate that the concepts are related to each other. Cross-referencing helps you organize information between different textbooks, reference books, or other classes or labs. The use of color can be a wonderful learning tool. Use color to help you identify, cross reference, or remember key concepts.
- **Read before you mark.** Completely read the passage, sentence, or paragraph. Think about what's important to mark or underline before actually marking.
- **Be consistent.** Standardize the use of your highlighting. Use the same color to represent the same level or importance in each chapter, passage, book, or notes.
- **Avoid the "coloring book syndrome."** Don't highlight everything on the page and don't use every color highlighter you own to mark your text. Using too many highlighter colors can be more confusing than helpful.
- **Avoid highlighting chapter headings.** The headings in your text are already bolded and color coded for you.
- **Be aware of colored legends and figures used in chapters.** Your text headings, subheadings, and clinical notations are already highlighted or

underlined for you. Learn what the text box colors mean. Use them as a guide while you read. There is no need to highlight them again.

- **Survey your textbook format.** Understand the color coding, highlighting, and use of graphics, charts, tables, boxed information, and "Best Practices" inserts to recognize important information discussed in the body of the text. Refer to the **Guide to Special Features** section, located in the front matter of *Medical-Surgical Nursing: Critical Thinking for Collaborative Care,* 5th Edition

- **Use standard abbreviations and symbols in the margins.** Be consistent and use the same abbreviations and symbols in all of your texts and notes to reduce confusion. The following abbreviations may be helpful as you develop a system that allows you to take notes quickly and accurately:

pt.	patient	**re:**	regarding
e.g.	for example	**rltnshp**	relationship
>	greater than	**w/o**	without
<	less than	**i.e.**	that is
↑	increase	**sgnft**	significant
↓	decrease	**mo**	month
f	frequency	**mos**	months
anlys	analysis	**etc.**	in addition

- **Use removable notes and/or page flags sparingly.** Having too many "stickies" on a page can make your text confusing to read.

- **Simplify your margin notes.** Don't attempt to write everything in the margins. Work to identify and mark key words and points. Consider taking notes from your text by creating "text notes" that are placed in your notebook. Organize these so your lecture notes and text notes are labeled, dated, and placed in the appropriate section of your notebook. When you pull them out of your binder for study, they can

easily be identified and later returned to their original location.

- **Create study cards or review sheets.** Attempt to pull out essential information from your text and notes when creating review materials. The process of creating these materials actually strengthens your memory and test-taking skills. Remember to be consistent with the use of color when creating these study tools. To make study cards, use mini (half size) standard 3- by 5-inch or 6- by 8-inch blank index cards. Write only on one side and label each card with the topic and card number (if you drop them or separate them, you can put them in order again). Write clearly and include key words. Carry these cards with you at all times and take advantage of "mini moments" in your day to quickly review essential information. An easy way to organize them is to punch a hole in the upper left hand corner and put them on a binder ring. These can be snapped open for adding or deleting cards. You can buy binder rings at any stationery store.

- **Be organized!** Keep your text notes in the same section as your class notes. When you review your notes, you'll have information on the same topic from a variety of sources. This might include class notes, text notes, handouts, or information regarding a nursing procedure.

- **Label each page with the date, text, topic, chapter number, and page numbers.** This helps organize your notes and makes it easier for review and test preparation.

- **Use both your class notes and text notes for studying.** If you've taken effective text notes and/or prepared study cards, you won't have to refer to your text again as you study for the test.

- **Be neat when you take notes from your text.** Take time to write clearly. If your handwriting is hard to read, consider printing.

- **Use colored paper.** Some students prefer to use another color of standard 8½- by 11-inch paper to differentiate their text notes from course notes. Several different pastel colors are available from school supply stores.
- **Use standard or legal-sized paper that is three-hole punched and that fits in your binder.**

Taking notes from your text is an important part of recording and remembering important information. If this technique is new to you, you may find it helpful in organizing and remembering key clinical information. The key to taking notes from your text is to pull out main ideas, major terms, or explanations that will help you recall information for use on exams or for use in a clinical setting. Try to create pictures, drawings, or symbols with your text notes. You can make some information even more memorable by creating a ridiculous picture, mnemonic, or memory trick. Some legal-sized paper has a wider margin on the left that allows you to write down key ideas. Corresponding details are written on the right side. This technique is sometimes called the Cornell Style of Note Taking. (See note-taking section.) The following is an example of how you can take Cornell style notes from your text.

Notes from Iggy Text P. 840

Myocardial Infarction
9/30/2005

Myocardial infarction	Happens when heart tissue is quickly and severely deprived of O_2
% blood flow reduced	80%-90% then <u>ischemia</u> develops. Can lead to necrosis of MI tissue if blood flow not restored
Result of MIs	atherosclerosis of coronary artery rupture of plaque thrombosis occlusion of blood flow
Other factors implicated	coronary artery spasm platelet aggregation emboli from mural thrombi
How MIs begin	Infarction (necrosis) of the subendocardial layer of cardiac muscle Cardial layer has longest myofibrils & greatest O_2 demand, poorest O_2 supply
2 zones around initial area of infarction	1. zone of injury 2. zone of ischemia
See figure 41-2 in text	
Summary see p. 841 re: zones	MI occurs when MC tissue is deprived of O_2. Ischemia devs. Most MIs result of atherosclerosis and other factors.

Becoming an effective listener and note taker will be essential to your success in the nursing program. You'll need to record information for future course and professional applications. If you haven't developed an effective style that you enjoy using, experiment using other styles. Your program advisor or counselor can help you select a style. Often, your note taking preference will reflect learning styles that you have developed or used throughout the years.

YOU'VE GOT STYLE

You've got style, all right—learning style, that is. We all have preferred ways of learning and retaining information. It's important that you become aware of your preferred style or styles of learning so you can better retain and use information from your classes. It's also important to know and accept that others, including your instructors, have preferred ways of learning and teaching. We use our learning styles to become aware of information around us. Some of us observe, reflect, think, hear, touch, do, or use our minds and bodies to identify or make sense of information. When we find ourselves naturally using a particular style, it's a signal that we're most comfortable learning in that mode. Many of us use more than one mode of learning, that is, *multimodal* or *multisensory learning*.

An easy way to start understanding how you learn best is to take a quick learning preference survey. There are many learning preference surveys and inventories that can help you identify your preferred ways of learning. Some are self-administered and quick; others require professional application and interpretation. You may have already experienced the opportunity to explore your learning preferences in a previous career or student success class. If so, review the information and put those preferences to work. When you learn in a preferred style, learning will take less effort and you'll remember more.

See your nursing advisor or counselors at your school to explore learning tools for identifying your learning styles. You can even access a variety of learning style inventories on the Internet. Look under "learning style inventories" and find

a survey that's interesting to you. (One popular example is the VARK questionnaire, which can be accessed at *http://vark-learn.com/english/page.asp?p=questionnaire*.) The inventories are easy to take and score. You'll be amazed at how much more you can learn when you study and use information in your preferred mode. Determine whether you like to study alone or with others, or if you like to study with food, music, bright light, dim light, noise, quiet, or a host of other study arrangements.

You've probably already become aware that there will be times when your learning style does not match those of your instructors, study group partners, or clinical teams. Instructors, clinicians, and others also have preferred ways of learning—and of teaching. Be patient and understanding of how you and others learn. Talk to your instructors outside of class. Talk with them about their preferred styles of teaching. Observe them as they teach and learn more about how they use their preferred learning styles to teach. As you meet with other students or study groups, discuss your preferred styles and develop a plan for completing class work. Just being aware that someone teaches or learns in a different style than your own is helpful. From there you can make decisions about how you might adapt your usual way of learning. For example, you might be asked to do an oral presentation in class. If your preference is to research and present a project by writing about it, you can talk with your instructor about doing both. Write out the project and use it as a preparation for delivering it orally in class. If given an assignment to write a paper about a particular topic and your preference is to present it verbally, consider talking into a tape recorder (your natural preference) then write down what you said.

You can become a more effective learner when you are aware of how you and others take in and use information. With practice, observations, and effort, you'll come to understand and successfully use your learning preferences to achieve greater learning—not to mention improved grades! Successful students take responsibility for what and how they learn. Being a "victim" to someone else's style won't help you succeed. You'll need to be flexible and understanding of each of your styles of learning and learning preferences. Understanding and using your learning preferences also has another advantage—you'll remember more. Many nursing students struggle with the vast amount of information presented to them in a variety of teaching styles in lectures, labs, and clinical classes. Remembering new terminology, lists, details, facts, procedures, and key concepts in nursing is a big challenge. The next section discusses memory tools and techniques that you can develop and use to improve your recall of important course and exam information.

IMPROVE YOUR MEMORY

We've all forgotten information we thought we knew—especially on exams. Recalling important information is largely a matter of developing a positive attitude about having a good memory. Many of us apologize because we think we don't have a good memory. The good news is that you do have a great memory—you just need to believe it. You'll also need to learn and apply specific memory techniques to the notes and text information you've written in your class notes. Fortunately this can be fun and easy to master. Here are some "memory tips" that will make it easier for you to recall information.

- Decide to remember.
- Organize the information (take, use, and file notes).
- Use specific memory strategies.
- Use memory tricks—mnemonics.
- Practice, practice, practice.
- Use your own words to recite, recite, recite!

Decide to Remember

You can remember more by "deciding to remember" and creating a positive attitude about developing a great memory. This might sound a bit odd but deciding that you want to remember can create the positive attitude that you need to retain and use information. Samuel Johnson once said that "The true art of memory is the art of attention." If you decide to remember more, pay attention, and focus on specific information of interest to you, you *will* remember more.

Memory is a process of using a variety of strategies to recall specific past events or information. Your job is to use your preferred learning style to learn the information, then use memory strategies to retrieve that information.

By establishing a positive approach to remembering more, you'll soon find yourself developing and using effective memory techniques that work for you. The result will be greater personal confidence, higher exam scores, and better grades.

Organize the Information

It's important to put all your collected notes, course materials, and study materials in some kind of order. By putting your course materials in one binder and labeling the sections, you can find anything you need. Your recall of information will increase when your mind "knows" where specific materials are stored. Some students organize their notes by color coding, highlighting, labeling, filing, or sequencing them for quick access and study.

Use Specific Memory Strategies

Try using some of the following strategies to enhance your learning:

- **Decide what you want to remember.** "Remember to remember." Make a conscious decision to remember specific information.
- **Develop a positive attitude!** How many of you tell others that you have a "terrible" memory and can't remember anything? Start telling people that you have an excellent memory! You'll start believing it too!
- **Stay alert and study in short sessions.** Study for 15 to 20 minutes, then take a break by standing, walking, drinking some water, or stretching. Research tells us that adult students can actively attend for about 15 to 20 minutes at a time. Complete a short study session then take a mini break. These short, focused sessions can be very effective for increasing your opportunities to remember more.

- **Reduce distractions.** "Turn off" common distractions like the TV, radio, or computer and "turn on" your attention. Try to concentrate on just one idea, concept, or procedure for a few minutes of focused studying. A few minutes of studying in a quiet place can be worth a few hours of studying in front of a TV or other distracters. Those of you with children know that this may be the only kind of studying you can do—short, focused study sessions while the children are playing or resting.
- **Use your preferred learning style or study method.**
- **Organize your information by creating mind maps or visual organizers.** Use colored index cards, a summary sheet, flash cards, or lists.
- **Be active and participate in your learning.** Don't just sit in class—take notes, ask questions. Form or join a study group. Get involved! Study groups, study partners, and other group tutoring offers students an opportunity to "hear" and "speak." Putting your ideas into your own words can improve your recall by 90%. The more active and involved you are while learning, the more you will be able to recall specific information.
- **Talk out loud to yourself.** You'll remember more when you're using more than one learning mode. Practice remembering information by *using your own words*.
- **Use as many learning modes as you can.** For example, while out walking, practice reciting the main point of a chapter. Consider tutoring a fellow student. You'll learn more because you're actively rehearsing and putting the ideas into your own words. Speak while you read; say important points while reading and highlighting in your textbook.
- **Ask yourself questions about what you've read in a text or heard in a lecture.**

- **Create visual associations.** Associate a new piece of information with a picture or image to help you create an association. For example, to remember the meaning of an aneurysm, think about a balloon.
- **Spark your interest in a subject.** When you get excited about a topic or idea, you tend to remember more about it.
- **Create and listen to audiotapes.** Tape record possible exam questions, leave a five second silence, and then say the answer. You'll be able to easily prepare practice tapes that you can listen to in your car or while walking or exercising. Endless loop tapes with different amounts of time are available at a variety of electronics stores.
- **Use note cards.** Frequent review of main points works. Consider drawing a diagram, describing a procedure, or putting a key point on each card.

Use Memory Tricks

Memory tricks or *mnemonics* can be used to help you remember long lists, dates, numbers, or terminology. Some of the most common forms follow:

Acronyms. Examples include:

SCUBA—**s**elf-**c**ontained **u**nderwater **b**reathing **a**pparatus

PEMDAS—**p**arentheses, **e**xponents, **m**ultiplication, **d**ivision, **a**ddition, and **s**ubtraction (the order of operations in math)

IPMAT—**i**nterphase, **p**rophase, **m**etaphase, **a**naphase, and **t**elophase (the stages of cell division)

ABC—**a**irway, **b**reathing, **c**irculation

Rhymes. Rhymes can be fun to compose and they're easy to remember. To remember the 12 cranial nerves (CNs), learn this rhyme: On Old Olympus Towering Tops A French and German Viewed Some Hops. Each upper case letter corresponds to the first letter of the 12 cranial nerves.

For example, CN I is *ol*factory, CN II is *oc*ulomotor, and so on.

Acrostics. The first letters of the words in the sentence "Every good boy does fine" helps us remember the music notes of the lines of the treble clef staff.

Association. Try to associate a memorable event with a date. For example, maybe 1995 was the year you graduated from high school. Or, you may remember a phone number because of the way it looks when you press the buttons on the keypad. For example, 321-3669 is easy to remember because when dialed, the buttons you push go across and down. That layout is a visual reminder of the phone number.

Memory cue. Choose specific information you want to remember, then create a cue or silly sentence. For example, if you want to remember the three main areas of genetics, that is, biochemical (molecular), mendelian, and population genetics, you could create a silly sentence like this: "Biochemical moles mend their population." It's easier to remember a sentence rather than a list. You could also create a memory cue to remember that a cubic foot of water weighs 95 lb: "At age 95, I drank a cubic foot of water."

Visualize a new piece of information in a ridiculous way. Exaggerate a mental picture of the information you want to learn or make it out of proportion. Then practice seeing that ridiculous picture mentally throughout the day. You'll remember it because it stands out in a unique way. For example, when you want to remember the Nutritional Checklist Warning Signs, described by the acronym "DETERMINE," create an image of a "*determined*" person whose "look" includes the characteristics in the list: **d**isease, **e**ating poorly, **t**ooth loss, **e**conomic hardship, **r**educed social contact, **m**ultiple medicines, **i**nvoluntary weight loss/gain, **n**eeds assistance in self care, **e**lder years older than age 80. "Seeing" that person in your mind associated with characteristics you want to remember will aid you in remembering that long list.

While reading your nursing text, look for opportunities to visualize the boxed features, charts, tables, or diagrams. Try to make them ridiculous. Make them stand out!

Practice, Practice, Practice

Review everyday! Short, frequent reviews can be more effective than sitting down to study for hours at a time.

Recite, Recite, Recite

Talk to yourself out loud. Summarize out loud. Discuss out loud. Sing about it. Talk about it. Be creative about practicing out loud. It works! Practice speaking as you write, create diagrams, draw mind maps, use charts, create lists, or practice clinical procedures.

Creating a positive attitude, organizing your information, using a variety of strategies, and frequently practicing out loud can help you remember more. Having a more effective memory is largely a matter of practice and using techniques that work for you. As you practice using some of these techniques, you'll find yourself relying on them for lifelong personal and professional applications in the field of nursing.

BE HEALTHY

You've made it into the nursing program! Now, you need to survive the demanding requirements to succeed! Maintaining your health and having enough energy to sustain the long class, lab, clinical practice, and study sessions will be extremely important. Actively listening, taking effective notes, participating, remembering incredible amounts of information, and studying daily are energy-draining tasks. Ask yourself if you are regularly eating nutritious foods, sleeping enough to be refreshed, resolving stress issues, and exercising. You'll need to maintain a balance between school and home demands. We all know about good health habits but we often need to be reminded about some of the simple methods for maintaining good health. Here are some tips to help you maintain good health.

- Eat a variety of nutritious foods that are home prepared (if possible) to control nutrient content and reduce costs.

- Be aware that you need to maintain regular and sufficient sleep.
- Use or develop strategies to reduce stress experienced at work, school, or home.
- Exercise to improve strength, manage your body weight, and maintain good cardiovascular health.

Many nursing students say they don't have enough time or money to regularly eat a variety of nutritious foods. Are you one of those who hurry to class without eating in the morning? Concentrating on an empty stomach during those long lecture, lab, or clinical classes can be very difficult. Sometimes students just suffer—waiting for a break at lunch. Some rely on vending machines to provide them with quick, generally nonnutritious, and often expensive candy bars, chips, or soft drinks. We all know these snacks are no substitute for healthy foods, so why not start the day with a "Power Smoothie"!

Jumpstart your day with a nutritious, easy-to-make, and low-cost breakfast that will provide you with enough energy to last until lunch. Consider making a Power Smoothie. A recent TV show featuring a member of the Stanford University Men's Swim Team talked about preparing a breakfast that helped team members compete successfully in and out of the pool. Here's the recipe. It doesn't require any special skill—just an interest in staying healthy. Try it for an easy and fun way to eat breakfast "on the go."

Equipment: blender

Ingredients: 1 to 2 cups juice, milk, water, or yogurt

1 banana (can be frozen)

1/2 to 1 cup oatmeal

Any ripe seasonal, frozen, or dried fruits

1/4 cup protein powder (any flavor, any brand)

Ice cubes

Extras: Cinnamon, honey, wheat germ, peanut butter, chocolate, etc.

Note: The amount of ingredients you use is up to you. You can add several pieces of fruit or just one or two. Include foods that appeal to you. Try to use fruits that are in season.

Method: The night before classes, set out your blender. Measure out the oatmeal, protein powder, dried fruits, or other nonliquid ingredients and place them in the blender. In the morning, just add fruits, liquid, ice, and extras. Turn on the blender. Mix for about 30 seconds to one minute. Add a straw and you've got breakfast in hand. You can even take it with you (although not recommended if you're driving). If you have a family at home, make an extra blender-full for them.

Almost any combination of the ingredients will do the job. You'll find that shopping for fruit and other smoothie ingredients once a week or so will take very little time and the cost will be minimal. Experiment with different fruits, ingredients, and amounts. You can't make a mistake! Enjoy a quick and nutritious way to start the day.

Other ways to keep your energy going throughout your long days—and sometimes nights—are to pack "trail mix" baggies with nuts, raisins, dried cranberries, and other dried fruits. These are also inexpensive to prepare. Select your favorite nuts, dried fruits, dried coconut, raisins, or other nutritious dried foods to take along for breaks between classes. And don't forget to take some water with you. Buy a "backpack" style water container. It won't leak, break, and can be put in the dishwasher. Fill it with water from home and take it with you. You'll always have something to drink—and it doesn't cost you anything compared to purchased, bottled water from vending machines.

Preparing nutritious meals and snacks isn't enough to survive your nursing program demands. Among other health factors, you'll need to be mindful of getting enough sleep.

ARE YOU GETTING ENOUGH SLEEP?

You may have seen this familiar scenario in your nursing classes. A student's eyes grow heavy… his head starts to bob…suddenly his head hits the desk. Although we might find this a little hu-

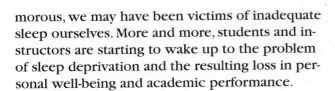

morous, we may have been victims of inadequate sleep ourselves. More and more, students and instructors are starting to wake up to the problem of sleep deprivation and the resulting loss in personal well-being and academic performance.

Here are some signs of sleep deficiency:

- Late arrival for class
- Inability to focus on tasks or assignments
- Reduced reasoning ability
- Increased forgetfulness
- Difficulty producing speech
- Immune system weakness (being sick)
- Higher level of anxiety
- Difficulty thinking creatively

According to the Sleep Medicine and Research Center in St. Louis, Missouri, adult sleep requirements can range from 4 to 10 hours per day.

The following questionnaire can help determine whether you're getting enough sleep.

1. Do you sleep less than 8 hours per night, on the average?
2. Do you have to nap during the day?
3. Do you fall asleep in class?
4. Do you have trouble organizing your thoughts for even simple tasks (like forgetting books or materials)?
5. Do simple assignments like homework seem overwhelming and extremely stressful, causing you to burst into tears or become depressed?
6. Do you overreact to situations then regret your actions the next day?
7. Do you have trouble being creative?
8. Are you excessively forgetful?
9. Are you late to your first class in the morning?
10. Do you have trouble falling asleep?

If you answered "yes" to any of these questions, you may be sleep deprived and not functioning at your fullest capacity. Try going to bed by 9 or 10 PM and getting at least 8 hours of sleep for 3 days. See how you feel. Just being mindful of your need for regular sleep is a start. Make a plan. Work it out with your family to arrange for sufficient sleep. You'll all benefit from your efforts.

With your busy and stressful life as a nursing student, you'll also need to consider the problems associated with your demanding work, class, and study schedules. Many of the problems resulting from stress include lack of proper exercise, improper posture, decreased endurance and strength, and, surprisingly, a poor self-image. We all know that we should routinely practice cardiorespiratory (aerobic) endurance exercises. Just 30 minutes four to five times a week of purposeful exercise can keep you in shape. What kind of exercise should you do? It's easy—just do something that you're willing to do! It might be walking the dog, going to a gym, performing yoga, stretching, running, dancing, swimming, or doing anything that will "make your back sweat" for 30 minutes. That's how much time you'll need to exercise to make a cardiovascular difference. While exercising during that 30 minutes, you should be able to talk. If you can't talk, your exercise workout is too strenuous.

Try to exercise early in the day—then it's done! But how can you find the time? One way is to study while you exercise. Try to find ways to make exercising a part of your day. For example, think about exercising with your study group. You can all walk together while discussing course topics. You'll feel more energized and healthy as a result. You can take a walk and carry your flash cards. Or, think about walking briskly while you listen to prepared audiotapes that contain course information. There are many ways to include purposeful exercise during the day. Be creative in discovering ways to be healthy. Make a decision to put these basic nutritional, rest, stress reduction, and exercise tips to work. You'll reduce stress, build strength, be more alert and energized, and be more able to successfully cope with the demands of your nursing program.

Developing and practicing effective strategies to actively learn, record, organize, and study course and text information can be a bit of work to put into place but once you're using these techniques, studying will become easier and more productive. Combine some of these tips with reading and mastering the information in your textbook and become a successful student—and nurse!

REFERENCES

Davis, B.G. (1993). *Tools for teaching.* San Francisco, CA: Jossey-Bass Publishers.

Downing, S. (2005). *On course: Strategies for creating success in college and in life.* Boston: Houghton Mifflin.

Ellis, D. (2003). *Becoming a master student.* Boston: Houghton Mifflin.

Ferrett, S.K. (1994). *Peak performance.* Burr Ridge, IL: Irwin Mirror Press.

Fleming, Neil. (2001). *VARK: A guide to learning styles.* [Electronic Version]. Retrieved June 23, 2004, from *http://vark-learn.com/english/page.asp?p=questionnaire* results.

Grunert, J. (1997). *The course syllabus: A learning-centered approach.* Bolton, MA: Anker Publishing.

Hopper, C.H. (2004). *Practicing college learning strategies.* New York: Houghton Mifflin.

Ignatavicius, D.D., & Workman, M.L. (2006). *Medical-surgical nursing: Critical thinking for collaborative care* (5th ed.). Philadelphia: W.B. Saunders.

Kanar, C. (2004). *The confident student.* Boston: Houghton Mifflin.

Laskey, M.L., & Gibson, P.W. (1997). *College study strategies.* Needham Heights, MA: Allyn & Bacon.

Nugent, P.M., & Vitale, B.A. (1993). *Test success: Test-taking techniques for beginning nursing students.* Philadelphia: F.A. Davis.

Pauk, W., & Owens, R.J.Q. (2005). *How to study in college.* Boston: Houghton Mifflin.

Pritchett, P. (N.D.). *The employee handbook of new work habits for a radically changing world: 13 ground rules for job success in the information age.* Dallas, TX: Pritchett.

Toft, D. (2005). *Master student guide to success.* New York: Houghton Mifflin.

Tools for teaching: Constructing knowledge. (2004). Albuquerque, NM: Albuquerque TVI Community College, Teaching and Learning Center.

Critical Thinking in the Role of the Medical-Surgical Nurse

LEARNING OUTCOMES

1. Explain why critical thinking is an essential part of medical-surgical nursing.
2. Compare and contrast common definitions of health.
3. Explain why some populations are more likely to experience health problems than others.
4. Explain the purpose of Healthy People 2010.
5. Differentiate the three levels of illness prevention and provide at least one example of each level.
6. Identify the major roles of the medical-surgical nurse.
7. Explain the relationship between critical thinking and evidence-based practice.
8. Assess factors that may affect the teaching-learning process.
9. Describe best practice interventions for promoting adult learning.
10. Review the key components of the nursing process.
11. Describe the difference between a nursing diagnosis and a medical problem.
12. Identify best practice interventions for clinical documentation.

LEARNING ACTIVITIES

1. Before completing the study guide exercises for this chapter, it is recommended that you review the following:
   - Concepts of health and health promotion, including Healthy People 2010
   - Consumer education and awareness
   - Teaching-learning process
   - North American Nursing Diagnosis Association (NANDA) current nursing diagnoses

2. Review the boldfaced terms and their definitions in Chapter 1 to enhance your understanding of the content.

STUDY/REVIEW QUESTIONS

Answers to the Study/Review Questions are provided on the companion Evolve Learning Resources Web site at http://evolve.elsevier.com/Iggy/.

1. List three characteristics of critical thinking:

    a. _____

    b. _____

    c. _____

2. Match the following origins of evidence with their associated levels of evidence (LOE).

Level of Evidence		Origin of Evidence	
_____ a.	LOE-1	1.	Well-conducted case control study
_____ b.	LOE-3	2.	Case studies
_____ c.	LOE-5	3.	Meta-analysis of multiple, well-designed, randomized controlled trials
_____ d.	LOE-8	4.	Well-designed trial without randomization

3. Name the three aspects of critical thinking and provide an example of each.

    a. _____

    b. _____

    c. _____

4. Explain the relationship between critical thinking and evidence-based practice.

5. What is the holistic view of health? How does it differ from the sociologic perspective?

6. Health reflects a person's biologic, psychologic, and sociologic states. Define these terms.

7. The Healthy People 2010 campaign has an aggressive plan to improve the nation's health. What are the two overall national health goals?

    a. _____

    b. _____

8. Identify at least three examples of practices that individuals can use to promote their health.

    a. _____

    b. _____

    c. _____

9. Match the following examples of preventive health behavior with their associated levels of intervention. Answers may be used more than once.

Preventive Health Behavior

_____ a.   Mammo-gram

_____ b.   Prevention of severe disability

_____ c.   Flu vaccine

_____ d.   Seat belts

_____ e.   Cardiac re-habilitation

_____ f.   Purified protein derivative (PPD)

Level of Intervention

1.   Primary
2.   Secondary
3.   Tertiary

10. Match the following role characteristics with their associated nursing roles. Answers may be used more than once.

Nursing Roles
1.   Caregiver
2.   Coordinator of care
3.   Continuing care planner
4.   Educator
5.   Advocate
6.   Change agent

Role Characteristics

_____ a.   Provides information

_____ b.   Arranges for home care

_____ c.   Conducts interdisciplinary clinical rounds

_____ d.   Arranges for post-hospitalization equipment

_____ e.   Performs collaborative functions

_____ f.   Works with legislators in effecting changes for better health care

_____ g.   Administers medications

_____ h.   Collaborates with other health care team members to assist client to meet expected outcomes

_____ i.   Provides physical care

_____ j.   Evaluates client's willingness to learn

_____ k.   Serves as role models and assists consumers in bringing about changes in work conditions

_____ l.   Explains implications of health care decisions

Questions 11 and 12 refer to the same client: a 60-year-old African-American woman who has recently been diagnosed with type II diabetes mellitus.

11. Your client requires teaching by the interdisciplinary team. List the important factors that could enhance or impede the teaching-learning process.

12. This client is anxious about the major lifestyle changes that having diabetes will require. Which approach may facilitate her learning?
   a.   Providing diabetes instruction in the evening hours in a large group setting with other people who have been newly diagnosed with diabetes
   b.   Directing the focus of the teaching to the daughter, who will then present the information to the client at a later time
   c.   Introducing small amounts of new information at a time and providing printed materials covering the same information
   d.   Presenting all information on diabetes care at one session and then repeating the same information 1 week later to determine retention

13. What are the three general types of hospital nursing units?

    a. _____

    b. _____

    c. _____

14. You have been considering a nursing position at a hospital. You thrive in crisis situations and work well under high stress. Which would be a good choice for your skills?
    a. Urology specialty unit
    b. Rehabilitation or transitional unit
    c. Shock trauma unit
    d. Orthopedic unit

15. How does the scientific method differ from the nursing process?

16. Identify the five steps of the nursing process.

    a. _____

    b. _____

    c. _____

    d. _____

    e. _____

17. Which of the following is an example of a medical diagnosis?
    a. Fever of unknown origin
    b. Impaired gas exchange
    c. Risk for infection
    d. Disturbed sleep pattern

18. Describe the difference between a nursing diagnosis and a collaborative problem.

19. Which of these activities would be included in a nursing assessment?
    a. Administering medications
    b. Determining client outcomes
    c. Analyzing client data
    d. Interviewing and taking a history

20. What is the end result of the data analysis step of the nursing process?
    a. Planning interventions based on problems
    b. Identifying actual or potential problems
    c. Determining data collection techniques for older adults
    d. Evaluating client response to plan

21. What are three critical functions of the planning step of the nursing process?

    a. _____

    b. _____

    c. _____

22. Expected client outcomes should have which of the following characteristics?
    a. Based on the Nursing Interventions Classification system
    b. Realistic for the client, measurable, and achievable
    c. Nurse- or health care provider-centered
    d. Focused on collaborative management activities

23. Match the following abbreviations to their definitions.

Abbreviations

_____ a.   NANDA

_____ b.   NIC

_____ c.   NOC

_____ d.   POC

_____ e.   DARE

Definitions

1. Classification for nursing outcomes
2. Interdisciplinary document, such as a critical pathway
3. The group that defines nursing diagnoses
4. Format used for Focus Charting
5. Classification system for nursing interventions

24. Which of the following statements about the collaborative client plan of care is correct?
    a. It is a means of communicating the nursing problems regarding client's care.
    b. It is an interdisciplinary document that outlines essential aspects of client care.
    c. It identifies exclusively the nursing interventions for client problems.
    d. It requires few modifications regardless of client's length of hospital stay.

25. Identify the four possible outcomes for the evaluation phase and the implications for further nursing actions.

    a. _____

    b. _____

    c. _____

    d. _____

26. Identify six important guidelines for nursing documentation.

    a. _____

    b. _____

    c. _____

    d. _____

    e. _____

    f. _____

27. Write an outcome objective that would indicate a positive result for your client for each of the nursing diagnoses below.
    a. Imbalanced nutrition, less than body requirements, related to nausea

    b. Disturbed sleep pattern related to pain

    c. Risk for aspiration related to impaired swallowing

Community-Based Care

LEARNING OUTCOMES

1. Explain the primary purpose of ambulatory care.
2. Identify the unique features of nursing primary care.
3. Discuss the growth of home care in the United States.
4. Describe the role of the nurse in home care.
5. Identify interventions for which Medicare typically pays in home care.
6. State the purpose of OASIS in home care.
7. Compare and contrast the common types of long-term care settings.
8. Differentiate assisted-living from other types of long-term care.
9. Describe the term *transitional care.*

LEARNING ACTIVITIES

1. Before completing the study guide exercises for this chapter, it is recommended that you review the concept of home care, long-term care, and acute care facilities as health providers.

2. Review the boldfaced terms and their definitions in Chapter 2 to enhance your understanding of the content.

STUDY/REVIEW QUESTIONS

Answers to the Study/Review Questions are provided on the companion Evolve Learning Resources Web site at http://evolve.elsevier.com/Iggy/.

1. What are the primary purposes of ambulatory care?

2. Identify four ambulatory settings in which clients may receive care.

   a. _____

   b. _____

   c. _____

   d. _____

3. Identify three major roles of nurses working in the ambulatory care setting.

   a. _____

   b. _____

   c. _____

4. List three examples of nursing primary health care providers.

   a. _____

   b. _____

   c. _____

5. List the factors that have contributed to the growth and acceptance of home care.

6. The major source of reimbursement for skilled home care services is which of the following?
   a. Private payment by the client
   b. Insurance companies
   c. Medicare
   d. Medicaid

7. Identify the differences between nursing in the home setting and nursing in an inpatient setting.

8. An older adult client has been discharged from the hospital after a stroke. The plan is to make a referral to a home care agency for physical therapy. Which home care agency would provide that service?
   a. A skilled home care service
   b. Private duty service
   c. Personal care service
   d. Home medical equipment service

9. An older adult client has dementia and the family wants a sitter to stay with her at night. Which home care agency would provide this service?
   a. A skilled home care service
   b. Home infusion therapy
   c. Private duty service
   d. Home medical equipment service

10. Medicare will pay for home care services if which of the following qualifying conditions is met?
    a. The client needs assistance with activities of daily living.
    b. The client is confined to the home.
    c. The health care provider writes an order for home care.
    d. The client needs follow-up care.

11. Once client eligibility has been established, which of the following services would be reimbursed by Medicare? *Mark all that apply.*

_____ a. Teaching a family member to manage a colostomy

_____ b. Transporting a client to get batteries for a hearing aid

_____ c. Preparing meals for an older client

_____ d. Providing wound care

_____ e. Management of a urinary catheter

_____ f. Homemaker services

12. Identify three advantages to computerized documentation in home care.

a. _____

b. _____

c. _____

13. In 1999, new regulations were instituted that require tracking outcome in Medicare-certified home care agencies by OASIS. Identify three benefits of this change.

a. _____

b. _____

c. _____

14. Why are nursing homes now accepting short-term residents for care?

15. For the client situations listed below, select the most appropriate placement from the following choices.
    a. Residential facility
    b. Nursing facility
    c. Chronic care facility
    d. Skilled nursing facility
    e. Transitional care unit

_____ A client is retired and is doing well but needs minor assistance with his activities of daily living.

_____ A client has sustained a severe head injury and requires ventilator support.

_____ A client has severe dementia and requires ongoing supervision.

_____ A client has a CVA and requires rehabilitative services and continuous heart monitoring for a potential rhythm disorder.

_____ A client has fractured her hip and needs short-term rehabilitative services.

16. Which of the following statements are true about nurses working in a nursing home? *Mark all that apply.*

_____ a. They are often in charge of a unit or shift.

_____ b. They require less training and fewer skills because the clients are medically stable.

_____ c. They must be familiar with laws that protect the clients.

_____ d. They are less autonomous than nurses working in the acute care setting.

_____ e. They must document carefully to meet regulations.

Introduction to Managed Care and Case Management

CHAPTER 3

LEARNING OUTCOMES

1. Explain the primary purpose of managed health care, including factors that drive concerns about cost and quality.

2. Contrast the fee-for-service and capitated reimbursement systems for health care.

3. Compare the health maintenance organization (HMO) with the preferred provider organization (PPO).

4. Delineate the overall goals of case management.

5. Explain the role of case management based on national standards.

6. Identify at least three certifications for case managers.

7. Clarify the differences and similarities between case management and disease management.

LEARNING ACTIVITIES

1. Before completing the study guide exercises for this chapter, it is recommended that you review the following:
   - Concepts of health and health promotion
   - Consumer education and awareness
   - Goals and standards of care for case management

2. Review the boldfaced terms and their definitions in Chapter 3 to enhance your understanding of the content.

STUDY/REVIEW QUESTIONS

Answers to the Study/Review Questions are provided on the companion Evolve Learning Resources Web site at http://evolve.elsevier.com/Iggy/.

1. The cost of health care in the United States has dramatically increased over the past 20 years and now accounts for _____ of the gross national product.
   a. 5%
   b. 8%
   c. 10%
   d. 15%

2. Discuss and contrast the fee-for-service arrangement and the capitated reimbursement system.

3. The primary purpose of managed care is to _____ _____.

4. In response to the managed care environment, an important role for the nurse is to:
   a. Focus care on the traditional disease-oriented approach.
   b. Learn to emphasize the curative process with client illnesses.
   c. Advocate for clients to ensure that they receive the necessary and appropriate care.
   d. Prepare clients for discharge after longer hospital stays.

5. Which statement about health maintenance organizations (HMOs) is true?
   a. They contract with primary physicians, hospitals, or other inpatient services to provide treatment.
   b. HMOs are the newest type of managed care organization.
   c. Clients can choose any hospital for their acute care.
   d. There is usually no charge or copayment for services.

6. The Joint Commission of Accreditation of Health Care Organizations (JCAHO) mandates that all accredited agencies must provide:
   a. Cost-effective, focused client care
   b. Collaborative, interdisciplinary care for clients
   c. Comprehensive and purely nursing-directed care
   d. Hospital-based comprehensive client care

7. Identify three certifications for case managers.
   a. _____
   b. _____
   c. _____

8. Name the four major roles of the case manager, and provide an example for each role.
   a. _____
   b. _____
   c. _____
   d. _____

9. List three goals of case management identified by the American Nurses Association (ANA).

10. In addition to the goals of case management listed in question 9, what additional goals are identified by the Case Management Society of America (CMSA)? Name at least four.

11. Internal case managers are focused on _____ care in a health care agency, whereas external case managers are focused on _____ of resources for insurance companies.

12. Many case managers in the United States practice disease state management. What is the purpose of this approach?

13. Which of the following statements about disease-specific case management are true? *Mark all that apply.*

   _____ a. Follows a disease-specific population during the acute phase of care

   _____ b. Focuses on care of clients with chronic disease or illness

   _____ c. Uses education to promote wellness

   _____ d. Focuses on resource utilization and cost of care

   _____ e. Is active across the continuum of care

14. The clinical pathway is a commonly used format for delineating the client's plan of care. There are other names for this interdisciplinary guideline. What are they?

Introduction to Complementary and Alternative Therapies in Nursing

CHAPTER

4

LEARNING OUTCOMES

1. Describe the purposes of the National Center for Complementary and Alternative Medicine (NCCAM).
2. Identify four examples of mind-body therapies.
3. Discuss the scope of complementary and alternative therapies with particular attention to the cultural aspects of their use.
4. Differentiate manipulative and body-based therapies from biologic-based therapies.
5. Provide examples of herbal therapies, their purpose, and adverse effects.
6. Identify selected complementary and alternative therapies that nurses can use in providing care to a variety of client populations.
7. Explain the purposes of commonly used therapies in nursing practice.
8. Discuss implications for care of clients using complementary and alternative therapies.

LEARNING ACTIVITIES

1. Before completing the study guide exercises for this chapter, it is recommended that you review the following:
   - Concepts of health and health promotion
   - Consumer education and awareness
   - Complementary and alternative therapy options

2. Review the boldfaced terms and their definitions in Chapter 4 to enhance your understanding of the content.

16 UNIT I   Health Promotion and Illness

STUDY/REVIEW QUESTIONS

Answers to the Study/Review Questions are provided on the companion Evolve Learning Resources Web site at http://evolve.elsevier.com/Iggy/.

1. Explain the difference among biomedicine, complementary therapies, and alternative therapies.

2. Puzzle: Complete each item by placing the correct answer in the appropriate number (across or down) in the puzzle.

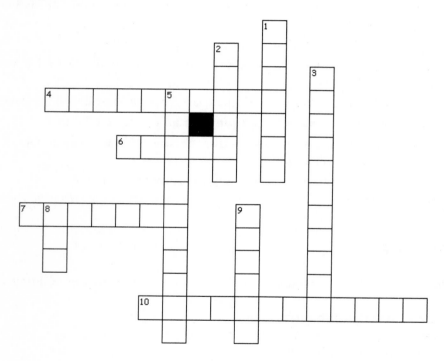

Across

4. A reflective therapy that is a tool for recording the process of one's life.
6. Therapeutic _____ is the use of the hands on or near the body with the purpose of healing.
7. Uses various strokes and pressure to manipulate soft tissues for therapeutic purposes.
10. Use of essential oils to promote relaxation and sleep.

Down

1. Uses the senses to form a mental representation of an object, place, event, or situation.
2. A mind-body exercise
3. Uses needles on various acupoints throughout the body to treat certain conditions.
5. Uses fingers to press certain points on the body to treat certain conditions.
8. Abbreviation for a therapy that uses animal companionship to promote positive health outcomes.
9. _____ preparations, plants used for medicinal purposes.

3. List the purposes of the National Center for Complementary and Alternative Medicine (NCCAM).

4. For each category of complementary therapy listed below, name at least two examples

   a. Systems of care _____

   _____

   b. Mind-body therapies _____

   _____

   c. Biologic-based therapies _____

   _____

   d. Manipulative and body-based therapies

   _____

   _____

   e. Energy therapies _____

   _____

5. Match the herbal preparation with its intended use or effect.

Herb		Intended Use or Effect
_____ a.	Ginkgo biloba	1. Mild to moderate depression
_____ b.	Echinacea	2. Memory problems
_____ c.	Garlic	3. Build immunity
_____ d.	St. John's wort	4. Anti-aging
_____ e.	Ginseng	5. Lower cholesterol

6. Match the herbal preparation with a caution or adverse effect. *Answers may be used more than once.*

Herb		Caution/Adverse Effect
_____ a.	Ginkgo biloba	1. Photosensitivity
_____ b.	Echinacea	2. May cause excessive bleeding if used with anti-coagulant drugs
_____ c.	Garlic	3. Should not be used for people with immune diseases
_____ d.	St. John's wort	

7. Although herbs are not classified as drugs in the United States, why is it important for clients to inform you concerning which herbs they are taking?

8. What should affect your decision to use touch therapy with your client?

9. Discuss the implications of complementary and alternative therapies for health professionals.

10. What conditions may be helped through the use of imagery?

11. Meditation has been used for what therapeutic purposes?

12. Name three benefits of massage therapy.

   a. _____

   b. _____

   c. _____

13. The nurse is preparing to give a massage to an older adult client who has been bedridden for 3 days. When the client's back is exposed, the nurse notes an area of redness on the sacrum that is about 6 cm in diameter. Which action is appropriate?

   a. Provide a vigorous massage over the area using long, flowing strokes.

   b. Provide a massage using light touch.

   c. Avoid massaging over an area of skin that is reddened or bruised.

14. Which of the following statements about aromatherapy are true? *Mark all that apply.*

   _____ a. Aromatherapy refers to the use of essential oils via smell.

   _____ b. Essential oils may be applied in compresses, used in baths, or applied to the skin.

   _____ c. Because essential oils are natural, they do not need to be diluted before being applied topically.

   _____ d. Lavender has been used for stimulation and to promote concentration.

   _____ e. Rose oil has been used to promote relaxation and sleep.

   _____ f. Allergies should be assessed before using essential oils.

15. Identify at least five considerations regarding the safety of herbal preparations that the nurse should keep in mind while considering herbal therapy.

   a. _____

   b. _____

   c. _____

   d. _____

   e. _____

Health Care of Older Adults

LEARNING OUTCOMES

1. Identify four subgroups of older adults.
2. Describe nursing interventions for relocation stress syndrome.
3. Discuss common health issues that may concern older adults.
4. Explain why older adults are often at high risk for falls.
5. State common interventions for older clients at high risk for falls.
6. Describe the nursing care required for clients who are restrained.
7. Explain the effects of drugs on the older adult.
8. Compare and contrast delirium and dementia.
9. Interpret the signs and symptoms of elder neglect or abuse.
10. Discuss potential economic issues for older adults.
11. Describe government and community resources that are available for older adults.

LEARNING ACTIVITIES

1. Before completing the study guide exercises for this chapter, it is recommended that you review the following:
   - Concepts of health and health promotion
   - Consumer education and awareness
   - Normal growth and development
   - Principles of sociology
   - Principles of developmental psychology

2. Review the boldfaced terms and their definitions in Chapter 5 to enhance your understanding of the content.

STUDY/REVIEW QUESTIONS

Answers to the Study/Review Questions are provided on the companion Evolve Learning Resources Web site at http://evolve.elsevier.com/Iggy/.

1. Which of the statements below about the health of older adults in the United States are true? *More than one answer may be correct.*

   _____ a. The fastest growing group is between 85 and 99 years of age.

   _____ b. Only 5% of older adults are in nursing homes.

   _____ c. The incidence of chronic illness increases with advanced age.

   _____ d. The lowest rate of suicide is in the older adult population.

2. Identify four interventions to reduce relocation stress in the older hospitalized client.

   a. _____

   b. _____

   c. _____

   d. _____

3. Which of the following statements would be included in an educational program on wellness behaviors for the older adult? *Mark all that apply.*
   a. Allow at least 10 to 15 minutes of sun exposure 2 to 3 times weekly.
   b. Take one aspirin twice a day.
   c. Obtain a yearly influenza vaccination.
   d. Create a hazard-free environment to prevent falls.
   e. Increase calcium intake to between 1000 and 1500 mg daily.
   f. Reduce dietary intake of complex carbohydrates and fiber.
   g. Take time alone at home and relax.

4. Which statement regarding how nutrition is affected in older adults is true?
   a. Changes in smell and taste can result in a decrease in use of sugar.
   b. Older adults need increased calorie intake to maintain ideal body weight.
   c. Loneliness and boredom may impact the older adult's incentive to eat.
   d. Obesity is the most common nutritional problem in nursing homes.

5. Identify six benefits of exercise in promoting and maintaining a high level of functioning.

   a. _____

   b. _____

   c. _____

   d. _____

   e. _____

   f. _____

6. How do losses experienced during one's older years affect one's self-concept?

7. Identify five of the factors that indicate a risk for falls in the older adult.

   a. _____

   b. _____

   c. _____

   d. _____

   e. _____

8. List at least four interventions for clients who are at high risk for falls.

   a. _____

   b. _____

   c. _____

   d. _____

9. Nursing interventions for the client requiring restraints must include (*more than one answer may be correct*):

   _____ a. Checking the client every 30 to 60 minutes

   _____ b. Releasing the restraint at least every 4 hours for repositioning and toileting

   _____ c. Turning on the television if the client is agitated to provide distraction

   _____ d. Placing the client in an area where he or she can be observed carefully

10. Which of the following types of psychoactive drugs is the *most* potent?
    a. Antidepressants
    b. Antipsychotics
    c. Antianxiety agents
    d. Sedative-hypnotics

11. Match the following physiologic changes affecting the drug use in older adults with their associated pharmacokinetic actions.

Pharmacokinetic Actions
1. Absorption
2. Distribution
3. Metabolism
4. Excretion

Physiologic Changes

_____ a. Increased gastric pH

_____ b. Reduced glomerular filtration

_____ c. Decreased cardiac output

_____ d. Decreased liver enzyme activity

12. Identify eight of the common adverse reactions to medications that may occur in older adults.

   a. _____

   b. _____

   c. _____

   d. _____

   e. _____

   f. _____

   g. _____

   h. _____

13. Which of the following statements are true? *More than one answer may be correct.*

   _____ a. Older adults have less reserve capacity in most organ systems.

   _____ b. Drug reactions are usually less severe in older adults due to reduced metabolism.

   _____ c. When prescribing medications for older adults, a policy of generalized "start high but taper quickly" is essential for safety.

   _____ d. All symptoms should be assessed for possible adverse reactions to medications in the older adult population.

14. Identify three common reasons why older adults may make mistakes when self-administering medications.

   a. _____

   b. _____

   c. _____

15. Which of these interventions is effective in helping to reorient a client suffering from delirium?
    a. Reorient the client frequently using a calm voice.
    b. Restrict visitors during periods of agitation.
    c. Remove personal items and store them safely.
    d. Apply wrist restraints to keep the client from pulling at tubing.

16. Which of the following may be signs and symptoms of depression in older adults? *More than one answer may be correct.*

    _____ a. Early morning insomnia

    _____ b. Reluctance to participate in social activities

    _____ c. Anger and aggressive behavior

    _____ d. Increased appetite and overeating

    _____ e. Excessive daytime sleeping

17. Differentiate dementia and delirium in older adults.

18. Which of the following statements regarding elder abuse is true? *More than one answer may be correct.*

    _____ a. The abuser is often a close family member.

    _____ b. Only physically dependent older adults are vulnerable to being victims of elder abuse.

    _____ c. Elder neglect is categorized as a type of elder abuse.

    _____ d. Approximately one-half of all cases involve physical force.

19. Match the type of elder abuse with its definition.

    Type of Abuse

    _____ a. Neglect

    _____ b. Physical abuse

    _____ c. Financial abuse

    _____ d. Emotional abuse

    Definition

    1. Mismanagement or misuse of an older client's property or resources.
    2. Intentional use of threats, humiliation, intimidation, and isolation.
    3. Examples include hitting, burning, pushing, and molesting the client.
    4. Failure to provide for basic needs, such as food and clothing.

20. Identify at least four factors that impact economic self-reliance in older adults.

    a. _____

    b. _____

    c. _____

    d. _____

21. Match the funding programs below with the governmental resources that support older adults.

    Governmental Resource
    1. Research on various aspects of aging
    2. Health care insurance
    3. Senior centers
    4. Retirement income

    Funding Program

    _____ a. Older Americans Act of 1965

    _____ b. Social Security Act

    _____ c. National Institute on Aging

    _____ d. Medicare and Medicaid

22. For each statement listed below, specify whether it describes Medicare or Medicaid.
    1. Medicare
    2. Medicaid

_____ a.   Federal program that provides health insurance to people 65 years of age or older.

_____ b.   Provides health insurance to qualified disabled people of any age.

_____ c.   Each state program determines its own criteria for eligibility.

_____ d.   Provides payment for medical services for the poor, including older adults who are poor.

_____ e.   Contains a Part B that is optional and requires a monthly premium that covers some outpatient costs.

CASE STUDY: MEDICATION USE IN OLDER ADULTS

Answer Guidelines for the Case Study questions are provided on the companion Evolve Learning Resources Web site at http://evolve.elsevier.com/Iggy/.

An 80-year-old client is brought to the emergency department after fainting at home. His serum digoxin level is 2.3 ng/mL. He is transferred to a medical-telemetry nursing unit. The next day the nurse asks the client to tell her about his routine for taking his daily digoxin tablets. He states that he was told to check his pulse every morning before taking a pill. He does this in his kitchen because the clock on the wall has big numbers and he can see the second hand go around. The nurse asks him how long he measures his pulse. He replies "I keep counting the beats until I get to 60. Sometimes it takes a long time. Then I take my heart pill." Later he tells you that he hates "having so many pills to take" and admits having trouble remembering to take his pills. He states that he sometimes can't remember which pills to take with breakfast and which to take at night.

1. Identify factors that may affect the client's understanding of digoxin self-administration.

2. What specific pharmacokinetic factor should be considered when giving digoxin to an older adult?

3. What can the nurse suggest to assist this client to take his multiple medications correctly?

4. Devise a teaching-learning plan to re-teach this client about taking digoxin at home.

5. Discuss how the nurse can validate whether the teaching plan has been effective.

Cultural Aspects of Health

LEARNING OUTCOMES

1. Define culture, cultural competence, cultural awareness, and ethnocentrism.
2. Explain the purpose and nursing implications of Healthy People 2010 as related to culture.
3. Identify common factors related to cultural assessment.
4. Describe three methods for cultural assessment.
5. Identify and describe three cultural groups that have often been neglected.
6. Discuss specific cultural practices, such as religion, nutrition, and folk medicine, that the nurse should consider when assessing a client's culture.
7. Describe ways that nurses can communicate sensitively with clients from various cultural groups.

LEARNING ACTIVITIES

1. Before completing the study guide exercises for this chapter, it is recommended that you review the following:
   - Difference between religion and spirituality
   - Community health nursing
   - Concepts of communication
   - Definitions of culture and cultural competence

2. Review the boldfaced terms and their definitions in Chapter 6 to enhance your understanding of the content.

STUDY/REVIEW QUESTIONS

Answers to the Study/Review Questions are provided on the companion Evolve Learning Resources Web site at http://evolve.elsevier.com/Iggy/.

Match the following terms with the appropriate definitions.

a. Culture
b. Subculture
c. Culture care preservation
d. Cultural competence
e. Culture care accommodation
f. Cultural assessment
g. Cultural restructuring
h. Transcultural nursing
i. Ethnocentrism
j. Cultural awareness

_____ 1. A way to help people of a particular culture retain or preserve relevant care values so they can maintain and/or preserve their well-being, recover from illness, or face handicaps and/or death

_____ 2. The ability of health care providers and organizations to understand and respond effectively to the cultural and linguistic needs that clients bring to the health care setting

_____ 3. An integrated pattern of human behavior, which is learned and transmitted to succeeding generations, that includes thought, speech, action, and artifacts

_____ 4. The judging of others through the exclusive lens of one's own cultural beliefs

_____ 5. An area of study and practice that focuses on the care, health, and illness patterns of people with similarities and differences in their cultural beliefs, values, and practices

_____ 6. Data collected or research conducted to learn about the culture of clients

_____ 7. Interventions that help clients to reorder or greatly modify their lifeways; providing a lifeway more beneficial or healthier than that practiced before the changes were co-established with the clients

_____ 8. The process through which one becomes respectful, appreciative, and sensitive to the values, beliefs, lifeways, practices, and problem-solving strategies of a client's culture

_____ 9. Part of a larger culture of the client

_____ 10. Professional actions and decisions that help people of a designated culture adapt to or negotiate with others for a beneficial or satisfying health outcome with professional care providers

11. Identify the three major methods for assessing the culture of a client and provide an example of each method.

    a. _____

    b. _____

    c. _____

12. Identify two ways a person can participate in a culture.

    a. _____

    b. _____

13. Identify three subcultures in our society that have been neglected often.

    a. _____

    b. _____

    c. _____

For Questions 14 through 20, read the statements and decide whether each is true or false. Write T for true or F for false in the blanks provided. If the statement is false, correct the statement to make it true.

_____ 14. Cultural practices that should be included as part of a cultural assessment include nutrition, family roles, pregnancy and childbirth, death rituals, and spirituality.

_____ 15. Transcultural nursing focuses on the care, health, and illness patterns of people with various cultural beliefs, values, and practices.

_____ 16. In the 2000 census, minorities accounted for 43.8% of the total population in the United States.

_____ 17. One goal of Healthy People 2010 is to eliminate disparities in health status experienced by racial and ethnic minorities.

_____ 18. All people within the same country have the same health care needs.

_____ 19. Garlic worn around the neck is thought to protect against cold and flu viruses in some cultures.

_____ 20. Pain is displayed the same way in all cultures.

21. Hypertension is referred to in some cultures as:
   a. High blood
   b. Low blood
   c. Hot blood
   d. Sour blood

22. Which of the following questions or statements reflects the best way to consider a client's religious or spiritual practice?
   a. "Do you have any dietary restrictions?"
   b. "Are you a Christian?"
   c. "Please tell me whether your religion allows you to accept blood products."
   d. "How can I help you in meeting any religious or spiritual needs you may have?"

23. You are the nurse for a client who does not speak your language. In choosing an interpreter, rank the following choices from 1 to 3, with 1 being the most preferable arrangement and 3 being the least preferable.

   _____ a. Use a friend or family member of the client.

   _____ b. Use a health care team member.

   _____ c. Use a person from the community or a local university.

24. The nurse is admitting an older woman who has cellulitis of her lower leg. She has been applying a homemade poultice to her leg for a week and refuses to remove it during the admission assessment. The nurse should:
   a. Remove the poultice in order to assess the lower leg.
   b. Inform the physician that the client won't remove the poultice.
   c. Ask the client about the poultice and how it has worked for her.
   d. Tell the client that her leg won't heal until she follows the doctor's orders.

CASE STUDY: ASSESSMENT OF A CULTURE

Answer Guidelines for the Case Study questions are provided on the companion Evolve Learning Resources Web site at http://evolve.elsevier.com/Iggy/.

The hospital where you are a nurse manager is opening an outreach clinic and has asked you to help set it up. The clinic is located in a community with many recent immigrants from Guatemala.

1. What do you need to know to be prepared to provide culturally appropriate care for your clients?

2. How will you find that information?

3. During a home visit, you discover that there is great concern in a family with a newborn infant because of a *mal ojo*. What could have caused this concern?

4. What are some ways to ensure proper communication when working with the Guatemalan clients in this clinic?

Pain: The Fifth Vital Sign

CHAPTER

7

LEARNING OUTCOMES

1. Define the concept of pain.
2. Identify three populations at high risk for undertreatment of pain.
3. Discuss the attitudes and knowledge of nurses, physicians, and clients regarding pain assessment and management.
4. Differentiate between addiction, tolerance, and physical dependence.
5. Compare and contrast the characteristics of the major types of pain.
6. Explain the transmission of pain.
7. Describe the components of a comprehensive pain assessment.
8. Describe the use of non-opioid analgesics in pain management.
9. Discuss and compare opioid analgesics, using an equianalgesic chart.
10. Explain the purpose of adjuvant medication in pain management.
11. Differentiate four routes of analgesic administration.
12. Identify special considerations for older adults related to pain assessment and management.
13. Identify physical and cognitive-behavioral therapies for clients experiencing pain.
14. Develop a teaching/learning plan for managing pain as part of community-based care for clients.
15. Describe the role of the nurse as an advocate in pain management.

LEARNING ACTIVITIES

1. Before completing the study guide exercises for this chapter, it is recommended that you review the following:
   • Anatomy and physiology of the peripheral and central nervous system
   • Actions and side effects of opioid analgesics and NSAIDs

2. Visit a health care facility's pain management department and review the institution's outcomes for pain management, including implementation of pain strategies and the evaluation of pain.

3. Review the boldfaced terms and their definitions in Chapter 7 to enhance your understanding of the content.

STUDY/REVIEW QUESTIONS

Answers to the Study/Review Questions are provided on the companion Evolve Learning Resources Web site at http://evolve.elsevier.com/Iggy/.

1. Read the following statements and decide whether each is true or false. *Write T for true or F for false in the blanks provided. If the statement is false, correct the statement to make it true.*

    _____ a. Pain is the number-one symptom or complaint that causes people to seek health care.

    _____ b. Pain alters the quality of life more than any other single health-related problem.

    _____ c. Over the years, there have been major advances in how pain is managed.

    _____ d. Unrelieved and untreated pain is a major public health problem in the United States.

    _____ e. The amount of pain a person feels and the response to it is a universal experience.

2. Name three factors that affect a client's perception of and response to pain.

    a. _____

    b. _____

    c. _____

3. Which of the following is not related to the gate control theory?
    a. It is an explanation of the relationship between pain and emotion.
    b. Perception of pain is influenced by physical and psychologic variables.
    c. Perception of pain occurs by way of the stimulus being transmitted directly to the gate in the brain.
    d. Interventions for pain management have been based on this theory.

4. The free nerve endings or receptors in the various body tissues that become activated by thermal, mechanical, or chemical stimuli to initiate the client's response to pain are called _____.

5. Briefly describe the following four categories relating to the location of pain:
    a. Localized pain

    b. Projected pain

    c. Radiating pain

    d. Referred pain

6. Differentiate chronic cancer pain and chronic noncancer pain.

7. Compare the structure, function, and sensation of the A delta and C fibers.

8. Differentiate neurotransmitters and neuromodulators that inhibit or facilitate the pain sensory input to the spinal cord.

9. Which of the following characteristics pertain to somatic pain? *Check all that apply.*

_____ a.   Sharp, burning or dull, aching, or cramping

_____ b.   Diffuse, deep, and stabbing

_____ c.   Painful numbness or shooting, burning, fiery

_____ d.   Poorly localized

_____ e.   Skeletal muscle spasms

_____ f.   Nerve compression

_____ g.   Insertion site of wound drain

_____ h.   Bladder spasms

_____ i.   Pancreatitis

_____ j.   Bony metastasis

10. Which of the following characteristics pertain to neuropathic pain? *Check all that apply.*

_____ a.   Sharp, burning or dull, aching, or cramping

_____ b.   Diffuse, deep, and stabbing

_____ c.   Painful numbness or shooting, burning, fiery

_____ d.   Poorly localized

_____ e.   Skeletal muscle spasms

_____ f.   Nerve compression

_____ g.   Insertion site of wound drain

_____ h.   Bladder spasms

_____ i.   Pancreatitis

_____ j.   Bony metastasis

11. Which of the following characteristics pertain to visceral pain? *Check all that apply.*

_____ a.   Sharp, burning or dull, aching, or cramping

_____ b.   Diffuse, deep, and stabbing

_____ c.   Painful numbness or shooting, burning, fiery

_____ d.   Poorly localized

_____ e.   Skeletal muscle spasms

_____ f.   Nerve compression

_____ g.   Insertion site of wound drain

_____ h.   Bladder spasms

_____ i.   Pancreatitis

_____ j.   Bony metastasis

12. "Age can be a factor that influences how pain is perceived and how it is assessed." Briefly summarize how this statement relates to pain and pain management in the older adult.

13. Identify the sources of the following three types of pain:
    a. Somatic pain

    b. Visceral pain

    c. Neuropathic pain

14. A client complains of a deep, localized cramping type of pain. These assessment findings indicate which type of pain?
    a. Somatic
    b. Psychosomatic
    c. Neuropathic
    d. Visceral

15. A client complains of a constant "achy" type of pain after abdominal surgery. This is an indication of which type of pain?
    a. Somatic
    b. Visceral
    c. Neuropathic
    d. Psychosomatic

16. For each of the characteristics listed, mark AP for acute pain, CP for chronic pain, or B for both.

    Characteristics   *AP = Acute pain*
                         CP = Chronic pain
                         B = Both

    _____ a. Duration greater than 3 months

    _____ b. Intensity ranges from mild to severe

    _____ c. May be accompanied by anxiety and restlessness

    _____ d. May be accompanied by depression, fatigue, and decreased functional ability

    _____ e. Begins gradually and persists

    _____ f. Cause may be well-defined

    _____ g. Reversible

17. Identify essential subjective data relevant to a pain assessment.

18. Identify clinical manifestations or physiologic changes in response to pain.

19. "The client's statement of pain is the only reliable indicator." Discuss why this is or is not true.

20. What is the best type of pain scale to use for clients who have language barriers or reading problems, or for children?
    a. 0 to 10 numeric rating scale
    b. FACES (smile to frown)
    c. Verbal description scales
    d. No type of scale

21. Identify possible nursing diagnoses of clients with pain other than acute pain or chronic pain.

22. Identify the three groups of medications used to manage pain and provide an example of each.

    a.   _____

    b.   _____

    c.   _____

23. A nurse would monitor for gastric irritation, signs of bleeding, and bruising as side effects of which pain medication? *Check all that apply.*

    _____ a.   Aspirin (non-opioid analgesic, NSAID)

    _____ b.   Acetaminophen (non-opioid analgesic)

    _____ c.   Ibuprofen (non-opioid analgesic, NSAID)

    _____ d.   Morphine (opioid analgesic)

24. A client with chronic bone pain as a result of osteoarthritis or rheumatoid arthritis may be prescribed which of the following agents? *Check all that apply.*

    _____ a.   Aspirin

    _____ b.   COX 2 inhibitor such as celecoxib (Celebrex)

    _____ c.   Opioid such as morphine

    _____ d.   Acetaminophen (Tylenol)

    _____ e.   NSAID such as ibuprofen (Motrin, Advil)

25. What are the routes of administration for opioid analgesics?

26. Read the following statements and decide whether each is true or false. *Write T for true or F for false in the blanks provided. If the statement is false, correct the statement to make it true.*

    _____ a.   The IM route is always the preferred route for most types of pain.

    _____ b.   The oral route is always the preferred route for most types of pain.

    _____ c.   The IV route is the most efficient route for pain management.

    _____ d.   The transdermal route provides quick pain relief.

27. The drug that can cause life-threatening seizures, particularly in the older adult, because of an accumulation of toxic metabolites is *(check all that apply)*:
    a.   Ibuprofen (Advil, Motrin)
    b.   Morphine
    c.   Meperidine (Demerol)
    d.   Acetaminophen (Tylenol)
    e.   Codeine

28. Identify the nursing interventions that should be performed when caring for a client receiving opioid analgesics.

29. Which of the following statements are true regarding the side effects of respiratory depression as a result of administering an opioid analgesic? *Mark all that apply.*
    a. Respiratory depression develops when opioid tolerance occurs.
    b. Monitor for respiratory depression in clients receiving opioids by IV administration, especially monitor opioid-naive adults.
    c. The pain, stress, and anxiety experienced by the client are potent respiratory stimulants that may override or negate the respiratory depression resulting from the drugs.
    d. Respiratory depression is less of a problem in the older adult.
    e. The drug used to reverse the respiratory depression is known as naloxone (Narcan).
    f. A one-time dose of naloxone (Narcan) is all that is needed to reverse the effects of the opioid.
    g. Sedation will occur before opioid-induced respiratory depression.

30. Which of the following statements about the adverse side effects of opioids is true?
    a. Bolus administration is less likely to produce central nervous system changes.
    b. Stimulants such as caffeine may counteract opioid-induced sedation.
    c. Opioid antagonists produce more respiratory depression than opioid agonists.
    d. Peripheral effects include vasoconstriction and elevated blood pressure.

31. Identify two factors that may influence a nurse's ability to manage a client's pain episodes successfully.

32. Match the following definitions of physiologic sequelae associated with opioid use with their correct terms. *Answers may be used more than once, and more than one term may apply to each sequela.*

Term

1. Physical dependency
2. Tolerance
3. Addiction

Physiologic Sequelae

_____ a. Persistent drug craving

_____ b. Withdrawal symptoms upon abrupt cessation

_____ c. Occurs in everyone who takes opioids over a period of time

_____ d. Gradual resistance to effect of the opioid

_____ e. Abuse for recreational purposes

_____ f. Higher doses needed to achieve pain relief

_____ g. A common fear in clients and health professionals

_____ h. A psychologic, not physical, phenomenon

_____ i. Problem with amount of medication given to a client with substance abuse

33. Is the following statement true or false? Explain your answer. "If a client reports pain relief after receiving a placebo, then the client is not experiencing real pain."

34. Read the following statements regarding patient-controlled analgesia (PCA) and decide whether each is true or false. *Write T for true or F for false in the blanks provided. If the statement is false, correct the statement to make it true.*

_____ a. Meperidine (Demerol) is the drug most commonly used for PCA therapy.

_____ b. The demand dose is ordered by the health care provider and is only available within specific intervals.

_____ c. During the lockout interval, a dose will be delivered if a client presses the button more than twice.

_____ d. Two nurses should program the dosing parameters into the PCA delivery device.

_____ e. Continuous or basal infusion of an opioid in addition to demand dosing causes overmedication.

_____ f. Use of a PCA system may result in the client needing less medication for pain than medication delivered by a nurse.

35. Which of the following statements are true regarding the use of epidural catheters for pain management? *Check all that apply.*

_____ a. It is an external catheter located in the lumbar or thoracic region near the spinal cord.

_____ b. It is used for hospitalized clients with postoperative pain.

_____ c. Morphine and hydromorphone (Dilaudid) may be used, along with a local anesthetic such as bupivacaine.

_____ d. The nurse monitors for nausea and vomiting, pruritus, and infection at the insertion site.

_____ e. Catheters are usually in place for 12 to 24 hours.

_____ f. Urinary retention and weakness in the legs can occur.

_____ g. Pain assessments can be performed less frequently while receiving pain medications through epidural catheters.

36. Name four various modalities of cutaneous stimulation that can be prescribed to control a client's acute or chronic pain.

37. What are the limitations of cutaneous stimulation as an effective measure to control a client's pain?

38. "Clients with a history of substance abuse should not receive opioids to treat their pain." Is this statement true or false? Give a rationale for your answer.

39. Briefly describe the use of a TENS unit to control pain.

40. Which of the following statements about the strategy of distraction is true?
    a. Distraction is effective for acute and chronic pain relief.
    b. Distraction influences the cause of pain directly.
    c. Distraction should be used instead of other pain control measures.
    d. Distraction alters the perception of pain.

41. In your role as a nurse, practice performing a complete pain assessment by using a pain assessment tool and a pain scale of your choice. As a result of your assessment, identify the type of pain the client is having and work collaboratively with other health care providers to determine a plan of care for the client to help relieve the pain.

42. "NSAIDs may cause renal toxicity; therefore, renal function blood tests should be routinely monitored with long-term therapy, especially in the older adult." Is this statement true or false?

43. Match the action or use with the corresponding adjuvant analgesic.

Adjuvant Analgesic

1. Topical preparations, such as Bio-Freeze gel
2. Oral local anesthetics, such as mexiletine (Mexitil)
3. Antianxiety agent clonazepam (Klonopin)
4. Antiepileptic drugs, such as topiramate (Topamax)
5. Antidepressants, such as sertraline (Zoloft)

Action/Use

_____ a. Used for neuropathy associated with diabetes mellitus

_____ b. Used for its sedative effects at bedtime

_____ c. Used for certain types of nerve injury pain

_____ d. Used for electric, shocklike, continuous pain

_____ e. Provides cryotherapy for muscle aches and pain

44. Identify two purposes of acupuncture.

    a. _____

    b. _____

45. Briefly describe the surgical procedure of a rhizotomy for the treatment of chronic pain.

46. What is the drug category of choice for the treatment of mild-to-moderate bone pain?
    a. NSAIDs
    b. Opioids
    c. Anticonvulsants
    d. Antianxiety agents

47. Match the following descriptions with their associated strategies for coping with pain. Answers may be used more than once.

Description		Associated Strategies
_____ a.	Massage	1. Imagery
_____ b.	Deep-breathing exercises	2. Relaxation
_____ c.	Going for a walk	3. Hypnosis
_____ d.	Mental experience of sensations or events	4. Distraction
_____ e.	Altered state of consciousness	
_____ f.	Focuses on pleasant or desirable feeling, sensation, or event	
_____ g.	Loses an overall sense of reality	

48. Define what is meant by the term *equianalgesic*. What would the equianalgesic dose of hydromorphone (Dilaudid) be for a client receiving 90 mg of morphine orally?

49. Identify the method that would be the recommended route for controlling pain of a hospice client with cancer who is unable to take oral medication.
    a. Intramuscular injection
    b. Continuous subcutaneous infusion
    c. Sublingual tablet
    d. Transdermal patch

50. Identify the two routes used to administer opioids via intraspinal medication for intractable pain. What is the purpose of using intraspinal medications? What are the methods for administration?

51. Read the following statements regarding fentanyl (Duragesic) patches and decide whether each is true or false. *Write T for true or F for false in the blanks provided. If the statement is false, correct the statement to make it true.*

    _____ a. Duragesic is available in patch doses of 25 mcg/hr, 50 mcg/hr, 75 mcg/hr, and 100 mcg/hr.

    _____ b. It is reserved for those clients with continuous and relatively stable pain.

    _____ c. It is supplemented by intermittent doses of pain medication for episodic or breakthrough pain.

_____ d.   It is an easy-to-use method for anyone in chronic pain because it is
easily titrated to control the pain.

_____ e.   When the patch is initially applied, it
may take up to 24 hours before pain
relief begins, so short-acting pain
medication must be administered
until the medication takes effect.

_____ f.   The patch is effective for 1 week;
then a new patch is applied.

_____ g.   The client's body temperature has
no effect on absorption of the medication.

52.   A temporary pain relief measure that involves localizing the nerve root by an anesthetic is called a _____.

53.   Identify at least three expected outcomes
for any client in pain.

1.   The client describes her pain as a "10" on a
scale of 1 to 10, deep, occasionally cramping, and sharp or stabbing. She waves her
hand over her chest and abdomen when
asked to pinpoint the location of the pain.
What kind of pain is she experiencing?

2.   During the pain assessment, the client has
difficulty identifying the location of her
pain. She says, "It just hurts all over!" What
can you do to help her specify the exact location of pain?

3.   During a discussion with the pain management nurse, it is suggested that the client
be given a Duragesic transdermal patch
for pain management. She comments, "Oh,
good! I know that will help make my pain
go away quickly." What should you say?

CASE STUDY: PAIN

_Answer Guidelines for the Case Study questions are pro-
vided on the companion Evolve Learning Resources Web
site at http://evolve.elsevier.com/Iggy/._

You are admitting a client to a medical unit. She
is 68 years of age, and has a history of ovarian
cancer. She had surgery 5 months ago and has
had pain ever since the surgery. She reports that
she has been taking Tylox tablets at home but
that the pain is "never gone."

4. After consideration of her history and her pain, the pain management specialist recommends that the client should receive patient-controlled analgesia (PCA). After discussing PCA therapy with her, an infusion is started with morphine as a basal infusion as well as interval self-dosing. The next morning, as you review the infusion notes, you see that she dosed herself four times during the night. She is awake and states that her pain is now at a "5" and that she feels "a bit of relief now." Later that afternoon, as you make rounds after lunch, you see that she is asleep and has not touched her meal. Her respiratory rate is 12, but she does not answer when you call her name. What should you do at this point?

5. During evening rounds, the client is found to be unresponsive, with respiratory rate of 7 breaths/min. Her son, who was staying with her, said that he "pushed the button a few times" while she was asleep because earlier she was complaining of hurting but wouldn't push it herself. What should you get ready to do now?

Substance Abuse

LEARNING OUTCOMES

1. Discuss substance abuse as a major health issue in the United States.
2. Explain the effects of substance abuse on the mental and physical health of individuals and society.
3. Describe the relationship between stress and substance abuse.
4. Identify assessment findings associated with use of nicotine, alcohol, stimulants, hallucinogens, depressants, opioids, inhalants, and steroids.
5. Prioritize care for clients who exhibit signs or symptoms of substance abuse.
6. Discuss recent biologic and genetic research in the etiology of substance abuse.
7. Identify symptoms that are indicative of emergency situations associated with the use of the following substances: alcohol, nicotine, stimulants, hallucinogens, depressants, opioids, inhalants, and steroids.
8. Identify the responsibilities of the nurse when a peer or other health care worker is suspected of abusing substances.
9. Identify common medication regimens that are used in the emergency treatment of drug withdrawal and adverse reactions to drugs and alcohol.
10. Prioritize nursing care for clients who are in alcohol withdrawal.

LEARNING ACTIVITIES

1. Before completing the study guide exercises for this chapter, it is recommended that you review the following:
    *   Cultural competence
    *   Stress and adaptation
    *   Coping
    *   The *ANA Code of Ethics*

2. Review the boldfaced terms and their definitions in Chapter 8 to enhance your understanding of the content.

STUDY/REVIEW QUESTIONS

Answers to the Study/Review Questions are provided on the companion Evolve Learning Resources Web site at http://evolve.elsevier.com/Iggy/.

1. In caring for a hospitalized client, the nurse recognizes that the client has a history of substance abuse. Answer the following questions.
   a. In your own words, described the terms *substance abuse* and *addiction*, and then compare your answers with the textbook definitions.

   b. In the table below, identify the six categories of substances most commonly abused, describe the action and effect on the body, and give examples of the abused substance for each category.

Categories	Action of Substance and Overall Effects on the Body	Examples

c. As stated in the text, the nurse must have a "firm awareness of self to avoid reactive behaviors to the client's beliefs or absence of personal convictions." Spend a little time now to think about your own viewpoints regarding substance abuse.

2. Read the following statements about substance abuse and decide whether each is true or false. *Write T for true or F for false in the blanks provided. If the statement is false, correct the statement to make it true.*

_____ a. In a recent study, the highest rates of illicit drug use were found among Asian Americans.

_____ b. Approximately 1 of 10 persons in the United States has a friend or family member with substance abuse problems.

_____ c. A plan of care for a client with substance abuse should be based only on the type of chemical used.

_____ d. Substance abuse only includes illicit or illegal drugs.

_____ e. Substance abuse is only related to teenagers and young adults.

_____ f. Any socioeconomic group is susceptible to substance abuse.

_____ g. Knowledge of the client's religious preference will influence the treatment modality.

_____ h. Older adults are at risk for substance abuse because of normal body changes related to the aging process.

_____ i. Women are generally susceptible to substance abuse because of biologic predisposition and stressors in the environment.

3. Which of the following statements regarding substance abuse, stress, and addiction are true? *Check all that apply.*

_____ a. Stress is a contributing factor for substance abuse.

_____ b. When the body experiences stress, the brain reacts by decreasing the level of stress hormones.

_____ c. Stress responses that are frequently triggered can result in a more sensitive response to the substance.

Questions 4 to 10 are related to the category of stimulants.

4. Identify the two stimulants that are prescribed therapeutically for attention deficit disorders, obesity, and narcolepsy.

a. _____

b. _____

5. What assessment finding would indicate to the nurse that the client is a chronic user of cocaine, particularly "crack" cocaine?

6. Cardiopulmonary arrest can occur with the first use of which stimulant?

7. A client withdrawing from stimulants should be assessed for which of the following?
a. Insomnia
b. Chills
c. Seizures
d. Fever

8. In order to measure the timing of the last ingestion of cocaine in a client who has been admitted with an overdose, which of the following would be ordered?
   a. Urine test
   b. Serum test
   c. Breath analysis
   d. Gastric pH

9. As stress increases, additional amounts of this substance are needed because the stress hormone corticosterone reduces its effect.
   a. Cocaine
   b. Nicotine
   c. Methamphetamine
   d. Amphetamine

10. Identify the stimulant that has both stimulant and sedative properties. Explain how this drug affects the body.

12. Which drug affects the serotonin- and dopamine-producing neurons in the brain?

13. Tolerance to what particular drug can develop so that an increased amount of the drug is needed to attain the same level of experience?

14. The priority of care in cases of ketamine overdose is _____.

15. Briefly explain why LSD is a dangerous health hazard with unpredictable results.

Questions 11 to 19 are related to the category of hallucinogens and related compounds.

11. True or false? *Write T for true or F for false in the blanks provided.*

   _____ a. Flashbacks are a common phenomenon when psychedelic drugs are used.

   _____ b. There are no therapeutic uses for hallucinogens that are acceptable for medical treatment.

   _____ c. Ketamine, or "Special K" is also known as the "date rape drug."

   _____ d. The effects of LSD can last up to 12 hours.

   _____ e. Addiction to hallucinogens is physical in nature, not psychological.

16. A client in the emergency department is suspected of using PCP. A key assessment finding that would indicate this diagnosis is which of the following?
   a. Violent behavior
   b. Shallow respirations
   c. Seizures
   d. Sedation

17. Briefly describe assessment findings in a client suspected of PCP abuse.

18. What drug is used experimentally to control chronic pain?

19. Briefly describe the effects of long-term or heavy use of marijuana.

Questions 20 to 28 are related to depressants.

20. The depressants that are medically used to treat anxiety and emotional disorders are _____ and _____.

21. Read the following statements and decide whether each is true or false. *Write T for true or F for false in the blanks provided. If the statement is false, correct the statement to make it true.*

_____ a. Abuse is present when the client continues to use benzodiazepines after clinical signs have subsided.

_____ b. Dependence on barbiturates takes a long time to occur.

_____ c. When medically indicated, older adults can tolerate only small doses of the barbiturate group.

_____ d. The safest method for withdrawing a client from depressants is to gradually reduce the dosage.

_____ e. Alcohol abuse occurs only when a person has a strong craving for alcohol.

22. Anxiety, restlessness, insomnia, irritability, and impaired attention are assessment findings for withdrawal from which drug?
   a. Barbiturates
   b. Benzodiazepines
   c. Opioids
   d. Alcohol

23. An assessment of a postoperative client with a history of substance abuse documents diaphoresis, agitation, elevated blood pressure, and tremors. These assessment findings are symptoms of:
   a. Benzodiazepine withdrawal
   b. Barbiturate withdrawal
   c. Alcohol withdrawal
   d. Amphetamine withdrawal

24. Alcohol withdrawal is evaluated by categories of severity. On a separate sheet of paper, briefly explain the assessment findings that would be monitored by the nurse for each of the following three alcohol withdrawal categories:
   a. Minor
   b. Major
   c. Life-threatening

25. A hospitalized client has a history of alcoholism. How soon after the client's last drink should the nurse monitor the client for withdrawal symptoms?
   a. 8 hours
   b. 24 hours
   c. 12 to 48 hours
   d. Up to 36 hours

26. A client is brought to the emergency department by a friend, who states that they had been at a party with "lots of booze." The friend claims to be the designated driver, but is concerned because the client passed out in the car and was unable to walk to his apartment. A blood alcohol level is drawn, and the results are 350 mg/dL. This level indicates:
   a. Mild to moderate intoxication
   b. Marked intoxication
   c. Severe intoxication
   d. Alcohol overdose

27. A client is in the rehabilitation unit for treatment of alcohol withdrawal. Which of the following drugs is used to prevent seizures and delirium tremens (DTs)?
    a. Thiamine
    b. Chlordiazepoxide (Librium)
    c. Disulfiram (Antabuse)
    d. Atenolol (Tenormin)

28. In the older adult, substance abuse can be a problem related to alcohol and which of the following?
    a. Stimulants
    b. Depressants
    c. Opioids
    d. Prescription and over-the-counter medications

Questions 29 to 33 are related to narcotics: opioids and morphine derivatives.

29. Opioids and morphine are drugs of addiction because of which effects?
    a. Analgesic and euphoric effects
    b. General numbing effect
    c. Stimulation effects
    d. Hallucinogenic effects

30. The opioid derivative that has no medical use is _____.

31. Briefly describe the effects heroin has on the body and why it is such a severe health hazard.

32. A client enters the emergency department and is diagnosed with opiate withdrawal grade 2. The assessment findings of this client would include:
    a. Increased vital signs, abdominal cramps, diarrhea, vomiting, and weakness.
    b. Drug craving, anxiety, and drug-seeking behavior.
    c. Dilated pupils, muscle twitching, and anorexia.
    d. Sweating, lacrimation, yawning, and rhinorrhea.

33. A client is admitted to the emergency department with a possible opioid overdose. She is semiconscious, has dilated pupils, and her respiratory rate is 8 breaths/min. The nurse prepares to give which of the following?
    a. Meperidine (Demerol)
    b. Midazolam (Versed)
    c. Disulfiram (Antabuse)
    d. Naltrexone (ReVia)

Questions 34 to 38 are related to inhalants and steroids.

34. The clients most likely to use inhalants are:
    a. Children
    b. Young adults
    c. Middle-aged adults
    d. Older adults

35. A young client states that solvents were inhaled. Examples of solvents are:
    a. Butane lighters, whipping cream aerosols, and spray paints
    b. Cyclohexanol nitrite and amyl nitrite
    c. Paint thinners, gasoline, glues, and paper correction fluid
    d. Hair or deodorant sprays, ether, and chloroform

36. True or false? *Write T for true or F for false in the blanks provided.*

_____ a.   A method to increase the effect of the inhalant is to dispense the substance from a paper bag to increase the concentration of the inhalant.

_____ b.   Early treatment is important for inhalant toxicity so that an antidote can be administered.

37. Reversible effects of inhalants include:
    a. Liver and kidney damage
    b. Hearing loss
    c. Limb spasms
    d. Bone marrow suppression

38. Anabolic steroids are abused for which of the following reasons?
    a. For euphoric effects
    b. To increase physical strength and performance
    c. To reduce aggressive tendencies
    d. To improve fertility in males

39. Match the substance with its toxic effects.

Toxic Effects
1. Respiratory depression, bradycardia, coma
2. Paranoid ideas, "hearing colors," brain damage, psychosis
3. Cardiopulmonary arrest, possibly with first use
4. Growth of facial hair, changes in menses, deepened voice
5. Chemical smell, red eyes, slurred speech, dazed appearance
6. Hyperthermia, convulsions, stroke

Substance

_____ a.   Inhalants

_____ b.   Anabolic steroids

_____ c.   Methamphetamines

_____ d.   Lysergic acid (LSD)

_____ e.   GHB or "liquid ecstasy"

_____ f.   Cocaine

End-of-Life Care

LEARNING OUTCOMES

1. Describe the pathophysiology of death.
2. Explain the purpose for advance directives.
3. Discuss the philosophies of palliative and hospice care.
4. Describe the role of the nurse and the interdisciplinary team in end-of-life care.
5. Interpret the common physical and emotional signs of impending death.
6. Identify common symptoms of distress near death.
7. Prioritize interventions for symptoms experienced by the client near death.
8. Describe common psychosocial issues for clients and their families near death.
9. Develop a plan of care to assist clients and families in coping with the dying process.
10. Explain how variations in culture and religious beliefs can impact the experience of dying and death.
11. Describe care of the client after death.
12. Discuss the ethical and legal obligations of the nurse with regard to end-of-life care.

LEARNING ACTIVITIES

1. Before completing the study guide exercises for this chapter, it is recommended that you review the following:
   - Concept of grief and loss
   - Death and dying
   - Concept of stress, coping, and adaptation
   - Pain management
   - Cultural diversity
   - Complementary and alternative therapies

2. Review the boldfaced terms and their definitions in Chapter 9 to enhance your understanding of the content.

STUDY/REVIEW QUESTIONS

Answers to the Study/Review Questions are provided on the companion Evolve Learning Resources Web site at http://evolve.elsevier.com/Iggy/.

1. Match the following terms related to loss with their correct definitions.

Term		Definition	
_____ a.	Death	1.	Reaction to loss
_____ b.	Dying	2.	Termination of life
_____ c.	Grieving	3.	The outward social expression of loss
_____ d.	Mourning	4.	A process leading to the end of life

2. A terminally ill client has been referred to hospice. The nurse explains to the client and family that hospice care differs from the care for a client expected to recover from an illness in that it has the following goals:

   a. _____

   b. _____

   c. _____

3. Which of the following statements regarding the approach to hospice/end-of-life care is correct?
   a. Hospice programs only provide provisions of care in the home.
   b. Admission to hospice is involuntary and directed by a physician's order.
   c. The focus is on the provision for facilitating a quality of life just for the dying client.
   d. An interdisciplinary team approach is used for the care of the client and family.

4. A client receiving nursing care in a home hospice program can expect which of the following?
   a. The use of high-technology equipment such as ventilators until time of death.
   b. To receive around-the-clock skilled direct nursing client care until time of death.
   c. To be provided pain and symptom management that will achieve the best quality of life.
   d. To be given complete relief of only distressing physical symptoms.

5. To qualify for hospice benefits, a criterion for admission is that the client's prognosis needs to be limited to:
   a. 2 weeks or less
   b. 3 months or less
   c. 6 months or less
   d. 1 year or less

6. Identify all of the following that apply when describing the concept of hospice:

   _____ a. Unit of care is client and the family

   _____ b. Preferred location is in the hospital setting

   _____ c. Control of symptoms

   _____ d. Ends with death

   _____ e. Palliative care in multiple settings

   _____ f. Available 24 hours a day, 7 days a week

   _____ g. A philosophy of care

   _____ h. Makes terminal illness pleasant

   _____ i. Interdisciplinary team approach

   _____ j. Support of family ends with client's death

   _____ k. Supports active euthanasia

   _____ l. Alleviates pain and suffering

   _____ m. Does not hasten death

   _____ n. Goal changes from curative to comfort

   _____ o. Control of disease process

7. Place in correct sequence the events that occur with multiple organ dysfunction syndrome (MODS).

　　_____　a.　Anaerobic metabolism, acidosis, hyperkalemia, and tissue ischemia

　　_____　b.　Release of toxic metabolites and destructive enzymes

　　_____　c.　Inadequate blood flow to body tissues and cells

8. In teaching the client and family about the dying process, the nurse discusses the emotional signs of approaching death. What are four common emotional signs and related interventions?

　　a.　_____

　　b.　_____

　　c.　_____

　　d.　_____

9. When performing an assessment of a terminally ill client, which of the following interventions is correct?
　　a.　Assess only the client; do not include the family's perception of the client's symptoms.
　　b.　When the client is unable to communicate, there is no need to assess symptoms of distress any longer.
　　c.　Assess clients who are unable to communicate distress by teaching the family to observe for objective signs of discomfort.
　　d.　The nurse only assesses the client for pain, dyspnea, agitation, nausea, and vomiting.

10. Identify two examples of transcultural differences when dealing with the dying process.

　　a.　_____

　　b.　_____

11. Identify the physical signs of death.

12. Which of the following interventions is correct when performing postmortem care?
　　a.　Place the head of the bed at 30 degrees.
　　b.　Remove pillows from under the head.
　　c.　Leave a Foley (indwelling) catheter in place in the bladder.
　　d.　Place pads under the hips and around the perineum.

13. Which of the following interventions after the death of a client are correct? *Mark all that apply.*

　　_____　a.　Remove the body to the morgue or funeral home immediately after death.

　　_____　b.　Follow agency policies to remove all tubes and lines from the body.

　　_____　c.　A death certificate must accompany the body to the funeral home.

　　_____　d.　Provide privacy for the family and significant others with the deceased.

　　_____　e.　Allow family and significant other to perform religious and cultural customs.

14. Differentiate the following terms, and state the American Nurses Association stand on each one.

 a. Active euthanasia

 b. Passive euthanasia

15. Match the term with its correct definition.

Definition

1. A legal document that appoints a person to make decisions regarding health care for someone else who becomes unable to make his or her own decisions.

2. A physician's order that specifies that a client has indicated that he or she does not want CPR.

3. A legal document that instructs health care providers and family members of what life-sustaining treatment one wants or does not want if that person becomes unable to make these decisions.

4. Requires that all clients admitted to health care agencies be asked if they have written Advance Directives.

Term

_____ a. Living will

_____ b. Durable power of attorney for health care

_____ c. Patient Self-Determination Act

_____ d. Do not resuscitate (DNR)

16. Briefly present your opinion about suicide. Include in the discussion your thoughts on whether this act is ever justifiable.

17. Give some thought to the following sentence: "Medical and scientific advances have contributed to longevity, but they have also contributed to prolonging dying." Participate in a discussion with your fellow students on how this impacts nursing care, and share your group's points with your clinical instructor.

18. The priority outcome for the client at the end of life is to achieve physical and psychological comfort until death. Identify the most common symptoms of distress of the terminally ill client.

19. Read the following statements regarding physically distressing symptoms of a terminally ill client and decide whether each is true or false. *Write T for true or F for false in the blanks provided. If the statement is false, correct the statement to make it true.*

_____ a. Anorexia is normal; however, clients should be forced to eat small, frequent meals.

_____ b. Cessation of food ingestion is a natural process and hydration with IV fluids can cause distressing respiratory symptoms.

_____ c. A client's sense of hearing is intact even though the client is withdrawn from the external environment.

_____ d. The most feared symptom of a terminally ill client is dyspnea.

_____ e. Pain is a not a universal problem although it is common and has many causes.

_____ f. The goals for a client with dyspnea are to relieve the primary cause and the psychological distress and autonomic response.

_____ g. *Dyspnea* is defined as the respiratory rate of less than 20 breaths/min. with observed labored breathing.

_____ h. Dyspnea is common in about 50% to 70% of clients and is considered by health care providers to be the worst symptom of distress when a client is near death.

_____ i. Nausea and vomiting occur in about 40% of terminally ill clients in the last week of life.

_____ j. There are a variety of causes of nausea and vomiting including constipation from opioid therapy.

_____ k. Nausea and vomiting are prevalent only in individuals with certain types of cancer.

_____ l. Agitation can result from either physical or spiritual distress.

20. The most common treatment of pain in a terminally ill client is administration of:
    a. Opioids
    b. Steroids
    c. Nonsteroidal anti-inflammatory agents
    d. Radiation treatments

21. A nursing diagnosis for a terminally ill client is Ineffective Breathing Pattern. On a separate sheet of paper, briefly discuss each of the following interventions for alleviating this distress.
    a. Opioids
    b. Diuretics
    c. Bronchodilators
    d. Anticholinergics
    e. Oxygen
    f. Sedatives
    g. Nonpharmacologic interventions

22. Assessment of a dying client and the family results in the nursing diagnosis of Deficient Knowledge related to dysphagia, pain, dyspnea, nausea and vomiting, agitation, and other common signs and symptoms. Develop a teaching plan for this client and family.

23. Define *palliative care*.

24. While caring for a Native American/American Indian client who is dying, the nurse should keep in mind which of the following?
    a. Traditional Native American/American Indian families are male-dominated.
    b. Expression of grief is open, especially among women.
    c. Families will not allow the client to die alone.
    d. Family members are likely to avoid visiting the terminally ill family member.

Rehabilitation Concepts for Acute and Chronic Problems

LEARNING OUTCOMES

1. Differentiate between impairment, disability, and handicap.
2. Identify the roles of each member of the interdisciplinary rehabilitation team.
3. Interpret physical and psychosocial assessment findings for the client in a rehabilitation program.
4. Describe the major components of a functional assessment.
5. Prioritize nursing diagnoses for the client in a rehabilitation program.
6. Develop a teaching plan for the rehabilitation client who has impaired physical mobility.
7. Explain the role of the interdisciplinary team in managing clients with self-care deficits.
8. Analyze risk factors for skin breakdown in clients who are in rehabilitation settings.
9. Differentiate bladder-training techniques for a client with spastic versus flaccid bladder.
10. Assess client outcomes of the interdisciplinary rehabilitation program.
11. Explain the primary concerns for clients being discharged to home after rehabilitation.

LEARNING ACTIVITIES

1. Before completing the study guide exercises for this chapter, it is recommended that you review the following:
   - Anatomy and physiology of the neurologic, muscular, cardiac, and respiratory systems
   - Techniques: urinary catheterization, bowel care, bowel and bladder training, principles of bathing, transferring, range of motion exercises, and ambulation
   - Hazards of immobility
   - Concept of body image
   - Concept of self-esteem
   - Concept of loss and grieving
   - Concept of adult development
   - Concept of human sexuality
   - Concepts of nutrition

2. If possible, visit a rehabilitation unit or facility and observe the care of clients with disabilities.

3. Review the boldfaced terms and their definitions in Chapter 10 to enhance your understanding of the content.

STUDY/REVIEW QUESTIONS

Answers to the Study/Review Questions are provided on the companion Evolve Learning Resources Web site at http://evolve.elsevier.com/Iggy/.

1. Interdisciplinary team meetings are held for planning client and family care. Match the interdisciplinary team member with the example of the type of work performed. *Answers can be used more than once, and there may be more than one answer for each example.*

Interdisciplinary Team Members

1. Physiatrist
2. Rehab nurse/case manager
3. Physical therapist
4. Occupational therapist
5. Speech-language pathologist
6. Recreational/activity therapist
7. Cognitive therapist
8. Social worker
9. Psychologist
10. Vocational counselor
11. Nursing or therapy assistant
12. Client

Types of Work Performed

_____ a. Screens, tests, and recommends feeding techniques for dysphagia

_____ b. Assists in job placement and seeking work-related training

_____ c. Works with clients in learning to feed, bathe, and dress themselves

_____ d. Teaches clients skills related to co-ordination such as picking up coins from a table

_____ e. Specializes in rehabilitation medicine

_____ f. Involved in client and family coping skills

_____ g. Identifies community resources

_____ h. Coordinates the team's plan of care

_____ i. Teaches client skills to achieve mobility

_____ j. Assists with care such as bathing and feeding

_____ k. Works directly with clients who have experienced head injuries and have difficulty with memory

_____ l. Assists clients in learning new interests or hobbies

_____ m. Involved in all aspects of restoration and maintenance of optimal health

_____ n. Teaches clients how to talk again, and works with swallowing problems

_____ o. Performs comprehensive physical, psychosocial, and spiritual assessments

_____ p. Discharge planning to determine adequacy of current situation and potential needs and how care will be provided to meet those needs

_____ q. Has final authority regarding teaching plan

2. Differentiate the following terms related to rehabilitation by defining these concepts in your own words.
   a. Rehabilitation

   b. Impairment

   c. Disability

   d. Handicap

e.   Chronic illness

f.   Disability condition

3.   As a result of a car accident, an adult client is unable to perform certain activities of daily living such as bathing without assistance. This is an example of which of the following terms? Explain why you chose your answer.
   a.   Rehabilitation
   b.   Impairment
   c.   Disability
   d.   Handicap

4.   The leading cause of disabling conditions in young adults and the third leading cause of death in adults 45 to 54 years of age is:
   a.   Stroke
   b.   Cancer
   c.   Arthritis
   d.   Accidents

5.   Identify the two primary goals of the rehabilitation team and give an example for each of those goals.

   a.   _____

   b.   _____

6.   Read the following statements regarding nursing care of the older adult in rehabilitation and decide whether each is true or false. *Write T for true or F for false in the blanks provided. If the statement is false, correct the statement to make it true.*

   _____ a.   Fatigue and physical complications often affect the length of time of a given workout session.

   _____ b.   Older adults are at increased risk for injury related to antihypertensive medications and orthostatic hypotension.

   _____ c.   Diarrhea is a risk factor because increased intestinal motility.

   _____ d.   Clients are at risk for ineffective coping related to a lack of family and significant other support systems.

   _____ e.   Assess for urinary problems present before illness or rehabilitation to determine effectiveness of a bladder training program.

   _____ f.   Turning the client every 2 hours is adequate for the skin type of the older adult.

   _____ g.   Encouraging ingestion of 2000 to 2500 mL of fluid per day is an important consideration in the prevention of complications from flaccid bladder and heart disease.

7. Identify the five categories of data that should be collected on all clients preparing for rehabilitation.

   a. _____

   b. _____

   c. _____

   d. _____

   e. _____

8. A client with Decreased Cardiac Output is entering a rehabilitation program. The nurse will expect to find which data during the assessment of this client?
   a. Has shortness of breath on activity
   b. Has the ability to ambulate without angina
   c. Feels rested upon awakening from sleep
   d. Uses an antihistamine for pollen allergies

9. Which of the following is a priority when assessing a paraplegic client who is entering a rehabilitation program?
   a. Family and cultural background
   b. Baseline hemoglobin and hematocrit measurements
   c. Habits of bowel elimination before illness
   d. Manual dexterity, muscle control, and mobility

10. A client with a neurogenic bladder is to be taught how to perform intermittent self-catheterization. Which of the following is essential for the nurse to assess before beginning the teaching-learning sessions?
    a. Motor function of both upper extremities
    b. The type of neurogenic bladder the client has
    c. The client's gender
    d. The age of the client

11. To maintain skin integrity of a client in a rehabilitation unit, the nurse assesses which of the following items? *Check all that apply.*

    _____ a. Amount of water or other fluids in a day

    _____ b. Type and amount of food

    _____ c. Sensation to the skin

    _____ d. Circulation of oxygen and elimination of waste

    _____ e. Ability to move extremities

    _____ f. Ability to feel pain from pressure

    _____ g. Ability to change position as needed

    _____ h. Ability to perform self-care activities

    _____ i. Respiratory status and oxygenation

12. Which of the following statements correctly describes the Functional Independence Measure (FIM)?

    _____ a. The FIM is a basic indicator of the severity of a disability.

    _____ b. The FIM tries to measure what a person should do, whatever the diagnosis or impairment.

    _____ c. The FIM tries to measure what the person actually does, whatever the diagnosis or impairment.

    _____ d. The assessment may be performed by any health care discipline.

    _____ e. Categories for assessment are self-care, sphincter control, mobility and locomotion, communication, and cognition.

    _____ f. Evaluations may be done at specified times during therapy to determine client progress.

13. For each of the activities listed, specify whether it is an Activity of Daily Living (ADL) or Independent Living Skill.

Activity

_____ a. Bathing

_____ b. Using the telephone

_____ c. Dressing

_____ d. Ambulating

_____ e. Shopping

_____ f. Preparing food

_____ g. Feeding

_____ h. Housekeeping

Type

1. Activity of daily living

2. Independent living skill

14. Nurses use the major body systems approach when performing a physical assessment of a client. Identify data collected for each of the following areas as they relate to the functional abilities of a client in rehabilitation and chronic illness.
    a. Cardiovascular assessment

    b. Respiratory assessment

    c. Gastrointestinal and nutritional assessment

    d. Renal and urinary assessment

    e. Neurologic assessment (motor, sensation, cognitive)

    f. Musculoskeletal assessment

    g. Skin assessment (risk for breakdown and actual breakdown)

15. What is the purpose of a vocational assessment for a client in rehabilitation?

16. The nurse reviews with the client the results of manual muscle testing performed by physical therapy. This procedure determines the client's:
    a. Body flexibility and muscle strength
    b. Range of motion and resistance against gravity
    c. Muscle strength and amount of pain on movement
    d. Voluntary versus involuntary muscle movement

17. A client is preparing for discharge from a rehabilitation facility. Identify and briefly explain the two methods that can be used to assess the readiness of the client and the home for this discharge.

    a. _____

    b. _____

18. A 24-year-old paraplegic client, as a result of a motor vehicle accident, is admitted to a rehabilitation unit after 6 weeks of hospitalization. On a separate sheet of paper, identify potential outcome(s) for each of the following problem areas and submit your answers for review to your clinical instructor. Use the outcome(s) in the "Planning: Expected Outcomes" section of your text as a guide.
    a. Impaired Physical Mobility
    b. Self-care Deficit
    c. Risk for Impaired Skin Integrity
    d. Total Urinary Incontinence
    e. Constipation
    f. Ineffective Individual Coping

19. When assisting a client with a hemiparesis to transfer or ambulate, the nurse instructs the client to:
    a. Lean the body weight backward.
    b. Use the weaker hand to assist.
    c. Lean the body weight toward the nurse.
    d. Use the strong hand to assist.

20. Which of the following items would be helpful to use when transferring a quadriplegic to a bed or chair? *Check all that apply.*
    a. Gait belt
    b. Sliding board
    c. "Quad" cane
    d. Long-handled reacher

21. A client with Impaired Physical Mobility must be monitored for which of the following early potential complications?
    a. Pressure ulcers
    b. Renal calculi
    c. Osteoporosis
    d. Fractures

22. The best ways to prevent pressure ulcers resulting from immobility is to teach the client and significant other which of the following? *Check all that apply.*

    _____ a. Change position often to relieve pressure on all bony prominences.

    _____ b. Maintain good skin care by keeping the skin clean and dry.

    _____ c. Inspect the skin at least once a day for problems such as reddened areas that do not fade readily.

    _____ d. Use pressure-relieving devices as a substitute for changing position.

    _____ e. Eat foods high in protein, carbohydrates, and vitamins for sufficient nutrition.

23. When assisting a client to perform range-of-motion (ROM) exercises, the nurse knows that ROM exercises should be performed:
    a. Only on the knees, hips, elbows, and shoulders
    b. On each joint three times per session
    c. Never beyond the point of inducing pain in the joint
    d. On each joint two times per day

24. A client in a rehabilitation unit has a nursing diagnosis of Risk for Falls related to the effects of orthostatic hypotension. Identify at least three nursing interventions to prevent falls and injuries.

    a. _____

    b. _____

    c. _____

25. Which of the following assistive-adaptive devices would be recommended to a client with a weak hand grasp?
    a. Gel pad
    b. Foam buildups
    c. Hook and loop fastener straps
    d. Buttonhook

26. When teaching a client with hemiplegia about energy conservation techniques, the nurse would include which of the following?
    a. Using a walker instead of a cane
    b. Scheduling physical therapy immediately before eating
    c. Using a bedside commode
    d. Scheduling recreational activities in afternoon or evening

27. Which of the following is true regarding the use of mechanical pressure-relieving devices?
    a. They effectively eliminate the need to turn clients.
    b. They still require repositioning clients regularly.
    c. They prevent pressure ulcers in debilitated clients.
    d. They have been shown to be ineffective against pressure ulcers.

28. A client has a lower motor neuron injury below T12. This injury results in which of the following types of neurogenic bladder?
    a. Reflex or spastic bladder
    b. Flaccid bladder
    c. Uninhibited bladder
    d. Inhibited bladder

29. A client with a flaccid bladder will have which of the following urinary elimination problems?
    a. Incontinence and inability to empty the bladder completely
    b. Incontinence caused by inability to wait until on a commode or bedpan
    c. Urinary retention and dribbling because of overflow of urine
    d. Incontinence due to loss of sensation

30. Match the bladder training intervention with the type of neurogenic bladder problem. Answers may be used more than once.

    Bladder Training Interventions

    Neurogenic Bladder Problem
    1. Reflex or spastic
    2. Flaccid
    3. Uninhibited

    _____ a. Credé maneuver

    _____ b. Facilitating/triggering

    _____ c. Intermittent catheterization

    _____ d. Medications

    _____ e. Consistent toileting schedule

    _____ f. Valsalva maneuvers

    _____ g. Regulation of fluid intake

    _____ h. Drinking fluids to promote an acidic urine

31. Which of the following are correct principles for performing an intermittent catheterization? *Check all that apply and correct the false answers.*

    _____ a. A catheter is inserted every 2 to 4 hours.

    _____ b. It is usually performed after the Valsalva or Credé maneuver.

    _____ c. A residual of less than 150 mL increases the interval between catheterization.

    _____ d. The maximum time interval between catheterizations is 6 hours.

    _____ e. The client uses sterile technique at home.

32. Which of the following medications would the client with a flaccid bladder most likely be given?
    a. Dantrolene sodium (Dantrium)
    b. Bethanechol chloride (Urecholine)
    c. Flavoxate hydrochloride (Urispas)
    d. Oxybutynin chloride (Ditropan)

33. The nurse is instructing a client and his family about which beverages to drink in order to create an acidic urine. Which of the following would *not* be included in this teaching?
    a. Citrus juices
    b. Prune juice
    c. Tomato juice
    d. Cranberry juice

34. Which of the following clients is most likely to have a flaccid bowel dysfunction?
    a. A 28-year-old client with a crushed pelvis
    b. A 54-year-old man with Guillain-Barré syndrome
    c. An 18-year-old woman with a displaced cervical fracture
    d. A 48-year-old woman who has multiple sclerosis

35. Digital stimulation of the anus as a method of re-establishing bowel control is most successful in the client who has had what problem?
    a. A myocardial infarction and is starting cardiac rehabilitation
    b. Chronic diarrhea resulting from radiation to the bowel
    c. Bowel incontinence resulting from a cerebrovascular accident
    d. A spinal cord injury resulting from a diving accident

36. What is the drug of choice for long-term management of bowel dysfunction?
    a. Milk of magnesia
    b. Senna concentrate (Senokot)
    c. Dulcolax or glycerin suppository
    d. Psyllium (Metamucil)

37. An example of a food that should be part of breakfast for the client with bowel dysfunction is:
    a. Dried apricots or plums
    b. White bread
    c. Cheddar cheese
    d. Sausage links

38. Lower motor neuron disease or injury results in which of the following bowel dysfunctions?
    a. Flaccid bowel pattern
    b. Reflex (spastic) bowel pattern
    c. Uninhibited bowel pattern
    d. Inhibited bowel pattern

39. A client with an uninhibited bowel pattern dysfunction has difficulty with:
    a. Defecation occurring suddenly and without warning.
    b. Defecation occurring infrequently and in small amounts.
    c. Frequent defecation, urgency, and complaints of hard stool.
    d. Intermittent constipation and diarrhea.

40. Match each intervention with the appropriate nursing diagnosis. The nursing diagnoses may be used more than once.

Nursing Diagnoses
1. Total urinary incontinence
2. Constipation
3. Risk for impaired skin integrity
4. Decreased cardiac output
5. Impaired physical mobility

Interventions

_____ a. Perform major tasks in the morning

_____ b. Complete the Braden Scale

_____ c. Credé maneuver

_____ d. Perform gait training

_____ e. Wheelchair "push-ups"

_____ f. Use a tilt table

_____ g. Digital stimulation

Genetic Concepts for Medical-Surgical Nursing

CHAPTER 11

LEARNING OUTCOMES

1. Describe the structure and forms of DNA.
2. List the events and processes involved in DNA replication.
3. Describe the relationship between genes and proteins.
4. Compare the concept of phenotype with that of genotype.
5. Compare the patterns of inheritance for single gene traits.
6. Explain how genetic variations can induce or affect adult health problems.
7. List 10 adult health problems that have a genetic basis.
8. Identify assessment questions that help obtain information for a genetic assessment.
9. Construct a three-generation pedigree.
10. Identify clients at risk for a genetic predisposition for health problems.
11. Explain how genetic testing is different from other laboratory tests.
12. Describe the role of the medical-surgical nurse in genetic counseling.

LEARNING ACTIVITIES

1. Before completing the study guide exercises for this chapter, it is recommended that you review the following:
   - Basic terms and concepts of genetics
   - Human Genome Project

2. Review the boldfaced terms and their definitions in Chapter 11 to enhance your understanding of the content.

STUDY/REVIEW QUESTIONS

Answers to the Study/Review Questions are provided on the companion Evolve Learning Resources Web site at http:// evolve.elsevier.com/Iggy/.

1. Puzzle: Complete each item by placing the correct answer in the appropriate number (across or down) in the puzzle.

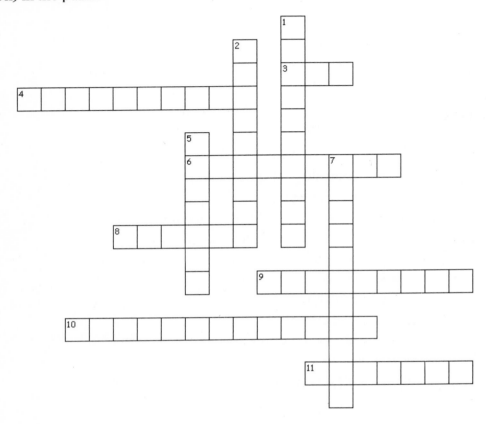

Across

3. Ribonucleic acid
4. The "pinched in" area of a chromosome where the two chromatids are joined.
6. The 22 pairs of human chromosomes that do not code for the sexual differentiation of the individual.
8. The complete set of genes for a species.
9. _____ siblings, two siblings that share a womb and are born at the same time, but are the result of different fertilized eggs.
10. The process of making a new strand of DNA.
11. The complete set of chromosome pairs found in all of the individual's somatic cells.

Down

1. Cellular DNA tightly condensed and coiled into a dense body.
2. The observed expression of any given single gene trait (such as blood type, hair color)
5. A set of chromosomes consisting of half of each pair.
7. _____ siblings, the product of one fertilized egg that split into two or more equal parts during embryogenesis.

2. Describe "genes." Where are they located? What do they do?

     d. G_2

     e.   M

6. Differentiate cytokinesis and nucleokinesis.

3. The text states that "all human cells with a nucleus each contain the entire set of human genes." What human cells are exceptions to this statement? Why?

7. Humans have _____ chromosomes that are divided into _____ pairs.

4. List the four bases in DNA.

8. Differentiate autosomes and sex chromosomes.

     a. _____

     b. _____

     c. _____

     d. _____

5. For each stage of the cell cycle, briefly describe what activity is occurring.

     a. G_0

9. Differentiate phenotype and genotype.

     b. G_1

     c.   S

10. Complete the following statements:
    a. When a person has homozygous alleles for a particular trait, the genotype and phenotype are the <u>same/different</u> *(circle one).*
    b. When a person has heterozygous alleles for a particular trait, the phenotype and the genotype are the <u>same/different</u> *(circle one).*
    c. For recessive traits, the phenotype and genotype are the <u>same/different</u> *(circle one).*

11. Which type of mutation is passed on to a person's children? Explain.

12. For each characteristic listed below, specify whether it is autosomal dominant (AD) or autosomal recessive (AR) pattern of inheritance, or both (B).
    _____ a. In order for a trait to be expressed, both alleles must be present.
    _____ b. A trait is expressed even when only one allele of the pair is dominant.
    _____ c. The trait is found equally in males or females.
    _____ d. The trait is found in every generation with no skipping.
    _____ e. The trait may not appear in all generations of any one branch of a family.
    _____ f. The risk for an affected person to pass the trait to his or her children is 50% with each pregnancy.

_____ g. The children of an affected mother and an affected father will always be affected (100% risk).

_____ h. The trait can be transmitted to children if one parent is an unaffected carrier and the other parent is either a carrier or is affected.

13. Which of the following statements about sex-linked recessive patterns of inheritance are true? *Write T for true or F for false in the blanks provided. If the statement is false, correct the statement to make it true.*

_____ a. X-linked recessive genes have a dominant expressive pattern of inheritance in males and a recessive expressive pattern of inheritance in females.

_____ b. The trait can be transmitted from father to son.

_____ c. Transmission of the trait is from father to daughters, who will be carriers.

_____ d. Female carriers have a 100% risk (with each pregnancy) of transmitting the gene to their children.

14. Which of the following statements best reflects the correct actions of the health care professional who is providing genetic counseling?
    a. "This test will help us to tell everything about you!"
    b. "We are going to perform this testing because you asked for it and it won't affect your family in any way."
    c. "The results of this genetic testing will be sent to your health insurance carrier immediately."
    d. "I'm here to provide information so that you can make an informed decision about genetic testing."

15. When assessing for genetic risks, which of the following are indicators that a client may have an increased genetic risk for a disease or disorder? *Mark all that apply.*

    _____ a. A close family member has an identified genetic problem.

    _____ b. A client tells you that he was exposed to a carcinogenic substance during a war.

    _____ c. A client has been diagnosed with two different types of cancer.

    _____ d. A client's sister had breast cancer at age 24.

16. Which of the following disorders has a genetic pattern of inheritance? *Mark all that apply.*

    _____ a. Malignant hyperthermia

    _____ b. Gallstones

    _____ c. Cystic fibrosis

    _____ d. Acute lymphocytic leukemia

    _____ e. Polycystic kidney disease

    _____ f. Sickle cell disease

17. For the following disorders, mark SLR for those that have a sex-linked recessive pattern of inheritance, and mark FC for those that have familial clustering.

    _____ a. Hemophilia

    _____ b. Hypertension

    _____ c. Alzheimer's disease

    _____ d. Red-green colorblindness

    _____ e. G6PD deficiency

    _____ f. Schizophrenia

18. Using your own family's information, construct a three-generation pedigree, using the symbols provided in Figure 11-21. Do you note any pattern of inheritance for a particular trait?

Emergency and Mass Casualty Nursing

LEARNING OUTCOMES

1. Describe the emergency department (ED) environment, including special populations, cultural considerations, and interdisciplinary team members.
2. Plan and implement best practices to maintain staff and client safety in the ED.
3. Explain the core competencies that nurses need to function in the ED.
4. Identify types of certification that ED nurses can obtain to demonstrate or develop their expertise.
5. Triage clients into emergent, urgent, and nonurgent categories.
6. Prioritize resuscitation interventions based on the primary survey of the ED client.
7. Describe the general process of admission through disposition of a client in the ED.
8. Contrast the triage process under usual conditions with triage in a mass casualty.
9. Identify the components of an Emergency Preparedness and Response Plan.
10. Compare the key personnel roles in an Emergency Preparedness and Response Plan.
11. Differentiate two types of debriefing that occur after a mass casualty incident.
12. Describe the general process that occurs in the ED when a client is suspected of having encountered a bioterrorism agent, such as anthrax.

LEARNING ACTIVITIES

1. Before completing the study guide exercises for this chapter, it is recommended that you review the following:
   - Concepts of emergency care
   - Basic principles of triage
   - Your area's Emergency Preparedness and Response Plan

2. Review the boldfaced terms and their definitions in Chapter 12 to enhance your understanding of the content.

STUDY/REVIEW QUESTIONS

Answers to the Study/Review Questions are provided on the companion Evolve Learning Resources Web site at http://evolve.elsevier.com/Iggy/.

1. Match the intervention with the Primary Survey category.

Category
1. Airway/cervical spine
2. Breathing
3. Circulation
4. Disability
5. Exposure

Intervention

_____ a. Maintain alignment of cervical spine.

_____ b. Re-evaluate level of consciousness frequently.

_____ c. Use direct pressure for external bleeding.

_____ d. Observe for chest wall trauma or other physical abnormalities.

_____ e. Establish patent airway.

_____ f. Remove all clothing to allow for thorough assessment.

_____ g. Maintain vascular access with a large-bore catheter.

_____ h. Prepare for chest decompression if needed.

2. How does triage under "usual conditions" differ from triage under "mass casualty conditions"?

3. Match the job description with the interdisciplinary team member.

Interdisciplinary Team Member
1. Forensic nurse examiner
2. Paramedic
3. Emergency medical technician
4. Psychiatric crisis nurse team

Job Description

_____ a. May work with clients involved with a sudden serious illness or death of a loved one

_____ b. Advanced life support provider who can perform advanced techniques, such as cardiac monitoring, advanced airway management and intubation, or giving intravenous drugs en route to the hospital

_____ c. Offers basic life support interventions such as oxygen, basic wound care, splinting, spinal immobilization, and may carry AEDs

_____ d. Obtains client histories, collects evidence, and offers counseling and follow-up for victims of rape, child abuse, and domestic violence

4. For each statement, name the certification described.
   a. This certification involves neonatal and pediatric resuscitation, and may be required in some areas:

   b. This certification is optional, and serves to validate core emergency nursing knowledge base:

   c. A required certification that involves noninvasive assessment and management skills for airway maintenance and CPR:

   d. This certification is usually required and involves invasive airway management skills, pharmacology and electrical therapies, and special resuscitation:

5. For the following individuals who have been injured due to a major explosion at an assembly plant, classify the triage priority according to the color-coded disaster triage tag system (green tag, yellow tag, red tag, or black tag).

_____ a. A client who has died of his injuries

_____ b. A client with a fractured ankle

_____ c. A client who is short of breath and has broken ribs and a hemothorax

_____ d. A client with an open fracture of the femur

_____ e. A client who has a weak pulse and is bleeding profusely from a severe arm laceration

_____ f. A client who has a 4-inch leg laceration that is oozing blood slowly

_____ g. A client who has fallen and sprained her shoulder

6. State the four most common reasons that clients seek emergency care.

a. _____

b. _____

c. _____

d. _____

7. Which age group has the highest emergency department visit rate?
   a. Newborn to 5 years
   b. 20 to 39 years
   c. 40 to 65 years
   d. 75 years and older

8. Which of the following statements are *true* regarding utilization of the emergency department?

_____ a. Some clients are labeled as "drug seekers."

_____ b. Some clients tend to use the emergency department for almost all their health care needs.

_____ c. Some clients use the emergency department as a means of establishing a relationship with a primary care provider.

9. For each safety consideration below, list two interventions that can be used to minimize risk.

a. Client identification
   1) _____
   2) _____

b. Injury prevention
   1) _____
   2) _____

c. Risk for errors and adverse effects
   1) _____
   2) _____

d. Injury prevention for staff
   1) _____
   2) _____

10. List at least four core competencies that are part of emergency nursing practice.

a. _____

b. _____

c. _____

d. _____

11. Each of the following patients has entered the emergency department's waiting room. Put them in order of priority, with 1 being the highest priority and 4 being the lowest priority.

    _____ a. A woman brings in her toddler who has an earache, had a temperature of 102.5° F at home, and is crying loudly.

    _____ b. A 65-year-old man is having crushing chest pain.

    _____ c. A 32-year-old woman who is complaining of severe abdominal pain.

    _____ d. A 16-year-old boy has a broken arm after falling while skateboarding.

12. Compare the "AVPU" mnemonic to the categories of the Glasgow Coma Scale.

13. Differentiate what occurs during the primary survey and the secondary survey in the emergency department setting.

14. Explain how the overall goal of triage in a mass casualty or disaster situation differs from the goal of triage in the emergency department of a hospital.

15. For each person listed below, describe the specific role during a mass casualty incident or disaster.
    a. Hospital incident commander

    b. Medical command physician

    c. Triage officer

16. Compare the two types of debriefing that occur after mass casualty incidents or disasters.

17. A client enters the emergency department and tells the nurse that he thinks that he has been exposed to anthrax. He opened an envelope that contained a white powder. Which of the following is the *first* thing the emergency department nurse should do?

    a. Have the client wait in the emergency department waiting room until the decontamination team arrives.

    b. Separate the client from others in the emergency department.

    c. Tell the client to go outside to wait until the decontamination team arrives.

    d. Ask the client for the envelope that contained the white powder.

18. When a client is seen in the emergency department, what is meant by "client disposition"?

19. Cite at least three examples of client and family education that may be done in the emergency department.

    a. _____

    b. _____

    c. _____

20. During the primary survey, what is the *highest* priority intervention?

21. When assessing breathing during the primary survey, what is included in this assessment?

22. By applying direct pressure on a client's arm, what type of hemorrhage is the nurse trying to control?

23. In a resuscitation situation, which is a quick way to estimate a client's blood pressure?

    a. Check for presence of a radial pulse.

    b. Check the blood pressure with an automated blood pressure machine.

    c. Check the blood pressure with a manual cuff and stethoscope.

    d. Check for the presence of a carotid pulse.

Interventions for Clients with Common Environmental Emergencies

LEARNING OUTCOMES

1. Assess clients for common types of heat-related injuries.
2. Teach clients how to prevent heat-related injuries.
3. Prioritize first aid interventions for clients who have heat-related injuries.
4. Prioritize first aid interventions for clients experiencing snakebites.
5. Differentiate care for clients who have arthropod bites and stings.
6. Develop a plan of care for a client who is allergic to bees and experiences a bee sting.
7. Teach clients how to prevent arthropod bites and stings.
8. Prioritize care for clients who have been struck by lightning.
9. Teach clients how to avoid cold injuries.
10. Explain the rationale for interventions when warming clients who have cold injuries.
11. Describe best practices for clients who are at risk for or experience altitude-related illnesses.
12. Develop a plan of care for a client with near-drowning.

LEARNING ACTIVITIES

1. Before completing the study guide exercises for this chapter, it is recommended that you review the following:
   - Principles of first aid
   - Basic principles of anaphylaxis and allergic response

2. Review the boldfaced terms and their definitions in Chapter 13 to enhance your understanding of the content.

STUDY/REVIEW QUESTIONS

Answers to the Study/Review Questions are provided on the companion Evolve Learning Resources Web site at http://evolve.elsevier.com/Iggy/.

1. Which of the factors listed below are predisposing factors associated with heat-related illness? *Check all that apply.*

   _____ a. High humidity

   _____ b. Low humidity

   _____ c. Obesity

   _____ d. Anemia

   _____ e. Seizures

   _____ f. Dehydration

   _____ g. Calcium channel blockers

   _____ h. Beta-adrenergic blockers

2. The nurse is providing client education about the prevention of heat-related illness. Which of the following statements is correct? For those that are not correct, rewrite to make them true.

   _____ a. Wear lightweight, dark-colored clothing when working outside.

   _____ b. Plan to limit activities at the hottest time of day.

   _____ c. Avoid fluids with electrolytes before, during, and after exercise.

   _____ d. Use a sunscreen with an SPF of at least 45.

3. The primary cause of heat exhaustion is _____ _____.

4. The main reason for exertional heat stroke is _____ _____.

5. Classic heat stroke results from _____ _____ _____.

6. An older adult woman has been found in her apartment after neighbors reported not seeing her for 2 days. The weather has been extremely hot for the last 2 weeks. Neighbors found that her windows were all shut, the air conditioner was not working, and she had no fans. The woman had a body temperature of 106° F, was weak, confused, and very upset. Her BP was 92/48, pulse 120, and respirations 32. She is suffering from which of the following conditions?
   a. Classic heat stroke
   b. Exertional heat stroke
   c. Heat exhaustion
   d. Dehydration

7. A television meteorologist has been doing a photo-shoot during a day when temperatures reached 110° F. Later in the day, he complains that he feels weak, has a headache, and feels nauseated and dizzy. He states that he had water with him but often forgot to drink it. His body temperature is 98.9° F. He is suffering from which of the following conditions?
   a. Classic heat stroke
   b. Exertional heat stroke
   c. Heat exhaustion
   d. Fluid overload

8. During a summer marathon at a beach resort city, a runner suddenly collapses after running in the race for 1 hour. The weather has been extremely hot during the race day, with temperatures of almost 100° F and high humidity. The runner's body temperature is 105.2° F, she is confused and sweating. She is suffering from which of the following conditions?
   a. Classic heat stroke
   b. Exertional heat stroke
   c. Heat exhaustion
   d. Dehydration

9. For the runner in question number 8, first aid interventions while waiting for an ambulance to arrive would include which of the following? *Check all that apply.*

    _____ a. Placing ice packs on the neck, axillae, chest, and groin.

    _____ b. Immersion in ice

    _____ c. Removing clothing

    _____ d. Oral fluids, especially electrolyte drinks

    _____ e. Wetting the body with tepid water, then fanning rapidly to cool by evaporation

    _____ f. Oral antipyretics, such as acetaminophen or aspirin

10. In the emergency department, what interventions are used to reduce the body temperature of the client with heat stroke, and what temperature is the immediate goal?

11. The nurse caring for the client with heat stroke should monitor closely for what three problems while implementing measures to reduce body temperature?

    a. _____

    b. _____

    c. _____

12. Name the two families of poisonous snakes that are found in North America, and name at least one example for each.

    a. _____

    b. _____

13. You are outside doing yard work when your neighbor calls you because he has just killed a snake that has bitten him on the arm while he was gardening. He does not know what kind of snake it is. What features would lead you to believe that this snake is poisonous? *Check all that apply.*

    _____ a. Triangular head

    _____ b. Two fangs that are curved

    _____ c. The snake hissed before biting.

    _____ d. A depression in the skin between each eye and nostril

    _____ e. A diamond pattern on its back

    _____ f. Black, red, and yellow bands of color on the snake (red bands next to black bands)

    _____ g. Black, red, and yellow bands of color on the snake (red bands next to yellow bands)

    _____ h. Puncture wounds in the skin

14. The snake in question number 13 is found to be a copperhead. What interventions for first aid should you implement after you call for an ambulance? List at least three.

15. For the client in question number 13, you are notified that the emergency medical service may not arrive for another hour or so because of an automobile accident. Which of the following actions are correct at this time?
    a. Apply ice to the wound.
    b. Incise the wound to allow the blood to flow freely.
    c. Place a constricting band, proximal to the wound, that does not impair venous drainage or arterial flow.
    d. Place a constricting band, proximal to the wound, that is tight enough to reduce arterial flow of the venom.

16. For each manifestation of envenomation from a poisonous snake, indicate whether the problem is seen with pit viper envenomation or coral snake envenomation, or both types.

Type of Envenomation
1. Pit viper envenomation
2. Coral snake envenomation
3. Both types

Manifestation
_____ a. Mild and transient pain at the bite site

_____ b. Severe pain, swelling, and bruising at the bite site

_____ c. Formation of vesicles or hemorrhagic bullae

_____ d. Cranial and peripheral nerve deficits

_____ e. Nausea and vomiting

_____ f. Coagulopathy

_____ g. Total flaccid paralysis

_____ h. Minty, rubbery, or metallic taste in the mouth

17. When administering antivenom medications, the nurse needs to monitor closely which common complication?
    a. Hemorrhage
    b. Neurologic impairment
    c. Anaphylactic shock
    d. Seizures

18. Complete the following puzzle, using the clues listed below.

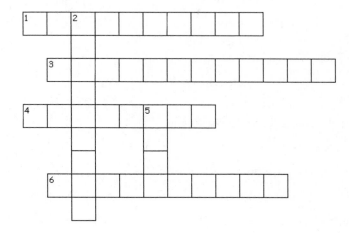

Across

1. The type of hairs launched by the spiders in 2 down that may induce a severe inflammatory reaction if they penetrate the eyes or skin.
3. This type of spider hides in areas that are dark and secluded, and are also known as fiddlebacks or violin spiders *(two words)*.
4. The type of bee that cannot sting repeatedly when disturbed.
6. The type of spider is often found in cool, damp areas such as outdoor log piles, under rocks, or in sheds or garages. The female has a red hourglass pattern on her ventral abdomen *(two words.)*

Down

2. The largest spiders in the arachnid class.
5. The venom of this type of scorpion is neurotoxic.

19. Match the first aid and hospital interventions with the appropriate spider bite. Some interventions may be appropriate for both types of spider bites.

Interventions

_____ a. Apply cold compresses.

_____ b. Elevate extremity.

_____ c. Administer opioid pain medications.

_____ d. Administer muscle relaxants.

_____ e. Administer oral dapsone.

_____ f. Administer tetanus prophylaxis.

_____ g. Monitor for seizures and rapidly rising BP.

_____ h. Antivenom is available for use.

_____ i. Debridement and skin grafting may be needed later for severe wounds to heal.

Spider Bites

1. Brown recluse spider

2. Black widow spider

20. Differentiate the appearance of a brown recluse spider bite and a black widow spider bite.

21. Define *lactrodectism*.

22. Your neighbor's teenage daughter told you that she would like to have a tarantula for a pet, but her mother is fearful of tarantula bites. What important information should you share with them before they buy a tarantula?

23. You are presenting a class to a group of Girl Scouts about prevention of arthropod bite and sting prevention. List at least four things that can be done to prevent such bites and stings.

24. Which way is the recommended method for removing the stinger after a bee sting?
    a. Remove the stinger with the fingers
    b. Remove the stinger with tweezers
    c. Gently scrape the stinger off with the edge of a knife blade or credit card.
    d. Using sticky tape, place the tape over the area and pull the tape off, repeating several times.

25. Read the following statements regarding bee and wasp stings and decide whether each is true or false. *Write T for true or F for false in the blanks provided. If the statement is false, correct the statement to make it true.*

_____ a. First aid for bee and wasp stings include quick removal of the stinger and application of warm compresses.

_____ b. Systemic effects develop if the individual is sensitive to the venom.

_____ c. An anaphylactic reaction results in respiratory distress, laryngeal edema, and hypotension.

_____ d. An "EpiPen" should be administered anytime a bee or wasp sting occurs.

_____ e. Subcutaneous (SC) epinephrine is recommended over the intramuscular (IM) route.

_____ f. An oral antihistamine should also be administered if an allergic reaction is suspected.

_____ g. Persons with a history of allergic reactions to bee or wasp stings should wear a medical alert tag.

26. According to the text, the best remedy for lightning injuries is _____.

27. When an individual is struck by lightning, several effects occur. List at least five of these effects, and note the one that is considered the most lethal initial effect.

28. You are leaving the beach because storm clouds are beginning to form, and suddenly, near the lifeguard stand, you see a bright flash of light. As you join the crowd of people to help, you notice three people lying on the sand. Which of the three should be given priority resuscitation measures? Explain your answer.
    a. A teenager who is motionless except for shallow respirations. He has a weak pulse.
    b. A woman who is pulseless and not breathing.
    c. A man who is moaning with a visible burn on his left arm.

29. Differentiate hypothermia and frostbite:

30. Which of the following measures are *correct* when rewarming a victim of deep frostbite? *Check all that apply.*

    _____ a. Rubbing the area helps speed the warming process.

    _____ b. Rapid rewarming in a 38° C to 41° C water bath will be required.

    _____ c. Rapid rewarming is avoided due to the possibility of seizures.

    _____ d. Rewarming does not cause pain due to damage to the peripheral nerves.

    _____ e. Opioid may be given because of the pain associated with rewarming.

    _____ f. Dry heat may be applied as needed to assist in the rewarming process.

    _____ g. After rewarming, the extremity should be elevated above the heart level.

    _____ h. Immunization for tetanus prophylaxis will be needed.

31. During a class for cold-weather hiking, which statement is correct when teaching about early recognition of frostbite? Hiking partners should observe each other frequently for:
    a. White, waxy appearance to exposed skin on the ears, nose, and cheeks
    b. Edema and redness over the exposed skin
    c. Coloring of the skin that is mottled
    d. Small blisters that contain dark fluid and areas that do not blanch

32. Define "frostnip" and how to treat it.

33. For each of the degrees of frostbite, describe the tissue damage that occurs.
    a. First degree

    b. Second degree

    c. Third degree

    d. Fourth degree

34. You are preparing for a ski trip. List at least five measures that should be taken to prevent hypothermia and frostbite during your time outdoors.

35. The physiologic consequence of increased altitude in humans is _____.

36. Match the characteristics with the type of clinical condition that may develop in people at high altitudes.

Clinical Conditions
(AMS) Acute mountain sickness
(HACE) High altitude cerebral edema
(HAPE) High altitude pulmonary edema

Characteristics

_____ a.   This is usually the first condition noticed.

_____ b.   The most frequent cause of death associated with high altitude.

_____ c.   Noted when ataxia without focal signs develops.

_____ d.   Persistent dry cough; cyanosis of lips and nail beds.

_____ e.   Confusion and impaired judgment.

_____ f.   Tachypnea and tachycardia noted at rest.

_____ g.   Feeling chilled, irritable, and apathetic.

_____ h.   Pink, frothy sputum is a late sign.

37. On a separate sheet of paper, describe the measures that should be taken to manage altitude-related illnesses:
    a.   AMS
    b.   HACE
    c.   HAPE

38. Differentiate the effects of fresh water and salt water aspiration into the lungs.

39. Explain how hypothermia and the diving reflex may actually assist a victim of near-drowning.

40. You are at the beach when a group of people pull a young girl from the water. Witnesses say she was body surfing and fell off the board, head first. What is a priority of care for this victim?
    a.   Begin airway management measures before she is removed from the water.
    b.   Perform abdominal thrusts to remove water from her lungs before attempting CPR.
    c.   Examine her neck and spine for obvious injuries before beginning CPR.
    d.   Take care to stabilize the spine before beginning airway management measures.

Fluid and Electrolyte Balance

LEARNING OUTCOMES

1. Explain why women and older adults have less total body water than do men and younger adults.
2. Interpret whether a client's serum electrolyte values are normal, elevated, or low.
3. Describe the expected blood volume responses when isotonic, hypertonic, or hypotonic intravenous fluids are infused.
4. Describe the expected blood osmolarity responses when isotonic, hypertonic, or hypotonic intravenous fluids are infused.
5. Explain the relationships between antidiuretic hormone, urine output volume, and osmolarity.
6. Analyze a client's hydration status on the basis of physical assessment findings.
7. Evaluate a client's food choices for sodium content.
8. Evaluate a client's food choices for potassium content.
9. Evaluate a client's food choices for calcium content.

LEARNING ACTIVITIES

1. Before completing the study guide exercises for this chapter, it is recommended that you review the following:
   - Normal anatomy and physiology
   - Fluid requirements of adults
   - Adult nutrition
   - Adult growth and development

2. Consult any fluid and electrolyte book for nursing.

3. Review the boldfaced terms and their definitions in Chapter 14 to enhance your understanding of the content.

STUDY/REVIEW QUESTIONS

Answers to the Study/Review Questions are provided on the companion Evolve Learning Resources Web site at http://evolve.elsevier.com/Iggy/.

1. What is homeostasis?
    a. The condition of being as close to normal as possible for proper body system functioning
    b. A balance of solvents and solutes for proper body functioning
    c. A balance of fluid and electrolytes to maintain proper body function
    d. The regulation of water and blood with other body substances

2. Indicate which of the following statements regarding water is true. *Write T for true or F for false in the blanks provided.*

    _____ a. Water is the solvent that delivers substances such as glucose, sodium, and potassium to organs, tissues, and cells.

    _____ b. Water is a passive member of the homeostatic regulatory mechanism.

    _____ c. Fluids, especially water, make up approximately 55% to 60% of total adult body weight.

    _____ d. For homeostasis of fluid and electrolytes, as the amount of solute increases, the volume of solvent must decrease.

    _____ e. When equilibrium occurs, net filtration of water stops because there is no hydrostatic pressure gradient.

    _____ f. In osmosis, the physiologic activity is one of movement from a lower to a higher concentration of molecules.

    _____ g. Lean muscle tissue is lower in water content than is fat.

    _____ h. The amount of body fat and the gender and age of the client affect total body water content.

3. Match the physiologic influences on fluids and electrolytes in the body with their descriptions.

Physiologic Influences
1. Diffusion
2. Filtration
3. Hydrostatic pressure
4. Osmolality
5. Osmolarity
6. Osmosis

Descriptions

_____ a. "Water-pushing" pressure

_____ b. The movement of electrolytes into or out of a cell

_____ c. The movement of water only (the solvent) through a selectively permeable membrane

_____ d. The unit of measure in a liter of solution that reflects the concentration of solutes

_____ e. The unit of measure in a kilogram of solution that reflects the concentration of solutes

_____ f. The movement of fluid through a membrane; usually occurs from capillaries to the interstitial space

4. Describe the two major functions of body fluids.

    a. _____

    b. _____

5. Describe the direction of fluid flow.
    a. When hypertonic fluids are infused

    b. When hypotonic fluids are infused

6. The major hypothalamic mechanism for stimulating fluid intake is _____ _____.

7. Identify the four areas a nurse must consider when assessing serum electrolyte values for significance and follow-up interventions.

    a. _____

    b. _____

    c. _____

    d. _____

8. Which of the following statements about the lymphatic system are true? *Check all that apply.*

    _____ a. Lymph fluid contains more protein than plasma.

    _____ b. Lymph flow is slower than blood flow.

    _____ c. Lymph flow is enhanced by a pump system.

    _____ d. Lymphatic vessels carry lymph fluid toward the heart.

    _____ e. Lymph fluid is filtered by lymph nodes.

    _____ f. The lymphatic system takes lymph to the kidneys for excretion.

9. How does active transport differ from diffusion and filtration?
    a. Energy is required.
    b. Solvent, rather than solute, is moved.
    c. It is more common in men than in women.
    d. Active transport moves cations and anions, whereas diffusion and filtration move only cations.

10. Match each electrolyte with the corresponding lab value and description. *Answers can be used more than once.*

Electrolytes
1. Sodium
2. Potassium
3. Calcium
4. Phosphorus
5. Magnesium
6. Chloride

Normal Lab Values and Descriptions

_____ a. Normal plasma value is 3.5 to 5.0 mEq/L.

_____ b. Major anion of extracellular fluid (ECF).

_____ c. Normal value is 98 to 106 mEq/L.

_____ d. Main cation in ECF of the cell that maintains ECF osmolarity.

_____ e. Works in balance with calcium.

_____ f. Normal plasma value is 136 to 145 mEq.

_____ g. Has more activity in the cell than in the blood.

_____ h. Major cation of intracellular fluid (ICF) in the cell.

_____ i. Maintains action potentials in excitable membranes.

_____ j. Functions include contraction of skeletal and cardiac muscle.

_____ k. Normal value is 3.0 to 4.5 mg/dL.

_____ l. Major intracellular anion.

_____ m. Free form is physiologically active in the body.

_____ n. Normal value is 1.3 to 2.1 mg/dL.

11. Identify two factors that primarily control the electrolyte balance within the body.

    a. _____

    b. _____

12. Identify three sources of body fluid intake and give the average daily amount of each for an adult.

    a. _____

    b. _____

    c. _____

13. Complete the following table regarding hormones that affect fluid and electrolyte balance.

Hormone	Effect on Renal Sodium Absorption	Effect on Renal Excretion of Water	Effect on Blood Osmolarity
Aldosterone			
Antidiuretic hormone (ADH)			
Natriuretic peptide			

14. Which statement about fluid and electrolyte changes associated with aging is correct?
    a. Over 60% of the body weight of an older adult is water.
    b. Changes in the renal function increase the risk of electrolyte imbalance.
    c. Skin turgor is a reliable measure of body fluid levels.
    d. Thirst sensation is the best indicator of body fluid balance.

15. Which statement regarding total body water in the older adult is correct?
    a. Decreased muscle mass results in decreased total body water.
    b. There is increased thirst and urination as a result of the aging process causing a loss of water.
    c. Loss of elasticity of the skin causes more evaporation of water from the skin.
    d. Older adults are susceptible to hypernatremia, which causes increased water retention.

16. When assessing for dehydration, what is the best location for assessing skin turgor on an older adult? How is this different than for other adults?

17. The potassium laboratory value of a 65-year-old client was 5.0 mEq/L. This value can be interpreted as
    a. High for the client's age
    b. Low for the client's age
    c. Normal for the client's age
    d. Dependent upon the medical diagnosis

18. Match the following cellular compartments with the descriptions. *Answers can be used more than once.*

Compartments
1. Extracellular compartment
2. Intracellular compartment

Cellular Descriptions

_____ a. Contains the largest amount of body fluid

_____ b. Contains plasma

_____ c. Contains interstitial fluid

_____ d. High in sodium and chloride content

_____ e. High in potassium and phosphorous content

_____ f. High in magnesium content

19. Identify and explain the four routes through which fluid is removed from the body.

20. The nurse assesses the urine specific gravity of 1.035 as an indication of
    a. Overhydration
    b. Dehydration
    c. Normal value for an adult
    d. Renal disease

21. Identify at least eight causes of fluid loss that may lead to a client's fluid imbalance.

    a. _____

    b. _____

    c. _____

    d. _____

    e. _____

    f. _____

    g. _____

    h. _____

22. A client is reviewing her dietary log with the nurse regarding maintenance of a low-sodium diet. Which of the following food items are high in sodium? *Check all that apply.*

    _____ a. Egg roll with soy sauce

    _____ b. White rice

    _____ c. Grilled cheese sandwich (American cheese)

    _____ d. Salads with oil and vinegar dressing

    _____ e. Bacon and eggs

    _____ f. Cottage cheese and tomato

    _____ g. Steak

    _____ h. Chicken breast

    _____ i. Soup with saltine crackers

    _____ j. Steamed vegetables

23. Identify common food sources for the following electrolytes:
    a. Sodium

    b. Potassium

    c. Calcium

    d. Phosphorus

    e. Magnesium

24. Which of the following best explains how antidiuretic hormone (ADH) affects urine output?
    a. It increases permeability to water in the tubules causing a decrease in urine output.
    b. It increases urine output as a result of water being absorbed by the tubules.
    c. Urine output is reduced as the posterior pituitary decreases ADH production.
    d. Increased urine output results from increased osmolarity and fluid in the extracellular space.

25. Identify three factors that affect the analysis of fluid and electrolyte assessment findings in the older adult.

    a. _____

    b. _____

    c. _____

26. Which of the following best explains the difference between men and women in relationship to total body water?
    a. Women excrete more water than men and have less body water.
    b. Men have less body fat and therefore less body water.
    c. Men retain more body water because they have more body fat.
    d. Men generally have less body fat than women do and more body water.

27. Which client would most likely have increased aldosterone secretion?
    a. Client who has excessive salt ingestion
    b. Client who drinks a lot of water
    c. Client who loses a lot of fluid and salt
    d. Client who loses potassium and water

28. Identify the two main hormones that regulate calcium absorption.

    a. _____

    b. _____

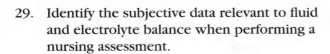
29. Identify the subjective data relevant to fluid and electrolyte balance when performing a nursing assessment.

30. Identify the objective data relevant to fluid and electrolyte balance when performing a nursing assessment.

31. Briefly discuss why psychosocial factors are important to an accurate fluid and electrolyte status assessment.

CASE STUDY: THE CLIENT WITH A FLUID IMBALANCE

Answer Guidelines for the Case Study questions are provided on the companion Evolve Learning Resources Web site at http://evolve.elsevier.com/Iggy/.

Your client is a 45-year-old man who had GI surgery 4 days ago. He is NPO, has a nasogastric tube, and IV fluids of D$_5$1/2 normal saline at 100 mL/hr. The nursing physical assessment includes the following: alert and oriented; fine crackles; capillary refill within normal limits (WNL); moving all extremities; complaining of abdominal pain, muscle aches, and "cottony" mouth; dry mucous membranes; bowel sounds hypoactive, last BM was 4 days ago; skin turgor is poor; 200 mL of dark green substance has drained from NG tube in last 3 hours. Voiding dark amber urine without difficulty. Intake for last 24 hours is 2500 mL. Output is 2000 mL including urine and NG drainage. Febrile and diaphoretic; BP 130/80; pulse 88; urine specific gravity 1.035; serum potassium 3.0 mEq/L; serum sodium 140 mEq/L; Cl 92 mEq/L; Mg 1.4 mg/dL.

1. Analyze the data in the case study. Do the findings indicate a fluid deficit or fluid excess problem? Support your answer with data from this client.

2. What factors could be contributing to a fluid deficit problem?

3. Evaluate this client's electrolyte values and give a rationale for the answer.

Interventions for Clients with Fluid Imbalances

CHAPTER 15

LEARNING OUTCOMES

1. Identify clients at risk for fluid imbalances.
2. Use laboratory data and clinical manifestations to assess fluid balance and imbalance.
3. Apply appropriate nursing techniques to promote comfort and safety in the client with dehydration.
4. Prioritize nursing care for the client with dehydration.
5. Explain why different types of intravenous fluids are used to treat different types of dehydration.
6. Develop a community-based teaching plan to prevent dehydration in the older client at continuing risk for fluid loss.
7. Analyze changes in clinical manifestations to determine the effectiveness of therapy for the client with dehydration.
8. Prioritize nursing care for the client with overhydration.
9. Analyze changes in clinical manifestations to determine the effectiveness of therapy for the client with overhydration.

LEARNING ACTIVITIES

1. Before completing the study guide exercises for this chapter, it is recommended that you review the following:
   - Normal nutrition for adults
   - Fluid and electrolyte requirements for adults

2. Consult any fluid and electrolyte book for nursing.

3. Review the boldfaced terms and their definitions in Chapter 15 to enhance your understanding of the content.

STUDY/REVIEW QUESTIONS

Answers to the Study/Review Questions are provided on the companion Evolve Learning Resources Web site at http://evolve.elsevier.com/Iggy/.

1. Which statement is true regarding dehydration in the adult?
   a. Dehydration may result from excessive sodium intake.
   b. Relative dehydration may be caused by fluid shifts.
   c. Persons older than 65 years of age have increased thirst mechanisms.
   d. Water loss is the primary reason for dehydration.

2. Match the type of dehydration with the corresponding pathophysiology. *Answers may be used more than once.*

Type of Dehydration
1. Isotonic dehydration
2. Hypertonic dehydration
3. Relative dehydration
4. Hypotonic dehydration

Pathophysiology
_____ a. Results from equal amounts of fluid and electrolyte loss
_____ b. Results when electrolyte loss is greater than water loss
_____ c. Results in cell shrinkage
_____ d. Plasma osmolality remains normal
_____ e. Fluid shifts without loss of total body water
_____ f. Results when water loss is greater than electrolyte loss

3. What serum laboratory values would you expect to see increased in hypertonic dehydration?

   a. _____
   b. _____
   c. _____
   d. _____
   e. _____

4. Which compensatory mechanism occurs as a result of hypertonic dehydration?
   a. Release of ANP from the heart
   b. Release of antidiuretic hormone (ADH) from the pituitary gland
   c. Fluid shift from the ECF (extracellular fluid) to the ICF (intracellular fluid)
   d. Increased aldosterone release from the adrenal gland

5. Identify four clinical symptoms that you might observe in a client with circulatory volume overload as a result of renal failure.

   a. _____
   b. _____
   c. _____
   d. _____

6. Which interventions would be effective for a client with fluid volume excess caused by congestive heart failure? *Identify all that apply.*

   _____ a. Sodium and fluid restriction
   _____ b. Slow infusion of hypotonic saline
   _____ c. Administration of potassium
   _____ d. Administration of loop diuretics
   _____ e. Position in semi-Fowler's to high Fowler's position
   _____ f. Monitor weight weekly

7. State the change (increase or decrease) for the following parameters seen in hypotonic overhydration.
   a. Serum sodium

   b. Blood pressure

   c. Intracellular fluid

   d. Hematocrit

8. Match the following clinical conditions to the most likely type of resulting fluid imbalances. *Answers can be used more than once.*

Resulting Fluid Imbalances
1. Hypertonic dehydration
2. Hypotonic dehydration
3. Isotonic dehydration
4. Hypotonic overhydration
5. Hypertonic overhydration
6. Isotonic overhydration

Clinical Conditions

_____ a. Vomiting

_____ b. Diabetes insipidus

_____ c. Hemorrhage

_____ d. Infusions of D_5/0.2% NS

_____ e. Infusions of 0.9% NS

_____ f. SIADH (syndrome of inappropriate antidiuretic hormone)

_____ g. Infusion of 3% NS

_____ h. Chronic malnutrition

_____ i. End-stage renal disease

_____ j. Unconsciousness

_____ k. Gastrointestinal suctioning

9. Explain why each of the following findings taken from a history of an older adult client are risk factors for dehydration.
    a. Age older than 70 years

    b. History of hypertension

    c. Weight loss of 4 pounds in 28 hours

d. Feelings of light-headedness

e. Change in cognition

10. A client at risk for fluid volume excess should be taught to
    a. Increase diuretic dose if swelling occurs.
    b. Limit the amount of free water in relation to sodium intake.
    c. Monitor his or her skin turgor.
    d. Weigh self each day on the same scale.

11. Which of the following manifestations is often the first indication of a fluid balance problem in an older adult?
    a. Fever
    b. Mental status changes
    c. Poor skin turgor
    d. Dry skin

12. Mild dehydration is best treated with
    a. Diuretics
    b. Intravenous fluid replacement
    c. Oral fluids
    d. Tube feedings

13. During rehydration with intravenous fluids for a client with severe dehydration, what are the *two* most important areas to monitor?
    a. Skin turgor
    b. Pulse rate
    c. Serum sodium levels
    d. Urine output
    e. Urine specific gravity
    f. Mucous membranes

14. Fill in the blanks with one of the following: *isotonic, hypotonic,* or *hypertonic*
    a. Isotonic dehydration is treated with
       _____ fluid solutions.
       Name two examples.

    b. Hypotonic dehydration is treated with
       _____ fluid solutions.
       Name two examples.

    c. Hypertonic dehydration is treated with
       _____ fluid solutions.
       Name one example.

15. When performing oral care for a client with dehydration, which of the following would be the best choice?
    a. Lemon glycerin swabs
    b. Rinsing with commercial mouthwash
    c. Frequent rinses with half-strength hydrogen peroxide
    d. Tap water or saline rinses ad lib

CASE STUDY: THE CLIENT WITH OVERHYDRATION

Answer Guidelines for the Case Study questions are provided on the companion Evolve Learning Resources Web site at http://evolve.elsevier.com/Iggy/.

A client is admitted to the hospital with a decreased serum osmolality and a serum sodium of 126 mEq/L. You recognize that dehydration or overhydration may accompany hypotonic conditions.

1. In further assessing the client, which of the following assessments would indicate that the client has fluid volume excess?
   a. Distended hand and neck veins
   b. Decreased urine output
   c. Decreased capillary refill
   d. Increased rate and depth of respirations

2. Which of the following assessments would indicate that the client has fluid volume excess? *Check all that apply.*
   _____ a. Increased, bounding pulse
   _____ b. Jugular venous distention
   _____ c. Diminished peripheral pulses
   _____ d. Presence of crackles
   _____ e. Thirst
   _____ f. Elevated blood pressure
   _____ g. Orthostatic hypotension
   _____ h. Skin pale and cool to touch

3. After determining by an in-depth clinical assessment that the client is not dehydrated, which of the following interventions would be appropriate to correct this hypotonic overhydration?
   a. Administration of 0.9% NS
   b. Restriction of free water
   c. Administration of antihypertensives
   d. Restriction of potassium

4. Which of the following would the nurse monitor for evidence of a worsening hypotonic condition?
   a. Mental status
   b. Urine output
   c. Skin changes
   d. Bowel sounds

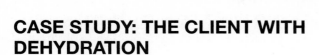

CASE STUDY: THE CLIENT WITH DEHYDRATION

Answer Guidelines for the Case Study questions are provided on the companion Evolve Learning Resources Web site at http://evolve.elsevier.com/Iggy/.

A client with a history of vomiting and diarrhea from the flu presents with a rapid pulse, orthostatic hypotension, urine output of 20 mL/hr, skin turgor poor with tenting, and increased respiratory rate.

1. Which type of dehydration do you suspect that this client has? Explain your answer.

2. In evaluating the client's laboratory values, would you expect the following values to be normal, elevated, or decreased?
   a. Urine specific gravity
   b. Urine volume
   c. Serum sodium
   d. Serum hematocrit and hemoglobin
   e. Blood urea nitrogen (BUN)
   f. Serum osmolality

3. The compensatory mechanism responsible for the client's rapid pulse is increased
   a. Circulation of angiotensin
   b. Sympathetic discharge
   c. Aldosterone production
   d. Renal reabsorption of sodium and water

4. Immediate interventions to correct this client's fluid volume imbalance would include which of the following?
   a. Rapid hydration with D_5W
   b. Administration of a loop diuretic
   c. Administration of an osmotic diuretic
   d. Rapid hydration with $D_5/0.45\%$ NS

5. Which of the following would be most important to monitor to determine the client's response to corrective interventions?
   a. Respiratory rate and depth
   b. Skin turgor
   c. Urinary output
   d. Weight

6. Which of the following would indicate that the client is having a negative response to fluid resuscitation?
   a. Increased blood pressure
   b. Urinary output of 40 mL/hr
   c. Presence of crackles
   d. Widening of pulse pressure

Interventions for Clients with Electrolyte Imbalances

LEARNING OUTCOMES

1. Identify clients at risk for imbalances of potassium.
2. Use laboratory data and clinical manifestations to assess potassium balance and imbalance.
3. Prioritize nursing care for the client with potassium imbalance.
4. Develop a community-based teaching plan to prevent deficiencies or excesses of potassium in the older adult client at risk for potassium imbalance.
5. Explain the effects of potassium imbalances on the activity of digoxin.
6. Differentiate diuretics that increase potassium loss from those that reduce potassium loss.
7. Analyze changes in clinical manifestations to determine the effectiveness of therapy for the client with potassium imbalance.
8. Identify clients at risk for imbalances of sodium.
9. Use laboratory data and clinical manifestations to assess sodium balance and imbalance.
10. Identify drugs that contain large amounts of sodium.
11. Prioritize nursing care for the client with sodium imbalance.
12. Develop a community-based teaching plan to prevent deficiencies or excesses of sodium in the older adult client at risk for sodium imbalance.
13. Analyze changes in clinical manifestations to determine the effectiveness of therapy for the client with sodium imbalance.
14. Identify clients at risk for imbalances of calcium.
15. Use laboratory data and clinical manifestations to assess calcium balance and imbalance.
16. Prioritize nursing care for the client with calcium imbalance.
17. Develop a community-based teaching plan to prevent deficiencies or excesses of calcium in the older adult client at risk for calcium imbalance.
18. Analyze changes in clinical manifestations to determine the effectiveness of therapy for the client with calcium imbalance.

LEARNING ACTIVITIES

1. Before completing the study guide exercises for this chapter, it is recommended that you review the following:
   - Fluids and electrolytes
   - Fluid requirements for adults

- Dietary information in any nutrition reference for foods high in potassium, sodium, calcium, phosphorus, and magnesium
- Nutrition requirements for adults
- Mechanism of action and nursing interventions for the drug digoxin

2. Review the boldfaced terms and their definitions in Chapter 16 to enhance your understanding of the content.

STUDY/REVIEW QUESTIONS

Answers to the Study/Review Questions are provided on the companion Evolve Learning Resources Web site at http://evolve.elsevier.com/Iggy/.

1. The laboratory value that refers to hypokalemia is
   a. Serum calcium level below 8.0 mg/dL
   b. Serum potassium level below 5.0 mEq/L
   c. Serum calcium level below 11.0 mg/dL
   d. Serum potassium level below 3.5 mEq/L

2. In addition to inadequate potassium intake, what type of clinical conditions would cause hypokalemia? Provide examples of the type of clients with these clinical conditions.

3. Which clinical finding indicates the effect of hypokalemia on the body?
   a. Hypertension, bounding pulses, and bradycardia
   b. Moist crackles, tachypnea, and diminished breath sounds
   c. General skeletal muscle weakness, lethargy, and weak hand grasps
   d. Increased specific gravity and decreased urine output

4. Older adults are at increased risk for developing hypokalemia mainly because they
   a. Often require medications that predispose them to hypokalemia
   b. Experience increased excretion of electrolytes through the urine
   c. Have an increased capacity for the kidney to concentrate urine
   d. Tend to consume large volumes of fluids leading to water intoxication

5. A client is to receive potassium supplements for treatment of hypokalemia. Indicate the nursing interventions for safely administering oral and intravenous medications.

6. The complication of rapid infusion of intravenous potassium is
   a. Pulmonary edema
   b. Cardiac arrest
   c. Postural hypotension
   d. Renal failure

7. Which of the following laboratory data are often found in association with hypokalemia?
   a. Decreased arterial blood $Paco_2$
   b. Elevated blood glucose levels
   c. Inverted urine sodium/potassium ratio
   d. Increased urine potassium levels

8. Which statement indicates the client understands the treatment of hypokalemia?
   a. "My wife does all the cooking. She shops for food high in calcium."
   b. "When I take the liquid potassium in the evening, I'll eat a snack beforehand."
   c. "I will avoid bananas, orange juice, and salt substitutes."
   d. "I hate being stuck with needles all the time to monitor how much sugar I can eat."

9. Which of the following statements about potassium and digoxin are true?
   a. Digoxin increases potassium loss through the kidneys.
   b. Digoxin toxicity can result if hypokalemia is present.
   c. Digoxin may cause potassium levels to rise to toxic levels.
   d. Hypokalemia causes the cardiac muscle to be less sensitive to digoxin.

10. Develop assessment criteria for a home care nurse to use with a cardiac client who was discharged from the hospital, is receiving loop diuretics, and is at risk for developing hypokalemia.

11. Which laboratory value refers to hyperkalemia?
    a. Serum calcium level above 8.0 mg/dL
    b. Serum potassium level above 3.5 mEq/L
    c. Serum calcium level above 11.0 mg/dL
    d. Serum potassium level above 5.0 mEq/L

12. In the hospitalized client, what is a common cause of hyperkalemia?
    a. Overuse of potassium-sparing diuretics
    b. Poor management of diabetes insipidus
    c. Too-rapid administration of intravenous fluids with potassium
    d. Administering blood with an 18-gauge or larger needle

13. If hyperkalemia results from dehydration, laboratory findings may include which of the following?
    a. Increased hematocrit and hemoglobin levels
    b. Decreased serum electrolyte levels
    c. Increased urine potassium levels
    d. Decreased serum creatinine

14. Which of the following is not an assessment finding associated with hyperkalemia?
    a. Wheezing on exhalation
    b. Numbness in hands, feet, and around the mouth
    c. Frequent, explosive diarrhea stools
    d. Irregular heart rate and hypotension

15. Identify nursing interventions that would be performed for clients with hyperkalemia.

16. Which of the following electrocardiogram (ECG) changes reflect hyperkalemia? How is this different from hypokalemia?
    a. Tall peaked T waves
    b. Narrow QRS complex
    c. Tall P waves
    d. Normal P-R interval

17. Which of the following clients are at risk for developing hyperkalemia or hypokalemia? Mark your answers with ↑ for hyperkalemia or ↓ for hypokalemia.

    _____ a. Severely malnourished older adult man

    _____ b. Client with chronic obstructive pulmonary disease (COPD) on prednisone

    _____ c. Client with short bowel syndrome on total parenteral nutrition

    _____ d. Client with gout

    _____ e. Older adult receiving high-dose gentamicin

    _____ f. Client with hypertension receiving Aldactone

    _____ g. Client with metabolic alkalosis

    _____ h. Client with an ileostomy

    _____ i. Client in early stage of severe burns

    _____ j. Client with respiratory acidosis

    _____ k. Client with diabetic ketoacidosis receiving intravenous insulin

    _____ l. Client with uncontrolled diabetes mellitus

    _____ m. Trauma client with crushed extremities

    _____ n. Client with congestive heart failure and taking loop diuretics

18. Compare and contrast subjective data for clients with hypokalemia and hyperkalemia in a nursing assessment.

19. Compare and contrast objective data for clients with hypokalemia and hyperkalemia in nursing assessment.

20. Match the following acid-balance imbalances with the associated conditions of hyperkalemia or hypokalemia.

    Imbalance

    _____ a. Metabolic acidosis
    _____ b. Metabolic alkalosis
    _____ c. Respiratory acidosis
    _____ d. Respiratory alkalosis

    Condition
    1. Hyperkalemia
    2. Hypokalemia

21. The part of the body that is the most sensitive to the early effects of hyperkalemia and hypokalemia is which of the following? Indicate the potential complication that can result and give a rationale for your answer.
    a. Heart
    b. Skeletal muscles
    c. Gastrointestinal tract
    d. Kidney

22. Hyponatremia refers to which of the following laboratory values?
    a. Serum sodium level below 136 mEq/L
    b. Serum chloride level below 95 mEq/L
    c. Serum sodium level below 145 mEq/L
    d. Serum chloride level below 103 mEq/L

23. Which statement is correct regarding the pathophysiology of hyponatremia?
    a. As the concentration of sodium falls in the extracellular fluid (ECF), it rises within the cell.
    b. Excitable membranes are more responsive during periods of hyponatremia.
    c. The nervous system tissues are the least affected by hyponatremia.
    d. Intracellular swelling may occur because of the shifts in osmotic pressure in the ECF.

24. Assessment findings of a client with hyponatremia include which of the following?
    a. Constipation and paralytic ileus
    b. Watery diarrhea with abdominal cramping
    c. Muscle cramping and spasticity
    d. Tachypnea and diminished breath sounds

25. Which of the following clients is at risk of developing hyponatremia?
    a. Diabetic client with a blood glucose of 430 mg/dL
    b. Febrile client with copious diarrhea
    c. Client with Cushing's syndrome
    d. Client with chronic obstructive pulmonary disease (COPD) taking high doses of steroids

26. The nurse would monitor for which of the following complications that can occur with hyponatremia?
    a. Proteinuria/prerenal failure
    b. Change in mental status/increased intracranial pressure
    c. Pitting edema/circulatory failure
    d. Possible stool for occult blood/gastrointestinal bleeding

27. Which of the following clients are at risk for developing hyponatremia? *Check all that apply.*
    _____ a. A postoperative client who has been NPO for 24 hours
    _____ b. Client with nephrotic syndrome
    _____ c. Client with high blood cholesterol
    _____ d. Client with overactive adrenal glands
    _____ e. Client playing tennis in 100° F weather
    _____ f. Client with gastrointestinal fistula draining copious fluids
    _____ g. Client on high-salt diet
    _____ h. Diabetic client with blood glucose of 250 mg/dL
    _____ i. Client with excessive intake of 5% dextrose solution
    _____ j. Client with no fluid intake for several days
    _____ k. Client with congestive heart failure
    _____ l. Febrile client with copious watery diarrhea
    _____ m. Client with massive systemic infection
    _____ n. Client with aldosterone deficiency
    _____ o. Client being given 0.9% normal saline at 100 mL/hr

28. When hyponatremia occurs with fluid deficit, the nurse can expect to administer
    a. Saline infusions
    b. 5% dextrose with saline
    c. 10% dextrose with saline
    d. Lactated Ringer's solution

29. Hypernatremia refers to
    a. Serum chloride level above 95 mEq/L
    b. Serum sodium level above 135 mEq/L
    c. Serum chloride above 103 mEq/L
    d. Serum sodium level above 145 mEq/L

30. What is the intervention of choice for a client with mild hypernatremia caused by excessive fluid loss?
    a. Intravenous infusion of 10 units of insulin in 50 mL of 10% dextrose
    b. Replacement of table salt with salt substitute
    c. Furosemide (Furoside; Lasix) 20 mg
    d. Increased water intake

31. Match the clinical situations with the resulting effect leading to hypernatremia. *Answers may be used more than once.*

Resulting Effects Leading to Hypernatremia
1. Inadequate water intake
2. Excess fluid loss
3. Excess sodium intake
4. Decreased sodium excretion

Clinical Situations

_____ a. Severe diarrhea

_____ b. Presence of fever

_____ c. Profound diaphoresis

_____ d. Primary hyperaldosteronism

_____ e. Kidney disease of the proximal tubule

_____ f. Confused and disoriented

_____ g. Multiple sodium bicarbonate injections

_____ h. Severe vomiting

_____ i. Restraints

32. Which problem/condition could result in a relative hypernatremia?
    a. Excessive sodium ingestion
    b. Inadequate sodium excretion
    c. Excessive water ingestion
    d. Inadequate water ingestion

33. Which of the following is the most common manifestation of a client with hypernatremia? Provide specific assessment findings.
    a. Gastrointestinal disorders
    b. Altered urinary elimination
    c. Impaired skin integrity
    d. Altered cerebral functioning

34. The nurse identifies the client most at risk for developing hypernatremia as one who
    a. Dislikes drinking milk and lacks calcium in the diet
    b. Is receiving total parental nutrition related to gastrointestinal surgery
    c. Is being seen in the emergency department with excessive diarrhea and vomiting from food poisoning
    d. Is an older adult client with decreased sensitivity to thirst

35. What precaution or intervention should you teach a client at continued risk for hypernatremia?
    a. Avoid salt substitutes.
    b. Avoid aspirin and aspirin-containing products.
    c. Read labels on canned or packaged foods to determine sodium content.
    d. Increase your average daily intake of caffeine-containing foods and beverages.

36. Compare and contrast objective data for clients with hyponatremia and hypernatremia in a nursing assessment.

37. As a result of hyponatremia or hypernatremia, a client is at risk for injury related to which of the following?
    a. Altered thought processes
    b. Spontaneous fractures
    c. Tetanic muscle contractions
    d. Painful paresthesia

38. Which of the following laboratory values indicates mild hypocalcemia?
    a. 5.0 mg/dL
    b. 8.0 mg/dL
    c. 10.0 mg/dL
    d. 12.0 mg/dL

39. Which of the following clinical conditions can result from hypocalcemia?
    a. Cardiac muscle contraction is stimulated.
    b. Intestinal and gastric motility are increased.
    c. Peripheral nerve excitability is decreased.
    d. Bone density is increased markedly.

40. Match the following clinical conditions that predispose a client to hypocalcemia with the etiologies. *Answers may be used more than once.*

Etiologies
1. Inhibited calcium absorption
2. Decreased ionized calcium
3. Endocrine disorder

Clinical Conditions

_____ a. Alkalosis

_____ b. Pancreatitis

_____ c. Inadequate calcium intake

_____ d. Lactose intolerance

_____ e. Parathyroidectomy

_____ f. Hyperphosphatemia

_____ g. Increased serum protein

_____ h. Celiac sprue

_____ i. Immobility

_____ j. Calcium-binding medications

_____ k. Inadequate vitamin D intake

41. Which of the following clients is at greatest risk of developing hypocalcemia?
    a. A 30-year-old Asian woman with breast cancer
    b. A 45-year-old Caucasian man with hypertension and diuretic therapy
    c. A 60-year-old African-American woman with a recent ileostomy
    d. A 70-year-old Caucasian man on long-term lithium therapy

42. Preventive measures for clients at risk for developing hypocalcemia include which of the following?
    a. Advising at-risk clients to increase the daily dietary calcium intake to 1000 mg.
    b. Encouraging clients to increase their intake of phosphorus.
    c. Applying a sunblock and wearing protective clothing whenever outdoors.
    d. Administering calcium-containing IV fluids to clients receiving multiple blood transfusions.

43. A client is at risk for developing hypocalcemia as result of a deficiency in
    a. Vitamin C
    b. Vitamin B_{12}
    c. Vitamin A
    d. Vitamin D

44. A client is at risk for hypocalcemia as a result of which of the following operations for an endocrine disorder?
    a. Thyroidectomy
    b. Adrenalectomy
    c. Pancreatectomy
    d. Gastrectomy

45. A typical nursing assessment finding of a client with hypocalcemia is
    a. Paresthesias and tingling followed by numbness
    b. Shortened ST segment, tachycardia, and hypertension
    c. Constipation and hypoactive bowel sounds
    d. Severe muscle weakness

46. Which of the following medication orders should the nurse clarify before administering the medication to a client with hypocalcemia? Explain why it should be questioned.
    a. Magnesium sulfate 1 g intramuscularly (IM) every 6 hours for four doses
    b. Aluminum hydroxide (AlternaGEL) 15 mL tid and hs PO
    c. Calcium carbonate 1000 mg pc and hs PO
    d. Calcium gluconate 5 mEq IV prn tetany

47. The nurse would implement which of the following in treatment of a client with hypocalcemia?
    a. Encourage activity by the client as tolerated, including weight-lifting.
    b. Encourage socialization with friends and family to avoid social isolation.
    c. Include a tracheostomy tray at the bedside for emergency use.
    d. Provide adequate intake of vitamin D and calcium-rich foods.

48. Which of the following foods provides both calcium and vitamin D for the client who needs supplemental diet therapy for hypocalcemia?
    a. Eggs
    b. Broccoli
    c. Milk
    d. Tofu

49. Which of the following electrolyte imbalances is often associated with hypocalcemia as a result of chronic renal failure?
    a. Hypophosphatemia
    b. Hyperphosphatemia
    c. Hyperkalemia
    d. Hyponatremia

50. Hypercalcemia refers to a serum calcium level greater than
    a. 5.0 mg/dL
    b. 8.0 mg/dL
    c. 10.5 mg/dL
    d. 12.0 mg/dL

51. Which of the following statements about the pathophysiology of hypercalcemia is true?
    a. Hypercalcemia has little effect on blood clotting.
    b. Hypercalcemia can lead to increased bone strength.
    c. Cardiac and nerve tissues are sensitive to various serum calcium levels.
    d. Excess ECF (extracellular fluid) calcium ions increase the responses of excitable tissues.

52. Which of the following conditions can cause an increase in bone resorption of calcium?
    a. Dehydration
    b. Lung cancer
    c. Renal failure
    d. Excessive oral intake of vitamin D

53. What is the relationship between excessive oral vitamin D intake and hypercalcemia?

54. A preventive intervention for clients at risk for developing hypercalcemia is
    a. Ensuring adequate hydration
    b. Discouraging weight-bearing activity such as walking
    c. Monitoring the client for fluid volume excess
    d. Administering multivitamin tablets twice per day

55. Which of the following assessment findings is related to hypercalcemia? *Check all that apply.*

    _____ a.   Bradycardia

    _____ b.   Paresthesia

    _____ c.   Leg cramping

    _____ d.   Hyperactive bowel sounds

    _____ e.   Ineffective respiratory movements

    _____ f.   Increased clot formation

    _____ g.   Hypertension

    _____ h.   Profound muscle weakness

    _____ i.   Changes in mental status

56. Which of the following are examples of nursing interventions related to clients with hypercalcemia? *Check all that apply.*

    _____ a.   Monitoring for a decreased urine output

    _____ b.   Assessing the client for a positive Homan's sign

    _____ c.   Measuring the abdominal girth

    _____ d.   Massaging calves to encourage blood return to the heart

    _____ e.   Monitoring for electrocardiogram (ECG) changes

    _____ f.   Providing adequate intake of vitamin D

    _____ g.   During treatment, monitoring for tetany

57. Treatment for hypercalcemia includes which of the following medications? *Check all that apply.*

    _____ a.   Magnesium sulfate

    _____ b.   Calcitonin

    _____ c.   Furosemide (Lasix)

    _____ d.   Calcitriol

    _____ e.   Calcium gluconate

    _____ f.   Aluminum hydroxide

    _____ g.   Plicamycin

58. Hypercalcemia can potentiate which of the following drug toxicities?
    a.   Tylenol
    b.   Gentamycin
    c.   Digoxin
    d.   Anticonvulsants

59. A preventive intervention for the client at risk for fracture related to decreased bone density is
    a.   Encouraging independent ambulation about the room
    b.   Using a lift sheet for moving the client up in bed
    c.   Reminding the client to shift position in bed frequently
    d.   Providing an overhead trapeze to assist with position changes

60. Compare and contrast subjective data relating to hypocalcemia and hypercalcemia.

61. Compare and contrast objective data relating to hypocalcemia and hypercalcemia.

62. A positive Trousseau's or Chvostek's sign demonstrates neuromuscular irritation resulting from
    a. Hypocalcemia
    b. Hypercalcemia
    c. Hyperkalemia
    d. Hypophosphatemia

63. Match each of the following assessment findings for hypocalcemia with the technique and positive result for that finding.

Assessment Findings
1. Trousseau's sign
2. Chvostek's sign

Technique and Positive Results

_____ a. Muscle twitching results when the facial nerve in front of the ear is tapped.

_____ b. Palmar flexion/contraction of the hand and fingers results upon inflation of a blood pressure cuff around the upper arm.

64. The immediate treatment of a client with a positive Trousseau's or Chvostek's sign is
    a. Intravenous calcium
    b. Calcitonin
    c. Intravenous KCl
    d. Large doses of oral calcium

65. Discuss the responsibilities of the nurse when administering intravenous calcium therapy.

66. A client with congestive heart failure is receiving a loop diuretic. The nurse should monitor for which three electrolyte imbalances?

    a. _____

    b. _____

    c. _____

67. Which of the following clients would the nurse monitor for hypocalcemia, hyperkalemia, and hypernatremia?
    a. Client with hypothyroidism
    b. Client with diabetes mellitus
    c. Client with chronic renal failure
    d. Client with adrenal insufficiency

68. The serum level of phosphorus exists in reciprocal balance with that of
    a. Magnesium
    b. Chloride
    c. Potassium
    d. Calcium

69. For the parathyroid hormone to regulate phosphate metabolism, which vitamin is necessary in adequate levels?
    a. Vitamin B_{12}
    b. Vitamin C
    c. Vitamin D
    d. Vitamin K

70. Hypophosphatemia refers to which serum level of phosphorus?
    a. 2.5 mg/dL
    b. 3.5 mg/dL
    c. 4.5 mg/dL
    d. 5.5 mg/dL

71. Match the following clinical conditions with their effects on serum phosphorus levels. *Answers are used more than once.*

Serum Phosphorus Levels
1. Hyperphosphatemia
2. Hypophosphatemia

Clinical Conditions

_____ a.   Aggressive cancer treatment

_____ b.   Malnutrition

_____ c.   Alcoholism

_____ d.   Hypoparathyroidism

_____ e.   Aluminum hydroxide–based antacids

_____ f.   Renal insufficiency

_____ g.   Respiratory alkalosis

_____ h.   Increased intake of phosphorus

_____ i.   Hyperparathyroidism

72. Indicate assessment findings for a client with hypophosphatemia.

73. Interventions for the client with hypophosphatemia include which of the following?
    a. Aggressive treatment with parenteral phosphorous
    b. Administering oral vitamin D and phosphorus supplements
    c. Concurrent administration of calcium supplements
    d. Eliminating beef, pork, and legumes from the diet

74. The nurse would monitor the client with hyperphosphatemia for which of the following accompanying electrolyte imbalances that potentially can cause life-threatening side effects?
    a. Hypercalcemia
    b. Hypocalcemia
    c. Hyponatremia
    d. Hyperkalemia

75. The normal range of serum magnesium levels is
    a. 0.5 to 1.0 mg/dL
    b. 1.2 to 2.0 mg/dL
    c. 2.4 to 4.0 mg/dL
    d. 4.5 to 6.0 mg/dL

76. List at least four clinical conditions that decrease intestinal absorption of magnesium causing hypomagnesemia.

    a. _____

    b. _____

    c. _____

    d. _____

77. List three conditions that increase renal excretion of magnesium causing hypomagnesemia.

    a. _____

    b. _____

    c. _____

78. Indicate the objective data in a nursing assessment of a client with hypomagnesemia.

79. Which of the following is correct in treating clients with hypomagnesemia? Why are the other answers incorrect?
    a. Administer intramuscular magnesium sulfate.
    b. Encourage eating foods such as fruits.
    c. Administer oral preparations of magnesium sulfate.
    d. Discontinue diuretic therapy and administer intravenous magnesium sulfate.

80. Manifestations of hypermagnesemia occur when serum magnesium levels exceed
    a. 1.2 mg/dL
    b. 2.0 mg/dL
    c. 3.0 mg/dL
    d. 4.0 mg/dL

81. The nurse monitors the effectiveness of magnesium sulfate by performing which assessment every hour?
    a. Assessment of deep tendon reflexes
    b. Assessment of vital signs
    c. Assessment of serum laboratory values
    d. Assessment of urine output

82. Give the objective data that would be noted in the assessment of a client with hypermagnesemia.

83. A client predisposed to hypermagnesemia is taught to limit what types of foods and medications?

CASE STUDY: THE CLIENT WITH A POTASSIUM IMBALANCE

Answer Guidelines for the Case Study questions are provided on the companion Evolve Learning Resources Web site at http://evolve.elsevier.com/Iggy/.

A male adult client is admitted for palpitations. His serum potassium level on admission is 5.4 mEq/L. Yesterday he ate two eggs, bacon, and toast for breakfast. For lunch he had a fresh fruit salad, and for dinner he ate baked halibut, baked potatoes, a salad, and spinach. He usually has a cola drink and dried fruit for a snack. He uses a salt substitute regularly. He tells you that he has been taking spironolactone 50 mg once daily for hypertension for 2 months, but missed his 1-month follow-up appointment.

1. Identify the foods in his diet that may be contributing to his hyperkalemia.

2. Which electrocardiogram (ECG) changes would be typical for a client such as this?

3. Formulate relevant nursing diagnoses for this client based on the above data.

6. Will the client continue to take the spirono-lactone? Explain.

7. Eventually this client recovers and is scheduled for discharge. Develop a teaching-learning plan for him including information about his diet, self-monitoring of his pulse, and the need for regular follow-up care.

This client states that he has had abdominal cramping and several very loose diarrhea stools since yesterday. The physician orders a sodium polystyrene sulfonate (Kayexalate) retention enema to be given stat.

4. Discuss the etiology of the client's symptoms.

5. Explain whether the nurse should clarify the physician's order before administering the enema.

CASE STUDY: THE CLIENT WITH SODIUM IMBALANCE

Answer Guidelines for the Case Study questions are provided on the companion Evolve Learning Resources Web site at http://evolve.elsevier.com/Iggy/.

The nurse is caring for a 77-year-old woman who was admitted after gardening on a hot summer day. Her daughter found her lying on the couch, slightly confused, and unable to get up to the bathroom. She is weak, anxious, and slightly confused to time and place. Her pulse is 110 beats/min; blood pressure is 108/58. Her skin is dry, and urine specific gravity is 1.028. The nurse notes that the client's deep tendon reflexes are slightly reduced.

1. Discuss whether this client's serum sodium would be elevated, decreased, or normal.

2. Develop a specific assessment plan for this client.

3. What treatment would you expect this client to receive at this time?

4. This client will be discharged to home care. Develop a teaching plan for her.

Infusion Therapy

LEARNING OUTCOMES

1. Categorize the purpose and types of intravenous (IV) infusion therapy.
2. Identify the types and characteristics of vascular access devices (VADs).
3. Evaluate clients for vascular access needs.
4. Distinguish the components of an infusion system.
5. Differentiate the types of rate control devices and nursing considerations for their use.
6. Prioritize nursing interventions for maintaining an infusion system.
7. Assess, prevent, and manage complications related to infusion therapy and VADs.
8. Determine special needs of older adults receiving IV therapy.
9. Identify nursing considerations for intra-arterial, intraperitoneal, subcutaneous, intraosseous, epidural, and intrathecal infusion therapy.

LEARNING ACTIVITIES

1. Before completing the study guide exercises for this chapter, it is recommended that you review the following:
    *   Fluid and electrolyte balance
    *   Anatomy and physiology of vascular system
    *   General principles of IV therapy

2. Review the standards of care regarding infusion therapy published by the Infusion Nurses Society (INS), a professional nursing organization for infusion therapy nurses.

3. Review the boldfaced terms and their definitions in Chapter 17 to enhance your understanding of the content.

STUDY/REVIEW QUESTIONS

Answers to the Study/Review Questions are provided on the companion Evolve Learning Resources Web site at http://evolve.elsevier.com/Iggy/.

1. The following questions are related to filters on an infusion administration set.
   a. What is the purpose of a filter?

   b. Briefly discuss the types of filters, how to select the proper filter, and their uses.

2. Match the following characteristics with either a pump or a controller infusion device.

Characteristic

_____ a. Delivers fluids under pressure

_____ b. Relies on gravity to create fluid flow

_____ c. Is pole-mounted or ambulatory and portable

_____ d. Is best for accurate infusion

_____ e. Counts drops to regulate flow

Device

1. Controller
2. Pump

3. Which of the following central venous catheters requires piercing of the skin each time the device is accessed?
   a. Broviac catheter
   b. Groshong catheter
   c. Hickman catheter
   d. MediPort implanted port

4. Identify four reasons why clients receive intravenous (IV) therapy.

   a. _____

   b. _____

   c. _____

   d. _____

5. Identify and describe the purpose of each component of an intravenous infusion system.

6. Identify special considerations to follow when initiating or maintaining peripheral IV therapy for the older adult.

7. Briefly explain the difference between tunneled and nontunneled catheters, and give an example of each.

8. Briefly explain the difference between an implanted port and a central venous catheter.

9. Which of the following is a recommended nursing intervention when inserting a peripheral IV? *Check all that apply.*

    _____ a. Use either an upper or lower extremity for the insertion site.

    _____ b. Start with more distal sites, such as the hand veins.

    _____ c. Start with more proximal sites, such as the forearm.

    _____ d. Choose the client's nondominant arm.

    _____ e. Choose the client's dominant arm.

    _____ f. Do not use the arm if a dialysis graft is present.

    _____ g. Avoid placing an IV over the palm side of the wrist.

    _____ h. Ensure that the vein is hard and cordlike before insertion.

10. Which of the following clients would receive intraperitoneal therapy?
    a. A client receiving total parental nutrition
    b. A client receiving blood and blood products
    c. A client receiving chemotherapy
    d. A client receiving medications for diagnostic tests

11. Identify responsibilities the nurse has when caring for a client who has an arterial catheter.

12. List three reasons for an arterial catheter.

    a. _____

    b. _____

    c. _____

13. What are the primary reasons a client would receive intraperitoneal therapy (IP therapy)?

14. Identify the complications of intraperitoneal therapy.

15. Identify the types of clients who might be candidates for continuous subcutaneous infusion.

16. A client with a total knee replacement is admitted to a general surgery floor with an epidural catheter for delivering pain medication.
    a. Briefly explain this method of pain medication delivery.

    b. What are the responsibilities of the nurse caring for a client with an epidural catheter?

    c. Identify medication-related complications for which the nurse assesses in clients receiving epidural pain medications.

17. Explain the difference between an epidural catheter and an intrathecal infusion.

18. Which of the following statements about intraosseous therapy (IO) are true? *Mark all that apply and correct the ones that are incorrect.*
    a. IO is only used in pediatric cases.

    b. IO should be used no longer than 24 hours.

    c. Possible sites include the distal or proximal tibia and distal femur.

    d. The sternum may be used in adults for IO.

    e. IO doses of medications and fluids are the same as for the intravenous route.

    f. Osteomyelitis may occur as a complication of IO.

19. Describe compartment syndrome, its possible consequences, and nursing interventions.

cate rhonchi over the lung fields bilaterally and a rash over his back and chest.
   a. What complication do these assessment findings indicate? Provide a rationale for your answer.
      (1) Infection in the blood
      (2) Allergic reaction
      (3) Speed shock
      (4) Circulatory overload

   b. Based on your conclusion as to the type of complication, what nursing interventions would be implemented?

20. A client's IV site is very edematous, the pump continues to infuse fluids, and the client is complaining of burning at the site. You notice a clear fluid leaking from the insertion site.
   a. Which of the following complications do these assessment findings indicate? Give a rationale for your answer.
      (1) Hematoma
      (2) Phlebitis
      (3) Infiltration
      (4) Infection

   b. Based on your conclusion as to the type of complication, what nursing interventions would be implemented?

22. A client having a central line inserted in the vena cava is at high risk for which of the following complications during this procedure?
   a. Pneumothorax
   b. Air embolism
   c. Circulatory overload
   d. Hydrothorax

23. The nurse is assisting a physician inserting a central line when the client develops chest pain and shortness of breath with decreased breath sounds and restlessness. The nurse would do which of the following?
   a. Tell the client to "Relax, the procedure will soon be over."
   b. Administer pain medication to minimize the pain of insertion.
   c. Administer oxygen and plan to assist with insertion of a chest tube.
   d. Monitor ongoing pulse oximetry and the client for respiratory changes.

21. A 65-year-old client has been receiving IV fluids at 100 mL/hr of D$_5$1/2% NS for the past 3 days, along with IV antibiotic therapy. Today the physician ordered a change in the client's medications. After giving the new antibiotic, the client complains of general itching and difficulty catching his breath, and you note audible wheezing and tearing of the eyes. Your assessment findings indi-

24. Immediately after a triple lumen catheter central line is inserted, the nurse would
   a. Start IV fluids but at a slower rate to prevent any fluid overload.
   b. Watch and wait for any complications before using the site.
   c. Get a portable chest x-ray immediately and hold IV fluids until after results are obtained.
   d. Assess vital signs and perform a complete assessment and, if client is stable, start IV fluids.

25. After a tubing change to the central line, the line is later found to be disconnected from the catheter. The client develops chest pain and restlessness, HR is 120, BP drops to 90/40, and pulse oximetry is 89%. The nurse performs which of the following interventions?
   a. Place client in Trendelenburg position on the left side, clamp the catheter, and notify the physician.
   b. Assess for patency of catheter, change the tubing, and resume IV fluids.
   c. Notify physician, remove the central line, apply pressure, and place the client in a semi-Fowler's position.
   d. Notify physician and administer urokinase to declot the catheter.

26. Which of the following nursing interventions is key to preventing an infection in a client with a central line?
   a. Administer antibiotics for at least a week in a timely manner.
   b. Use aseptic technique during dressing changes, administering medications, and tubing changes.
   c. Change the catheter every 72 hours and tubing every 24 hours.
   d. Monitor the client's temperature for any elevation and give acetaminophen as needed.

27. A client needs a 2-month course of antibiotics to treat a resistant infection. Which device would be chosen for this therapy?
   a. Short peripheral catheter
   b. Midline catheter
   c. Nontunneled percutaneous central catheter
   d. Peripherally inserted central catheter (PICC)

28. Which nursing intervention is appropriate when caring for the client with an implanted port? *Check all that apply.*
   _____ a. A noncoring needle is used to access the port before an infusion.
   _____ b. The port must be flushed daily with saline when not in use.
   _____ c. The external catheter requires dressing changes every other day.
   _____ d. A topical anesthetic cream may be used before accessing the port.
   _____ e. Careful palpation is required before accessing the septum.

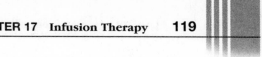

29.   Complete the following puzzle by answering the questions regarding complications of IV therapy.

Across

1.   During a central line dressing change, the nurse notes redness and swelling at the catheter insertion site, and a small amount of purulent drainage. The nurse suspects _____ at the insertion site.

3.   During rounds, the nurse notes that the client's IV site is swollen, cool, and that the IV has stopped infusing. The client complains of tenderness at the IV site. The nurse suspects what?

4.   The client is receiving an infusion of chemotherapy, and the nurse monitors the IV infusion and site closely because the medication may cause tissue damage if it escapes into the subcutaneous tissue. The medication is known as a/an _____.

8.   After multiple IV start attempts, the nurse finally starts a peripheral IV infusion. However, that evening, the area is swollen, tender, red at the site, and the vein looks engorged. The infusion has stopped. The nurse suspects a/an _____ at the IV site.

Down

2.   If the medication in question 4 across infuses into the subcutaneous tissue, it is known as _____ and may result in tissue sloughing.

5.   Two days after a peripheral IV infusion has been discontinued, the client calls the clinic because he noticed a red, cordlike vein on his forearm above the old IV site. The nurse suspects _____.

6.   A client receiving heparin has accidentally dislodged his IV catheter. A new IV has been started, but the old site is slightly swollen, bruised, and very tender.

7.   After a dose of IV penicillin, the client complains of itching, and has a rash across his back. Slight wheezes are audible. This is a/an _____ reaction.

9.   After hanging an IVPB antibiotic, the nurse steps out when called by another client. The nurse returns after a few minutes to find that the IV antibiotic has completely infused. The client is complaining of dizziness, chest tightness, and has an irregular pulse and a flushed face. The nurse suspects _____.

CASE STUDY: THE CLIENT RECEIVING INTRAVENOUS THERAPY

Answer Guidelines for the Case Study questions are provided on the companion Evolve Learning Resources Web site at http://evolve.elsevier.com/Iggy/.

Your client is an older adult resident at a skilled nursing facility. She is receiving IV antibiotics and fluids for pneumonia via a peripheral site. She complains that her arm is hurting where she is receiving the IV, especially when the antibiotic is given.

1. What would be the nurse's best action at this time?

2. What possible complications may explain her discomfort?

After examining her site, you decide to discontinue the IV. It is restarted in her other arm, and the infusion set at 50 mL/hr as ordered. When you recheck her in an hour, you see that the entire 1000 mL bag of normal saline has infused. The client is complaining of shortness of breath, and you see that she has puffiness around her eyes and engorged neck veins. Assessment of breath sounds reveals crackles over both lower lobes, and her blood pressure is 154/96.

3. Another nurse tells you that the client is experiencing speed shock because the saline went in too fast. Do you agree? Explain your answer.

4. What should you do at this time?

Acid-Base Balance

LEARNING OUTCOMES

1. Describe the relationship between free hydrogen ion level and pH.
2. Explain the role of bicarbonate in the blood.
3. Explain the concept of compensation.
4. Compare the role of a buffer in conditions of acidosis and alkalosis.
5. Compare the roles of the respiratory system and the renal system in maintaining acid-base balance.
6. Describe the role of oxygen in maintaining acid-base balance.
7. Interpret whether the client's arterial blood gas values are normal, elevated, or low.

LEARNING ACTIVITIES

1. Before completing the study guide exercises for this chapter, it is recommended that you review the following:
   - Principles of acid and base solutions from basic chemistry
   - Normal anatomy and physiology of the lungs and kidneys

2. Review the boldfaced terms and their definitions in Chapter 18 to enhance your understanding of the content.

STUDY/REVIEW QUESTIONS

Answers to the Study/Review Questions are provided on the companion Evolve Learning Resources Web site at http://evolve.elsevier.com/Iggy/.

1. Which of the following statements regarding acid-base balance is true?
   a. Acid-base balance is mainly a function of cellular metabolism.
   b. pH is equal to the logarithm of hydrogen ion concentration.
   c. Arterial blood pH is slightly more acid than venous blood.
   d. Hydrogen ion reflects acid production and elimination.

2. Identify four ways that the hydrogen ion is produced by the body:
   a. _____
   b. _____
   c. _____
   d. _____

3. Match the following terms with their associated functions and substances.

Associated Statements		Terms
_____ a.	Accepts hydrogen ion	1. Acid
_____ b.	Donates hydrogen ion	2. Base
		3. Buffer
		4. pH
_____ c.	Formed in the body as a result of metabolism	
_____ d.	Releases or binds hydrogen ions	
_____ e.	Measure of the body's free hydrogen ion level	
_____ f.	H_2CO_3	
_____ g.	Increases as the amount of base increases	
_____ h.	HCO_3^-	
_____ i.	Hemoglobin	

4. A pH of 7.40 in the body reflects a ratio of bicarbonate to carbonic acid as
   a. 50:50.
   b. 1:1.
   c. 1:20.
   d. 20:1.

5. Use arrows ($\leftarrow$ or $\rightarrow$) to indicate the direction the carbonic anhydrase equation shifts when excess carbon dioxide is produced.

$$CO_2 + H_2O \underline{\hspace{1cm}} H_2CO_3 \underline{\hspace{1cm}} H^+ + HCO_3^-$$

6. a. For the equation in question 5, does the hydrogen ion concentration increase or decrease?

   b. For the equation in question 5, does the pH increase or decrease?

7. Under the following conditions, will the plasma pH increase or decrease?
   a. Increase in CO_2

   b. Decrease in HCO_3^-

   c. Increase in lactic acid

   d. Increase in HCO_3^-

   e. Decrease in CO_2

8. Identify four sources of bicarbonate ions.
   a. _____
   b. _____
   c. _____
   d. _____

9. The immediate binding of excess hydrogen ions would primarily occur where?
   a. In the red blood cell
   b. In the renal tubule
   c. In the pulmonary capillary
   d. In the capillary microbed

10. Match the buffer system with the statements.

Buffer Systems
1. Chemical
2. Respiratory
3. Renal
4. Protein

Statements

_____ a. Chemoreceptor response to increase in CO_2

_____ b. Secretion of hydrogen ions to form H_2PO_4

_____ c. Reabsorbs HCO_3^-

_____ d. Binds H^+ with HCO_3^-

_____ e. Binds H^+ with hemoglobin

_____ f. Response occurs within minutes

11. Which buffer system will respond to acid-base imbalances most likely to occur from a metabolic origin?

12. Which of the following statements is true regarding compensation?
    a. The lungs compensate for acid-base imbalances of respiratory origin.
    b. Renal compensation is the most powerful and rapid.
    c. Compensation occurs as the body attempts to maintain a pH of 7.35 to 7.45.
    d. Compensation is the result of carbonic acid elimination.

13. Determine whether the following arterial blood values would indicate an acid or alkaline condition.

    a. Pa_{CO_2} = 66 mm Hg _____

    b. Bicarbonate = 16 mEq/L _____

    c. pH = 7.55 _____

    d. pH = 7.32 _____

14. When assessing a client for acid-base imbalances, the nurse should keep in mind which of the following?
    a. The nurse must be familiar with the client's baseline assessment because acid-base imbalances can occur quickly.
    b. Mental status changes rarely occur with acid-base imbalances.
    c. Laboratory data results are the most important parts of the assessment for acid-base imbalances.
    d. The focus of the assessment should be on the lungs and kidneys, not neuromuscular or gastrointestinal function.

15. Identify two physiologic changes that occur in the lungs with aging that contribute to the older adult's risk for acid-base imbalances.

    a. _____

    b. _____

16. Identify the physiologic changes that occur in the kidneys with aging that contribute to the older adult's risk for acid-base imbalances.

    a. _____

    b. _____

17. Which of the following medications increases the older adult client's risk for acid-base imbalances?
    a. Carbamazepine (Tegretol)
    b. Conjugated estrogen (Premarin)
    c. Furosemide (Lasix)
    d. Metoclopramide (Reglan)

18. The serum pH value is
    a. Directly related to the concentration of carbon dioxide
    b. Directly related to the concentration of hydrogen ion
    c. Inversely related to the concentration of hydrogen ion
    d. Inversely related to the concentration of bicarbonate

19. Which of the following is correct about pH?
    a. A solution with a pH of 6.5 is a weak base and has more hydrogen ions than a solution with a pH of 6.9.
    b. A solution with a pH of 7.0 is neutral and has fewer hydrogen ions than a solution with a pH of 6.8.
    c. A solution with a pH of 7.5 is a weak acid and has fewer hydrogen ions than a solution with a pH of 7.8.
    d. A solution with a pH of 8.7 is a strong base and has more hydrogen ions than a solution with a pH of 8.5.

20. Which of the following processes might be responsible for an increase in pH?
    a. Hypoventilation
    b. Ketoacidosis
    c. Nasogastric suction
    d. Diarrhea

21. Which of the following processes might be responsible for a decrease in bicarbonate?
    a. Pancreatitis
    b. Hypoventilation
    c. Vomiting
    d. Emphysema

22. A $Paco_2$ of 55 mm Hg will most likely result in:
    a. A pH of 7.45.
    b. $Paco_2$ of 60 mm Hg.
    c. A pH of 7.55.
    d. HCO_3^- of 34 mEq/L.

23. A main cause of increased bicarbonate levels is
    a. Respiratory elimination of acid.
    b. Albumin binding with hydrogen ion.
    c. Renal reabsorption.
    d. Intracellular uptake of hydrogen ion.

24. When assessing a client with an acid-base balance problem, which of the following Gordon's Functional Health Patterns are affected *most*? *Check all that apply.*
    _____ a. Values/beliefs
    _____ b. Activity-exercise
    _____ c. Health perception–health management
    _____ d. Elimination
    _____ e. Sleep–rest
    _____ f. Cognitive–perceptual
    _____ g. Coping–stress tolerance

25. Which of the following is a major extracellular fluid (ECF) buffer?
    a. Carbon dioxide
    b. Bicarbonate
    c. Ammonium
    d. Phosphate

26. The acid released by the lungs to regulate pH is
    a. Bicarbonate
    b. Phosphate
    c. Hydrogen
    d. Carbon dioxide

27. Which of the following statements about the neural regulatory control of acid-base balance is correct?
    a. Baroreceptors in the ECF are sensitive to bicarbonate.
    b. Chemoreceptors in the ECF are sensitive to carbon dioxide.
    c. Chemoreceptors in the brain are sensitive to carbon dioxide.
    d. Baroreceptors in the brain are sensitive to bicarbonate.

28. When the respiratory rate slows, pH
    a. Increases
    b. Decreases
    c. Is unchanged
    d. Fluctuates

29. The kidney regulates pH by controlling:
    a.   Urea
    b.   Bicarbonate
    c.   Carbon dioxide
    d.   Hemoglobin

30. Which of the following statements about the role of chemical buffers in regulating acid-base balance is correct?
    a.   They are able to correct the imbalance permanently.
    b.   They are present in the body fluids and act immediately.
    c.   They constitute the largest store of buffers in the body.
    d.   They can correct the underlying problems that led to the imbalance.

31. Identify, in order of sequence, the three regulatory mechanisms that the body uses to control acid-base balance.

    a.   _____

    b.   _____

    c.   _____

32. Ammonia, a normal by-product of protein metabolism, is converted to ammonium in the kidney by the addition of
    a.   Urea
    b.   Nitrogen
    c.   Hydrogen
    d.   Phosphate

33. Describe a situation in which the renal system is used to compensate for acid-base imbalance.

34. Describe a situation in which the respiratory system is used to compensate for acid-base imbalances.

35. Briefly describe full compensation and partial compensation.

36. Identify four changes in the body that would occur if the pH was not closely regulated.

    a.   _____

    b.   _____

    c.   _____

    d.   _____

37. Which of the following blood pH values is within normal limits?
    a.   7.27
    b.   7.37
    c.   7.47
    d.   7.5

Interventions for Clients with Acid-Base Imbalances

LEARNING OUTCOMES

1. Identify clients at risk for acidosis.
2. Use laboratory data and clinical manifestations to determine the presence of acidosis.
3. Analyze arterial blood gases to determine whether acidosis is respiratory or metabolic in origin.
4. Analyze arterial blood gases to determine whether respiratory acidosis is acute or chronic.
5. Prioritize nursing care for the client with acute acidosis.
7. Develop a community-based teaching plan to prevent acidosis in the client at continuing risk for acid-base imbalances.
8. Identify clients at risk for alkalosis.
9. Use laboratory data and clinical manifestations to determine the presence of alkalosis.
10. Analyze arterial blood gases to determine whether alkalosis is respiratory or metabolic in origin.
11. Prioritize nursing care for the client with alkalosis.
12. Develop a community-based teaching plan to prevent alkalosis in the client at continuing risk for acid-base imbalances.

LEARNING ACTIVITIES

1. Before completing the study guide exercises for this chapter, it is recommended that you review the following:
    * Acid-base balance
    * Normal anatomy and physiology of the lungs and kidneys

2. Review the boldfaced terms and their definitions in Chapter 19 to enhance your understanding of the content.

STUDY/REVIEW QUESTIONS

Answers to the Study/Review Questions are provided on the companion Evolve Learning Resources Web site at http://evolve.elsevier.com/Iggy/.

1. Which condition would cause acidosis resulting from excess production of hydrogen ion?
   a. Renal failure
   b. Emphysema
   c. Seizures
   d. Diarrhea

2. Which of the following statements regarding acidosis is true?
   a. Acidosis may result from a base deficit.
   b. Acidosis always occurs when excess hydrogen ion is produced.
   c. Acidosis is reflected by HCO_3^-.
   d. Acidosis results in an increased ratio of HCO_3^- to H_2CO_3.

3. Match the following etiologies of metabolic acidosis to the resulting state of pathophysiology.

Etiology of Metabolic Acidosis
1. Hydrogen ion production
2. Hydrogen ion elimination
3. Base elimination
4. Base production

Pathophysiology State
_____ a. Diabetic ketoacidosis
_____ b. Renal failure
_____ c. Dehydration
_____ d. Seizures
_____ e. Pancreatic insufficiency
_____ f. Diarrhea

4. Respiratory acidosis occurs as a result of
   a. Hyperventilation
   b. Hypoventilation
   c. Renal reabsorption of bicarbonate
   d. Renal secretion of hydrogen ion

5. Match the pathophysiologic causes of respiratory failure with the associated conditions.

Associated Conditions
1. Respiratory depression
2. Inadequate chest expansion
3. Airway obstruction
4. Altered alveolar capillary diffusion

Pathophysiology
_____ a. Asthma
_____ b. Muscular dystrophy
_____ c. Morphine infusion
_____ d. Pulmonary embolus
_____ e. Bronchiolitis
_____ f. Ascites
_____ g. Stroke
_____ h. Flail chest
_____ i. Hemothorax
_____ j. Hyperkalemia
_____ k. Pneumonia

6. Which laboratory value would indicate that a client was acidotic?
   a. $Paco_2 = 55$ mm Hg
   b. $HCO_3^- = 25$ mEq/L
   c. Lactate = 2.5 mmol/L
   d. pH = 7.30

7. Identify four common medications that may be administered to decrease bronchial constriction.

   a. _____

   b. _____

   c. _____

   d. _____

8. Which of the following nursing assessment findings would indicate a worsening of the respiratory acidosis?
   a. Decreased respiratory rate
   b. Decreased blood pressure
   c. Use of accessory respiratory muscles
   d. Pale nail beds

9. State whether each of the following signs and symptoms would be seen in metabolic acidosis or respiratory acidosis.
    a. Kussmaul respirations
    b. Shallow, rapid respirations
    c. Warm, flushed skin
    d. Skin pale to cyanotic
    e. Elevated Pa_{CO_2}
    f. Decreased bicarbonate

10. Which of the following statements made by a client might indicate that he has an alkaline condition?
    a. "I am more and more tired and can't concentrate."
    b. "I have tingling in my fingers and toes."
    c. "My feet and ankles are swollen."
    d. "I am short of breath all of the time."

11. The most important intervention for a client with ketoacidosis is to
    a. Administer bicarbonate.
    b. Give furosemide.
    c. Administer insulin.
    d. Administer potassium.

12. Which of the following is likely to result in metabolic alkalosis as a result of base excess?
    a. Thiazide diuretics
    b. Nasogastric suction
    c. Severe vomiting
    d. Massive blood transfusions

13. Respiratory alkalosis is likely to occur as a result of
    a. Lactic acidosis.
    b. Hypoventilation.
    c. Hyperventilation.
    d. Antacid administration.

14. Metabolic alkalosis may result in which electrolyte imbalance?
    a. Hyperkalemia
    b. Hypophosphatemia
    c. Hyperchloremia
    d. Hypocalcemia

15. Tall peaked T waves on an electrocardiogram (ECG) of a client who has metabolic acidosis is most likely the result of
    a. An increase in ionized calcium
    b. A shift of glucose from the extracellular fluid (ECF) to the intracellular fluid (ICF)
    c. A shift of potassium from the ICF to the ECF
    d. A decrease in serum magnesium

16. A nursing intervention to correct metabolic alkalosis would include
    a. Maintenance of fluid restriction
    b. Administration of potassium
    c. Administration of antiemetics
    d. Administration of bicarbonate

17. Match each statement with its associated acid-base condition. *Answers may be used more than once.*

Acid-Base Condition
1. Respiratory acidosis
2. Metabolic acidosis
3. Respiratory alkalosis
4. Metabolic alkalosis

Statements

_____ a. May occur as a result of anxiety

_____ b. Results from bicarbonate loss

_____ c. Caused by hypoventilation

_____ d. May be a result of blood transfusions

_____ e. May be caused by diarrhea

_____ f. Associated with Kussmaul respiration

_____ g. Associated with ingestion of antacids

_____ h. Results in hypocalcemia

_____ i. Compensation occurs through renal reabsorption of bicarbonate

_____ j. Compensation occurs through hyperventilation

_____ k. Compensation occurs through hypoventilation

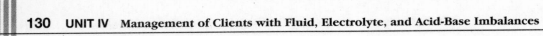

18. Which two conditions account for most of the clinical manifestations seen with metabolic alkalosis?

    a. _____

    b. _____

19. Describe the difference between acidosis and acidemia.

20. Describe the difference between alkalosis and alkalemia.

State whether the following arterial blood gases reflect metabolic acidosis, respiratory acidosis, metabolic alkalosis, respiratory alkalosis, or normal values. Determine which values indicate partial or complete compensation, and give a condition that may cause the abnormality.

21. pH 7.35, $Paco_2$ 66, bicarbonate 38, Pao_2 70

22. pH 7.52, $Paco_2$ 45, bicarbonate 36, Pao_2 95

23. pH 7.55, $Paco_2$ 24, bicarbonate 20, Pao_2 95

24. pH 7.28, $Paco_2$ 24, bicarbonate 15, Pao_2 95

25. pH 7.35, $Paco_2$ 24, Bicarbonate 15, Pao_2 95

26. pH 7.45, $Paco_2$ 50, Bicarbonate 42, Pao_2 80

27. pH 7.46, $Paco_2$ 41, HCO_3 25, Pao_2 97

28. Identify the three major causes of acidosis and alkalosis.

    a. _____

    b. _____

    c. _____

29. Which of the following electrolyte balances is likely to be disrupted in acidemia?
    a. Sodium
    b. Potassium
    c. Chloride
    d. Calcium

30. The cause of respiratory acidosis is
    a. Overexcretion of hydrogen and bicarbonate ions from the kidney
    b. Underelimination of carbon dioxide from the lungs
    c. Overelimination of carbon dioxide from the lungs
    d. Underelimination of metabolic waste products from the gastrointestinal tract

31. Inadequate chest expansion, which leads to respiratory acidosis, is most likely to be caused by
    a. Lordosis
    b. Emphysema
    c. Prolonged bedrest
    d. First-trimester pregnancy

32. Interference with alveolar-capillary diffusion results in
    a. Carbon dioxide retention and acidemia
    b. Hydrogen ion elimination and acidemia
    c. Hydrogen ion depletion from water vapor loss
    d. Aerobic metabolism and lactic acid buildup

33. One cause of metabolic acidosis is
    a. Aspirin poisoning
    b. Overuse of antacids
    c. Prolonged nasogastric suction
    d. Potassium-sparing diuretics

34. Arterial Pao_2
    a. Decreases in respiratory acidosis and alkalosis
    b. Increases in metabolic acidosis and alkalosis
    c. Increases in respiratory and combined acidosis
    d. Is unchanged in alkalosis

35. The hallmark of metabolic acidosis is
    a. Increased bicarbonate and normal carbon dioxide levels
    b. Decreased bicarbonate and normal carbon dioxide levels
    c. Increased bicarbonate and increased carbon dioxide levels
    d. Decreased bicarbonate and increased carbon dioxide levels

36. The hallmark of chronic respiratory acidosis is
    a. Elevated bicarbonate and increased arterial $Paco_2$ levels
    b. Elevated bicarbonate and normal arterial $Paco_2$ levels
    c. Decreased bicarbonate and normal arterial $Paco_2$ levels
    d. Decreased bicarbonate and increased arterial $Paco_2$ levels

37. The hallmark of metabolic alkalosis is
    a. Increased bicarbonate and normal arterial $Paco_2$ levels
    b. Increased bicarbonate and rising arterial $Paco_2$ levels
    c. Increased bicarbonate and decreased arterial $Paco_2$ levels
    d. Decreased bicarbonate and falling arterial $Paco_2$ levels

38. The hallmark of respiratory alkalosis includes
    a. Decreased bicarbonate and decreased arterial $Paco_2$ levels
    b. Increased bicarbonate and arterial $Paco_2$ levels
    c. Decreased bicarbonate and normal arterial $Paco_2$ levels
    d. Decreased bicarbonate and increased arterial $Paco_2$ levels

39. The safest way to administer oxygen to a client with chronic respiratory acidosis is by
    a. High-volume intermittent positive pressure
    b. Low-flow oxygen (2 L/min) via nasal cannula
    c. High-flow 40% oxygen via face mask
    d. Hyperbaric pressure chamber

40. Which of the following assessments indicates that a client with chronic respiratory acidosis is responding favorably to treatment?
    a. Nail beds pale, extremities cool
    b. Respiratory stridor with inspiration
    c. Expectorating clear, thin mucus
    d. Diffuse crackles auscultated bilaterally

41. The diet of a client with chronic respiratory acidosis should include
    a. Whole-grain breads
    b. Raw fruits and vegetables
    c. Chicken noodle soup (low-sodium)
    d. Carbonated soft drinks and juices

42. Discharge instructions for the client with chronic respiratory acidosis should include
    a. Discussing how to plan for periods of increased activity
    b. Teaching about low-protein, low-carbohydrate diet
    c. Demonstrating exercises to increase vital capacity
    d. Encouraging participation in activities such as jogging

43. Interventions for the client with metabolic alkalosis include
    a. Intravenous infusion of lactated Ringer's solution
    b. Administration of bolus intravenous calcium gluconate
    c. Siderails padded and kept in the "up" position
    d. Administration of insulin and fluid hydration

44. Which of the following interventions is appropriate for the client with metabolic acidosis?
    a. Administer bicarbonate to reduce the level of hydrogen ions.
    b. Administer bicarbonate only if serum bicarbonate levels are low.
    c. Give glucose to correct altered levels of potassium.
    d. Compensation occurs when high-volume oxygen is delivered.

45. Which of the following statements about combined metabolic and respiratory acidosis is true?
    a. Uncorrected acute metabolic acidosis always leads to respiratory acidosis.
    b. Combined metabolic and respiratory acidosis is best treated with immediate oxygen therapy.
    c. Combined acidosis is less severe than either metabolic acidosis or respiratory acidosis alone.
    d. Combined acidosis is more severe than either metabolic acidosis or respiratory acidosis alone.

CASE STUDY: THE CLIENT WITH RESPIRATORY ACIDOSIS

Answer Guidelines for the Case Study questions are provided on the companion Evolve Learning Resources Web site at http://evolve.elsevier.com/Iggy/.

Your client is a 75-year-old man with a history of emphysema. He is admitted to the hospital with pneumonia.

1. Which of the following assessments would indicate that this client has impaired gas exchange?
    a. Decreased urine output
    b. Lethargy
    c. Decreased chest excursion
    d. Hypotension

2. Which of the following arterial blood gas values indicates that this client is a CO_2 retainer?
    a. Pa_{CO_2} = 40 mm Hg
    b. Pa_{CO_2} = 60 mm Hg
    c. Bicarbonate = 42
    d. Pa_{O_2} = 60 mm Hg

3. The client's baseline arterial blood gases are: pH 7.36; Paco$_2$ 60 mm Hg, Pao$_2$ 52 mm Hg, bicarbonate 42 mEq/L. Which of the following would most likely indicate that he is having a negative response to the administration of oxygen?

   a. pH 7.35; Paco$_2$ 64, Pao$_2$ 60, bicarbonate 42 mEq/L

   b. pH 7.36, Paco$_2$ 60, Pao$_2$ 60, bicarbonate 42 mEq/L

   c. pH 7.36, Paco$_2$ 60, Pao$_2$ 58, bicarbonate 38 mEq/L

   d. pH 7.33, Paco$_2$ 66, Pao$_2$ 66, bicarbonate 42 mEq/L

4. Based on the answer for question 3, is the client's respiratory acidosis compensated or uncompensated? Explain your answer.

5. What immediate interventions are needed for this client?

6. Later in the shift, you note that his oxygen is set at 5 L/minute. The client says that he asked the nursing assistant to turn up his oxygen because he was having trouble breathing. What actions, if any, should you take at this time?

CASE STUDY: THE CLIENT WITH METABOLIC ACID-BASE IMBALANCE

Answer Guidelines for the Case Study questions are provided on the companion Evolve Learning Resources Web site at http://evolve.elsevier.com/Iggy/.

A 65-year-old woman with a recent history of cellulitis is admitted to the hospital with fever, shortness of breath, and hypotension. She has had a 2-day history of diarrhea related to the flu. Her ABG reveals a pH of 7.30, Paco$_2$ of 28, Pao$_2$ of 88, bicarbonate of 17 mEq/L.

1. This client's symptoms are most likely a result of

   a. Metabolic acidosis

   b. Respiratory acidosis

   c. Metabolic alkalosis

   d. Respiratory alkalosis

2. The bicarbonate level of 17 mEq/L is the result of

   a. Respiratory hypoventilation

   b. Overelimination of bicarbonate

   c. Respiratory compensation

   d. Underelimination of hydrogen ions

3. Which of the following symptoms would indicate a worsening acidotic condition?
   a. Increased blood pressure
   b. Anxiety
   c. Rising Pa_{CO_2}
   d. Increased urinary output

4. Which of the following interventions would be critical in reversing this client's condition?
   a. Administration of fluids
   b. Administration of oxygen
   c. Administration of bicarbonate
   d. Administration of potassium

5. Explain whether or not bicarbonate would be given to this client to correct her condition.

6. What other laboratory values would be important to monitor at this time? Explain.

Interventions for Preoperative Clients

LEARNING OUTCOMES

1. Differentiate among the various types and purposes of surgery.
2. Identify personal factors that increase the client's risk for complications during and immediately following surgery.
3. Use effective communication when teaching clients and family members about what to expect during the surgical experience.
4. Assume the role of client advocate.
5. Perform an accurate preoperative assessment of the client's physical and psychosocial status.
6. Identify laboratory value changes that may affect the client's response to drugs, anesthesia, and surgery.
7. Describe the legal implications and proper procedures for obtaining informed consent.
8. Explain the purposes and techniques commonly used for client preoperative preparation.
9. Prioritize teaching needs for the client preparing for surgery.
10. Recognize client conditions or issues that need to be communicated to the surgical and postoperative teams.

LEARNING ACTIVITIES

1. Before completing the study guide exercises for this chapter, it is recommended that you review the following:
   - Principles of teaching and learning in client care
   - Normal laboratory values
   - Normal ranges for vital sign measurements

2. Review the boldfaced terms and their definitions in Chapter 20 to enhance your understanding of the content.

STUDY/REVIEW QUESTIONS

Answers to the Study/Review Questions are provided on the companion Evolve Learning Resources Web site at http://evolve.elsevier.com/Iggy/.

1. Which of the following statements best describes the preoperative period?
   a. The preoperative period begins when the client makes the appointment with the surgeon to discuss the need for surgery.
   b. The preoperative period is the time during which the client receives education and testing related to the impending surgery.
   c. The preoperative period is a time during which the client's need for surgery is established.
   d. The preoperative period begins when the client is scheduled for surgery and ends at the time of transfer to the surgical suite.

2. Match each description with the category of surgery.

Category of Surgery
1. Palliative
2. Diagnostic
3. Restorative
4. Cosmetic
5. Curative

Definition

_____ a. Performed to alter or enhance personal appearance

_____ b. Performed to improve a client's functional ability

_____ c. Performed to resolve a health problem by repairing or removing the cause

_____ d. Performed to determine the origin or cause of a disorder

_____ e. Performed to relieve symptoms of a disease process, but does not cure

3. Name at least one example of a condition or surgical procedure for each category of surgery listed in Question 2.

   a. _____

   b. _____

   c. _____

   d. _____

   e. _____

For Questions 4 through 6, specify whether the urgency of the surgery is elective, urgent, or emergent.

4. A 22-year-old nursing student is scheduled for an appendectomy.

5. A 77-year-old woman is scheduled for a total knee replacement.

6. A 55-year-old man is scheduled for a colon resection due to a small bowel obstruction.

7. The nurse screens the preoperative client for conditions that may increase the risk for complications during the perioperative period. Which of the following conditions are possible risk factors?
   a. The client is 70 years old and obese.
   b. The surgical procedure planned is a bunionectomy.
   c. The client is 5 feet tall and weighs 100 pounds.
   d. The surgery is planned as an ambulatory/same day surgery procedure.

For Questions 8 through 14, read the following statements regarding preoperative care and decide whether each is true or false. Write T for true or F for false in the blanks provided. If the statement is false, correct the statement to make it true.

_____ 8.   The nurse functions as the client advocate by reporting to the surgeon and anesthesiology personnel any abnormalities found on the physical assessment.

_____ 9.   Throughout the physical assessment, the nurse focuses on the problem areas identified from the client's history that are limited to body systems affected directly by the surgical procedure.

_____ 10.   In the preoperative setting, the nurse is functioning as a client advocate when the client's home environment, self-care capabilities, and support systems are assessed and used in the discharge planning process.

_____ 11.   As a client advocate, the nurse can provide the client with educational materials appropriate to the client's ability to learn.

_____ 12.   The nurse has an awareness of factors that can influence coping and will use this knowledge when providing preoperative care.

_____ 13.   When the nurse evaluates preoperative laboratory test values, only abnormal values related to the surgery need to be reported to the surgeon and anesthesiology personnel.

_____ 14.   Clients who have had minor outpatient surgery do not usually require discharge planning.

15.   The preoperative diagnostic assessment may include a variety of tests. List seven of the most common tests.

a.   _____

b.   _____

c.   _____

d.   _____

e.   _____

f.   _____

g.   _____

16.   Which of the following statements is true regarding the client who has given consent for a surgical procedure?
a.   Information necessary to understand the nature of and reason for the surgery has been provided.
b.   Information about length of stay in the hospital has been preapproved by the managed care provider.
c.   Information about the surgeon's experience has been provided.
d.   The client has read all preoperative materials presented in the surgeon's office.

17. Which answer best describes the collaborative roles of the nurse and surgeon when obtaining the informed consent?
    a. The nurse is responsible for having the informed consent form on the chart for the physician to witness.
    b. The nurse may serve as a witness that the client has been informed by the physician before surgery is performed.
    c. The nurse may serve as witness to the client's signature after the physician has the consent form signed before preoperative sedation is given and before surgery is performed.
    d. The nurse has no duties regarding the consent form if the client has signed the informed consent form for the physician, even if the client then asks additional questions about the surgery.

18. A client is in the holding area in preparation for a left breast biopsy. Describe how the nurse will ensure that the correct site is identified before surgery.

19. A client is scheduled for surgery in the morning. Which of the following drugs do you expect to be held in the morning of surgery?
    a. Oral antidiabetic drug
    b. Antidepressant drug
    c. Anticonvulsant drug
    d. Bronchodilator

20. Complete the following chart regarding aspects of preoperative teaching about postoperative procedures and exercises.

Procedure/Exercise	Purpose
Breathing exercises and incentive spirometry	a.
b.	Performed along with deep breathing. Helps to expel secretions, keep the lungs clear, promote full aeration of the lungs, and prevent pneumonia and atelectasis.
Antiembolism stockings and elastic wraps	c.
d.	Devices that provide intermittent periods of compression to the lower leg, thus preventing venous stasis and enhancing venous flow.
Early ambulation	e.
f.	Passive or active, these help prevent joint rigidity and muscle contracture.

CASE STUDY: THE PREOPERATIVE CLIENT

Answer Guidelines for the Case Study questions are provided on the companion Evolve Learning Resources Web site at http://evolve.elsevier.com/Iggy/.

Your client is a 42-year-old woman who is scheduled for a total hysterectomy under general anesthesia this morning. She is admitted to the preoperative area in the same-day surgery admitting area. During the admission assessment, the client mentions to the nurse that her last menses was 2 months ago and that the bleeding was heavier than usual, which she assumes is why her surgeon is recommending the surgery. When asking her about medications that she takes, the client denies taking any prescription medicines but does mention taking a baby aspirin a day and assorted herbal medicines for the bleeding.

1.   What assessment should the nurse make to determine this client's nutritional status and potential risk from the preoperative preparation and surgery?

2.   What laboratory results of this client's should the nurse review? State the rationales for doing so.

3.   Prioritize teaching needs for this client before surgery.

4.   Develop a teaching-learning plan for this client's postoperative care.

5.   Identify any client conditions or information that is to be shared with the surgeon or anesthesiologist.

6.   The client states that she doesn't know whether her hysterectomy will be done vaginally or abdominally. Recognizing that the client is in need of more information, what would the nurse do?

7. The client asks if she will lose a lot of blood in surgery and, if so, can her daughter donate blood that she can receive if needed. What teaching would you give the client concerning blood donations?

8. Identify which category of surgery is related to each aspect of this client's impending surgery.
   a. Reason:

   b. Urgency:

   c. Degree of risk of surgery:

   d. Extent of surgery:

9. While this client is waiting in the preoperative area, she begins to cry, saying she is fearful of the surgery and "going under." What interventions could be used to reduce the client's anxiety?

10. The client is about to be sent to the operating room. What items on a final checklist should be evaluated before leaving the preoperative area?

Interventions for Intraoperative Clients

LEARNING OUTCOMES

1. Discuss nursing interventions to reduce client and family anxiety.
2. Explain procedures to ensure the identity of the client and the accuracy of the planned surgical procedure.
3. Describe the roles and responsibilities of various intraoperative personnel.
4. Identify interventions to ensure the client's safety and dignity during an operative procedure.
5. Identify nursing responsibilities for management of clients receiving anesthesia.
6. Select nursing interventions to prevent skin breakdown for older adult clients during surgery.
7. Recognize the clinical manifestations of malignant hyperthermia.
8. List interventions for the client with malignant hyperthermia.
9. Discuss the potential adverse reactions and complications of specific anesthetic agents.
10. Assess clients for specific problems related to positioning during surgical procedures.

LEARNING ACTIVITIES

1. Before completing the study guide exercises for this chapter, it is recommended that you review the following:
   - Principles of sterile technique
   - Principles of skin care
   - Normal ranges for vital sign measurements
   - Normal laboratory values
   - The role of the nurse anesthetist in the perioperative setting

2. Review the boldfaced terms and their definitions in Chapter 21 to enhance your understanding of the content.

STUDY/REVIEW QUESTIONS

Answers to the Study/Review Questions are provided on the companion Evolve Learning Resources Web site at http://evolve.elsevier.com/Iggy/.

1. Which of the following nursing interventions can reduce the preoperative client's anxiety?
   a. Provide a climate of privacy, comfort, and confidentiality when caring for the client.
   b. Instruct the client that after the preoperative medication has taken effect, the anxiety will go away.
   c. Avoid discussing the activities taking place around the client while in the holding area.
   d. Assist members of the surgical team readying the operating room suite.

2. Match the perioperative personnel with the descriptions of duties in the perioperative area.

Duties
1. Coordinates, oversees, and participates in the client's nursing care while the client is in the operating room
2. Assumes responsibility for the surgical procedure and any surgical judgments about the client
3. Manages the client's care while the client is in this area and initiates documentation on a perioperative nursing record
4. Educated in a particular type of surgery and responsible for intraoperative nursing care specific to clients needing that type of surgery
5. Sets up the sterile field, assists with the draping of the client, and hands sterile supplies, sterile equipment, and instruments to the surgeon
6. Physician who specializes in the administration of anesthetic agents

Personnel
_____ a. Surgeon
_____ b. Holding area nurse
_____ c. Anesthesiologist
_____ d. Circulating nurse
_____ e. Scrub nurse
_____ f. Specialty nurse

3. During surgery, anesthesia personnel monitor, measure, and assess which of the following? *Check all that apply.*

   _____ a. Intake and output
   _____ b. Vital signs
   _____ c. Cardiopulmonary function
   _____ d. Level of anesthesia

4. How does the anesthesiologist monitor, assess, and measure the client's cardiopulmonary function?

5. Define the term *anesthesia*.

6. What is the purpose of anesthesia?

7. Match the following nursing interventions with the stage of general anesthesia.

Nursing Interventions	Stages of Anesthesia
_____ a. Prepare for and assist in treatment of cardiovascular and/or pulmonary arrest. Document in record.	Stage 1 Stage 2 Stage 3 Stage 4
_____ b. Shield client from extra noise and physical stimuli. Protect the client's extremities. Assist anesthesia personnel as needed. Stay with client.	
_____ c. Close operating room doors and control traffic in and out of room. Position client securely with safety belts. Maintain minimal discussion in operating room.	
_____ d. Assist anesthesia personnel with intubation of client. Place the client in position for surgery. Prep the client's skin in area of operative site.	

8. What anesthetic agents are known most commonly to trigger a malignant hyperthermia (MH) crisis?

9. Which of the following clinical features are found in an MH crisis? *Check all that apply. Correct the answers that are incorrect.*

_____ a. Sinus tachycardia

_____ b. Tightness and rigidity of the client's jaw area

_____ c. Lowering of the blood pressure

_____ d. A decrease in the end-tidal carbon dioxide level with a profound increase in oxygen saturation

_____ e. Skin mottling and cyanosis

_____ f. An extremely elevated temperature, as high as 111.2° F (44° C) early into the crisis.

_____ g. Tachypnea

10. The surgical team understands that time is crucial in recognizing and treating an MH crisis. Once recognized, what is the treatment of choice?
    a. Danazol gluconate
    b. Dilantin sodium
    c. Diazepam sulfate
    d. Dantrolene sodium

11. *True or false?* In an MH crisis, an extremely elevated and uncontrollable body temperature is one of the early signs of a problem.

12. Identify five of the best practices for a client with malignant hyperthermia.

    a. _____

    b. _____

    c. _____

    d. _____

    e. _____

13. Positioning of the client during surgical procedures is important in preventing postoperative problems. Match the following nursing interventions with the potential complications, which can be prevented with appropriate positioning and monitoring.

Interventions

1. Support the wrist with padding; do not overtighten wrist straps.
2. Place pillow or foam padding under bony prominences; maintain good body alignment; slightly flex joints and support with pillows, trochanter rolls, and pads.
3. Place a safety strap above the ankle; do not place equipment on lower extremities.
4. Pad the elbow; avoid excessive abduction; secure the arm firmly on an arm board positioned at shoulder level.
5. Place a safety strap above or below the area. Place a pillow or padding under the knees.

Anatomic Area/Complications

_____ a. Brachial plexus/paralysis; loss of sensation

_____ b. Radial nerve/wrist drop

_____ c. Medial or ulnar nerves (hand deformities); peroneal nerve (foot drop)

_____ d. Tibial nerve/loss of sensation on the plantar surface of the foot

_____ e. Joints/stiffness; pain; inflammation

14. Differentiate assisted respiration and controlled respiration during anesthesia.

15. Match the anesthetic agent with the appropriate characteristic.

Characteristic
1. Used for local or regional anesthesia.
2. A barbiturate; low incidence of postoperative nausea and vomiting.
3. Emergence reactions, such as hallucinations, unpleasant dreams, and restlessness, are common.
4. Excellent postoperative analgesia, but may cause significant respiratory depression.
5. Short acting; client becomes responsive quickly postoperatively.
6. Sweet smell makes it easy to use in children.
7. May cause coughing and excitement during induction.
8. Needs addition of other agents for longer procedures.

Agent

_____ a. Halothane

_____ b. Nitrous oxide

_____ c. Desflurane

_____ d. Thiopental sodium

_____ e. Ketamine HCl

_____ f. Propofol

_____ g. Fentanyl

_____ h. Tetracaine

16. Discuss how benzodiazepines are used during anesthesia.

17. What is important for the nurse to remember when the client is receiving opioid analgesics during and after surgery?

18. Describe the purpose of neuromuscular blocking agents, and differentiate nondepolarizing and depolarizing blocking agents. Cite examples of each.

19. Match the type of anesthesia with the appropriate definition.

Definition

1. Injection of the anesthetic agent into the epidural space; the spinal cord areas are never entered. Used for lower extremity surgeries, as well as anorectal, vaginal, perineal, and hip surgeries.
2. Injection of anesthetic agent into or around a nerve or group of nerves, resulting in blocked sensation and motor impulse transmission. Used to prevent pain during a procedure or to identify the cause of pain. A type of regional anesthesia.
3. Agents applied directly to the area of skin or mucous membrane to be anesthetized. Onset is within 1 minute; duration is up to 30 minutes.
4. Injection of an anesthetic agent directly into the tissue around an incision, wound, or lesion. Blocks peripheral nerve function at its origin.
5. Also called intrathecal block; injection of anesthetic agent into the cerebrospinal fluid in the subarachnoid space. Used for lower abdominal and pelvic surgery.

Type of Anesthesia

_____ a.   Topical anesthesia

_____ b.   Local infiltration

_____ c.   Nerve block

_____ d.   Spinal anesthesia

_____ e.   Epidural anesthesia

20. Which client would be a candidate for conscious sedation? *Check all that apply.*

_____ a.   Endoscopy

_____ b.   Caesarean section delivery

_____ c.   Closed fracture reduction

_____ d.   Cardiac catheterization

_____ e.   Suturing a laceration

_____ f.   Abdominal surgery

_____ g.   Cardioversion

CASE STUDY: THE INTRAOPERATIVE CLIENT

Answer Guidelines for the Case Study questions are provided on the companion Evolve Learning Resources Web site at http://evolve.elsevier.com/Iggy/.

A 71-year-old man is scheduled to receive orthopedic surgery in 3 hours. The nurse in the holding area has assessed the client and begins to prepare him for the surgical procedure.

1.   This client has his intravenous catheter inserted and has a surgical shave performed before surgery. The client is expected to be free of injury during surgery. Identify nursing diagnoses that would be appropriate for this client.

2.   While this client is in the holding area, members of the surgical team are preparing the surgical suite. Identify factors related to physical safety in the surgical suite and give the rationale for each.

3.   Identify three factors related to what the surgical team does to minimize risk of surgical infection for the client; also identify the rationale for each.

4.   The client sees the surgical team scrubbing their hands and arms and states "Oh, it makes me feel good to know that their hands are going to be sterile for my surgery." Evaluate this statement.

5.   This client is having regional anesthesia for surgery because of a family history of malignant hyperthermia (MH). Which of the following statements is true about epidural anesthesia?
   a.   Regional anesthesia is used when a Certified Registered Nurse Anesthetist (CRNA) will be administering the anesthetic.
   b.   The circulating nurse does not have to monitor the client's reactions to the anesthetic.
   c.   There is no risk of pulmonary complications with regional anesthetics.
   d.   An advantage of regional anesthesia is the ability to retain the epidural catheter for postoperative pain management.

6. The surgeon, nurse, and anesthesiologist have discussed anesthesia options with the client, who agrees that an epidural anesthetic will be a good choice for him. What are potential complications the surgical team should be aware of with this choice? What are the symptoms of these potential complications?

8. As the surgical team closes the operative wound, what type of skin closures would you expect to see?

7. What will the circulating nurse's role be for this client during the intraoperative period? *Check all that apply.*

_____ a. Offers information and reassurance before anesthesia is implemented

_____ b. Monitors the client's vital signs during surgery

_____ c. Observes for breaks in sterile technique

_____ d. Holds the retractors during surgery to improve viewing of the operative site

_____ e. Positions the client safely

_____ f. Sets up the sterile field and drapes the client

_____ g. Anticipates the client's and surgical team's needs

_____ h. Documents care, events, findings, and counts

Interventions for Postoperative Clients

LEARNING OUTCOMES

1. Describe the ongoing head-to-toe assessment of the postoperative client.
2. Prioritize nursing interventions for the client recovering from surgery and anesthesia during the first 24 hours.
3. Prioritize nursing care for the client who has respiratory depression after surgery.
4. Discuss the criteria for determining readiness of the client to be discharged from the postanesthesia care unit.
5. Use proper technique for wound assessment and dressing changes.
6. Recognize wound complications after surgery.
7. Describe steps to take when a client has a surgical wound dehiscence or evisceration.
8. Compare the actions, side effects, and nursing implications for different types of drug therapy for pain management after surgery.
9. Develop a community-based teaching plan for clients after surgery.

LEARNING ACTIVITIES

1. Prior to completing the study guide exercises for this chapter, it is recommended that you review the following:
   - Assessment and care of the client having pain
   - The principles of fluid and electrolyte balance
   - Principles of sterile technique
   - Principles of skin care
   - Normal ranges for vital sign measurements
   - Normal laboratory values
   - Principles of teaching and learning in client care

2. Review the boldfaced terms and their definitions in Chapter 22 to enhance your understanding of the content.

STUDY/REVIEW QUESTIONS

Answers to the Study/Review Questions are provided on the companion Evolve Learning Resources Web site at http://evolve.elsevier.com/Iggy/.

1. Which of the following describes the beginning of the postoperative period?
   a. Completion of the surgical procedure and arousal of the client from anesthesia
   b. Discharge planning initiated in the preoperative setting
   c. Closure of the client's surgical incision
   d. Completion of the surgical procedure and transfer of the client to the postanesthetic care unit (PACU) or intensive care unit

2. What is the primary purpose of a PACU?
   a. Follow-through on the surgeon's postoperative orders
   b. Ongoing critical evaluation and stabilization of the client
   c. Prevention of lengthened hospital stay
   d. Arousal of client following the use of conscious sedation

3. In the list below, which are considered postoperative complications? *Check all that apply.*
   _____ a. Sedation
   _____ b. Dysrhythmia
   _____ c. Incisional pain
   _____ d. Pulmonary embolism
   _____ e. Vomiting
   _____ f. Hypothermia
   _____ g. Hyperthermia
   _____ h. Wound evisceration
   _____ i. Sleepiness
   _____ j. Wound infection

4. Identify at least five risk factors in a client that may slow wound healing.
   a. _____
   b. _____
   c. _____
   d. _____
   e. _____

5. If a client experiences a wound dehiscence, which of the following describes what is happening with the wound?
   a. Purulent drainage is present at incision site because of infection.
   b. Extreme pain is present at incision site.
   c. A partial or complete separation of outer layers is present at incision site.
   d. The inner and outer layers of the incision are separated.

6. When a client describes being able to see "internal organs" at the incision site, what is he describing?
   a. An infection
   b. Evisceration
   c. Poor wound healing
   d. Split skin sutures

7. During PACU care, part of the nursing assessment includes the dressing. What characteristics will the nurse be noting?
   a. How much adhesive is in place upon admission into the PACU
   b. The size of the drain used
   c. Amount, color, odor, and consistency of drainage on the dressing
   d. The appearance of the wound under the dressing

8. Identify the types of information that should be included on the report of the client's status upon arrival in the PACU.

Match the following assessment findings that may be noted for clients in the PACU with their corresponding body systems. Answers may be used more than once. More than one body system may be involved in a finding.

Body Systems

a. Respiratory
b. Cardiovascular
c. Fluid and electrolyte balance
d. Neurologic
e. Renal/urinary
f. Gastrointestinal
g. Integumentary

Assessment Findings

_____ 9. Eyes open on command
_____ 10. Symmetrical chest wall expansion
_____ 11. Foley catheter to facilitate drainage
_____ 12. Absent dorsalis pedis pulsations
_____ 13. Use of accessory muscles
_____ 14. Large amount of sanguineous drainage
_____ 15. Negative Homans' sign
_____ 16. IV infusion of dextrose 5% Ringer's lactate
_____ 17. States name when asked
_____ 18. Rounded, firm abdomen
_____ 19. Exhalation felt from nose or mouth
_____ 20. Decreased blood pressure
_____ 21. Wound edges approximated
_____ 22. Dry mucous membranes
_____ 23. Vomiting
_____ 24. Pupils constrict equally
_____ 25. Sternal retraction
_____ 26. Nasogastric tube in place
_____ 27. Evisceration
_____ 28. Dullness over symphysis pubis
_____ 29. Tenting
_____ 30. Faint heart sounds
_____ 31. Wound dressing dry
_____ 32. Absent bowel sounds
_____ 33. Vesicular crackles
_____ 34. Hand grips equal
_____ 35. Simultaneous apical and radial pulsations
_____ 36. Dehiscence
_____ 37. Snoring

38. Airway assessment is completed immediately upon arrival to the PACU to establish a patent airway and adequate respiratory exchange. Identify the key points in the respiratory assessment.

39. The client arrives at the PACU and the nurse notes a respiratory rate of 10, with sternal retractions. The report from anesthesia personnel indicated that the client had received fentanyl during surgery. Number from 1 to 7 the following nursing interventions to be performed in order of first to last.

_____ a. Continue to monitor the client for effects of naloxone for at least 1 hour.

_____ b. Have suction available.

_____ c. Closely monitor vital signs and pulse oximetry readings until the client responds.

_____ d. Do not leave the client unattended until he or she is able to respond fully.

_____ e. Observe for significant reversal of anesthesia.

_____ f. Administer oxygen as ordered.

_____ g. Maintain an open airway.

40. Identify three common nursing diagnoses and collaborative problems for a client in the PACU.

a. _____

b. _____

c. _____

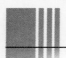

41. The health care team determines the client's readiness for discharge from the PACU by noting a postanesthesia recovery score of at least 10. After determining that all criteria have been met, the client is discharged to the hospital unit or home. Review the following client profiles after 1 hour in the PACU. Number the clients in order of anticipated discharge from the PACU area.

_____ a.   10-year-old girl, tonsillectomy, general anesthesia. Duration of surgery 30 minutes. Immediate response to voice. Alert to place and person. Able to move all extremities. Respirations even, deep, rate of 20. VS are within normal limits. IV solution is D₅RL. Has voided on bedpan. Eating ice chips. Complaining of sore throat.

_____ b.   35-year-old woman, cesarean section, epidural anesthesia. Duration of surgery 27 minutes. Awake and alert. Able to bend knees and lift lower extremities. Respirations 16 breaths/min and unlabored. Foley draining 300 mL urine. IV of RL infusing. VS are within normal limits.

_____ c.   55-year-old man, repair of fractured lower left leg. General anesthesia. Duration of surgery 1 hour, 30 minutes. Drowsy, but responds to voice. Nausea and vomiting twice in PACU. No urge to void at this time. IV infusing D₅NS. Pedal pulses noted in both lower extremities. VS: T 98.6° F; P 130; R 24; BP 124/76.

_____ d.   24-year-old man, reconstruction of facial scar. General anesthesia. Duration of surgery 2 hours. Sleeping, groans to voice command. VS are within normal limits. Respirations 10 breaths/min. No urge to void. IV of D₅RL infusing. Complains of pain in surgical area.

_____ e.   42-year-old woman, colonoscopy. IV conscious sedation. Awake and alert. Up to bathroom to void. IV discontinued. Resting quietly in chair. VS are within normal limits.

42. You are caring for a client who has had abdominal surgery. After a hard sneeze, the client complains of pain in his surgical area, and you immediately see that he has a wound evisceration. What should you do? Include in your answer the timing of the interventions.

43. Which of the following interventions for postsurgical care of the client is correct?
    a.   When positioning the client, use the knee gatch of the bed to bend the knees and relieve pressure.
    b.   Gentle massage on the lower legs and calves helps promote venous blood return to the heart.
    c.   Encourage bedrest after surgery to prevent complications.
    d.   The client should splint the surgical wound for support and comfort when getting out of bed.

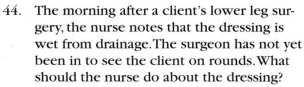

44. The morning after a client's lower leg surgery, the nurse notes that the dressing is wet from drainage. The surgeon has not yet been in to see the client on rounds. What should the nurse do about the dressing?
    a. Remove the dressing and put on a dry, sterile dressing.
    b. Reinforce the dressing by adding dry, sterile dressing material on top of the existing dressing.
    c. Lift up the dressing and apply dry, sterile dressing material to the wound, then retape the original dressing.
    d. Do nothing to the dressing but call the surgeon to evaluate the client immediately.

45. Differentiate serous, sanguineous, and serosanguineous drainage.

CASE STUDY: POSTOPERATIVE CARE

Answer Guidelines for the Case Study questions are provided on the companion Evolve Learning Resources Web site at http://evolve.elsevier.com/Iggy/.

A 30-year-old woman is admitted to the recovery area following a laparoscopy for an ovarian cyst removal. She is a small woman: 5 feet 1 inch and 103 pounds. Her surgery lasted 1 hour and 45 minutes, and the circulating nurse reported that she had a severe hemorrhage from the surgical site during that time. Upon admission to the postanesthesia care unit, the client's blood pressure is 112/62, pulse range is 84 to 92, and respirations are 20 and shallow. She is groggy but answers when asked questions. An intravenous infusion of 1000 mL of D_5 Ringer's lactate is infusing at a rate of 200 mL per hour, and 800 mL remains in the bottle. During surgery, 100 mL of D_5 Ringer's lactate and 500 mL of normal saline were infused. An endotracheal tube (ET) is in place.

1. What assessments should the nurse perform before removing the ET?

2. How often should the nurse monitor the client's vital signs?

A very slight amount of drainage is present on her dressing. Her blood pressure has been rising slowly and is now 20 mm Hg higher than the last time recorded, which was during surgery. She is restless and her respirations are 24 per minute.

3. After reviewing the above data, the nurse performs further assessment. What additional parameters should be assessed and why?

4. The nurse contacts the surgeon who orders the intravenous rate be reduced to 100 mL per hour. What is the reason for this order?

5. The client's condition stabilizes and she is transferred to the postsurgical nursing unit. Discuss the information that the PACU nurse should report to the unit nurse.

Concepts of Inflammation and the Immune Response

LEARNING OUTCOMES

1. Describe the concept of self-tolerance.
2. Explain the differences between inflammation and infection.
3. Compare and contrast the cells, purposes, and features of inflammation and immunity.
4. Describe the basis for the five cardinal manifestations of inflammation.
5. Interpret a white blood cell count with differential to indicate no immune problems, an acute bacterial infection, a chronic bacterial infection, or an allergic reaction.
6. Explain how complement activation and fixation assists in protection from infection.
7. Compare the cells, function, and protective actions of antibody-mediated immunity and cell-mediated immunity.
8. Compare the different types of antibody-mediated immunity for their protection effectiveness and duration of immunity.
9. Describe how the immune system responds to the presence of transplanted tissues or organs.
10. Explain the actions and short- and long-term side effects of immunosuppressive drugs.

LEARNING ACTIVITIES

1. Before completing the study guide exercises in this chapter, it is recommended that you review the following:
   - Anatomy and physiology of the immune system
   - Process of inflammation
   - Process of immunity
   - White blood cells and their activities in the process of inflammation, immunity, and rejection
   - Sequence of the inflammatory response
   - Types of immunity
   - Transplant rejection and management
   - Immunosuppressive drug therapy

2. Review the boldfaced terms and their definitions in Chapter 23 to enhance your understanding of the content.

STUDY/REVIEW QUESTIONS

Answers to the Study/Review Questions are provided on the companion Evolve Learning Resources Web site at http://evolve.elsevier.com/Iggy/.

1. Which of the following statements about the purpose of the immune system are true? *Check all that apply.*

   _____ a. The immune system provides protection from and eliminates or destroys microorganisms.

   _____ b. The immune system is able to identify non-self protein and cells.

   _____ c. The immune system removes foreign proteins and other substances.

   _____ d. The immune system protects against allergic/anaphylactic reactions.

2. Explain self-tolerance:

3. Identify five factors that affect immune function.

   a. _____

   b. _____

   c. _____

   d. _____

   e. _____

True or False? Write T for true or F for false in the blank provided.

_____ 4. Most immune cells originate in the bone marrow and are released in the blood at maturity.

_____ 5. The immune system cells are the only body cells capable of determining self from non-self.

_____ 6. The presence inflammation always indicates that an infection is present.

7. Identify the three processes or components of immunity needed for full immunocompetence.

   a. _____

   b. _____

   c. _____

8. Identify the important actions of leukocytes that provide protection.

   a. _____

   b. _____

   c. _____

   d. _____

   e. _____

   f. _____

   g. _____

9. Which of the following statements about the inflammatory response is true?
   a. Response is different with each incident.
   b. Response is the same whether the insult to the body is a burn or otitis media.
   c. Response depends on the location in the body.
   d. Response is specific to the cell type invaded or injured.

10. The inflammatory response is present in which of the following conditions? *Choose all that apply.*

    _____ a. Sprain injuries to joints

    _____ b. Surgical wounds

    _____ c. Poison ivy

    _____ d. Scalding burn injury

    _____ e. Appendicitis

11. Which cell types are associated with the inflammatory response that participate in phagocytosis?
    a. Neutrophils and eosinophils
    b. Macrophages and neutrophils
    c. Macrophages and eosinophils
    d. Eosinophils and neutrophils

12. The body produces the most of which type of white blood cell?
    a. Macrophages
    b. Eosinophils
    c. Neutrophils
    d. Band neutrophils

13. Match the cell characteristics with the types of cells. *Answers may be used more than once.*

Characteristics

_____ a. 12- to 18-hour life span

_____ b. 1% to 2% of total WBCs

_____ c. Contains chemicals such as histamine

_____ d. Can participate in multiple episodes of phagocytosis

_____ e. When mature, capable of phagocytosis

_____ f. Clinical sign of left shift indicates not enough mature cells being produced

_____ g. Liver and spleen have greatest concentration

_____ h. Vascular leak syndrome

_____ i. The number in circulation increases during an allergic response

Cell Types

1. Neutrophil
2. Macrophage
3. Basophil
4. Eosinophil

14. Which of the following statements about phagocytosis are true? *Check all that apply.*

_____ a. It is a process that engulfs invaders and destroys them by enzymatic degradation.

_____ b. It rids the body of debris and destroys foreign invaders.

_____ c. It is done in a predictable manner.

_____ d. It is a function of all leukocytes.

15. When an injury or invasion occurs, which of the following functions will the phagocytic cell perform? *Check all that apply.*

_____ a. Release chemotaxins or leukotaxins.

_____ b. Initiate repair of damaged tissue.

_____ c. Generate specific antibodies.

_____ d. Gain direct contact with the antigen or invader.

16. Describe opsonization:

17. When stimulated, complement activation and fixation is a mechanism of opsonization and phagocytic adherence that includes 20 different inactive protein components that will
    a. Cause individual complement proteins to activate, join together, surround the antigen, and adhere.
    b. Join together, cause individual complement proteins to activate, surround the antigen, and adhere.
    c. Cause individual phagocytic cells to clump together, forming a barrier to an invader.
    d. Stimulate the bone marrow to increase production of macrophages.

18. Phagocytes are capable of
    a. Making antibodies
    b. Ingesting cells
    c. Secreting complement
    d. Producing insulin

19. Identify the five cardinal signs of inflammation for which the nurse should assess.

    a. _____

    b. _____

    c. _____

    d. _____

    e. _____

20. All the signs of inflammation are present in which stage?
    a. Stage I
    b. Stage II
    c. Stage III
    d. Stage IV

21. What occurs in the body at the time of inflammation is a colony-stimulating factor that stimulates which of the following?
    a. Bone marrow to produce leukocytes in less time
    b. Bone marrow to produce immature leukocytes
    c. Bone marrow to release immature leukocytes
    d. Bone marrow to synthesize immunoglobulins

22. The substance commonly called *pus* is produced by exudate in which stage of inflammation?
    a. Stage I
    b. Stage II
    c. Stage III
    d. Stage IV

23. Neutrophils attack and destroy foreign material and remove dead tissue through which process?
    a. Phagocytosis
    b. Adherence
    c. Cytokines
    d. Fixation

24. B-lymphocytes, part of the antibody-mediated immunity (AMI) response, become sensitized to an antigen, and then
    a. Release colony-stimulating factors.
    b. Cause leukocytes to aggregate.
    c. Generate specific antibodies.
    d. Suppress phagocytosis.

25. List the seven special actions, in sequence, that take place when a person is exposed to an antigen.

    a. _____

    b. _____

    c. _____

    d. _____

    e. _____

    f. _____

    g. _____

26. What cells interact in the presence of an antigen to start antibody production?
    a. Macrophages, T-helper/inducer cells, B-lymphocytes
    b. Neutrophils, T-helper/inducer cells, B-lymphocytes
    c. Macrophages, T-suppressor cells, B-lymphocytes
    d. Neutrophils, T-suppressor cells, B-lymphocytes

27. Which of the following statements about B-lymphocytes and sensitizing to one antigen is true?
    a. Once sensitized, always sensitized to that antigen.
    b. Plasma cells produce the antigen.
    c. The plasma cell lies dormant until next exposure.
    d. Memory cells prevent plasma cells from oversecreting antibodies.

28. In what way is antibody-mediated immunity (AMI) different from cell-mediated immunity (CMI)?
    a. AMI is more powerful than CMI.
    b. AMI can be transferred from one person to another; CMI cannot.
    c. CMI requires constant re-exposure for "boosting;" AMI does not.
    d. CMI requires inflammatory actions for best function; AMI function is independent of inflammatory actions.

29. Match the following actions with the antibody-binding reactions.

Antibody-binding Reactions
1. Agglutination
2. Lysis
3. Precipitation
4. Inactivation (neutralization)
5. Complement fixation

Actions

_____ a. Cell membrane destruction

_____ b. Large, insoluble antibody molecules

_____ c. Clumping-like antibody action

_____ d. Activated by IgG and IgM

_____ e. Covers antigen's active site

30. Which of the following statements is true of innate-native immunity?
    a. Innate-native immunity is genetically determined, nonspecific, and cannot be transferred.
    b. Innate-native immunity adapts to individual exposure and invasion.
    c. Innate-native immunity cannot be altered by environmental or physiologic changes.
    d. Innate-native immunity requires a special interaction with antibody-mediated immunity for activation.

31. Explain how active and passive immunities are different.

32. Identify an example of each of the following types of immunity:

    a. Natural active immunity: _____

    _____

    b. Artificial active immunity: _____

    _____

    c. Natural passive immunity: _____

    _____

    d. Artificial passive immunity: _____

    _____

33. Identify the three T-lymphocyte subsets that are critically important to cell-mediated immunity (CMI).

    a. _____

    b. _____

    c. _____

34. What statement best describes the function of CD4+ (cluster of differentiation 4, or T4+) cells?
    a. They participate in specialized episodes of phagocytosis directed against cancer cells.
    b. They provide a frame or lattice for tissue repair and regeneration after inflammatory events.
    c. They secrete lymphokines that can enhance the activity of other WBCs.
    d. They deliver a "lethal hit" of lytic substance to a target cell in response to antibody-dependent lysis.

35. Match each type of cell with its function. *Answers may be used more than once.*

Cell Type
1. Suppressor cell
2. Natural-killer cell
3. Helper/inducer T cell
4. Cytotoxic/cytolytic T-cell

Function

_____ a.   Prevents overreaction

_____ b.   Binds with infected cell's antigen that results in death of affected cell

_____ c.   Secretes lymphokines that stimulate activities of other cells of the immune system

_____ d.   Exerts cytotoxic effect without first undergoing period of sensitization

_____ e.   Regulates variety of inflammatory and immune responses

True or False? Write T for true or F for false in the blank provided.

_____ 36.   Cancer prevention is assisted by cell-mediated immunity through its surveillance system.

37. The action of which cell type must be suppressed to prevent acute rejection of transplanted organs? *Check all that apply.*

_____ a.   Eosinophils

_____ b.   Suppressor T-cells

_____ c.   Natural killer cells

_____ d.   Cytotoxic/cytolytic T-cells

38. Identify three types of graft rejection.

a. _____

b. _____

c. _____

39. Match the descriptors with the types of rejection. *Answers may be used more than once.*

Descriptors

Types of Rejection
1. Hyperacute rejection
2. Acute graft rejection
3. Chronic rejection

_____ a.   Immediate

_____ b.   Includes both cellular and antibody-mediated mechanisms

_____ c.   Rejection cannot be stopped

_____ d.   Occurs within 1 week to 3 months

_____ e.   Leads to organ destruction

_____ f.   Does not mean loss of transplant

_____ g.   Accelerated graft atherosclerosis

_____ h.   Triggers blood clotting cascade

_____ i.   Fibrotic and scarlike tissue

_____ j.   Major cause of death in heart transplant clients

_____ k.   Is antibody-mediated

40. What precaution or intervention has the highest priority for the client going home on maintenance drugs after receiving a kidney transplant?
    a. Monitoring for bacterial and fungal infections
    b. Avoiding the use of table salt
    c. Measuring abdominal girth daily
    d. Avoiding blood donation

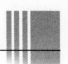

41. Match each antibody characteristic with the correct antibody type.

Characteristic

_____ a. Mediates ABO incompatibility reactions in blood transfusions

_____ b. Mediates many types of allergic reactions

_____ c. Present in body secretions such as tears, mucus, saliva

_____ d. Has the highest percentage in the blood

Antibody

1. IgA
2. IgE
3. IgG
4. IgM

42. Complete the following table:

Drug	Use
Cyclosporine	a.
Tacrolimus FK506 (Prograf)	b.
Corticosteroids	c.
Daclizumab (Zenapax)	d.
Muromonab-CD3 (Orthoclone OKT3)	e.

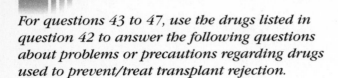

For questions 43 to 47, use the drugs listed in question 42 to answer the following questions about problems or precautions regarding drugs used to prevent/treat transplant rejection.

43. Induction of capillary leak syndrome is common; may require premedication with corticosteroids.

44. Immunosuppression is more profound than what occurs with other agents.

45. There is a high incidence of flu-like symptoms.

46. Drug may also be used as a rescue agent in kidney rejection.

47. Drug may stimulate hyperglycemia, increase body and facial hair, and cause gingival hyperplasia.

48. Which of the following drugs should not be given with grapefruit juice?
    a. Sirolimus (Rapamune)
    b. Mycophenolate Sodium (Myfortic)
    c. Basiliximab (Simulect)
    d. Antithymocyte globulin (Atgam)

Interventions for Clients with Connective Tissue Disease and Other Types of Arthritis

LEARNING OUTCOMES

1. Compare and contrast the pathophysiology and clinical manifestations of osteoarthritis (OA) and rheumatoid arthritis (RA).
2. Prioritize collaborative interventions for clients with OA and RA.
3. Determine common nursing diagnoses for postoperative clients having total joint replacement surgery.
4. Evaluate the expected outcomes for clients having total joint replacement surgery.
5. Interpret laboratory findings for clients with rheumatoid disease.
6. Identify the nursing implications associated with drug therapy for clients with rheumatoid arthritis.
7. Identify educational needs for clients with arthritis.
8. Differentiate between discoid lupus erythematosus and systemic lupus erythematosus.
9. Describe the priority nursing interventions for clients who have progressive systemic sclerosis.
10. Discuss the treatment of gout based on knowledge of pathophysiology.
11. Explain the differences between polymyositis, systemic necrotizing vasculitis, polymyalgia rheumatica, ankylosing spondylitis, Reiter's syndrome, and Sjögren's syndrome.
12. Describe interventions that clients can use to prevent Lyme disease.
13. Identify the primary concern in care for clients with Marfan's syndrome.
14. Describe current treatment strategies for clients with fibromyalgia.

LEARNING ACTIVITIES

1. Before completing the study guide exercises in this chapter, it is recommended that you review the following:
   - Anatomy and physiology of the musculoskeletal system
   - Process of inflammation
   - Normal laboratory values related to immune system
   - Assessment of the musculoskeletal system
   - Postoperative care
   - Hazards of immobility
   - Principles of teaching/learning

2. Review the boldfaced terms and their definitions in Chapter 24 to enhance your understanding of the content.

STUDY/REVIEW QUESTIONS

Answers to the Study/Review Questions are provided on the companion Evolve Learning Resources Web site at http://evolve.elsevier.com/Iggy/.

1. Identify these abbreviations commonly used in relation to connective tissue disease.

   CTD _____

   DJD _____

   OA _____

   HRT _____

   ESR _____

   TJR _____

   TJA _____

   DVT _____

   CPM _____

   RA _____

   TMJ _____

   PSS _____

   SLE _____

2. A rheumatic disease is any condition or disease of the
   a. Blood
   b. Bone marrow
   c. Skin and heart
   d. Musculoskeletal system

3. Connective tissue diseases are characterized by which of the following? *Check all that apply.*

   _____ a. Chronic pain

   _____ b. Dry skin

   _____ c. Decreased function

   _____ d. Joint deterioration

4. Identify the two pathophysiologic characteristics of osteoarthritis.

   a. _____

   b. _____

5. What are the most common sites for osteoarthritis?
   a. Hands, back, hips, and knees
   b. Hands, elbows, and pelvis
   c. Hands, back, and pelvis
   d. Knees, hips, and back

6. During erosion of the cartilage associated with osteoarthritis, which of the following also occurs?
   a. Excessive formation of scar tissue
   b. Widening of the joint space and "filling in" with osteoclasts
   c. Nerve degeneration resulting in joint paresthesias
   d. Bone cyst formation and joint subluxation

7. Identify three types of factors that may contribute to development of osteoarthritis.

   a. _____

   b. _____

   c. _____

8. In what way does obesity influence the development of osteoarthritis?
   a. The obese person has a reduced inflammatory response with less joint swelling than a normal-weight person.
   b. The high body fat levels of the obese client lubricate joints and improve mobility in osteoarthritis.
   c. The extra weight of obesity increases the degeneration rate of hip and knee joints.
   d. Obesity has no positive or negative influence on development of osteoarthritis.

9. Osteoarthritis is a universal problem that
   a. Increases with age
   b. Has a very high incidence in women
   c. Has a very high incidence in men
   d. Is most common in thin people

10. How would a client describe crepitus?
    a. As spasms of surrounding muscles
    b. As pain with motion
    c. As a continuous grating sensation
    d. As protruding bony lumps

11. Which characteristic is associated with Heberden's nodes?
    a. Found at the distal interphalangeal joints
    b. Found at the proximal interphalangeal joints
    c. Usually appear unilaterally
    d. Found primarily in lower-extremity joints with osteoarthritis

12. The presence of fluid in the knees may be diagnosed as
    a. Subcutaneous swelling
    b. Joint nodules
    c. Joint effusions
    d. Joint deformities

13. Osteoarthritis affecting the spine may present as
    a. Localized pain at L3-4, bone spurs, stiffness, and muscle spasm
    b. Radiating pain at L3-4, C4-6, stiffness, muscle spasms, and bone spurs
    c. Localized pain at T6 to T12, stiffness, and muscle atrophy
    d. Radiating pain throughout the spine, stiffness, and muscle spasms

14. Which response from a client with advanced osteoarthritis alerts you to a problem coping with the image and role changes necessitated by disease progression?
    a. "I used to volunteer at my child's school as a playground assistant; now I work with children who need help with their reading skills."
    b. "I must be getting younger. I used to tie my shoes, and now I am using Velcro closures, just like my kids."
    c. "I find it easier to do my ironing sitting down rather than standing up."
    d. "I try to avoid public places so no one will see my ugly hands."

15. To determine an alteration in a client's body image and self-esteem, what should the nurse assess? *Check all that apply.*

    _____ a. Church affiliation

    _____ b. Personal care of self

    _____ c. Demeanor as happy or sad

    _____ d. Expression of feeling of reacting to change

    _____ e. Number of years the client has been married

16. Identify and prioritize at least five nursing diagnoses for the client with osteoarthritis.

    a. _____

    b. _____

    c. _____

    d. _____

    e. _____

17. For your client with osteoarthritis, identify types of analgesia medication and explain their actions.

18. Identify treatments other than medication that this client may receive for arthritis.

    a. _____

    b. _____

    c. _____

    d. _____

    e. _____

19. When educating a client regarding total joint replacement, what would the nurse do first?
    a. Ask the client whether he or she has insurance.
    b. Review instructions.
    c. Assess the client's knowledge and begin education if needed.
    d. Ask the client if the doctor has explained the procedure.

20. During the surgery for total joint replacement, the nurse will expect the client to receive which of the following? *Check all that apply.*

    _____ a. An intravenous antibiotic

    _____ b. Blood transfusion

    _____ c. An antibiotic in the cement

    _____ d. Local anesthetic

    _____ e. Immunosuppressant drug therapy

True or False? Write T for true or F for false in the blank provided.

_____ 21. Polymethyl methacrylate is a fixer that holds new prostheses in place but will most likely need replacement in several years.

_____ 22. After a total hip replacement, subluxation or total dislocation can occur if the legs are in the abducted position.

23. Which of the following are contraindications total joint arthroplasty? *Check all that apply.*

    _____ a. Infection

    _____ b. Severe pain

    _____ c. Advanced osteoporosis

    _____ d. Severe inflammation

24. After total hip replacement, what are the signs of dislocation?
    a. Hip pain, shortening of leg, and leg rotation
    b. Swelling in hip, hip pain, and leg rotation
    c. Swelling of leg, shortening of leg, and leg rotation
    d. Swelling of hip, shortening of leg, and leg rotation

25. What is the treatment for dislocation of a total hip replacement?
    a. Manipulation and bedrest
    b. Bedrest and pain medication
    c. Manipulation and immobilization
    d. Manipulation and continuation of previous care

26. Which of the following should be reported to the physician as a possible sign of infection following a total hip replacement?
    a. Confusion and excessive or foul drainage
    b. Swelling of the foot and bruising
    c. Diaphoresis and lowered blood pressure
    d. Pain in surgical area

True or False? Write T for true or F for false in the blanks provided.

_____ 27. The most potentially life-threatening complication following TJR is venous thromboembolism.

_____ 28. A TJR client's ESR is elevated, which may indicate infection at the site.

_____ 29. Initial drainage from the surgical site of the TJR is most likely to be about 250 mL.

30. After total joint replacement, how are the drains removed that were placed during surgery?
    a. By the surgeon
    b. By allowing them to fall out
    c. At the first dressing change
    d. By the physical therapist when weight-bearing has started

31. After total joint replacement, when is hemoglobin and hematocrit monitored?
    a. On the operative day only
    b. Only after a transfusion
    c. Only if there is drainage on the dressings
    d. 2 to 3 days postoperatively

32. Which of the following are used to reduce the chance of having a blood transfusion reaction? *Check all that apply.*

    _____ a. Autologous transfusions

    _____ b. NSAIDs

    _____ c. Epoetin alfa administration

    _____ d. Hypotensive neuroaxial anesthesia

    _____ e. Blood salvage

33. How does a "pain buster" device work?
    a. By continuously infusing intravenous opioids
    b. By continuously infusing a local anesthetic into the surgical site
    c. By continuously circulating cold liquids within a wrap around the incision site
    d. By continuously stimulating vibration-sensitive receptors in the incision area to "close the gate" on pain

34. What problems do older clients sometimes have who have undergone total joint replacement?
    a. Disorientation and delirium
    b. Inability to sleep
    c. Very high pain threshold
    d. Very low pain threshold

35. Postoperative total hip replacement clients can develop numerous complications. How can these be prevented?
    a. Bedrest with pillow between the legs
    b. Adequate diet and fluid intake
    c. Getting out of bed on the first postoperative day
    d. Sitting on the side of the bed

36. Which postoperative complication occurs more frequently among clients who have total hip replacements than among clients who have total knee replacements?
    a. Deep vein thrombosis
    b. Joint dislocation
    c. Acute pain
    d. Infection

37. For clients who have total joint replacements, the risk of deep vein thrombosis is high. Which of the following statements are true? *Check all that apply.*

    _____ a. Older adults are at high risk for DVT because of age and compromised circulation.

    _____ b. Thin clients are more at risk than obese clients.

    _____ c. Clients with a history of DVT are at high risk for recurrence.

    _____ d. Leg exercises are started in the immediate postoperative period.

38. Identify three measures used in the hospital to prevent a DVT.

    a. _____

    b. _____

    c. _____

39. To prevent a DVT, several types of anticoagulant medications can be ordered. Which is the most commonly used during hospitalization?
    a. Oral or parenteral aspirin
    b. Warfarin
    c. Intravenous tPA
    d. Subcutaneous low–molecular weight (LMW) heparin

40. It is important to monitor which laboratory test for clients on anticoagulant therapy with LMW heparin after total joint arthroplasty? *Check all that apply.*

    _____ a. Prothrombin time and international normalized ratio (INR)

    _____ b. Oxygen saturation

    _____ c. Complete blood count

    _____ d. Activated partial thromboplastin time

    _____ e. Platelet count

41. Develop a teaching plan for your client with a total hip replacement who is being discharged.

42. Postoperative care for total knee replacement may include which of the following? *Check all that apply.*

    _____ a. Hot compresses to the incisional area

    _____ b. Continuous passive motion (CPM) used immediately or several days postoperatively

    _____ c. Ice packs or cold packs to the incisional area

    _____ d. The use of a CPM machine in the daytime and an immobilizer at night

    _____ e. Maintaining abduction

43. What position or actions should the client with a total knee replacement avoid postoperatively?

    a. _____

    b. _____

44. What is the most common problem associated with a total shoulder replacement postoperatively?

45. Identify the major problem associated with total elbow replacement and why it occurs.

46. Postoperative care following finger and wrist replacements includes which of the following? *Check all that apply.*

    _____ a. Traction

    _____ b. Joint wrapped in a bulky dressing

    _____ c. Splint, brace, or cast

    _____ d. Abduction pillow

    _____ e. Elevation of the arm to prevent edema

    _____ f. CPM machine

47. Identify the nursing diagnosis and major interventions that would be used for joint replacements.

    Nursing Diagnosis:

    a. _____

    Interventions:

    b. _____

48. What is an important health teaching point in client education for a client with total joint replacement?
    a. "Do as much as you can."
    b. "Try to reach beyond what the physical therapist has asked."
    c. "Protect the joint."
    d. "No pain, no gain."

49. Because arthritis is not curable, many "cures" are marketed to clients with the disease. What should the nurse encourage the client to do?
    a. Take advantage of clinical trials or experimental therapy.
    b. Check with the Arthritis Foundation for appropriate modalities.
    c. Buy special liniments and creams.
    d. Take herbals and vitamins.

50. When evaluating client outcomes for arthritis and total joint replacement, the nurse should assess what three things?

    a. _____

    b. _____

    c. _____

51. Which of the following statements regarding rheumatoid arthritis (RA) are true? *Check all that apply.*

    _____ a. RA is a chronic, progressive, systemic inflammatory process.

    _____ b. RA primarily affects the synovial joints.

    _____ c. RA is known to have periods of remission.

    _____ d. RA occurs most often in older men and women.

52. Because of the inflammatory process in RA, a pannus forms in the joint. What is a pannus?
    a. Scar tissue
    b. Vascular granulation tissue
    c. Necrotic tissue
    d. Fluid

53. The articulator cartilage erodes and destroys the bone in clients with RA. Identify the resulting four bone changes:

    a. _____

    b. _____

    c. _____

    d. _____

54. The client with rheumatoid arthritis who has lost bone density has secondarily developed _____.

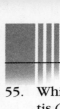

55. Which of the following is rheumatoid arthritis (RA) considered to be, even though the etiology of RA is unknown?
    a. An autoimmune disease
    b. Associated with aging
    c. More common in men then in women
    d. The result of joint misuse

56. For the following manifestations of rheumatoid arthritis, specify whether they are early (E) or late (L) manifestations.
    _____ a. Joint deformities
    _____ b. Joint inflammation
    _____ c. Osteoporosis
    _____ d. Vasculitis
    _____ e. Subcutaneous nodules
    _____ f. Paresthesias
    _____ g. Low-grade fever
    _____ h. Anemia

57. Your client comes to the office with the following complaints and you suspect rheumatoid arthritis. Which of these complaints would be typical?
    a. "My hands are stiff, swollen, and tender."
    b. "My right hand is weak."
    c. "My left hand is stiff and swollen."
    d. "My knees are swollen and stiff."

58. When a client has rheumatoid arthritis of the temporomandibular joint, what is the major complaint?
    a. Pain on chewing and opening the mouth
    b. Headache at the temple
    c. Toothache
    d. Earache

59. What is the most common area of involvement of rheumatoid arthritis in the spine?
    a. Lumbar spine
    b. Sacral spine
    c. Cervical spine
    d. Thoracic spine

60. Complications of spinal involvement in RA may be seen as which of the following? *Check all that apply.*
    _____ a. Compression of the phrenic nerve that controls the diaphragm
    _____ b. Resulting subluxation of the first and second vertebrae
    _____ c. Becoming quadriplegic or quadriparetic
    _____ d. Bilateral sciatic pain in the legs

61. In clients with rheumatoid arthritis, where might Baker's cysts be located?
    a. Ankle
    b. Wrists
    c. Popliteal bursae
    d. Achilles tendon

62. In late rheumatoid arthritis, the client may have systemic involvement called "flares." How are these described?
    a. Moderate-to-severe weight loss
    b. Fever and fatigue
    c. Muscle atrophy
    d. Joint contractures

63. Which of the following is not consistent with a client with rheumatoid arthritis?
    a. Ischemia
    b. Malfunctional joints
    c. Small brownish spots in the nail beds
    d. Subcutaneous nodules

64. What are the respiratory complications of advanced rheumatoid arthritis?

    a. _____

    b. _____

    c. _____

    d. _____

65. What are the two cardiac complications of advanced rheumatoid arthritis?

    a. _____

    b. _____

66. What are two ocular complications of advanced rheumatoid arthritis?

    a. _____

    b. _____

67. In clients with advanced rheumatoid arthritis, Sjögren's syndrome may develop. What are the manifestations?
    a. Dry eyes, dry mouth, and dry vagina
    b. Obstruction of secretory glands and ducts
    c. Nodules in the lungs
    d. Enlarged spleen and liver

68. What might a psychosocial examination of a client with advanced rheumatoid arthritis reveal? *Check all that apply.*

    _____ a. Role changes

    _____ b. Poor self-esteem and body image

    _____ c. Grieving and depression

    _____ d. Loss of control and independence

69. Which test is most specific for diagnosing rheumatoid arthritis?
    a. Latex agglutination
    b. Antinuclear antibodies
    c. Rheumatoid factor test
    d. Rose-Waaler test

70. Which of the following may be present for a client with an elevated "sed rate," or ESR? *Check all that apply.*

    _____ a. Inflammation or infection in the body

    _____ b. Pregnancy

    _____ c. Vasculitis and organ damage

    _____ d. Anemia

71. What CBC laboratory values would a nurse expect for a client with rheumatoid arthritis? *Circle high or low for each value.*
    a. Hemoglobin: High   Low
    b. Hematocrit: High   Low
    c. RBC: High   Low
    d. WBC: High   Low
    e. Platelets: High   Low

72. *True or False? If false, correct the statement to make it true.* The presence of only *one* hot, swollen, painful joint (out of proportion to the other joints) is a key diagnostic marker of rheumatoid arthritis.

73. Arthrocentesis being done on a client with rheumatoid arthritis may reveal which of the following in the synovial fluid of the joint?
    a. Glucose and glycogen
    b. Inflammatory cells and immune complexes
    c. Protein, such as albumin
    d. Platelet aggregation

74. The common side effect of chronic salicylate and NSAID therapy is _____
    _____.

75. Match each drug with the possible side effect for which the nurse should be aware in clients with RA. *Side effects may be used more than once.*

Drugs

1. Salicylates
2. NSAIDs
3. Steroids
4. Plaquenil (Antimalarial)
5. Methotrexate (Rheumatrex)
6. Minocycline
7. Analgesics
8. Etanercept (Enbrel)
9. Gold salts
10. Leufonamide (Arava)

Side Effects

_____ a. Headache, dizziness, drowsiness

_____ b. Diabetes, infection, hypertension

_____ c. Gastrointestinal problems

_____ d. Bone marrow suppression, mouth sores

_____ e. Rash, blood dyscrasias, renal involvement

_____ f. Red, itchy rash at injection site

_____ g. Retinal toxicity

_____ h. Low incidence of adverse effects and resistance

_____ i. Hair loss, diarrhea, decreased WBCs and platelets

76. Identify at least five complementary and alternative therapies that can be used to relieve pain in the client with rheumatoid arthritis.

   a. _____

   b. _____

   c. _____

   d. _____

   e. _____

77. Identify signs and symptoms the nurse would note in the client with rheumatoid arthritis and fatigue.

78. Identify the nurse's care plan for the client with rheumatoid arthritis and fatigue.

For questions 79 to 82, choose the answers from the following list of drugs:

a. NSAIDs
b. Aspirin
c. Methotrexate
d. Biologic response modifiers
e. Gold therapy

_____ 79. Which drug is the first choice for the treatment of mild rheumatoid arthritis?

_____ 80. Which drug is the first choice for the treatment of moderate to severe rheumatoid arthritis?

_____ 81. Which drug is used less commonly now and requires a test dose before the first injection?

_____ 82. Which drug requires that a purified protein derivative (PPD) test be performed to rule out the presence of tuberculosis?

83. Identify the two types of lupus and describe their differences.

   a. _____

   b. _____

84. What can be expected for a client with recently diagnosed systemic lupus erythematosus (SLE)?
    a. An acute inflammatory disorder
    b. Spontaneous remission and exacerbations
    c. Symptoms limited to arthritis
    d. Symptoms limited to skin lesions

85. What is the most common cause of death in clients with SLE?
    a. Cardiac failure
    b. Skin involvement
    c. Central nervous system involvement
    d. Renal failure

86. The clinical manifestations of SLE are many and varied. Describe the clinical manifestations of SLE.

87. Discoid lupus can be diagnosed only by doing a _____.

88. Rheumatoid arthritis and systemic lupus erythematosus (SLE) are treated with like medications and client teaching. Identify two important differences that a client with SLE should know and practice.

    a. _____

    b. _____

89. Review Chart 24-11 to compare symptoms of systemic lupus erythematosus (SLE) and progressive systemic sclerosis (PSS).

90. PSS, or "scleroderma," affects the _____ system the most, but death from PSS is usually caused by _____ involvement.

91. Identify the CREST syndrome that is seen in progressive systemic sclerosis clients with the worst prognosis.

    a. _____

    b. _____

    c. _____

    d. _____

    e. _____

92. A client with scleroderma may have which of the following problems? *Check all that apply.*
    _____ a. Dysphagia, esophageal reflux
    _____ b. Smooth tongue
    _____ c. Malabsorption problems causing malodorous diarrhea stools
    _____ d. Butterfly lesions on the face and nose

93. Raynaud's phenomenon in the client with scleroderma may present as which of the following? *Check all that apply.*
    _____ a. Digit necrosis
    _____ b. Excruciating pain
    _____ c. Autoamputations of digits
    _____ d. Periungual lesions

94. What are characteristics of primary gout? *Check all that apply.*
    _____ a. Results from medications such as diuretics
    _____ b. Is sodium urate deposited in the synovium
    _____ c. Affects large joints most commonly
    _____ d. Affects middle-aged and older men
    _____ e. Peak time of onset after age 50

True or False? Write T for true or F for false in the blank provided.

_____ 95. For clients with secondary gout, it is important to treat the underlying disorder.

96. Identify the four stages of primary gout.

a. _____

b. _____

c. _____

d. _____

97. What part of the body is first affected by gout?
   a. Fingers
   b. Knees
   c. Great toe
   d. Shoulder

True or False? Write T for true or F for false in the blanks provided.

_____ 98. A client with acute gout cannot tolerate having the joint touched or moved.

_____ 99. The client with chronic gout may have tophi on the outer ear.

100. Identify the two medications most commonly ordered for acute gout.

a. _____

b. _____

101. A client with polymyositis that has a heliotrope rash with periorbital edema is diagnosed with _____.

102. Clients with dermatomyositis have weakness and muscle atrophy demonstrated as difficulty swallowing and talking, but they also have high incidences of _____ _____.

103. Polymyalgia rheumatica and temporal arteritis present with which of the following? *Check all that apply.*

_____ a. Stiffness, weakness, and arthralgias

_____ b. Low-grade fever

_____ c. Decreased ESR

_____ d. Polycythemia

104. Clients with ankylosing spondylitis have the threat of which of the following?
   a. Compromised respiratory function
   b. Cardiac involvement
   c. Hip pain
   d. Dysphagia

105. Identify the three common findings associated with Reiter's syndrome.

a. _____

b. _____

c. _____

106. Which manifestation is expected in a client with Marfan's syndrome?
   a. Obesity
   b. Shortened hands and feet
   c. Short swollen fingers
   d. Excessive height

107. Lyme disease is identified early by which of the following? *Check all that apply.*

_____ a. Known bite from deer tick

_____ b. Bull's-eye rash at onset

_____ c. Facial paralysis

_____ d. Dysphagia

True or False? Write T for true or F for false in the blanks provided.

_____ 108. Lyme disease is treated with antibiotics over an extended period of time (10 to 21 days).

_____ 109. Pseudo gout is a mimic of gout depositing uric crystals in the joints.

110. Identify the five primary manifestations of fibromyalgia.

   a. _____

   b. _____

   c. _____

   d. _____

   e. _____

111. Clients with fibromyalgia may need which category of drugs to get adequate rest?

112. Match the disease or condition with its definition.

Disease/Condition
1. Polyarthralgia
2. Polymyositis
3. Polymyalgia rheumatica
4. Giant cell arteritis
5. Ankylosing spondylitis
6. Sjögren's syndrome
7. Lyme disease

Definition

_____ a. Systemic infectious disease that is caused by the spirochete *Borrelia burgdorferi*

_____ b. Affects the vertebral column and causes spinal deformities

_____ c. A diffuse, inflammatory disease of skeletal (striated) muscle

_____ d. A systemic vasculitis that affects large and midsized arteries

_____ e. Aching around multiple joints

_____ f. A clinical syndrome characterized by stiffness, weakness, and aching of the proximal musculature

_____ g. Inflammatory condition in which secretory ducts and glands are obstructed

Interventions for Clients with HIV/AIDS and Other Immunodeficiencies

LEARNING OUTCOMES

1. Compare primary and secondary immunodeficiencies for cause and onset of problems.
2. Explain the differences in nursing care required for a client with a pathogenic infection versus a client with an opportunistic infection.
3. Distinguish between the conditions of human immunodeficiency virus (HIV) infection and acquired immunodeficiency syndrome (AIDS) for clinical manifestations and risks for complications.
4. Describe the ways in which HIV is transmitted.
5. Identify techniques to reduce the risk for infection in an immunocompromised client.
6. Develop a teaching plan for condom use among sexually active, non–English-speaking adults.
7. Prioritize nursing care for the client with AIDS who has impaired gas exchange.
8. Identify teaching priorities for the HIV-positive client receiving highly active antiretroviral therapy.
9. Develop a community-based teaching plan for the client with immunodeficiency living at home.
10. Plan a week of meals for the client who has protein-calorie malnutrition.
11. Identify drug therapy categories that have the potential to reduce immune function.
12. Describe the infections that adult clients with congenital immunodeficiencies are at greatest risk for developing.
13. Describe the nursing actions and responsibilities for administration of IV immunoglobulin.

LEARNING ACTIVITIES

1. Before completing the study guide exercises in this chapter, it is recommended that you review the following:
    - Anatomy and physiology of the immune system
    - Infection
    - Complete physical assessment
    - Grief and loss
    - Death and dying
    - Self-concept
    - Therapeutic communication
    - Nutrition

2. Review the boldfaced terms and their definitions in Chapter 25 to enhance your understanding of the content.

STUDY/REVIEW QUESTIONS

Answers to the Study/Review Questions are provided on the companion Evolve Learning Resources Web site at http://evolve.elsevier.com/Iggy/.

1. Which of the following statements about immunodeficiency is *true*?
    a. Immunodeficiency causes a decrease in the client's risk for infection.
    b. Immunodeficiency is always acquired.
    c. Immunodeficiency occurs when a person's body cannot recognize antigens.
    d. Immunodeficiency is the same as autoimmunity.

2. Match the descriptions with the types of immunodeficiencies.

Types of Immunodeficiencies
1. Primary
2. Secondary
3. HIV
4. AIDS
5. Immunodeficiency

Descriptions

_____ a. Last and most serious stage of HIV infection

_____ b. Disease/deficiency present since birth

_____ c. Chronic infection with immunodeficiency virus

_____ d. Disease/deficiency acquired as a result of viral infection, contact with a toxin, or medical therapy.

_____ e. Deficient immune response as a result of impaired or missing immune components

True or False? Write T for true or F for false in the blank provided.

_____ 3. Everyone who has AIDS has HIV infection, and everyone who has HIV infection has AIDS.

4. Using Table 25-1 in the textbook, identify the HIV/AIDS clinical classification (a, b, or c) for the following symptoms and diagnoses:

    _____ Bacterial endocarditis

    _____ Toxoplasmosis

    _____ Kaposi's sarcoma

    _____ Persistent generalized lymphadenopathy

    _____ Herpes zoster

    _____ Idiopathic thrombocytopenic purpura

    _____ Fever and diarrhea lasting over a month

    _____ Cytomegalovirus retinitis

    _____ Severe cervical dysplasia

5. Define *retrovirus* and describe its actions.

6. Which immune function abnormality is a result of HIV infection?
    a. Lymphocytosis
    b. CD4+ cell depletion
    c. Increased CD8+ cell activity
    d. Long macrophage life span

7. Which of the following groups is experiencing the highest increase in the number of HIV infections?
    a. Men having sex with other men
    b. IV drug users
    c. Women
    d. Asians

8. Which of the following are characteristics of a nonprogressor? *Check all that apply.*

    _____ a. Has been infected for 10 years

    _____ b. Is asymptomatic

    _____ c. Has no CD4 or T-lymphocytes

    _____ d. Is immunocompetent

9. Which of the following conditions may occur in women with HIV? *Check all that apply.*

    _____ a. Vaginal candidiasis

    _____ b. Bladder infections

    _____ c. Cervical neoplasia

    _____ d. Pelvic inflammatory disease (PID)

10. Which statement regarding HIV/AIDS among older adults is true?
    a. The risk for HIV infection after exposure is minimal for older adults.
    b. Older men are more susceptible to HIV infection than are older women.
    c. It is not necessary to assess an older adult for a history of drug abuse.
    d. Older adults who participate in high-risk behaviors are susceptible to HIV infection.

11. What is the most important means of preventing HIV spread or transmission?
    a. Engineering
    b. Education
    c. Isolation
    d. Counseling

12. HIV can be transmitted by what routes?
    a. Viral contact, sexual contact, and parenteral contact
    b. Parenteral contact, airborne contact, and perinatal contact
    c. Sexual contact, parenteral contact, and perinatal contact
    d. Perinatal contact, sexual contact, and viral contact

13. HAART (highly activated antiretroviral therapy) causes which of the following?
    a. Reversal of a client's antibody status
    b. Decrease of the viral load
    c. Increase of the viral load
    d. More detectable HIV

14. Describe the procedure for teaching IV drug users to care for equipment.

    a. _____

    b. _____

    c. _____

15. Which practice is recommended by the CDC to prevent sexual transmission of HIV?
    a. Use of latex condoms
    b. Use of natural membrane condoms
    c. Use of oral contraceptives
    d. Use of an intrauterine device

16. Identify seven of the most common symptoms of HIV.

    a. _____

    b. _____

    c. _____

    d. _____

    e. _____

    f. _____

    g. _____

17. Which of the following opportunistic infections can be observed in AIDS? *Check all that apply.*

    _____ a. Protozoan

    _____ b. Viral

    _____ c. Bacterial

    _____ d. Fungal

18. A client with *Pneumocystis carinii* pneumonia usually presents with which of the following symptoms?
    a. Dyspnea, tachypnea, persistent dry cough, and fever
    b. Cough with copious thick sputum, fever, and dyspnea
    c. Low-grade fever, cough, and shortness of breath
    d. Fever, cough, and vomiting

19. A client presenting with toxoplasmosis may have which of the following signs and symptoms? *Check all that apply.*

    _____ a. Difficulty with speech and headaches

    _____ b. Headaches, confusion, and lethargy

    _____ c. Cyanosis, cough, and bruising

    _____ d. Visual changes and difficulties with gait

20. Cryptosporidiosis is a form of gastroenteritis in which diarrhea that can amount to a loss of how many liters per day?
    a. 1 to 2
    b. 3 to 5
    c. 5 to 8
    d. 15 to 20

21. Where can candidiasis be found in the body? *Check all that apply.*

    _____ a. Mouth

    _____ b. Esophagus

    _____ c. Vagina

    _____ d. Nose

    _____ e. Ears

True or False? Write T for true or F for false in the blanks provided.

_____ 22. Cryptococcosis is a type of meningitis.

_____ 23. Histoplasmosis is a localized respiratory infection.

_____ 24. *Mycobacterium avium-intracellulare* complex (MAC) is the most common bacterial infection among people with HIV/AIDS.

25. Define *anergy* and the situation in which it is clinically significant.

26. Where in the body can cytomegalovirus (CMV) present with symptoms? *Check all that apply.*

    _____ a. Eyes, causing visual impairment

    _____ b. The kidneys as glomerulonephritis

    _____ c. Respiratory tract, causing pneumonitis

    _____ d. Gastrointestinal tract, causing colitis

27. How does the herpes simplex virus (HSV) manifest itself in clients with HIV and AIDS? *Check all that apply.*

    _____ a. As malignant vesicles that can metastasize

    _____ b. As a chronic ulceration when vesicles rupture

    _____ c. As vesicles located in the perirectal, oral, and genital areas

    _____ d. As numbness and tingling occurring before the vesicle forms

28. Varicella-zoster virus (VZV) leaves the nerve endings and appears as _____, which is very painful.

29. Lymphomas associated with AIDS include which of the following? *Check all that apply.*

    _____ a. Non-Hodgkin's B-cell lymphomas

    _____ b. Immunoblastic lymphoma

    _____ c. Hodgkin's lymphoma

    _____ d. Burkitt's lymphoma

30. Identify the nine most common nursing diagnoses and collaborative problems associated with AIDS.

    a. _____

    b. _____

    c. _____

    d. _____

    e. _____

    f. _____

    g. _____

    h. _____

    i. _____

31. Which of the following are ways to boost the immune system? *Check all that apply.*

    _____ a. Radiation therapy

    _____ b. Bone marrow transplantation

    _____ c. Lymphocyte transfusion

    _____ d. Administration of interleukin-2

32. Pentamidine isethionate can be administered to a client with *Pneumocystis carinii* pneumonia (PCP) by which of the following routes? *Check all that apply.*

    _____ a. Orally

    _____ b. Intravenously

    _____ c. Intramuscularly

    _____ d. Inhalation (by aerosol)

33. Which of the following cause severe pain in HIV disease and AIDS? *Check all that apply.*

    _____ a. Enlarged organs

    _____ b. Peripheral neuropathy

    _____ c. Tumors

    _____ d. High fevers

34. What methods or agents are used to treat Kaposi's sarcoma? *Check all that apply.*

    _____ a. Radiotherapy

    _____ b. Chemotherapy

    _____ c. Antibiotics

    _____ d. Cryotherapy

    _____ e. Surgery

35. Describe the care required for HSV abscesses.

36. Keeping a client oriented can be done by which of the following actions? *Check all that apply.*

    _____ a. Repeating person, place, and time

    _____ b. Using clocks and calendars

    _____ c. Giving the MMSE screening test

    _____ d. Having familiar items present

37. List at least five factors that contribute to malnutrition in the client with advanced AIDS.

    a. _____

    b. _____

    c. _____

    d. _____

    e. _____

38. Corticosteroids perform which of the following actions? *Check all that apply.*

    _____ a. Block the movement of neutrophils and monocytes through cell membranes.

    _____ b. Increase cell production in the bone marrow.

    _____ c. Reduce the number of circulating T-cells, resulting in suppressed cell-mediated immunity.

    _____ d. Decrease intracranial pressure.

    _____ e. Constrict blood vessels.

True or False? For questions 39 to 48, write T for true or F for false in the blanks provided. For those that are false, correct the statements to make them true.

_____ 39. The higher the degree of blood concentration of HIV, the greater the risk of sexual transmission.

_____ 40. The person with HIV infection can transmit the virus to others at all stages of disease.

_____ 41. Lesions resulting from Kaposi's sarcoma are painful and have purulent drainage.

_____ 42. Opportunistic infections are usually prevented by a properly functioning immune system of the HIV client.

_____ 43. AIDS dementia complex (ADC) is caused by infection of the cells in the central nervous system by HIV.

_____ 44. Clients with HIV should know that as CD4+ counts lower, clinical manifestations decrease.

_____ 45. A client is leukopenic if the WBC is less than 3500 cell/mm^3 and lymphopenic if lymphocytes are less than 1500 cell/mm^3.

_____ 46. The viral load test measures the presence of HIV genetic material in the client's blood and helps with monitoring the disease progression.

_____ 47. Antiretroviral drug therapy kills the virus before it is able to replicate.

_____ 48. HIV is more easily transmitted from infected female to uninfected male than vice versa.

49. Which of the following are means of transmitting HIV? *Check all that apply.*

    _____ a. Sexual intercourse

    _____ b. Household utensils

    _____ c. Breast milk

    _____ d. Toilet facilities

    _____ e. Mosquitoes

50. Which two methods are the only absolutely safe methods of preventing HIV infection through sexual contact?

    a. _____

    b. _____

51. Rank the following in order of risk for transmission of HIV from highest to lowest risk (with 1 being highest risk and 4 being lowest risk).

    _____ a. Intravenous drug use

    _____ b. Blood and blood product transfusions

    _____ c. Sexual exposure

    _____ d. Perinatal transmission from mothers with AIDS

52. For each of the following laboratory tests, indicate whether the presence of HIV will increase, decrease, or cause no change in the levels.

    a. CD4+

    b. CD8+

    c. WBC

    d. Lymphocytes

53. Complete the following chart regarding drug therapy for HIV.

Drug	Classification	Therapeutic Use	Nursing Intervention
Pentamidine isethionate			
Metronidazole (Flagyl)			
Zidovudine (Retrovir)			
Ritonavir (Norvir)			
Enfuvirtide (Fuzeon)			
Nevirapine (Viramune)			
Fluconazole (Diflucan)			

54. Name the two goals of HAART therapy:

    a. _____

    b. _____

55. What is the purpose of counseling when testing for HIV?

Interventions for Clients with Immune Function Excess: Hypersensitivity (Allergy) and Autoimmunity

LEARNING OUTCOMES

1. Compare the bases and manifestations of allergy and autoimmunity.
2. Discuss anaphylaxis prevention measures.
3. Discuss the nursing responsibility for a client with anaphylaxis.
4. Identify the common drugs, dosages, and side effects used as therapy for anaphylaxis.
5. Describe allergy testing techniques.
6. List the defining characteristics of type I, type II, type III, type IV, and type V hypersensitivity reactions.
7. Explain the differences in mechanisms of action between antihistamines and mast cell stabilizers.
8. Develop a community-based teaching plan for the client who has severe allergic reactions.

LEARNING ACTIVITIES

1. Before completing the study guide exercises in this chapter, it is recommended that you review the following:
   - Anatomy and physiology of the immune system
   - Process of allergens
   - Anaphylactic shock
   - Assessment of inflammation and infection
   - Drug therapy for anaphylaxis

2. Review the boldfaced terms and their definitions in Chapter 26 to enhance your understanding of the content.

STUDY/REVIEW QUESTIONS

Answers to the Study/Review Questions are provided on the companion Evolve Learning Resources Web site at http://evolve.elsevier.com/Iggy/.

1. The most dramatic and life-threatening example of a type I hypersensitivity reaction is known as _____.

2. "Overreactions" to invaders or foreign antigens can be the result of which of the following? *Check all that apply.*
   _____ a. Hypersensitivity
   _____ b. Allergic response
   _____ c. An autoimmune response
   _____ d. Phagocytosis

3. Which of the following best describes allergy or hypersensitivity?
   a. Excessive response to the presence of an antigen
   b. Excessive response against self cells and cell products
   c. Failure of the immune system to recognize self cells as normal
   d. Failure of the immune system to recognize foreign cells and microbial invaders

4. Match the type of hypersensitivity to a clinical example. *Types may be used more than once.*

Type of Hypersensitivity
1. Type I: Immediate
2. Type II: Cytotoxic
3. Type III: Immune Complex-Mediated
4. Type IV: Delayed
5. Type V: Stimulated

Clinical Example
_____ a. Autoimmune hemolytic anemia
_____ b. Poison ivy
_____ c. Hay fever
_____ d. Graves' disease
_____ e. Serum sickness
_____ f. Anaphylaxis
_____ g. Myasthenia gravis
_____ h. Graft rejection
_____ i. Allergic asthma
_____ j. Vasculitis

5. Identify four ways allergens can be encountered. Provide at least one example of each.

   a. _____

   _____

   b. _____

   _____

   c. _____

   _____

   d. _____

   _____

6. Describe allergy desensitization.

7. Match the body's reactions with their corresponding cause.

Causes
1. Allergen
2. Leukotriene
3. Histamine
4. Rhinorrhea

Reactions

_____ a. Increases capillary permeability, nasal and conjunctival mucous secretions, and itching

_____ b. Promotes allergic responses mediated by IgE

_____ c. Runny nose, clear drainage, and pink mucosa

_____ d. Responsible for secondary phase of type I hypersensitivity reactions

8. Which of the following are used for allergy management? *Check all that apply.*

   _____ a. Avoidance

   _____ b. Desensitization

   _____ c. Conization

   _____ d. Antibiotics

9. Identify which of the following methods are used for testing for allergies. *Check all that apply.*

   _____ a. Topical serums

   _____ b. Scratch

   _____ c. Intravenous

   _____ d. Intradermal

10. Match the following drug types with their corresponding actions:

Drug Types
1. Decongestant
2. Antihistamine
3. Corticosteroids
4. Mast cell stabilizers
5. Leukotriene antagonist

Actions

   _____ a. Competes for histamine at histamine receptor sites

   _____ b. Causes vasoconstriction, reducing edema; may be combined with anticholinergics

   _____ c. Decreases inflammation and immune response in a short time

   _____ d. Prevents mast cells from opening when allergen binds with IgE

   _____ e. Prevents leukotriene synthesis and blocks leukotriene receptors

11. Identify the most common complaints of a client experiencing anaphylaxis.

   a. _____

   b. _____

   c. _____

   d. _____

   e. _____

   f. _____

12. A client in anaphylaxis who is going into respiratory failure will demonstrate which of the following symptoms? *Check all that apply.*

   _____ a. Laryngeal edema

   _____ b. Hypoxemia

   _____ c. Hypocapnia

   _____ d. Dehydration

   _____ e. Crackles

   _____ f. Wheezing

   _____ g. Dry mouth

13. As nurse for the client with anaphylaxis described above, you would expect to find which of the following?
   a. Hypertension and rapid, weak pulse
   b. Hypotension and rapid, weak pulse
   c. Hypertension and rapid, bounding pulse
   d. Hypotension and rapid, bounding pulse

True or False? For questions 14 to 23, write T for true or F for false in the blanks provided. If the question is false, rewrite it to make it true.

   _____ 14. Rhinitis may or may not be an allergic response.

_____ 15. Desensitization therapy can last 5 years.

_____ 16. After the proper dose of epinephrine is administered to a client having an anaphylactic reaction, the nurse must wait 60 minutes before repeating the dose.

_____ 17. The body's response to epinephrine is constriction of the blood vessels, increased myocardial contractions, and dilation of bronchioles.

_____ 18. The anaphylactic client should be observed for fluid overload.

_____ 19. Latex allergies are confined to the skin, so latex-free gloves are the only necessary precaution for those with a latex allergy

_____ 20. A person who is allergic to bananas must be aware of the possibility that he or she could develop a latex allergy.

_____ 21. In a type III immune complex reaction, the deposited immune complex activates complement, and tissue and vessel damage results.

_____ 22. Benadryl is the oral drug of choice for type IV delayed hypersensitivity reactions.

_____ 23. Clients with a history of allergy to bee-stings should carry a prescription for injectable epinephrine at all times. Clients with bee sting allergies should carry the actual kit that contains injectable epinephrine for immediate treatment as needed.

24. What is the cause of a hemolytic transfusion reaction?

25. Your client is experiencing a cytotoxic reaction to an intravenous drug. As the nurse, what is your _first_ intervention?

26. Identify clinical manifestations of systemic lupus erythematosus that are caused by immune complex reaction.
    a. Vasculitis, nephritis, arthritis
    b. Hypertension, anemia
    c. Destruction of mucus-producing glands, such as lacrimal and salivary
    d. Increased urinary output, cystitis

27. Serum sickness occurs less frequently than in the past for what reason?
    a. Vaccines are no longer made from horse and rabbit serum.
    b. Clients have become less allergic.
    c. Penicillin and related drugs and some animal serums are antitoxins.
    d. Manufacturing techniques produce vaccines that contain fewer impurities.

28. Identify the type IV delayed hypersensitivity reactions. _Check all that apply._

    _____ a. Positive PPD test for tuberculosis

    _____ b. Anaphylaxis after insect sting

    _____ c. Thrombocytopenic purpura

    _____ d. Contact dermatitis

29. Define *type V stimulating response* and identify the common form of hyperthyroidism.

30. What is the most important aspect of treating type V stimulating reactions?
    a. Medication management and observation for adverse effects
    b. Removing stimulated tissue to return the organ to normal functioning
    c. Monitoring for other organ involvement
    d. Surgical removal of secondary immune tissue

31. Define *autoimmunity*.

32. Identify which of the following are types of autoimmune diseases. *Check all that apply.*
    _____ a. Polyarteritis nodosa
    _____ b. Systemic lupus erythematosus
    _____ c. Hypothyroidism
    _____ d. Rheumatic fever
    _____ e. Hashimoto's thyroiditis

33. Autoimmune diseases occur mostly in which group of women?
    a. African-American
    b. Asian-American
    c. White
    d. Hispanic

34. In whom does Sjögren's syndrome mostly appear?
    a. Men 35 to 40 years of age
    b. Women younger than 25 years of age
    c. Women 35 to 40 years of age
    d. Men and women 35 to 40 years of age

35. What is the most common cause of Sjögren's syndrome thought to be?
    a. A bacterial infection
    b. A viral infection
    c. Inflammation
    d. An allergic reaction

36. As the nurse, you suspect Sjögren's syndrome because the client has which of the following complaints? *Check all that apply.*
    _____ a. Increased tooth decay
    _____ b. Burning and itching of the eyes
    _____ c. Painful intercourse
    _____ d. Nosebleeds

37. As the nurse, you would expect the lab results on a client with Sjögren's syndrome to include which of the following? *Check all that apply.*
    _____ a. Increased presence of general antinuclear antibodies.
    _____ b. Elevated levels of IgM rheumatoid factor.
    _____ c. Decreased presence of anti-SS-A or anti-SS-B antibodies.
    _____ d. Decreased erythrocyte sedimentation rate.

38. Match each symptom with the appropriate intervention/treatment. *Some treatments are used for more than one symptom.*

Treatments

_____ a. Water-soluble lubricants

_____ b. Artificial tears

_____ c. Systemic pilocarpine

_____ d. Room humidifiers

_____ e. Artificial saliva

_____ f. Blocking tear outflow duct

_____ g. NSAIDs

Symptoms

1. Dry eyes
2. Dry mouth
3. Vaginal dryness
4. Pain control

39. The autoimmune disorder Goodpasture's syndrome is a disorder of autoantibodies against which of the following?
    a. Skin cells and vascular tissue
    b. Hepatic support cells and RBCs
    c. Glomerular basement membrane and neutrophils
    d. Capillary walls

40. The symptoms of Goodpasture's syndrome include which of the following? *Check all that apply.*

    _____ a. Hemoptysis

    _____ b. Increased urine output

    _____ c. Bradycardia

    _____ d. Shortness of breath

    _____ e. Weight loss

    _____ f. Generalized edema

41. The cause of death in Goodpasture's syndrome is usually _____ _____.

42. The main form of drug therapy for Goodpasture's syndrome is usually what?

43. Explain how plasmapheresis may be useful in the treatment of immune disorders.

44. What is an important intervention that should be done before giving any drug or therapeutic agent?

For questions 45 to 50, name the specific condition and its classification described by the mini-cases.

45. During an annual physical examination, a 45-year-old woman reports dry eyes, painful joints, and states that for the last two months, she has had painful intercourse due to vaginal dryness.

46. After injection with dye for an intravenous pyelogram, the client complains of feeling anxious, itchy all over, and having difficulty breathing.

47. In a screening clinic, a nurse notes induration and redness at a the injection site of a purified protein derivative (PPD) test.

48. After a slumber party at a friend's house, a teenage girl comes home with a runny nose with clear drainage, watery eyes, and a scratchy throat. The teenager tells her mother that her friend owns three long-haired cats.

49. A teenage boy is taken to the emergency department with shortness of breath, hemoptysis, a rapid heart rate, and generalized edema. His mother tells you that he has not urinated since early that morning.

50. After a lengthy surgery, a client has a transfusion reaction after receiving two units of packed red blood cells.

CASE STUDY: THE CLIENT WITH HYPERSENSITIVITY

Answer Guidelines for the Case Study questions are provided on the companion Evolve Learning Resources Web site at http://evolve.elsevier.com/Iggy/.

A 62-year-old woman is admitted for total knee replacement surgery. Following surgery, cefazolin sodium (Ancef), 2 g, was ordered to be given IVPB every 8 hours for 24 hours. She received her first dose when she arrived at the orthopedic unit after surgery. Vital signs upon arrival: BP 136/84, P 88, R 12, T 98.8° F.

1. This client has a history of allergy to penicillins. With this history, what type of hypersensitivity reaction is this client most likely to experience?

Thirty minutes after the medication was started, the client calls the nurse and reports "itching all over" and difficulty breathing. The nurse notes facial edema and audible wheezing. The client's skin is red with large, swollen blotches over her arms, trunk and back. Her systolic blood pressure is 118/78, pulse 108, and respirations 24. The IVPB antibiotic bag has infused about three fourths of the dose.

2. What should the nurse's *first* action be?

3. The nurse stays with the client to monitor her condition. What must the nurse observe for during this time?

4. What medications and by what route should the nurse expect the physician to prescribe? Explain the rationale for the medications used in this situation. What other interventions should follow?

5. What precautions should have been taken by health care providers to prevent this problem?

Altered Cell Growth and Cancer Development

LEARNING OUTCOMES

1. Explain why causes of cancer can be hard to establish.
2. Compare the features of benign and malignant tumors.
3. List three cancer types associated with tobacco use.
4. Identify cancer types for which primary prevention is possible.
5. Compare the cancer development processes of initiation and promotion.
6. Describe the TNM system for cancer staging.
7. Explain the differences between a "low-grade" cancer and a "high-grade" cancer.
8. Discuss the roles of oncogenes and suppressor genes in cancer development.
9. Identify four common sites of distant metastasis for cancer.
10. Discuss the role of immunity in protection against cancer.
11. Identify which cancer types arise from connective tissues and which types arise from glandular tissues.
12. Describe how genetic predisposition can increase a person's risk for cancer development.
13. Identify behaviors that reduce the risk for cancer development and cancer death.
14. Identify specific issues about genetic testing for cancer predisposition.

LEARNING ACTIVITIES

1. Before completing the study guide exercises in this chapter, it is recommended that you review the following:
   • Anatomy and physiology of the immune system
   • Types of prevention
   • Normal cell growth and development

2. Consult your area's local chapter of the American Cancer Society to obtain demographic information about the types and incidences of cancers in your area.

3. Review the boldfaced terms and their definitions in Chapter 27 to enhance your understanding of the content.

STUDY/REVIEW QUESTIONS

Answers to the Study/Review Questions are provided on the companion Evolve Learning Resources Web site at http://evolve.elsevier.com/Iggy/.

1. Identify the cancers being targeted in Healthy People 2010:
   a. Testicular, colorectal, cervical, throat, skin, and alcohol- and tobacco-related
   b. Alcohol- and tobacco-related, cervical, breast, skin, colorectal, and testicular
   c. Colorectal, cervical, skin, throat, breast, and alcohol- and tobacco-related
   d. Lung, liver, throat, breast, colorectal, testicular, skin, and cervical

2. Which of the following statements is true regarding hypertrophy and hyperplasia?
   a. They are the same, except that one is in an organ and the other is in tissue.
   b. Hypertrophy is the expansion of cells; hyperplasia is an increased number of cells.
   c. Hypertrophy is an increase in the number of cells; hyperplasia is the expansion of cells.
   d. Hypertrophy is a decrease in the number of cells; hyperplasia is the shrinkage of cells.

3. Which of the following are characteristics of neoplasia? *Check all that apply.*

   _____ a. Is new or continued cell growth that is not needed for tissue replacement

   _____ b. Is always malignant

   _____ c. Has a parent cell that was normal

   _____ d. Typically leads to death

   _____ e. Is always abnormal

   _____ f. Some cause no harm

4. State the two purposes of cell mitosis.

   a. _____

   b. _____

True or False? For questions 5 to 11, write T for true or F for false in the blanks provided. For the false answers, rewrite to make the statements true.

_____ 5. Normal body cells are recognized by their appearance, size, and shape.

_____ 6. Each cell in the body performs one special function that contributes to homeostasis.

_____ 7. All cells produce fibronectin, which binds them closely together so they do not migrate.

_____ 8. All cells capable of mitosis have a specific pattern or cycle they follow.

_____ 9. Most cells in the body spend their existence in a reproductive resting state or M phase of the cell cycle.

_____ 10. Embryonic cells are aneuploid.

_____ 11. Cell division (mitosis) happens throughout our lives at a well-controlled rate to maintain the tissues and organs.

12. Explain what is meant by the terms *pluripotency, multipotency,* or *totipotency* regarding embryonic cell.

13. When a gene is "turned on," it is which of the following?
    a. Repressed
    b. Suppressed
    c. Expressed
    d. Depressed

14. Characteristics of benign cells include which of the following? *Check all that apply.*

    _____ a. Being tissue unnecessary for normal function

    _____ b. Resembling the parent tissue

    _____ c. Having a small nucleus

    _____ d. Performing their differentiated function

    _____ e. Invading other tissues

    _____ f. Being nonmigratory

    _____ g. Being aneuploid

15. Which of the following statements is true of cancer cells? *Check all that apply.*

    _____ a. They are slow-growing.

    _____ b. Cancer cells divide nearly continuously.

    _____ c. They are harmful to the body.

    _____ d. They are abnormal.

    _____ e. Cancer cells contain a small nucleus.

    _____ f. They have an unlimited life span.

16. Why do cancer cells spread throughout the body? *Check all that apply.*

    _____ a. They make little fibronectin.

    _____ b. They are able to metastasize.

    _____ c. They are persistent in their growth.

    _____ d. Cell division occurs under adverse conditions.

17. The actions of carcinogens include which of the following? *Check all that apply.*

    _____ a. Damaging the DNA.

    _____ b. Changing the activity of a cell.

    _____ c. Turning on proto-oncogenes.

    _____ d. Creating allergic reactions.

True or False. For questions 18 to 22, write T for true or F for false in the blanks provided. For the false answers, rewrite to make the statements true.

_____ 18. If growth conditions are right, widespread metastatic disease can develop from just one cancer cell.

_____ 19. In carcinogenesis and oncogenesis, a normal cell undergoes malignant transformation.

_____ 20. Initiators start nonreversible mutations in a normal cell.

_____ 21. Once a cell has been initiated, it is a recognizable tumor.

_____ 22. As the tumor cells grow, there are changes within the tumor cells themselves allowing for "selection advantages."

23. Which of the following is the initiated cell's response to the promoter? *Check all that apply.*

    _____ a. Promoted or enhanced cell growth

    _____ b. Shortened latency period

    _____ c. Lengthened latency period

    _____ d. Metastasis

24. Promoters may include which of the following? *Check all that apply.*

    _____ a. Chemicals

    _____ b. Hormones

    _____ c. Drugs

    _____ d. Antibodies

25. Primary tumors located in vital organs can do which of the following?
    a. Increase the organ's rate of cell division
    b. Decrease the organ's response to injury
    c. Interfere with the organ's functioning
    d. Increase function of the organ initially

26. Which of the following statements correctly describes metastatic tumors?
    a. They are caused by cells breaking off the primary tumor.
    b. They become less malignant over time.
    c. They are usually less harmful than a primary tumor.
    d. They become the tissue of the organ where they spread.

27. During metastasis, which of the following actions take place? *Check all that apply.*

    _____ a. Tumor vascularization results in blood supply to the tumor.

    _____ b. Enzymes open up pores in client's blood vessels.

    _____ c. Clumps of the cells break off for transport.

    _____ d. Cells stop circulating and then invade.

True or False? Write T for true or F for false in the blank provided.

_____ 28. Brain tumors usually metastasize only within the central nervous system.

_____ 29. During metastasis, local seeding takes place near the primary site.

_____ 30. Lymphatic spread is usually to primary sites with few lymph nodes.

31. Which of the following describes a "high-grade" tumor? *Check all that apply.*

    _____ a. It barely resembles the parent cell.

    _____ b. It is slow-growing.

    _____ c. It rapidly metastasizes.

    _____ d. It is the easiest to cure.

32. Which information can be obtained from grading a tumor?
    a. Cause of the cancer
    b. Location of metastasis
    c. Cell differentiation
    d. How long the cancer has been present

33. Which of the following are performed during clinical staging of suspected cancer? *Check all that apply.*

    _____ a. Clinical tests

    _____ b. Biopsy

    _____ c. Major surgery

    _____ d. Evaluation of manifestations

34. What are the primary factors influencing the development of cancer? *Check all that apply.*

    _____ a. Environmental exposure to carcinogens

    _____ b. Gender of the client

    _____ c. Genetic predisposition

    _____ d. Immune function

35. Indicate whether cancer arises commonly (C) or rarely (R) from each of the following tissues or organs in adults.

    _____ a. Heart muscle

    _____ b. Bone marrow

    _____ c. Skin

    _____ d. Nerve tissue

    _____ e. Lining of the gastrointestinal tract

    _____ f. Lining of the lungs

    _____ g. Skeletal muscle

36. Match the environmental carcinogen with the associated site of cancer. *Sites may be used more than once.*

Carcinogen	Site of Cancer
_____ a. Anabolic steroids	1. Colon
_____ b. Asbestos	2. Eyes
_____ c. Sunlight	3. Liver
_____ d. Alcoholic beverages	4. Lung
_____ e. Tobacco	5. Mouth
_____ f. Pesticides	6. Pancreas
	7. Skin

37. Which of the following can naturally contain radiation? *Check all that apply.*

_____ a. Radon

_____ b. Uranium

_____ c. Soil

_____ d. Water

38. The most common form of radiation is _____ radiation.

39. A few viruses are known as *oncoviruses* because they do what? *Check all that apply.*

_____ a. Infect the cell.

_____ b. Break the DNA chain.

_____ c. Insert their own genetic material.

_____ d. Grow slowly.

40. How does the immune system protect the body from cancer? *Check all that apply.*

_____ a. By using cell-mediated immunity

_____ b. By using natural killer cells

_____ c. By using antibody-mediated immunity

_____ d. By using helper T-cells

41. Name three types of clients who have a higher incidence of developing cancer due to immunosuppression.

a. _____

b. _____

c. _____

42. The single most important risk factor for developing cancer is _____.

43. For which type of cancer is risk modifiable? *Check all that apply.*

_____ a. Breast cancer

_____ b. Colon cancer

_____ c. Ovarian cancer

_____ d. Prostate cancer

_____ e. Cervical cancer

_____ f. Lymphatic

44. Using Table 27-14 in the textbook, identify four cancers that have genetic predisposition.

a. _____

b. _____

c. _____

d. _____

45. Which of the following cultures has the highest rate of incidence and death rate, and the largest increase in incidence of cancer?
a. Whites
b. Hispanics
c. African-Americans
d. Asian-Americans

46. Which client would have the best prognosis for survival based on the TNM staging classification listed?
a. $T_{IS}N_0M_0$
b. $T_xN_xM_x$
c. $T_2N_1M_0$
d. $T_2N_3M_1$

47. The American Cancer Society reports that the cancer incidence and survival rate are related to which of the following? *Check all that apply.*

_____ a. Gender

_____ b. Availability of health care services

_____ c. Early health care

_____ d. Age

48. List the seven warning signs of cancer:

a. _____

_____

b. _____

_____

c. _____

_____

d. _____

_____

e. _____

_____

f. _____

_____

g. _____

_____

49. Name at least three dietary measures that may help reduce the risk of cancer.

a. _____

b. _____

c. _____

50. Which of the following measures are considered secondary prevention for cancer? *Check all that apply.*

_____ a. Yearly mammography for women over age 40

_____ b. Avoidance of tobacco

_____ c. Yearly fecal occult blood testing in adults

_____ d. Removing colon polyps

_____ e. Using sunscreen when outdoors

_____ f. Colonoscopy at age 50 and then every 10 years

_____ g. Chemoprevention with vitamin therapy

General Interventions for Clients with Cancer

LEARNING OUTCOMES

1. Identify the goals of cancer therapy.
2. Distinguish between cancer surgery for cure and cancer surgery for palliation.
3. Discuss how the nursing care needs for the client undergoing cancer surgery compare to those for the client undergoing any other type of surgery.
4. Compare the purposes and side effects of radiation therapy and chemotherapy for cancer.
5. Prioritize nursing care for the client with radiation-induced skin problems.
6. Develop a community-based teaching plan for the client receiving external beam radiation.
7. Compare the personnel safety issues for working with clients receiving teletherapy radiation versus those receiving brachytherapy radiation.
8. Identify nursing interventions to promote safety for the client experiencing chemotherapy-induced anemia or thrombocytopenia.
9. Develop a community-based teaching plan for the client receiving chemotherapy.
10. Prioritize nursing care for the client with chemotherapy-induced neutropenia.
11. Prioritize nursing care for the client with mucositis.
12. Explain the rationale for hormonal manipulation therapy.
13. Discuss the uses of biological response modifiers as supportive therapy in the treatment of cancer.
14. Explain the basis of targeted therapy for cancer.
15. Identify clients at risk for oncologic emergencies.
16. Prioritize nursing care needs for clients experiencing oncologic emergencies.

LEARNING ACTIVITIES

1. Before completing the study guide exercises in this chapter, it is recommended that you review the following:
   - Altered cell growth
   - Immunity and inflammation response in the body
   - Hematologic norms
   - Anatomy and physiology of the immune system
   - Principles of infection
   - Fluid and electrolytes

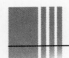

- Normal cell growth and development
- Principles of a complete physical assessment
- Drug therapy for clients with cancer

2. Review the boldfaced terms and their definitions in Chapter 28 to enhance your understanding of the content.

STUDY/REVIEW QUESTIONS

Answers to the Study/Review Questions are provided on the companion Evolve Learning Resources Web site at http://evolve.elsevier.com/Iggy/.

1. Which type of cancer puts clients at greatest increased risk for infection?
   a. Breast cancer
   b. Leukemia
   c. Lung cancer
   d. Prostate cancer

2. Cancer invading the bone marrow can cause which of the following? *Check all that apply.*
   _____ a. Decreased potassium and sodium
   _____ b. Suppressed production of RBCs, WBCs, and platelets
   _____ c. Pathologic fractures
   _____ d. Degenerative joint disease

3. Cachexia describes which of the following?
   a. Electrolyte imbalance in the client with cancer
   b. Decreased cognition
   c. Extreme body wasting and malnutrition
   d. Chemotherapy-induced nausea and vomiting

4. Which statement about gastrointestinal function and cancer is true?
   a. Only cancers within the gastrointestinal system alter gastrointestinal function.
   b. Gaining weight during cancer therapy indicates successful treatment.
   c. A low-fat diet improves survival rates for people with cancer.
   d. The liver is a common site of cancer metastasis.

5. Invasion of the bone usually is caused by metastases from which of the following? *Check all that apply.*
   _____ a. Prostate cancer
   _____ b. Brain cancer
   _____ c. Breast cancer
   _____ d. Lung cancer

6. Cancer metastases to the brain can cause problems in which of the following? *Check all that apply.*
   _____ a. Sensory areas
   _____ b. Motor areas
   _____ c. Cognitive areas
   _____ d. Autonomic areas

7. Differentiate the different types of diagnostic biopsies/surgeries that may be performed when cancer is suspected.

8. What problem may occur with each type of diagnostic/biopsy surgery for cancer?

True or False? For questions 9 to 13, write T for true or F for false in the blanks provided. For the false answers, rewrite to make the statements true.

_____ 9. Pain is present with all cancers.

_____ 10. Clients with lung cancer can develop pulmonary edema and dyspnea.

_____ 11. The primary goal of cancer treatment is to cure the client.

_____ 12. Surgery for a cancer client may be a part of diagnosis or treatment.

_____ 13. The purpose of "second-look" therapy is to determine the status of the disease and the course of treatment for the cancer client.

14. Which factors determine the type of therapy for cancer? *Check all that apply.*

_____ a. Type and location of cancer

_____ b. Overall health of the client

_____ c. Whether the cancer has metastasized

_____ d. The type of health insurance the client has

15. Which of the following is an example of appropriate prophylactic cancer surgery?

_____ a. Tonsillectomy following numerous episodes of "strep throat"

_____ b. Removing part of a tumor to provide pain relief

_____ c. Removal of a mole that is often irritated by the client's waistband

_____ d. Breast reconstruction after a mastectomy

16. What is the purpose of cytoreductive surgery for cancer?

a. Cancer prevention by removal of "at-risk" tissue

b. Cancer control by reducing the size of the tumor

c. Cancer cure by removing all gross and microscopic tumor tissue

d. Cancer rehabilitation by improving the function or appearance of a previously treated body area

17. Which of the following are reasons for performing palliative surgery? *Check all that apply.*

_____ a. Relieving pain

_____ b. Relieving an obstruction

_____ c. Curing the cancer

_____ d. Diagnostic staging

18. Reconstructive surgery is for cancer survivors who may need which of the following? *Check all that apply.*

_____ a. Breast reconstruction

_____ b. Revision of scars and release of contractures

_____ c. Bowel reconstruction

_____ d. Pain relief

19. What is an appropriate nursing diagnosis for a postsurgical client who has lost a body part?

a. Anticipatory Grieving

b. Disturbed Body Image

c. Anxiety

d. Chronic Sorrow

20. Differentiate the terms *exposure* and *dose* as they pertain to radiation therapy.

True or False? For questions 21 to 29, write T for true or F for false in the blanks provided. For the false answers, rewrite to make the statements true.

_____ 21. Cell damage occurs with any exposure to radiation, which may cause the cell to die or lose the ability to divide.

_____ 22. The dosage of radiation is commonly determined by cell cycle.

_____ 23. Normal cells are not damaged during radiation therapy.

_____ 24. Each cell has its own response to radiation, such as dying, becoming sterile, or repairing self.

_____ 25. The goal of radiation therapy is to administer enough treatment to kill all of the cancer cells.

_____ 26. Brachytherapy uses isotopes and is placed on or near the cancer tissue, making the client hazardous to others.

_____ 27. Unsealed radiation sources can be given orally, intravenously, or as an instillation in a body cavity, making clients and their excrement radioactive for 48 hours.

_____ 28. Needles and seeds for sealed radiation sources make the client and his or her excrement radioactive.

_____ 29. Teletherapy is also called beam therapy.

30. What is the meaning of the "inverse square law" for radiation exposure?
   a. The further away a person is from a radiation source, the less radiation is absorbed.
   b. When chemotherapy is added to the treatment regimen, less radiation is needed.
   c. As the distance from the radiation source increases, more tumor cells are killed.
   d. Less radiation is needed if natural sources are used.

31. Which factors are used to determine a cancer client's absorbed radiation dose? *Check all that apply.*

   _____ a. Intensity of radiation exposure

   _____ b. Proximity of radiation source to the cells

   _____ c. Duration of exposure

   _____ d. Age of the client

32. Why is the therapeutic dose of radiation fractionated for cancer treatment?
   a. To reduce total treatment cost
   b. To ensure a higher cancer cell kill with less damage to normal cells
   c. To prevent profound bone marrow suppression with resulting anemia
   d. To allow time for chemotherapy to first reduce the tumor size

33. At what point is the client receiving radiation treatment by teletherapy radioactive and a potential danger to other people?
   a. The client is never radioactive.
   b. When the linear accelerator is turned on.
   c. For the first 24 to 48 hours after treatment.
   d. Until the radiation source has decayed by at least one half-life.

34. What are the systemic side effects of radiation?
    a. Altered taste sensation and fatigue
    b. Skin changes and permanent local hair loss
    c. Diarrhea and tooth loss
    d. Immunosuppression and weight gain

35. For the client undergoing external radiation therapy, the nurse's instruction should include which of the following? *Check all that apply.*

    _____ a. Do not remove the markings.

    _____ b. Do not use lotions or ointments.

    _____ c. Avoid direct skin exposure to sunlight for up to a year.

    _____ d. Use soap and water on the affected skin.

36. Why should the nurse wear a dosimeter when providing care to a client receiving brachytherapy?
    a. To indicate special expertise in radiation therapy
    b. To protect the nurse from absorbing radiation
    c. To determine the amount of radiation exposure experienced
    d. To ensure that the radiation source remains active

37. What is the rationale for chemotherapy as a cancer treatment?
    a. Chemotherapy is less expensive and safer than radiation therapy.
    b. Chemotherapy decreases the client's risk for life-threatening complications.
    c. Chemotherapy is systemic treatment for cancer cells that may have escaped from the primary tumor.
    d. Chemotherapy concentrates in secondary lymphoid tissues and prevents widespread metastasis.

38. Match each type of chemotherapy with the corresponding action.

Chemotherapy
1. Antimitotic agents
2. Topoisomerase inhibitor
3. Antimetabolites
4. Alkylating agent

Type of Action

_____ a. "Counterfeit" chemicals that fool cancer cells into using them, but prevent cell division

_____ b. Causes major damage to DNA and RNA synthesis

_____ c. Cross-links DNA; prevents RNA synthesis

_____ d. A plant source that interferes with formation of microtubules

39. What is the lowest level of bone marrow activity and WBCs called?
    a. Anemia
    b. Nadir
    c. Leukopenia
    d. Immunosuppression

40. Each chemotherapeutic agent has a specific nadir. What is it important to do when giving combination therapy?
    a. Give two agents with like nadir.
    b. Avoid giving agents with like nadirs at the same time.
    c. Allow for one agent's nadir to recover before giving another agent.
    d. Give two agents from the same drug class.

41. Drug dosage is based on total body surface area (TBSA); therefore it is important for the nurse to do which of the following?
    a. Ask the client's height and weight.
    b. Weigh and measure the client.
    c. Assess body mass index.
    d. Measure abdominal girth.

42. A course of chemotherapy normally includes which of the following? *Check all that apply.*

    _____ a. Rounds every week for a total of 6 weeks

    _____ b. Variance with clients' responses to therapy

    _____ c. Timed dosing of the therapy to minimize normal cell damage

    _____ d. A concurrent dose of radiation

43. Most chemotherapy is administered intravenously. What, then, is the major potential complication?
    a. Electrolyte imbalance
    b. Bruising
    c. Extravasation
    d. Thrombus formation

44. Which side effect of chemotherapy is most serious?
    a. Nausea and vomiting
    b. Peripheral neuropathy
    c. Bone marrow suppression
    d. Dry desquamation of the skin

45. The nurse administering a vesicant must be prepared for complications and must have knowledge of which of the following?
    a. The antidote
    b. The pH of the vesicant
    c. How to use hot or cold packs
    d. The type of available dressings

46. Indicate which chemotherapeutic agents are vesicants (V) and which are irritants (I).

    _____ a. Daunorubicin

    _____ b. Mitomycin C

    _____ c. Bleomycin

    _____ d. Vincristine

    _____ e. Paclitaxel

47. When thinning or loss of hair is a known side effect of a drug being administered, the nurse should do which of the following? *Check all that apply.*

    _____ a. Have the client use gentle hair shampoo.

    _____ b. Help the client select wigs, turbans, or scarves.

    _____ c. Instruct the client that hair loss is permanent.

    _____ d. Remind the client to avoid hair washing.

48. Which of the following is true regarding nausea and vomiting related to chemotherapy administration? *Check all that apply.*

    _____ a. It is a common side effect of emetogenic agents.

    _____ b. It usually lasts for 1 to 2 days after administration.

    _____ c. It lasts as long as 3 weeks after administration.

    _____ d. It is purely psychosomatic.

49. Explain the difference between mucositis and stomatitis.

50. Because of the rapid cell division in the gastrointestinal tract, chemotherapy
    a. Kills off the cells immediately
    b. Prevents the body from replacing cells
    c. Causes cells to be killed more rapidly than they can be produced
    d. Helps to increase cell division

51. Oral care for a client with stomatitis should include which of the following? *Check all that apply.*

    _____ a.   Observation

    _____ b.   Hard-bristled brush

    _____ c.   Saline mouthwash

    _____ d.   Glycerin swabs

    _____ e.   Commercial mouthwashes

    _____ f.   Petrolatum jelly to lips after each mouth care

52. Bone marrow suppression will cause which of the following to occur? *Check all that apply.*

    _____ a.   Decreased leukocytes

    _____ b.   Decreased electrolytes

    _____ c.   Decreased erythrocytes

    _____ d.   Decreased platelets

53. What clinical manifestations should you expect in a client who has chemotherapy-induced bone marrow suppression? *Check all that apply.*

    _____ a.   Alopecia

    _____ b.   Fatigue

    _____ c.   Bleeding gums

    _____ d.   Dry skin

    _____ e.   Diarrhea

    _____ f.   Pallor

True or False? Write T for true or F for false in the blank provided.

_____ 54.   Biological response modifier drugs stimulate the immune system to produce cells.

_____ 55.   The most important role of biological response modifiers is the prevention of cancer development.

56. The nurse is responsible for teaching both the immunosuppressed client and the family about health promoting activities. The most important activity is which of the following?
    a.   Handwashing
    b.   Isolation
    c.   Boiling dishes
    d.   Wearing masks

57. Match each biological response modifier to its action.

Modifier
1.   Interleukin
2.   Interferons
3.   Monoclonal antibodies

Action

_____ a.   Binds with cell and prevents cell division

_____ b.   Helps immune system recognize and destroy cancer cells

_____ c.   Helps cancer cells revert to original characteristics

58. The biological response modifiers have which positive effect on the client receiving chemotherapy?
    a.   Less risk of life-threatening infections
    b.   Reduced incidence of alopecia
    c.   Reduced severity of nausea
    d.   Euphoria and increased libido

59. Side effects of interleukin therapy can be dramatic. The client may need to be treated in a critical care unit for which of the following side effects? *Check all that apply.*

    _____ a.   Fluid shifts

    _____ b.   Severe inflammatory reaction

    _____ c.   Capillary leak

    _____ d.   Nausea and vomiting

60. What are common immediate reactions to biological response modifier therapy?

   _____ a. Fever, chills, nausea and vomiting, malaise

   _____ b. Fever, chills, rigor, malaise

   _____ c. Hypertension, constipation

   _____ d. Hives, diarrhea, low back pain

61. A client with cancer tells you she has numbness and weakness in her legs. What is your best response?
   a. "Are you having any back pain?"
   b. "Have you been exercising vigorously?"
   c. "When was your last dose of pain medication?"
   d. "Don't worry. This is a normal response to chemotherapy."

62. Which manifestation and/or piece of laboratory data alerts you to the possibility of SIADH in the client who has cancer?
   a. Tall T-waves on ECG and hyperkalemia
   b. Positive Chvostek's sign and hypocalcemia
   c. Kussmaul respirations and hypochloremia
   d. Weight gain of 6 pounds and hyponatremia

63. Name the major dose-limiting side effect of cancer chemotherapy.

64. Match the colony stimulating factor (CSF) agent with the type of cell affected.

Cell Type		CSF Agent	
_____ a.	Erythrocytes	1.	Sargramostim (Leukine)
_____ b.	Neutrophils	2.	Epoetin alfa (Epogen, Procrit)
_____ c.	Platelets	3.	Filgrastim (Neupogen)
_____ d.	Monocytes and macrophages	4.	Oprelvekin (Neumega)

65. Name each complication described below.
   a. A client with lymphoma wakes up with severe facial edema, tightness of the collar of her nightgown, and epistaxis.

   b. A client who has received chemotherapy now has an infection from organisms that have entered the bloodstream.

   c. The client in "b" is also experiencing severe bleeding from his IV sites, as well as dyspnea and tachycardia.

   d. A client with bone cancer complains of fatigue, loss of appetite, and constipation.

   e. A client with advanced breast cancer complains of severe back pain and leg weakness.

CASE STUDY: THE CLIENT RECEIVING CHEMOTHERAPY

Answer Guidelines for the Case Study questions are provided on the companion Evolve Learning Resources Web site at http://evolve.elsevier.com/Iggy/.

A 63-year-old woman is seen in the cancer therapy unit for her first round of chemotherapy for breast cancer. She had a lumpectomy 2 months ago and a double-lumen PICC line inserted at that time. Her medications include 5-fluorouracil (Adrucil), ifosfamide (IFEX), and mesna (MESNEX). Ondansetron (Zofran) is ordered for nausea.

1. Describe the action of each chemotherapeutic agent listed. If appropriate, note the timing of the medication's nadir.

2. How does the drug mesna differ from the other agents?

3. What precautions are needed for handling these agents?

4. Before giving the chemotherapy, the nurse prepares to give the ondansetron. The client asks why she is getting that medication "when I'm not even nauseated." How should the nurse answer the client?

After 10 days, the client comes to the office for follow-up laboratory work. The results are as follows:

- Sodium: 135 mEq/L
- Potassium: 3.7 mEq/L
- Hemoglobin: 8.5 g/dL
- Hematocrit: 25%
- Red blood cells: 2.3 million/mm³
- White blood cells: 2.8 mm³
- Platelets: 45,000 mm³/mL

5. Which laboratory values are expected at this time? What is the cause of these altered laboratory values?

6. What, if anything, can be done to protect this client during this period? What other medications may be ordered at this time?

Interventions for Clients with Infection

LEARNING OUTCOMES

1. Explain the chain of infection.
2. Describe the principles of infection control in inpatient and community-based settings.
3. Identify the Centers for Disease Control and Prevention (CDC) hand hygiene recommendations for health care workers.
4. Differentiate the four types of transmission-based precautions.
5. Identify the major causes and results of inadequate antimicrobial therapy.
6. Assess the common clinical manifestations of infection.
7. Interpret laboratory test findings related to infections and infectious diseases.
8. Evaluate nursing interventions for management of the client with an infection.
9. Develop a teaching plan for clients who have an infection or infectious disease.

LEARNING ACTIVITIES

1. Before completing the study guide exercises in this chapter, it is recommended that you review the following:
   - Anatomy and physiology of the immune system
   - Process of inflammation
   - Process of immunity
   - Process of inflammation

2. Review the boldfaced terms and their definitions in Chapter 29 to enhance your understanding of the content.

STUDY/REVIEW QUESTIONS

Answers to the Study/Review Questions are provided on the companion Evolve Learning Resources Web site at http://evolve.elsevier.com/Iggy/.

1. Match terms and definitions related to infection.

Terms
1. Communicable
2. Reservoirs
3. Pathogen
4. Pathogenicity
5. Colonization
6. Susceptible host
7. Virulence
8. Normal flora

Definitions

_____ a.   Cause agent

_____ b.   Infection recipient

_____ c.   Ability to cause disease

_____ d.   Degree of communicability

_____ e.   Characteristic bacteria

_____ f.   Pathogenic microbes present but no symptoms

_____ g.   Sources of infectious agents

_____ h.   Transmitted from person to person

2. Using Figure 29-1 in the textbook, review the chain of infection. Describe the two types of animate and inanimate reservoirs.

a.   _____

b.   _____

3. Match each type of pathogen with its description.

Pathogen
1. Toxin
2. Exotoxin
3. Endotoxin

Description

_____ a.   Substances produced and released by certain bacteria, such as tetanus and diphtheria, into the surrounding environment

_____ b.   Substances produced in cell walls of certain bacteria, such as typhoid, and released by cell lysis

_____ c.   Protein molecules released by bacteria to affect host cells at distant sites

4. Which factors increase a client's susceptibility to infection? *Check all that apply.*

_____ a.   Alcohol consumption

_____ b.   Steroid use

_____ c.   Diabetes mellitus

_____ d.   Nicotine use

_____ e.   Oral contraceptives

_____ f.   High-protein diet

_____ g.   Advanced age

5. Explain how medical interventions can increase a client's susceptibility to infection.

6. Match the portal of entry with the method of transmission. *Answers may be used more than once.*

Method of Transmission

_____ a. Droplet

_____ b. Ingestion

_____ c. Intravascular device

_____ d. Insect bite

_____ e. Catheterization

_____ f. Laceration

Portal of Entry

1. Bloodstream
2. Skin/mucous membrane
3. GU tract
4. GI tract
5. Respiratory tract

7. Match the contact site for infection to the mode of transmission. *Answers may be used more than once.*

Contact Site

_____ a. Skin-to-skin

_____ b. Contaminated needle

_____ c. Sneezing

_____ d. Contaminated food

_____ e. Lyme disease

Mode of Transmission

1. Airborne
2. Vehicle
3. Vector
4. Direct
5. Indirect

8. Name three ways that intact skin acts as a barrier to infection:

a. _____

b. _____

c. _____

9. Name two ways that the mucous membranes act as a barrier to infection:

a. _____

b. _____

10. Name three ways that the respiratory tract acts as a barrier to infection:

a. _____

b. _____

c. _____

11. Identify the two sources of nosocomial infections.

a. _____

b. _____

12. What is the other term for "nosocomial" infection? _____

13. Identify the three primary goals of infection control in the community.

a. _____

b. _____

c. _____

True or False? For questions 14 to 19, write T for true or F for false in the blank provided. For the false answers, rewrite the statement to make it true.

_____ 14. The portal of exit for an infection may be the same as the portal of entry.

_____ 15. The body's skin is the best barrier or defense against infection.

_____ 16. Phagocytosis decreases a client's risk for infection.

_____ 17. The use of gloves eliminates the need to wash your hands.

_____ 18. Artificial nails have a low risk of spreading infection.

_____ 19. Nosocomial infection means that the infection was caused by health care.

20. Describe effective handwashing.

21. What situations call for soap and water handwashing instead of use of an alcohol-based hand rub?

22. Match each precaution with an example of its use.

Precaution
1. Contact precautions
2. Droplet precautions
3. Standard precautions
4. Airborne precautions

Use

_____ a. All body secretions and excretions, most membranes and tissue, excluding perspiration, are potentially infectious

_____ b. Uses negative airflow rooms, high-efficiency particulate air (HEPA) filters, or ultraviolet (UV) lights

_____ c. Infection transmitted by droplet; an example is meningitis

_____ d. Transmission by touch of client or environment; examples are methicillin-resistant *Staphylococcus aureus* (MRSA) and vancomycin-resistant *Enterococcus* (VRE)

23. Complications of infection are usually caused by which of the following? *Check all that apply.*

_____ a. Incorrect choice of antibiotic

_____ b. Poor client compliance

_____ c. Client unable to afford medication

_____ d. The client's overall health condition

24. Differentiate sterilization and disinfection.

25. Local symptoms of infection may include: *Check all that apply.*

_____ a. Pain and redness

_____ b. Swelling and pus

_____ c. Cool and clammy skin

_____ d. Fever and chills

26. Match each diagnostic test with its description.

Test

1. Biopsy
2. Scanning
3. Ultrasonography
4. Radiographic studies
5. Erythrocyte sedimentation rate
6. Complete blood count
7. Culture
8. Sensitivity

Description

_____ a. Pathogen is isolated for identification

_____ b. Pathogen is tested for antibiotic reactions

_____ c. Checks WBC, neutrophils, lymphocytes, monocytes, eosinophils, and basophils

_____ d. Measures rate of RBC fall through plasma; increased rate indicates infection or inflammation

_____ e. X-ray films used to monitor infection

_____ f. Noninvasive procedure: used particularly for diagnosing heart valve problems

_____ g. Use of radioactive agents to determine presence of inflammation

_____ h. Tissue specimen obtained for tissue culture

27. Explain what is meant by a "shift to the left" when reviewing the differential count.

True or False? For questions 28 to 31, write T for true or F for false in the blank provided. For the false answers, rewrite the statement to make it true.

_____ 28. Antibiotic therapy should not begin until after the culture specimen is obtained.

_____ 29. Clients with a temperature greater than 100° F are considered to have a systemic infection.

_____ 30. Older adult clients may have a severe infection with no fever.

_____ 31. A superinfection is an infection with an extremely resistant microbe.

32. Identify two nursing diagnoses for a client with infection.

a. _____

b. _____

33. In a client with an infection, interventions to reduce fever may include which of the following? _Choose all that apply._

_____ a. Antipyretic drugs such as aspirin or acetaminophen

_____ b. External cooling, cooling blankets, cool compresses

_____ c. Fluid administration, oral and IV

_____ d. Antimicrobial therapy with antibiotic, antiviral, or antifungal agents

34. Name the antimicrobials that correspond to each drug action listed below.
a. Inhibits reproduction

b. Injures the cytoplasmic membrane

c. Inhibits nucleic acid synthesis

d. Inhibits cell wall synthesis

35. Discuss the four components of effective antimicrobial therapy and why they must be present.

36. Match the organism to its disease manifestation.

Organism

1. *Escherichia coli*
2. *Plasmodium* sp.
3. Pinworm
4. *Streptococcus* sp.
5. *Pneumocystis carinii*
6. *Entamoeba histolytica*
7. Rickettsiae
8. Rhinovirus
9. *Candida albicans*

Disease Manifestation

_____ a. Rocky Mountain spotted fever

_____ b. Thrush

_____ c. Diarrhea

_____ d. Common cold

_____ e. Malaria

_____ f. Urinary tract infection

_____ g. Anal pruritus

_____ h. Pharyngitis

_____ i. Pneumonia

37. Name three organisms, and the resultant diseases, that have a portal of entry via the gastrointestinal tract.

a. _____

b. _____

c. _____

38. Name three organisms and the resultant diseases that have a portal of entry via the bloodstream.

a. _____

b. _____

c. _____

39. Which of the following body fluids are *likely* to transmit bloodborne diseases? *Check all that apply.*

_____ a. Feces

_____ b. Blood

_____ c. Vomitus

_____ d. Semen

_____ e. Vaginal secretions

_____ f. Sputum

_____ g. Breast milk

_____ h. Sweat

_____ i. Cerebrospinal fluid

_____ j. Urine

_____ k. Saliva

40. For each situation described below, name the infectious agent that is responsible for the symptoms.
    a. A week after returning from a refugee camp mission, the client experiences fever, chills, swollen glands in his groin and axillary areas, and headache. He has several flea bites over his legs.

b.   The client has had the flu and was feeling better yesterday, but woke up today with severe dyspnea, tachycardia, fever, and diaphoresis.

c.   After eating canned foods in an old cabin while camping, the client has severe vomiting and diarrhea and is experiencing symmetrical flaccid paralysis but is still alert.

d.   In a temporary hospital set up to serve an area where severe flooding occurred, several clients come in complaining of severe headaches. They have high temperatures, and a papular rash over their faces and extremities, including the palms of their hands. Some of the skin lesions are vesicular and pustular.

Assessment of the Respiratory System

LEARNING OUTCOMES

1. Compare the structures and functions of the upper airways to those of the lower airways.
2. Distinguish between normal and abnormal (adventitious) breath sounds.
3. Describe the respiratory changes associated with aging.
4. Calculate the pack-year smoking history for the client who smokes or who has ever smoked cigarettes.
5. Demonstrate proper technique when using observation and auscultation to assess the respiratory system.
6. Demonstrate proper technique when using palpation and percussion to assess the respiratory system.
7. Interpret arterial blood gas values to assess the client's respiratory status.
8. Prioritize educational needs for the client undergoing pulmonary function tests.
9. Prioritize nursing care needs for the client after bronchoscopy or open lung biopsy.

LEARNING ACTIVITIES

1. Before completing the study guide exercises in this chapter, it is recommended that you review the following:
   - Anatomy and physiology of the respiratory tract
   - Process of respiration
   - Principles of diffusion, perfusion, and ventilation
   - Techniques for performing a physical assessment
   - Principles of blood gas analysis
   - Normal and adventitious breath sounds

2. Review the boldfaced terms and their definitions in Chapter 30 to enhance your understanding of the content.

STUDY/REVIEW QUESTIONS

Answers to the Study/Review Questions are provided on the companion Evolve Learning Resources Web site at http://evolve.elsevier.com/Iggy/.

1. Match each function/description of the airway with the corresponding location.

Location of Airway
1. Upper airway
2. Lower airway

Function/Description of Airway Segment

_____ a. Traps particles not filtered by nares

_____ b. Traps organisms entering nose and mouth

_____ c. Trachea

_____ d. Contains cilia to move mucus to trachea

_____ e. Composed of alveoli for gas exchange

_____ f. Pharynx, or throat

_____ g. Place where the trachea divides into the right and left bronchi

_____ h. Larynx

_____ i. Dividing point where solid foods and fluids are separated from air

_____ j. Epiglottis

_____ k. Pleura

_____ l. Alveoli

2. What are the three main functions of the nose and sinuses?

a. _____

b. _____

c. _____

3. What is surfactant and where is it found in the lower airway? What are three purposes of surfactant in the respiratory process?

4. What is the difference between the pulmonary and bronchial circulatory systems?

5. Match each of the following processes of respiration with its description.

Process
1. Diffusion
2. Perfusion
3. Ventilation

Description

_____ a. Movement of air in and out of the lungs

_____ b. Exchange of oxygen and carbon dioxide in the capillary-alveolar network

_____ c. Pumping of oxygenated blood through the body

6.   Develop a concept map relevant to the respiratory system using the following outline:

	Subjective data	Objective data
Physiologic factors		
Psychosocial factors		
Developmental factors		

Questions 7 to 10 relate to a 64-year-old woman.

7.   In obtaining a smoking history, this client reports that she smoked a pack of cigarettes a day for 9 years, quit for 2 years, then smoked 2 packs a day for the last 30 years. Calculate pack-years for this client.
   a.   39 years
   b.   69 years
   c.   19.5 years
   d.   41 years

8.   As a result of the client's history of smoking and complaints of dyspnea and chronic cough, she is scheduled for pulmonary function tests (PFTs). She calls the office and asks to speak to the nurse to learn more about this procedure. Develop a Deficient Knowledge related to PFT plan for this client.

9.   Which of the following will not be reported in the PFT test results?
   a.   Flow volume curves
   b.   Diffusion capacity
   c.   Muscle fatigue factor
   d.   Lung volumes

10. Match the following PFTs with their descriptions.

Pulmonary Function Test

_____ a.   FEV (forced expiratory volume)

_____ b.   FRC (functional residual capacity)

_____ c.   FVC (forced vital capacity)

_____ d.   RV (residual volume)

_____ e.   TLC (total lung capacity)

_____ f.   VC (vital capacity)

_____ g.   Diffusion

Description
1.   Maximal amount of forced air that can be exhaled after maximal inspiration
2.   Amount of air in lungs at the end of maximal inhalation
3.   Amount of air remaining in lungs after normal exhalation
4.   Maximal amount of air that can be exhaled over a specific time
5.   Amount of air remaining in lungs at the end of full, forced exhalation
6.   Measure of carbon monoxide uptake across alveolar-capillary membrane
7.   Maximum amount of gas that can be exhaled after maximal inspiration

11. Which PFT result for this client will more than likely show a decline as a result of aging and/or respiratory disorders and why?

12. This client is having difficulty with discolored sputum and was scheduled to have a bronchoscopy. She was NPO for several hours before the test. Now, a few hours after the test, she states that she is hungry and would like a meal. You, as a nurse, would do which of the following?
    a. Order a meal because she is now alert and oriented.
    b. Check a pulse oximetry to be sure oxygen saturation has returned to normal.
    c. Check for a gag reflex before allowing her to eat.
    d. Assess for nausea as a result of the medications she received for the test.

13. After the bronchoscopy, the client's sputum from her cough contains blood. What is the most appropriate nursing intervention?
    a. Take vital signs and notify the physician of this change in her sputum.
    b. Monitor client to see if blood in the sputum continues.
    c. Send the sputum for cytology for possible lung cancer.
    d. Tell the client this is a normal response after a bronchoscopy.

14. The nurse would perform a respiratory assessment and monitor for a pneumothorax after which of the following procedures?
    a. Bronchoscopy
    b. Laryngoscopy
    c. Computed tomography of lungs
    d. Percutaneous lung biopsy

15. At what reading of pulse oximetry should immediate intervention be started?
    a. 98%
    b. 93%
    c. 89%
    d. 85%

16. What would the nursing intervention be in the previous question?
    a. Place client in high Fowler's position.
    b. Start oxygen via nasal cannula at 2 L/min.
    c. Notify physician for a stat ABG.
    d. Encourage coughing and deep breathing exercises.

17. Describe the physiologic changes that usually occur in the respiratory function of the following when assessing an older adult.
    a. Chest wall

    b. Alveoli

    c. Lungs

    d. Pharynx and larynx

    e. Pulmonary vasculature

    f. Exercise tolerance

    g. Respiratory muscle strength

    h. Immune system

18. The need for vigorous coughing and deep breathing exercises when an older adult is confined to bed is most likely related to which of the following physiologic changes?
    a. Decreased elasticity of lungs
    b. Decreased alveolar surface and elastic recoil
    c. Decreased effectiveness of cilia
    d. Increase of slackness in vocal cords

19. Analyze the physiologic changes in the older adult shown in Chart 30-1 of the textbook. Which of the following results would the nurse anticipate to be normal arterial blood gases in a 76-year-old client?
    a. Normal pH, normal Pao_2, normal $Paco_2$
    b. Normal pH, decreased Pao_2, normal $Paco_2$
    c. Decreased pH, decreased Pao_2, normal $Paco_2$
    d. Decreased pH, decreased Pao_2, decreased $Paco_2$

20. Match the following adventitious and normal breath sounds with their descriptions. *Breath sounds may have more than one answer.*

Breath Sounds

_____ a.   Bronchial

_____ b.   Bronchophony

_____ c.   Bronchovesicular

_____ d.   Egophony

_____ e.   Pleural friction rub

_____ f.   Crackles

_____ g.   Rhonchi

_____ h.   Vesicular

_____ i.   Wheezes

_____ j.   Whispered pectoriloquy

_____ k.   Rales

Descriptions

1.   Popping sound as air moves through moisture in small airways
2.   Normal sounds heard over lung periphery
3.   Grating, scratching sound with respiration
4.   Musical, squeaky sounds related to narrowing of airway
5.   Normal sounds heard over bronchi; abnormal when heard elsewhere in the lung
6.   Normal sound heard over trachea
7.   Vocalized "A" is heard as "E" with stethoscope
8.   Abnormal loud transmission of "99" during auscultation
9.   Snoring, rattling sound; coarse, in large airways
10.   Loud sound when client softly says "1, 2, 3."
11.   Rattling sounds that change with coughing or suctioning

21. Answer the following three questions related to the nursing diagnosis of Ineffective Airway Clearance.

a.   Which of the following is not an etiology for the nursing diagnosis of Ineffective Airway Clearance for the older adult?
   (1)   Loss of elastic recoil of the lungs
   (2)   Weakened vocal cords
   (3)   Diminished ciliary action
   (4)   Decreased muscle strength and cough

b.   What other indications would cause the nursing diagnosis of Ineffective Airway Clearance?

c.   What are potential nursing interventions related to this nursing diagnosis for the older adult?

22. What is the best position in which to place the client when performing a physical assessment of the respiratory system?
   a.   Side-lying
   b.   Semi-Fowler's
   c.   Supine
   d.   Sitting upright

23. Upon performing a lung sound assessment of the anterior chest, the nurse hears moderately loud sounds on inspiration that are equal in length with expiration. Where in the airway would this lung sound be considered normal?
   a.   Trachea
   b.   Primary bronchi
   c.   Lung fields
   d.   Larynx

24. The name that describes the particular lung sound in the previous question is which of the following?
    a. Bronchial
    b. Bronchovesicular
    c. Vesicular
    d. Basilar

25. What is the lung sound that should be heard throughout the lung fields in the smaller bronchioles and the alveoli?
    a. Bronchial
    b. Bronchovesicular
    c. Vesicular
    d. Basilar

26. Relating to the previous question, which of the following is characteristic of the normal lung sound heard throughout the lung fields?
    a. Short inspiration, long expiration, loud, harsh
    b. Soft sound, long inspiration, short quiet expiration
    c. Mixed sounds of harsh and soft, long inspiration and long expiration
    d. Loud, long inspiration and short, loud expiration

27. Upon assessing the lungs, the nurse hears short, discrete popping sounds in the lower lobes. This assessment would be documented as which of the following?
    a. Rhonchi in bilateral lower lobes
    b. Wheezes in bilateral lower lobes
    c. Fine crackles in bilateral lower lobes
    d. Coarse crackles in bilateral lower lobes

28. Provide a rationale for why the three incorrect answer options in the previous question are wrong.

29. When the nurse reports that the client is short of breath upon lying down, it would be documented as which of the following terms? What are assessment findings for the incorrect answers?
    a. Orthopnea
    b. Paroxysmal nocturnal dyspnea
    c. Bradypnea
    d. Tachypnea

30. On the diagram below, indicate the correct sequence for percussion and auscultation for the anteroposterior assessment of the lungs.

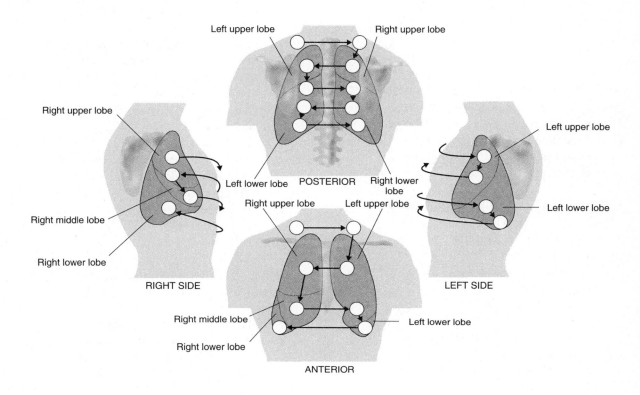

31. Identify the three areas of the body that are assessed during a physical examination of the respiratory system.

    a. _____

    b. _____

    c. _____

32. Which of the following clients has an increased risk of respiratory system problems?
    a. A 45-year-old man who breeds and raises racing pigeons
    b. An 18-year-old who enjoys body surfing in the ocean
    c. A 68-year-old woman who does needlework for relaxation
    d. A 56-year-old man who ties flies for trout fishing

33. The following is a partial client history. On a separate sheet of paper, discuss the significance these data have as an assessment of the respiratory system.

    White man, 36 years old; married with two children. History of cigarette smoking for the past 20 years, one pack per day. Works as a machinist in a factory, manufacturing metal tools and molds for tool-making. In his current job for 17 years. Completed vocational high school. Hobbies include making model airplanes and model railroading. Denies allergies to any medications. Suffers from seasonal allergies (rhinitis, sneezing). No difficulty with ADLs.

34. Using the data in the previous question, document a physical assessment of the respiratory system on a separate sheet of paper.

35. What observations would be made when assessing the lungs and thorax?

   a. _____

   b. _____

   c. _____

36. Which of the following data is an objective sign of chronic oxygen deprivation?
   a. Complaints of shortness of breath
   b. Paroxysmal nocturnal dyspnea
   c. Chest pain with deep inspiration
   d. Clubbing of fingernails

37. Palpation of the chest is used to assess for which of the following?
   a. Retractions or bulging
   b. Tactile fremitus
   c. Accessory muscle use
   d. Friction rub

38. Decreased levels of which of the following laboratory data is associated with chronic airflow limitations?
   a. Hemoglobin
   b. Neutrophils
   c. Eosinophils
   d. Arterial oxygen

39. The nurse determines there is uneven symmetry on the client's thoracic expansion. What steps would the nurse use to palpate this finding?

   a. _____

   b. _____

   c. _____

   d. _____

40. Upon inspection, the nurse would assess an increase in anteroposterior (AP) diameter of the chest when which of the following occurs?
   a. There is unequal movement from side to side of the chest.
   b. The client cannot take a deep breath because of changes in aging.
   c. Ratio of the depth of the chest to the width of the chest is equal.
   d. The ribs are horizontal and not sloping downward.

41. Which of the following abnormal findings does percussion determine?
   a. Tracheal deviation
   b. Hyperresonance
   c. Barrel chest
   d. Friction rub

42. Which of the following characteristics best describe the sound heard in hyperresonance?
   a. High-pitched, loud, and musical
   b. Thud-like, medium sound
   c. Normal sound over lung tissue in periphery
   d. Very loud, long duration, and high pitched

43. The best position for the client during a thoracentesis is which of the following?
   a. Side-lying, affected side exposed, head slightly raised
   b. Lying flat with arm on affected side across the chest
   c. Sitting up, leaning forward on over-bed table
   d. On stomach with arms above the head

44. After which of the following procedures or tests would the nurse observe for signs and symptoms of a pneumothorax?
   a. Thoracocentesis
   b. PET scan
   c. Lung angiogram
   d. Ventilation-perfusion scan ($\dot{V}/\dot{Q}$ scan)

45. A client is admitted for a deep vein thrombosis (DVT) and later becomes short of breath. A pulmonary embolus is suspected. What test would be ordered to confirm this diagnosis?
    a.   Pulse oximetry
    b.   Ventilation and perfusion scanning (V̇/Q̇ scan)
    c.   Magnetic resonance imaging (MRI)
    d.   Chest x-ray

46. Upon inspection, the color of the client's sputum is yellow. Which of the following is this an indication of?
    a.   Infection
    b.   Normal color sputum
    c.   Obstruction
    d.   Unknown problem

47. The nurse observes the following signs: dusky skin, pale mucous membranes, decreased capillary refill, and poor respiratory rate and chest movement. What is the nursing diagnosis?
    a.   Ineffective Airway Clearance
    b.   Ineffective Tissue Perfusion
    c.   Activity Intolerance
    d.   Anxiety related to procedure

48. When caring for a client, the nurse would assess early signs of decreased oxygenation by using which of the following assessment findings?
    a.   Cyanosis
    b.   Unexplained restlessness
    c.   Cool, clammy skin
    d.   Paleness, shortness of breath

49. Demonstrate to your clinical instructor the proper technique for auscultation, palpation, and percussion in a respiratory assessment. Report and document your assessment findings. Validate the findings with your clinical instructor. Complete the remaining steps of the nursing process regarding your assessment findings.

50. A nurse has received a client from the recovery room on hospital unit. The pulse oximetry has dropped from 95% to 90%. Which of the following is the nursing intervention to be accomplished at this time?
    a.   Administer oxygen at 2 L by nasal cannula, then reassess.
    b.   Have client perform coughing and deep breathing exercises, then reassess.
    c.   Administer Narcan to reverse narcotic sedation effect.
    d.   Withhold narcotic pain medication to reduce sedation effect.

True or False? Write T for true or F for false in the blank provided. If false, correct the statement.

_____ 51. Pulse oximetry, or Pao$_2$ can determine adequate oxygenation of a client regardless of cardiac status or underlying clinical problems.

52. Which of the following medications warrants further inquiry when collecting subjective data for the respiratory system?
    a.   Erythromycin (E-Mycin) for chronic recurrent otitis media
    b.   Warfarin sodium (Coumadin) for management of thrombophlebitis of the leg
    c.   Lithium carbonate (Lithobid) for management of bipolar disorder
    d.   Lovastatin (Mevacor) for hypercholesterolemia

53. In preparing a client for a ventilation-perfusion scan, the nurse explains to the client which of the following? Correct the wrong answers.
    a. Being NPO before the examination is necessary to prevent aspiration of the dye.
    b. After the test, the client will be in isolation for 8 hours because of the radioactive dye.
    c. Allergy to iodine must be assessed because of the radioactive dye.
    d. The test is only a screening test for pulmonary embolus; a CT scan will follow if needed.

54. A nurse uses a pulse oximeter to measure which of the following?
    a. Oxygen perfusion in the extremities
    b. Mixed venous saturation
    c. Carbon dioxide saturation of the blood
    d. Oxygen saturation in the red blood cells

55. Match the pulmonary function capacities and functions with the correct corresponding assessment findings.

Pulmonary Assessment Findings

_____ a. Reduced in clients with obstructive disease and increased with exercise or CHF

_____ b. Air left in lung after a forced exhalation

_____ c. Largest amount of air the lungs can hold

_____ d. After a maximum deep breath, amount of air quickly exhaled

_____ e. Not used to measure larger airway obstructions

_____ f. After a maximum deep breath, the maximum amount of air exhaled in the first 1 second

Pulmonary Function Capacities and Functions
1. FVC: forced vital capacity
2. FEV_1: forced expiratory volume in 1 sec
3. FEF: forced expiratory flow
4. FRC: functional residual capacity
5. TLC: total lung capacity
6. RV: residual volume
7. DLCO: diffusion capacity of carbon monoxide

56. In pulmonary function testing, which of the following would be considered a normal result in the older adult?
    a. Increased forced vital capacity
    b. Decline in forced expiratory volume in 1 second
    c. Decrease in diffusion capacity of carbon monoxide
    d. Increased functional residual capacity

57. In the older adult, as a result of loss of elastic recoiling of the lung and decreased chest wall compliance, the nurse may observe which of the following on physical examination?
    a. Thoracic area becomes shorter
    b. Finger clubbing
    c. Increase in anteroposterior ratio
    d. Severe shortness of breath

58. In the older adult, there is a decreased number of functional alveoli; this change in the lungs will result in which of the following?
    a. Decreased Pao_2
    b. Increased Pao_2
    c. False elevation in pulse oximetry
    d. False low value in the pulse oximetry

59. A nurse explains to a client the changes cigarette smoking makes on the lower respiratory tract. Which of the following statements is true?
  a. Clients are more susceptible to respiratory infection because of the damage to the cilia.
  b. Cigarette smoke affects the ability to effectively cough secretions from the lungs.
  c. Cigarette smoke improves the oxygen saturation of the alveoli.
  d. Clients notice that smoking dilates the large and small airways to increase Pao_2.

60. A client with a pulse oximetry of 80% and a blood gas result of Pao_2 of 62 was started on continuous oxygen therapy. Describe what assessment findings would indicate that the client is having a positive response to oxygen therapy.

61. A nursing diagnosis for a client is Activity Intolerance, with a pulse oximetry of 99%. Which of the following laboratory tests contributes to this problem and is related to oxygenation? Would oxygen therapy help this client?
  a. Eosinophils count of 0.6
  b. WBC count of 8.0
  c. Hemoglobin of 9
  d. Glucose 120

62. When performing a respiratory assessment including pulse oximetry, which of the following clients or situations may cause an artificially low reading? *Mark Y for yes or N for no, and provide a rationale for your answer.*

  _____ a. Client with peripheral arterial disease

  _____ b. Client with anemia

  _____ c. Client with sickle cell disease

  _____ d. Client with a fever

  _____ e. Client receiving oxygen via nasal cannula

  _____ f. Client in severe shock

  _____ g. Client receiving narcotic pain medication

  _____ h. African-American client

  _____ i. Female clients versus male clients

  _____ j. Client with history of respiratory diseases such as cystic fibrosis or TB

  _____ k. Client with allergies

63. A client who has had neck surgery complains after the operation of being restless, "not being able to breathe very well," with decreased chest movement and elevated pulse. Which of the following tests may be performed by the physician to determine the etiology of this problem? Explain why the other answers are incorrect.
    a. Mediastinoscopy
    b. Direct laryngoscopy
    c. Gastroscopy
    d. Bronchoscopy

64. The nurse prepares the client in the previous question for a bronchoscopy. What client education should the nurse provide?

65. The client returns to the unit after the bronchoscopy. In addition to a respiratory assessment, which of the following would be most important to monitor in order to prevent aspiration?
    a. Sore throat
    b. Position
    c. Chest discomfort
    d. Gag reflex

66. A nurse assesses fine crackles in a lung assessment of a client immediately postoperative. This would more than likely be an indication of which of the following? Explain why the other answers are incorrect. What nursing intervention would help relieve this respiratory problem?
    a. Pneumonia
    b. Atelectasis
    c. Thick secretions
    d. Bronchospasms

67. Which of the following signs of a respiratory assessment is considered the principal, or main, sign of respiratory disease? What questions would the nurse ask in a respiratory assessment regarding this sign?
    a. Sputum production
    b. Cough
    c. Chest movement
    d. Respiratory rate

68. When performing a respiratory assessment, the nurse inquires about the color of the sputum. Which of the following would indicate to the nurse that the client has an infection of the respiratory tract?
    a. Sputum is tan.
    b. Sputum is green.
    c. Sputum is white or clear.
    d. Sputum is gray.

69. A client was admitted for complaints of a sudden onset of sharp pain after sneezing and had a history of a fever and cough. Lung sounds were diminished over the left upper lobe. These clinical assessment findings indicate which of the following?
    a. Bronchitis
    b. Asthma
    c. Tuberculosis
    d. Pneumothorax

70. Which of the following pathologies is significant to the respiratory system when assessing the family history?
    a. Kyphoscoliosis
    b. Genital herpes simplex
    c. Fibrocystic breast disease
    d. Rheumatoid arthritis

71. During a respiratory assessment for tactile fremitus, the nurse requests the client to do which of the following?
    a. Breathe deeply three times.
    b. Cough hard.
    c. Whisper.
    d. Say "ninety-nine."

72. State the definition of dyspnea.

73. For a healthy adult, the respiratory rate per
     minute is usually defined as which of the
     following?
     a.   10 to 12
     b.   12 to 15
     c.   12 to 20
     d.   20 or more

CASE STUDY: RESPIRATORY TRACT ASSESSMENT

*Answer Guidelines for the Case Study questions are pro-
vided on the companion Evolve Learning Resources Web
site at http://evolve.elsevier.com/Iggy/.*

Your adult client reports to the pulmonary
clinic with complaints of a productive cough
that "won't go away." She is a 62-year-old married housewife whose children are grown. She
smoked two packs of cigarettes per day for
20 years, but she has not smoked for the past
10 years. She contracted a "virus" 4 weeks ago,
which "settled in her chest." Her usual remedies
have not resulted in improvement in her status.

1. What additional subjective data should the
    nurse elicit from this client?

2. What physical assessments should the nurse
    perform on this client?

3. What effect does this client's 10 years of
    not smoking have on the condition of her
    lungs?

4. The physician orders a chest x-ray and a
    sputum specimen. What should the nurse
    tell this client about these tests?

After 1 week, this client reports no improvement,
and the chest x-ray results also indicate that there
is no change. A bronchoscopy is scheduled to be
done in the outpatient surgical unit the following
day. (The physician would prefer to do an MRI
scan, but the client has an inner-ear implant.)

5. Prepare a teaching-learning plan for this cli-
    ent regarding the bronchoscopy. Consider
    restrictions related to breathing during the
    procedure.

6. When the client reports to the outpatient
    surgical unit the next morning, what assess-
    ments should the nurse make?

7. Both the client and her husband are very anxious. Describe interventions that the nurse should implement to assist the client and her spouse.

10. What special actions must the nurse take after the procedure is completed and the client is taken to the PACU?

Thirty minutes before the procedure, the client is given atropine sulfate 0.6 mg IM. An intravenous infusion is begun with $D_5 1/2$ NS, and diazepam (Valium) 10 mg IV is given.

11. What equipment should be available when she arrives?

8. Why have these medications been ordered?

12. What are the reasons for having this equipment available?

9. A topical anesthetic agent is applied to the pharynx immediately before the bronchoscopy is to begin. What is the purpose of this agent?

Interventions for Clients Requiring Oxygen Therapy or Tracheostomy

LEARNING OUTCOMES

1. Compare the uses and nursing care issues of oxygen delivery by nasal cannula with oxygen delivery by mask.
2. Explain the problems of oxygen therapy for those clients whose respiratory efforts are controlled by the hypoxic drive.
3. Analyze changes in clinical manifestations to determine the effectiveness of therapy for the client receiving oxygen.
4. Use laboratory data and clinical manifestations to determine the presence of hypoxemia or hypercarbia.
5. Develop a community-based teaching plan for the client receiving supportive oxygen therapy at home.
6. Prioritize nursing care needs for the client with a new tracheostomy.
7. Identify techniques to reduce the risk for aspiration when helping the client with a tracheostomy to eat.
8. Develop a community-based teaching plan for the client with a tracheostomy living at home.

LEARNING ACTIVITIES

1. Before completing the study guide exercises in this chapter, it is recommended that you review the following:
    *   Principles of sterile technique
    *   Assessment of the respiratory system
    *   Acid-base balance
    *   Concept of respiratory failure
    *   Care of a client receiving enteral feedings
    *   Assessment of the respiratory system

2. Review the boldfaced terms and their definitions in Chapter 31 to enhance your understanding of the content.

STUDY/REVIEW QUESTIONS

Answers to the Study/Review Questions are provided on the companion Evolve Learning Resources Web site at http://evolve.elsevier.com/Iggy/.

1. The following words are used when discussing the care of clients needing oxygen therapy. Briefly describe, in your own words, the meaning of each of the following words.

   a. Hypoxemia

   b. Hypoxia

   c. Hypercarbia

   d. Pulse oximetry

   e. Pao_2

   f. Fio_2

2. Which of the following is not a clinical indication for the use of oxygen therapy?
   a. Decreased arterial Po_2 levels, as in pulmonary edema
   b. Increased cardiac output, as in client with valve replacement
   c. Decreased blood oxygen-carrying capacity, as in anemia
   d. Increased oxygen demand, as in sustained fever

3. *True or False? Read the following statements regarding oxygen therapy and decide whether each is true or false. Write T for true or F for false in the blanks provided. If the statement is false, correct the statement to make it true.*

   _____ a. Oxygen therapy is needed when the normal 21% oxygen in the air is inadequate and causes hypoxemia and hypoxia.

   _____ b. Examples of conditions that can increase the body's need for more oxygen are infection in the blood, increase in body temperature such as 101° F, Hgb of 9.0, or sickle cell disease.

   _____ c. Hypoxemia and hypoxia can be measured by low Pao_2 and low pulse oximetry.

   _____ d. In order to improve breathing, supplemental oxygen is based on analysis of the client's symptoms.

   _____ e. The primary drive for breathing in most clients is the amount of oxygen in arterial blood.

   _____ f. Oxygen is a fire hazard because it can spontaneously ignite when in use.

4. When a client is requiring oxygen by nasal cannula or mask, which of the following statements should the nurse know regarding oxygen administration?
   a. Adult clients require 2 to 6 L/min by nasal cannula in order for oxygen to be effective.
   b. A minimum of 40% oxygen is used with the Venturi mask.
   c. Nurses should be familiar with why the client is receiving oxygen, expected outcomes, and complications.
   d. When administering oxygen, the nurse should know that the goal is the highest Fio_2 possible for the particular device being used.

5. The normal mechanism of the body that stimulates breathing and causes an increase in the respiratory rate is which of the following?
   a. The increase in the CO_2 level as sensed by chemoreceptors in the brain (medulla)
   b. The decreased amount of oxygen saturation in the blood as sensed by the brain (medulla) chemoreceptors
   c. The low levels of carbon dioxide as sensed by the brain (medulla)
   d. The brain recognizes the hypoxemia that occurs with decreased respiration

6. A client with chronic lung disease is admitted to the hospital with oxygen-induced hypoventilation. The nurse needs to be aware that the stimulus to breathe for these clients is which of the following? Provide an explanation for that answer.
   a. Excessively high carbon dioxide (60 to 65 mm Hg) levels in the blood that rose over time
   b. The low level of oxygen concentration in the blood, as sensed by the chemoreceptors in the brain
   c. The low level of oxygen concentration in the blood, as sensed by the peripheral chemoreceptors
   d. CO_2 narcosis in which an elevation of carbon dioxide in the blood turns off the normal mechanism

7. When a nurse administers oxygen to a client who is hypoxic and has chronic high levels of carbon dioxide, the nurse must know that which of the following prevents a decrease in respiratory effort?
   a. F_{IO_2} higher than the usual 2 to 4 L/min nasal cannula is needed.
   b. Venturi mask of 40% is used only to deliver oxygen.
   c. Lower concentration of oxygen (1 to 2 L/min) is provided to minimize worsening of the hypercarbia.
   d. Variable F_{IO_2} via nasal cannula or mask is used as the client's condition changes.

8. The nurse should perform which of the following interventions for a client who is at high risk or unknown risk for oxygen-induced hypoventilation? Indicate why the other answers are incorrect.
   a. Monitor signs of nonproductive cough, chest pain, crackles, and hypoxemia every 1 to 2 hours.
   b. Monitor change in color from pink, to gray, to cyanotic in the first 30 minutes of administering oxygen.
   c. Monitor for signs and symptoms of hypoventilation rather than hypoxemia.
   d. Monitor for changes in level of consciousness, apnea, improvement in color, and pulse oximetry in the first 30 minutes.

9. When administering a high concentration of oxygen to a client, the nurse must be aware of which of the following and why?
   a. Lungs should be auscultated 1 to 2 hours for oxygen toxicity.
   b. Audible wheezes from bronchospasms can occur as a result of absorption atelectasis.
   c. Monitoring the client every 15 to 30 minutes is necessary for observation of side effects.
   d. Crackles and diminished lung sounds can be signs of absorption atelectasis.

10. Increased risk for oxygen toxicity is related to which of the following? *Check all that apply.*

    _____ a. Continuous delivery of oxygen at greater than 50% concentration.

    _____ b. Delivery of a high concentration of oxygen over 24 to 48 hours.

    _____ c. The severity and extent of lung disease.

    _____ d. Neglecting to monitor the client's status and reducing oxygen concentration as soon as possible.

    _____ f. Excluding measures such as CPAP or PEEP

11. Which of the following is a classic indication of chronic hypoxemia?
    a. Finger clubbing
    b. Adventitious lung sounds
    c. Anteroposterior ratio increase
    d. Weight gain with even muscle development

12. Humidified oxygen places the client at high risk for which of the following nursing diagnoses?
    a. Risk for Injury related to the moisture in the tube
    b. Risk for Infection related to the condensation in the tubing
    c. Risk for Infection related to the nasal prongs or mask
    d. Risk for Impaired Skin Integrity related to the mask

13. The organism that causes an infection in clients with humidified oxygen is which of the following?
    a. *Escherichia coli*
    b. *Streptococcus*
    c. *Staphylococcus*
    d. *Pseudomonas*

14. Nursing interventions to prevent infection in clients with humidified oxygen would include which of the following?
    a. Use normal saline to provide moisture.
    b. Drain condensation into the humidifier to conserve moisture.
    c. Remove condensation into a water trap without disconnecting the tubing.
    d. Maintain the smallest flow rate possible.

15. Which of the following is not a hazard of oxygen therapy?
    a. Increased combustion
    b. Oxygen-induced hyperventilation
    c. Oxygen toxicity
    d. Absorption atelectasis

16. Which of the following correctly describes the proper care of the client who is receiving oxygen therapy?
    a. Only the respiratory therapist should be familiar with the devices and techniques used.
    b. Only the nurse should be familiar with the devices and techniques used.
    c. The nurse and the respiratory therapist rely on the physician to be familiar with the devices used.
    d. The nurse must be familiar with the devices and techniques used in order to provide proper care.

17. A client with an oxygen delivery device would like to ambulate to the bathroom but the tubing is too short. Extension tubing is added. What is the maximum length of the tubing that can be added in order to deliver the amount of oxygen needed for that device?
    a. 25 feet
    b. 35 feet
    c. 45 feet
    d. 50 feet

18. Briefly describe the difference between a low-flow and high-flow oxygen delivery system.

19. List oxygen delivery systems by flow types.

Low-flow systems

High-flow systems

20. A client is being discharged from the hospital with home oxygen therapy. As this client's nurse, what nursing interventions would you perform before discharge and what interventions will be ongoing for this client?

21. Indicate the goal for providing discharge planning and teaching for a client receiving home oxygen therapy.

22. Identify and describe the three ways oxygen can be provided to a client on home oxygen therapy.

23. What effect does a reservoir-type nasal cannula have on oxygen flow?
    a. Humidification is necessary for any rate of flow.
    b. The oxygen flow must be increased by 25%.
    c. The oxygen flow may be decreased by 50%.
    d. Humidification is necessary only at flow rates of 2 L per minute or less.

24. Complete this chart on the oxygen delivery systems:

Oxygen Delivery System	Description and Amount of Oxygen Concentration Delivered to the Client	When Used and Types of Clients Using This System	Key Nursing Interventions
Nasal cannula			
Simple face mask			
Partial rebreather mask			
Non-rebreather mask			
Venturi mask			
Tent and aerosol mask			

25. Which of the following is the correct critical nursing intervention for a client with a non-rebreather mask? Correct the wrong answers.
   a. Maintain liter flow so that the reservoir bag is up to one-half full.
   b. Maintain 60% to 75% FIO_2 at 6 to 11 L/min.
   c. Ensure that valves and rubber flaps are patent, functional, and not stuck.
   d. Assess for effectiveness of oxygen and switch to partial rebreather for more precise FIO_2.

26. A client with a face mask at 5 L/min is able to eat. Which of the following nursing interventions would be performed at mealtimes?
   a. Change the mask to a nasal cannula of 6 L/min or more.
   b. Have the client work around the face mask as best as possible.
   c. Obtain a physician order for a nasal cannula at 5 L/min.
   d. Obtain a physician order to remove the mask at meals.

27. A client with respiratory difficulty is using noninvasive positive-pressure ventilation (NPPV). Which of the following statements is correct about this delivery system? Correct the wrong answers.
    a. Only used as an oxygen delivery method.
    b. Used to keep the alveoli open and improve gas exchange.
    c. A form of airway intubation.
    d. A system that only uses bilevel positive airway pressure (BiPAP) delivery method.

28. Describe the difference between the two NPPV systems of BiPAP and nasal continuous positive airway pressure.

29. A physician orders transtracheal oxygen therapy for a client with respiratory difficulty. What does this type of oxygen delivery method do?
    a. Delivers oxygen directly into the lungs
    b. Can be inserted into the trachea by any health care provider
    c. Is used in place of an endotracheal tube
    d. Does not require any client home care education

30. A nursing diagnosis for a client receiving oxygen therapy is Risk for Impaired Skin Integrity. Nursing interventions related to prevention include which of the following? Check all that apply and correct the false statements.

    _____ a.   Assess the client's ears, back of neck, and face at least every 4 to 8 hours for irritation.

    _____ b.   Apply padding on tubing to prevent pressure on skin.

    _____ c.   Use petroleum jelly on nostrils, face, and lips to relieve dryness.

    _____ d.   Assess nasal and mucous membranes for dryness and cracks.

    _____ e.   Obtain an order for humidification when oxygen is being delivered at 6 L/min or more.

    _____ f.   Provide mouth care every 8 hours and as needed.

    _____ g.   Position tubing so it will not pull on client's ears.

31. A client is receiving oxygen therapy for respiratory problems. According to NIC interventions for administration and monitoring of its effectiveness, a nurse does which of the following?
    a. Monitors the effectiveness of oxygen therapy at least once every 8 hours
    b. Monitors for signs of oxygen toxicity and absorption atelectasis
    c. Instructs the client to replace the oxygen mask when the device is removed
    d. Delegates monitoring the oxygen liter flow and equipment management to respiratory therapist

32. The nurse observes a client with "stridor." This indicates which of the following respiratory etiologies?
    a. Pneumonia
    b. Tuberculosis
    c. Atelectasis
    d. Partial obstruction of trachea or larynx

33. Which of the following would be used for a client needing long-term airway maintenance?
    a. Tracheostomy
    b. Nasal trumpet
    c. Endotracheal tube
    d. Continuous positive airway pressure (CPAP)

34. A client is receiving preoperative teaching for a total laryngectomy and will have a tracheostomy postoperatively. The nurse explains to the client that a tracheostomy is which of the following?
    a. An opening in the trachea that enables breathing
    b. A surgical incision into the trachea
    c. A tube that is inserted into an opening in the trachea
    d. An opening in the neck for placement of an endotracheal tube

35. Identify the types of clients you would anticipate needing a tracheostomy.

36. Immediately postoperative, the nurse would monitor for which of the following complications of a tracheostomy?
    a. Pneumothorax from the displacement of the tube in the trachea
    b. Septic shock as a result of the secretions and suctioning
    c. Subcutaneous emphysema related to the opening in the trachea
    d. Dislodgment of the tracheostomy tube causing air to enter the tissues

37. Identify possible complications associated with a tracheostomy. Develop a chart with assessment findings and collaborative management with prevention strategies related to the complications.

38. A client with a tracheostomy develops increased coughing, inability to expectorate secretions, and difficulty breathing. These are assessment findings related to which of the following?
    a. Airway obstruction
    b. Tracheoesophageal fistula
    c. Cuff leak and rupture
    d. Tracheal stenosis

39. Which of the following is false as relates to postoperative nursing intervention for a client with an artificial airway?
    a. Assuring the tube placement
    b. Auscultating breath sounds bilaterally
    c. Suctioning via a nasotracheal approach
    d. Observing for chest wall movement

40. To prevent accidental extubation of a tracheostomy tube when the client is not on a ventilator, the nurse should implement which of the following interventions?
    a. Continuously restrain the client's arms.
    b. Secure the tube in place using ties or fabric fasteners.
    c. Allow some flexibility in motion of the tube while coughing.
    d. Instruct the client to hold the tube with a tissue while coughing.

41. Equipment that should be kept at the bedside of a client who has a tracheostomy includes which of the following?
    a.   A pair of wire cutters
    b.   Chest tube with water seal drainage collection device
    c.   Code cart
    d.   A tracheostomy tube with obturator

42. Match each of the following terms related to a tracheostomy tube with their descriptions.

Terms

_____ a.   Cuff

_____ b.   Double-lumen tracheostomy tube

_____ c.   Faceplate

_____ d.   Fenestrated tracheostomy tube

_____ e.   Inner cannula obturator

_____ f.   Outer cannula obturator

_____ g.   Single-lumen tracheostomy tube

_____ h.   Talking tracheostomy tube

_____ i.   Tracheostomy button

Descriptions

1.   Plastic or metal tube with blunted end used during insertion of tracheostomy tube
2.   Single-cannula tracheostomy tube
3.   Maintains stoma patency while client is in transition from mechanical ventilation to spontaneous breathing
4.   Prevents aspiration when inflated
5.   Consists of inner and outer tubes and an obturator
6.   Provides a means for communication
7.   Fits into outer cannula and facilitates cleaning and suctioning
8.   Part of outer cannula that anchors tube into the trachea
9.   Has precut opening in outer cannula that facilitates speech
10. Fits into the tracheostomy and keeps airway open

43. Why should tracheostomy cuffs be deflated?
    a.   To allow the client to speak
    b.   To permit suctioning more easily
    c.   To enable the client to eat or drink
    d.   To provide access for tracheostomy care

44. Which of the following is a nursing intervention to prevent obstruction of a tracheostomy tube? Identify other nursing measures that can be taken.
    a.   Provide tracheal suctioning
    b.   Provide oxygen with humidification
    c.   Inflate the cuff to maximum pressure
    d.   Suction with a Yankauer catheter

45. After 72 hours, a client experiences decannulation of the tracheostomy tube. When this occurs, the nurse performs which of the following? What is the nursing intervention if decannulation occurs the first 72 hours?
    a.   Ventilate the client and notify the physician because this is a medical emergency.
    b.   Quickly and gently replace the tube with a clean cannula kept at the bedside.
    c.   Insert the obturator, administer oxygen, and call the physician.
    d.   Call the code team and prepare for CPR.

46. Briefly discuss the following possible complications of a tracheostomy tube.
    a.   Pneumothorax

    b.   Subcutaneous emphysema

    c.   Bleeding

    d.   Infection

47. Humidification and warming of air are essential for the client with an artificial airway because humidification helps do which of the following?
    a. Prevent tracheal damage
    b. Promote thick secretions
    c. Dry out the airways
    d. Warm the air

48. Which of the following is not a complication related to tracheal suctioning?
    a. Hypoxia
    b. Tissue trauma
    c. Infection
    d. Bronchodilation

49. Indicate the sequence the nurse would follow when suctioning a client with an artificial airway by marking the steps 1 through 14.

    _____ a. Explain procedure to the client.

    _____ b. Pour sterile saline into sterile container.

    _____ c. Preoxygenate the client.

    _____ d. Check suction source for low suction.

    _____ e. Assemble the necessary equipment.

    _____ f. Keep catheter sterile; attach to suction.

    _____ g. Wash hands.

    _____ h. Insert catheter into trachea without suctioning.

    _____ i. Assess need for suctioning.

    _____ j. Lubricate catheter tip in sterile saline solution.

    _____ k. Open suction kit.

    _____ l. Withdraw catheter, applying suction and twirling catheter.

    _____ m. Put on sterile gloves.

    _____ n. Document procedure after discarding supplies used and washing hands.

50. Briefly describe how to ensure that a tracheostomy tube is never dislodged during tracheostomy care.

51. Indicate the sequence for administering tracheostomy care by marking steps 1 through 16.

    _____ a. Remove old dressing and excess secretions.

    _____ b. Wash hands.

    _____ c. Suction tracheostomy tube.

    _____ d. Put on sterile gloves.

    _____ e. Reinsert inner cannula into outer cannula.

    _____ f. Open tracheostomy kit and pour peroxide into one side of container and saline into another.

    _____ g. Assemble necessary equipment.

    _____ h. Clean stoma site and plate.

    _____ i. Explain procedure to client.

    _____ j. Rinse inner cannula in sterile saline.

    _____ k. Remove inner cannula.

    _____ l. Change tracheostomy ties if needed.

    _____ m. Place inner cannula in peroxide solution.

    _____ n. Position client.

    _____ o. Place new tracheostomy dressing.

    _____ p. Use brush to clean inner cannula.

52. Nursing interventions for the client with a tracheostomy include which of the following? Indicate why the other answers are incorrect.
    a. Changing the tracheostomy ties daily
    b. Suctioning continuously for 10 to 15 seconds
    c. Providing oral hygiene with glycerin swabs
    d. Cleaning the incision with hydrogen peroxide

53. Discharge instructions for the client with a tracheostomy include teaching about which of the following?
    a. Sterile suction technique
    b. Tap water instillations
    c. Decreasing humidity in the home
    d. Wearing a medical alert bracelet

54. A client with a permanent tracheostomy is interested in developing an exercise regimen. Which of the following activities is not appropriate for this client?
    a. Aerobics
    b. Tennis
    c. Golf
    d. Swimming

55. Describe the difference between a tracheostomy collar and a T-piece, both of which are used to deliver oxygen therapy. What are the nursing interventions for clients with these devices?

56. A nurse provides oral hygiene for a client with a tracheostomy by doing which of the following?
    a. Cleansing the mouth with glycerin swabs
    b. Encouraging the use of mouth washes that alter pH of the oral cavity
    c. Mixing hydrogen peroxide and sterile water
    d. Using toothettes or a soft-bristled brush moistened in water

57. When the client is able to speak and is not on mechanical ventilation, the nurse would expect the client to have which type of tracheostomy tube and why?
    a. Standard cuffless tube
    b. Standard cuffed tube
    c. Cuffed fenestrated tube
    d. Talking tracheostomy tube

58. Match each type of tracheostomy tube with its description.

Descriptions of Tracheostomy Tubes

_____ a. Used with clients who can speak while on a ventilator for a long-term basis

_____ b. Has a cuff that seals airway when inflated

_____ c. Used for long-term management of clients not on mechanical ventilation or at high risk for aspiration

_____ d. Has three parts—outer cannula, inner cannula, and obturator

_____ e. Used for permanent tracheostomy

_____ f. Used often with clients with spinal cord paralysis or muscular disease who do not require a ventilator all the time

_____ g. Has no inner cannula and is used for clients with long or extra thick necks

_____ h. Used when weaning a client from a ventilator; allows the client to speak

Types of Tracheostomy Tubes
1. Double-lumen tube
2. Single-lumen tube
3. Cuffed tube
4. Cuffless tube
5. Fenestrated tube
6. Cuffed fenestrated tube
7. Metal tracheostomy tube
8. Talking tracheostomy tube

59. How does a nurse determine when the cuff is inflated or deflated on a tracheostomy tube?

60. To prevent tissue damage of the tracheal mucosa of a client with a cuffed tracheostomy tube without a pressure relief valve, the nurse would do which of the following?
    a. Deflate the cuff every 2 to 4 hours and maintain as needed
    b. Change the tracheostomy tube every 3 days or per hospital policy.
    c. Assess and record cuff pressures each shift using the occlusive technique.
    d. Assess and record cuff pressures each shift using minimal leak technique.

61. Other than high cuff pressure, what other factors should the nurse monitor to prevent tissue damage? What nursing interventions would help minimize the chance of this problem occurring?

62. According to NIC interventions, which of the following interventions is appropriate regarding nursing care of a client with an artificial airway?
    a. Before deflating the cuff, suction the oropharynx and secretions from the top of the tube.
    b. Monitor the cuff pressures every 4 to 8 hours on inspiration.
    c. Provide trachea care once every 24 hours and maintain as needed.
    d. Monitor for signs and symptoms of pulmonary edema and fluid overload.

63. To assess whether the client is aspirating food or fluids, the nurse would perform which of the following?
    a. When client is coughing, monitor for increased amount of secretions.
    b. Add food coloring to fluids or enteral feedings and monitor the color of the secretions.
    c. Position the client in high Fowler's position and monitor for signs of aspiration.
    d. Obtain an order for a chest x-ray to determine the presence of aspiration pneumonia.

64. To prevent aspiration during swallowing, the nurse would perform which of the following interventions? Correct the wrong answers and identify other interventions.
    a. Hyperextend the head to allow food to enter the stomach and not the lungs.
    b. Have the client drink thin liquids because they are the easiest to swallow.
    c. Encourage the client to "dry swallow" after each bite to clear residue from the throat.
    d. Maintain a high Fowler's position during eating and 2 hours afterward.

65. Indicate five nursing interventions to prevent hypoxia in a client with a tracheostomy tube.

    a. _____

    b. _____

    c. _____

    d. _____

    e. _____

66. While being suctioned, a client demonstrated vagal stimulation by a drop in heart rate to 54 and a drop in blood pressure to 90/50. Upon assessment of this client, the nurse would do which of the following?
    a. Inflate the cuff and "bag" the client with 100% oxygen.
    b. Call a code and be ready to perform CPR.
    c. Stop suctioning, oxygenate with 100% oxygen, and monitor the client.
    d. Stop suctioning and monitor blood pressure and heart rate.

67. Describe how aspiration may occur with a cuffed tracheostomy tube.

68. When the client with a tracheostomy is unable to speak, what nursing interventions can be performed to facilitate communication?

69. Upon discharge from the hospital, the client should be able to perform tracheostomy care, nutritional care, suctioning, and have means for communication. Identify additional information the client with a tracheostomy tube will need to know.

Interventions for Clients with Noninfectious Problems of the Upper Respiratory Tract

LEARNING OUTCOMES

1. Prioritize nursing care needs for the client after a nasoseptoplasty.
2. Compare the manifestations and care needs of a client with an anterior nosebleed with those of a client with a posterior nosebleed.
3. Prioritize nursing care needs for a client with facial trauma.
4. Describe the pathophysiology and the potential complications of sleep apnea.
5. Develop a plan of communication for a client who has a disruption of speech and cannot read.
6. Use clinical manifestations and laboratory data to determine airway adequacy in a client with laryngeal or neck injury.
7. Identify the risk factors for head and neck cancer.
8. Explain the psychosocial consequences of surgery for head and neck cancer.
9. Develop a community-based teaching plan for the client who is getting ready to go home after undergoing a complete laryngectomy.

LEARNING ACTIVITIES

1. Before completing the study guide exercises in this chapter, it is recommended that you review the following:
   - Anatomy and physiology of the respiratory system
   - Principles of oxygen therapy
   - Concept of body image
   - Perioperative nursing management
   - Assessment of the respiratory system
   - Concept of respiratory failure
   - Care of clients with trauma or injuries
   - Tracheostomy care

2. Review the boldfaced terms and their definitions in Chapter 32 to enhance your understanding of the content.

STUDY/REVIEW QUESTIONS

Answers to the Study/Review Questions are provided on the companion Evolve Learning Resources Web site at http://evolve.elsevier.com/Iggy/.

1. Review the various anatomic structures and their function in the upper respiratory system.

2. The nurse would assess and be prepared for potential interventions in what three primary areas of care for clients with upper respiratory system problems?

    a. _____

    b. _____

    c. _____

3. The nursing priority for the client with any problems of the upper airway is to assess which of the following?
    a. Thickness of nasal and oral secretions and encourage ingestion of oral fluids or performing suction
    b. Anxiety and pain. Provide comfort measures such as sedation and NSAIDs
    c. Adequacy of oxygenation and ensure an unobstructed air passageway
    d. For spinal cord injuries and trauma, and obtain order for x-rays

4. A woman states to the physician that she is concerned that her overweight husband who is a heavy smoker has sleep apnea because of his heavy snoring. Changing sleeping positions and losing weight does not seem to be of help. What other indications would be obtained from the client's history that would lead to a diagnosis of sleep apnea and the need for further testing?

5. The man in the previous question is to have a polysomnograph. The client and his wife are unfamiliar with this study. As the nurse, explain to the client and family the purpose of the test, how it will be performed, and how long it will take to complete.

6. To be diagnosed as having sleep apnea, the client would need to have which of the following criteria?
    a. Apnea for 5 seconds or longer, occurring a minimum of 10 times a night
    b. Apnea for 5 seconds or longer, occurring a minimum of 5 times an hour
    c. Apnea for 10 seconds or longer, occurring a minimum of 10 times a night
    d. Apnea for 10 seconds or longer that occurs a minimum of 5 times an hour

7. The need for diagnosing sleep apnea is related to the complications of which of the following?
    a. Side effects of hypoxemia, hypercapnia, and sleep deprivation
    b. Increase in arterial carbon dioxide levels and sleep deprivation
    c. Respiratory alkalosis with retention of carbon dioxide
    d. Irritability, obesity, enlarged tonsils, or adenoids

8. Various devices are used at home to prevent airway obstruction during sleep. These devices would include which of the following?
   a. CPAP and NPPV breathing assistive device
   b. Oxygen via face mask to prevent hypoxia
   c. Neck brace to support the head in a certain position to facilitate breathing
   d. Nebulizer treatments with bronchodilators

9. When nasal devices are used to treat apnea, what intervention would be of help to the client to prevent dryness of nasal mucosa?
   a. Encourage ingestion of fluids to 3000 mL per day.
   b. Intermittently use the device to decrease irritation.
   c. Use medicated nasal sprays routinely.
   d. Moisturize the nasal mucosa with normal saline sprays.

10. When playing football, a client injured his nose and he suspects there is a simple fracture. The best intervention at this time would be for the client to do which of the following?
    a. Seek medical attention for a stent placement to keep the airway open.
    b. Monitor the injury for at least 24 hours for swelling and bleeding and apply ice to see whether medical attention is necessary.
    c. Seek medical attention for correction within 24 hours to minimize further complications.
    d. Monitor the symptoms for 24 hours to determine whether medical attention for plastic surgery and nose reconstruction is needed.

11. Briefly explain the term *moustache dressing* and when a client would need this type of dressing. Describe what observations the nurse and client would make when having this type of dressing.

12. After a client has a rhinoplasty, a family member is instructed by the nurse to monitor the client for postnasal drip by using a flashlight. If bleeding is noticed, the client should be instructed to do which of the following?
    a. Place ice packs on nose and back of neck, and apply pressure on the nose to immediately stop the bleeding.
    b. Hyperextend the neck to facilitate draining the blood, and apply pressure and ice packs as needed.
    c. Notify the physician to seek medical attention for the bleeding problem.
    d. Continue to monitor, and notify the physician if the bleeding continues for more than 24 hours.

13. Clients should be taught that after rhinoplasty, their appearance will be altered by which of the following?
    a. A very large dressing on the nose
    b. Bruising of the eyes, nose, and face
    c. Swelling that will cause loss of sense of smell
    d. The nose being three times its normal size for 3 weeks

14. A client with a history of nosebleeds is admitted to the emergency department. The nurse attempts to stop the nosebleed by which of the following methods?
    a. Administering sedation/relaxation medication; applying ice packs and pressure to the nose; monitoring respiratory status
    b. Immediately packing nose; applying ice packs; having client sit with head forward; monitoring amount of bleeding.
    c. Relaxing client; having client sit with head forward; monitoring color and amount of blood; monitoring vital signs; applying ice pack and pressure to nose
    d. Applying pressure and ice; having client blow nose hard to remove obstruction of clots; administering humidified oxygen

15. A client's nosebleed is not subsiding with the interventions performed in the emergency department. The physician has determined that the bleeding originated in the posterior region and the client needs further intervention. Describe how this intervention will be performed by the physician.

16. After being treated in the emergency department for posterior nosebleed, the client is admitted to the hospital. The nursing assessment and interventions for this client would be based on which of the following priority nursing diagnoses?
    a. Risk for Impaired Gas Exchange
    b. Risk for Imbalanced Nutrition
    c. Risk for Anxiety
    d. Acute Pain

17. Briefly compare and contrast nursing care and discharge instructions for the client with packing from a posterior nosebleed and the client in the emergency department with an anterior nosebleed.

18. Short answer:
    a. Anterior packing involves packing nose with _____.
    b. Which produces more risk for respiratory failure, anterior or posterior packing?

    c. Clients are hospitalized for what type of packing: posterior, anterior, or both?

    d. Are NSAIDs used to control the pain from inflammation? Why or why not?

    e. How long does packing remain in place?

    f. After removing posterior packing, the nose may be cleaned and lubricated with _____.
    g. After posterior packing is removed, the client should avoid what activities for several weeks?

    h. The nursing diagnosis Risk for Infection relates to which type of packing?

19. After a client has a rhinoplasty, postoperative instructions should be given to the client and family. Which of the following should be included in the instructions provided by the nurse?
    a. Avoid constipation the first few days after surgery to prevent pressure on the incision and other complications.
    b. Resume food and fluids as tolerated. Minimize fluids to decrease nasal secretions.
    c. Mild analgesics only, such as Tylenol, Excedrin with Aspirin, and Motrin, should be needed for discomfort.
    d. Swelling and discoloration should be relieved quickly with ice packs placed over the surgical site, eyes, and face.

20. Obstruction of airflow and interference with sinus drainage may result from a deviated septum. The client would require which type of procedure to correct this problem?
    a. Rhinoplasty
    b. Nasoseptoplasty
    c. Open repair of the submucous
    d. Open repair of the deviated septum

21. Nursing care of a client after surgery for a deviated septum would include which of the following interventions?
    a. Apply ice to the nasal area and eyes to decrease swelling and pain.
    b. Encourage deep breathing and coughing exercises to prevent atelectasis and clear secretions.
    c. Administer aspirin, NSAIDs, or Tylenol every 4 to 6 hours for pain relief and elevated temperature.
    d. Apply moist heat and humidity to the nasal area to promote comfort and circulation, and drainage.

22. Facial trauma requires emergent care that includes the nurse assessing the following three areas:

    a. _____

    b. _____

    c. _____

23. The nurse monitors a client in the emergency department for signs and symptoms of upper airway obstruction. What signs and symptoms would indicate an upper airway obstruction? Why is early recognition essential?

24. What additional findings, other than upper airway obstruction, would the nurse assess in a client with facial trauma?

25. In addition to clients with facial trauma, identify other types of clients who may experience upper airway obstruction.

26. Management of upper airway obstruction includes which of the following?
    a. Repositioning the head and neck so that the head is slightly flexed
    b. Using Heimlich maneuver on the client with a partial airway obstruction
    c. Performing a cricothyroidotomy and inserting a hollow tube to maintain patency
    d. Inserting a nasal airway and administering oxygen by nasal cannula

27. A client with facial trauma has undergone surgical intervention to wire the jaw shut. Which of the following would be included in discharge teaching and why?
    a. Bleeding, oral care and nutrition, pain control, and activity
    b. Oral care, nutrition, pain, communication, and aspiration prevention
    c. Prevention of airway obstructions, bleeding and oral infection, and pain control
    d. Activity, diet, communication, bleeding, and shock

28. Which of the following symptoms in a client with facial trauma should be reported to the physician immediately?
    a. Asymmetry of the mandible
    b. Bloody drainage from both nares
    c. Nonparallel extraocular movements
    d. Pain upon palpation over the nasal bridge

29. Which of the following foods should be encouraged in the diet of a client who has an inner maxillary fixation?
    a. Milk shakes
    b. Cheeseburgers
    c. Carbonated beverages
    d. Tuna and noodle casserole

30. A client enters the emergency department with dyspnea, inability to produce sounds, hoarseness, and subcutaneous emphysema. These clinical findings indicate which of the following?
    a. Vocal cord polyps
    b. Cancer of the vocal cords
    c. Laryngeal trauma
    d. Vocal cord paralysis

31. A client involved in a motor vehicle accident had a neck injury that resulted in laryngeal trauma. The client is being treated in the emergency department with humidified oxygen and is being monitored every 15 to 30 minutes for respiratory distress. Which of the following assessment findings may indicate the need for further intervention?
    a. Respiratory rate 24, Pao_2 80 to 100, no difficulty with communication
    b. Pulse oximetry 96%, anxious, fatigued, blood in sputum, abdominal breathing
    c. Confused and disoriented because of air hunger, difficulty producing sounds, pulse oximetry 80%
    d. Anxious, respiratory rate 20, talking rapidly about the accident, color pink, warm to touch

32. The client in the emergency department with laryngeal trauma has developed shortness of breath with stridor, decreased level of consciousness, restlessness, and decreased oxygen saturation. The nurse should prepare the client and family for which of the following procedures?
    a. Oral or nasal airway
    b. Tracheostomy
    c. Endotracheal tube
    d. Laryngoscopy

33. Identify those who are at risk for developing vocal cord nodules. Compare these people with those at risk for developing polyps.

34. Clients with vocal cord nodules or polyps should be advised to do which of the following?
    a. Drink plenty of cold liquids.
    b. Talk in a whisper.
    c. Discontinue treatment of allergies because that can exacerbate the problem.
    d. Humidify the air they breathe.

35. Which of the following statements about nasal polyps is correct?
    a. They occur more often in clients with intestinal polyps.
    b. They are removed by application of liquid nitrogen.
    c. They arise more often in clients with viral rhinitis.
    d. They contribute to an increased risk of airway obstruction.

36. Which of the methods of treatment listed below would the nurse expect to perform when treating a client with hypertrophy of the turbinates?
    a. Inhalation
    b. Topical
    c. Oral
    d. Transdermal

37. A postoperative cervical diseconomy client has developed laryngeal edema. The nurse would assess for which of the following?
    a. Eupnea
    b. Crackles
    c. Laryngeal stridor
    d. Cheyne-Stokes respirations

38. The nurse notifies the physician stat of the assessment of laryngeal edema. Why is this a medical emergency?

39. Which of the following structures in the neck is treated with a tracheostomy if this site is damaged?
    a. Cricoid bone
    b. Thyroid cartilage
    c. Cricoid cartilage
    d. Thyroid gland

40. Initial emergency management for upper airway obstruction as a result of foreign body aspiration includes which of the following?
    a. Several sharp blows between the scapulae
    b. Cardiopulmonary resuscitation
    c. Nasotracheal suctioning
    d. Abdominal thrusts (Heimlich maneuver)

41. Identify three causes of neck trauma.

    a. _____

    b. _____

    c. _____

42. As a result of neck trauma, the nurse must monitor for problems related to which of the following? *Check all that apply.*

    _____ a. Esophagus

    _____ b. Cervical spine

    _____ c. Carotid artery

    _____ d. Frontal lobe of the brain

43. Clients with head and neck trauma or surgery are unable to verbally communicate. Identify at least four methods that such a client can use to communicate.

    a. _____

    b. _____

    c. _____

    d. _____

44. The type of tumor that most commonly affects the head and neck area is which of the following carcinomas?
    a. Adenocarcinoma
    b. Basal cell carcinoma
    c. Squamous cell carcinoma
    d. Melanoma

45. Which of the following statements regarding head and neck cancer is correct?
    a. Metastasizes often to the brain
    b. Usually develops over a short time
    c. Often seen as red edematous areas
    d. Often seen as white patchy mucosal lesions

46. When performing a nursing history, the nurse would assess for what risk factors that would relate to head and neck cancer? What are the two highest risk factors?

47. Which of the following clients is at risk for developing, specifically, cancer of the larynx?
    a. A 57-year-old male alcoholic
    b. An 18-year-old marijuana smoker
    c. A 28-year-old female school teacher
    d. A 34-year-old male who snorts cocaine

48. Identify at least five warning signs of head and neck cancer.

   a. _____

   b. _____

   c. _____

   d. _____

   e. _____

49. To facilitate comfort and breathing for a client with a laryngeal tumor, the nurse would use which type of positioning?
   a. Sims'
   b. Supine
   c. Fowler's
   d. Trendelenburg

50. The one surgical procedure that does not put the client at risk postoperatively for aspiration is which of the following and why?
   a. Total laryngectomy
   b. Transoral cordectomy
   c. Supraglottic laryngectomy
   d. Partial laryngectomy

51. The nurse would teach the client to be aware that aspiration can occur as a result of which procedure for treating laryngeal cancer? Indicate other procedures for which the client is at risk for aspiration.
   a. Transoral cordectomy
   b. Laser surgery
   c. Radiation therapy
   d. Supraglottic laryngectomy

52. The client asks the nurse why there is a risk for aspiration as a result of supraglottic laryngectomy. What would be her answer?

53. Explain to a client the steps in performing the supraglottic method of swallowing.

54. Which of the following regarding aspiration precautions is false?
   a. Administer pills as whole tablets; they are easier to swallow.
   b. Aspiration with a nasogastric tube is a risk because of an incompetent LES.
   c. Keep head of bed elevated 30 to 45 minutes after feeding.
   d. Follow routine reflux precautions when an NG tube is in place.

55. If frequent aspiration occurs as result of supraglottic laryngectomy, what measures must be taken?

56. Which of the following tests is performed to determine a client's ability for swallow rehabilitation and aspiration precautions?
   a. Chest x-ray of the neck and chest
   b. CT scan of head and neck
   c. Barium swallow under fluoroscopy
   d. Direct and indirect laryngoscopy

57. Carotid precautions following radical neck dissection surgery include which of the following?
    a. Performing physical therapy exercise
    b. Monitoring the flap using a Doppler
    c. Moving the client to an observation bed
    d. Applying wet-to-dry dressings to the flap

58. What measures are available to the client for speech rehabilitation as a result of a total laryngectomy? Indicate what elements need to be in place for these measures.

59. A client is being evaluated by a speech therapist for either esophageal speech or tracheoesophageal fistula. Explain the difference between these two methods.

60. Which of the following is true regarding a radical neck dissection?
    a. Wound drainage tubes are not necessary for this type of surgery because a tracheostomy is in place.
    b. There will not be a permanent tracheostomy tube or stoma opening.
    c. Swallowing will not resume. Client is left with a permanent nasogastric or gastrostomy tube.
    d. Clients will have shoulder muscle weakness and limited range of motion resulting from nerve damage.

61. *Read the following statements regarding head and neck cancers and decide whether each is true or false. Write T for true or F for false in the blanks provided. If the statement is false, correct the statement to make it true.*

    _____ a. Head and neck cancers can be cured when treated early.

    _____ b. Diagnosis is usually not made until the disease is advanced.

    _____ c. Signs and symptoms of the disease are related to the location of the cancer.

    _____ d. Red velvety patches are called leukoplakia.

    _____ e. Many diagnostic tests are performed. CT scan aids in finding the exact location of a tumor, whereas MRI defines soft tissue invasion.

    _____ f. Radiation treatments are the preferred treatment for all locations and sizes of head and neck cancers.

    _____ g. Physical therapy is for postoperative radical neck surgery clients only.

    _____ h. Discharge teaching for all partial or total laryngectomy clients will include tracheostomy care.

    _____ i. Clients may have tubes removed before they are discharged from the hospital.

    _____ j. Discharge teaching for a total laryngectomy client will include stoma care, which combines wound and airway care.

62. The treatment of small specific tumors and/or early malignancies is which of the following? Develop a client teaching plan for this procedure.
   a. Radical neck dissection
   b. Radiation
   c. Chemotherapy
   d. Partial laryngectomy

63. Which of the following statements regarding client education and radiation therapy is true?
   a. The client's voice will initially be hoarse but should improve over time.
   b. There are no side effects other than a hoarse voice.
   c. Dry mouth after radiation therapy is temporary and short-term.
   d. The throat is unlikely to feel the effects of radiation because it is not directly affected by radiation.

64. A client with a partial laryngectomy should be prepared postoperatively for which of the following?
   a. Clients will have permanent swallowing problems after surgery.
   b. Because of postoperative swelling, the client will have a tracheostomy tube and nasogastric tube for feeding.
   c. Voice conservation measures can protect verbal communications after the tracheostomy tube is removed.
   d. The tracheostomy is always permanent and is referred to as a laryngectomy stoma.

65. Complete the table regarding each of the surgical procedures for laryngeal cancer.

Surgical Procedures	Description	Resulting Voice Quality
Laser surgery		
Transoral cordectomy		
Supraglottic partial laryngectomy		
Hemilaryngectomy		
Total laryngectomy		

66. Which of the following topics would not be included in preoperative teaching for a client scheduled for a total laryngectomy and why?
    a. Airway tube and suctioning
    b. Compensatory method of communication
    c. Drains and tubes
    d. Reconstruction using tissue "flaps"

67. Discharge teaching for clients with tracheotomies includes self-care instructions related to which of the following?
    a. Esophageal speech
    b. Using a table mirror for visibility when suctioning
    c. Never being able to shower again
    d. Not being able to eat solid foods

68. Develop a discharge teaching plan related to a client with total laryngectomy that includes all of the following items. Show your plan to your clinical instructor.
    a. Tracheostomy and stoma care
    b. Method of communication
    c. Activities of daily living
    d. Nutritional support
    e. Psychosocial issues

Interventions for Clients with Noninfectious Problems of the Lower Respiratory Tract

LEARNING OUTCOMES

1. Explain the differences in pathophysiology between asthma from bronchospasm and asthma from inflammation.

2. Prioritize educational needs for the client at step III of stepped therapy for asthma.

3. Interpret peak expiratory rate flow (PERF) readings for the need for intervention.

4. Discuss the complications of chronic oral steroid therapy for treatment of chronic airflow limitation (CAL).

5. Compare the pathophysiology and clinical manifestations of asthma, bronchitis, and emphysema.

6. Identify risk factors for chronic obstructive pulmonary disease (COPD).

7. Prioritize educational needs for the client with COPD who is receiving oxygen therapy at home.

8. Describe the mechanisms of action, side effects, and nursing implications for pharmacologic management of COPD.

9. Describe interventions for energy conservation for the client with COPD.

10. Prioritize nursing care needs for the client immediately following lung volume reduction surgery.

11. Explain the nutritional needs for the client with COPD.

12. Use laboratory data and clinical manifestations to determine the effectiveness of therapy for impaired gas exchange in a client with obstructive or restrictive breathing problems.

13. Identify the risk factors for lung cancer.

14. Compare the side effects of radiation treatment for lung cancer with those of chemotherapy for lung cancer.

15. Explain how to troubleshoot the chest tube drainage system in a client 1 day after a thoracotomy.

16. Develop a community-based teaching plan for a client getting ready to go home after a pneumonectomy.

LEARNING ACTIVITIES

1. Before completing the study guide exercises in this chapter, it is recommended that you review the following:
    - Anatomy and physiology of the lower respiratory tract
    - Assessment of the respiratory system including pulse oximetry
    - Process of respiration
    - Principles of diffusion, perfusion, and ventilation
    - Perioperative nursing management
    - Concept of body image
    - Pulmonary function studies
    - Grief and loss
    - Signs and symptoms of respiratory failure
    - Acid-base balance

2. Review the boldfaced terms and their definitions in Chapter 33 to enhance your understanding of the content.

STUDY/REVIEW QUESTIONS

Answers to the Study/Review Questions are provided on the companion Evolve Learning Resources Web site at http://evolve.elsevier.com/Iggy/.

1. Match each of the following lower respiratory tract structures with the corresponding function.

Lower Respiratory Tract Structures

_____ a.   Alveolus

_____ b.   Bronchus

_____ c.   Bronchioles

_____ d.   Carina

_____ e.   Cilia

_____ f.   Hilum

_____ g.   Lung

_____ h.   Parietal pleura

_____ i.   Surfactant

_____ j.   Trachea

_____ k.   Visceral pleura

Lower Respiratory Tract Functions

1. Point where trachea bifurcates
2. Propels mucus for lower airways to trachea
3. Reduces surface tension in the alveoli
4. Carries air to each lobe of lungs
5. Elastic organs that allow for ventilation and air diffusion
6. Carries air from bronchi to alveolar ducts
7. Carries air from larynx to bronchi
8. Covers lung surfaces to decrease friction
9. Lines inside of thoracic cavity to decrease friction with respiration
10. Gases are exchanged in this basic unit
11. Forms the roof of the lungs

2. If problems arise in the lower respiratory tract, they would involve mainly what two principles of respiration?

    a. _____

    b. _____

3. A client has been diagnosed with a chronic airflow limitation (CAL) problem. Which of the following is not a disease of CAL?
    a. Bronchiectasis
    b. Bronchial asthma
    c. Chronic bronchitis
    d. Pulmonary emphysema

4. Which of the following statements best characterizes the long-term effect of asthma and COPD as chronic diseases of the lower respiratory system?
    a. Asthma and COPD result in acute reversible airway respiratory distress episodes with no permanent alveoli damage.
    b. Asthma and COPD cause acute episodes that result in permanent alveoli damage that worsen over time causing respiratory failure.
    c. Asthma results in acute reversible airway distress with no permanent alveoli damage. COPD causes permanent alveoli damage that worsens over time.
    d. Asthma causes permanent alveoli damage that worsens over time. COPD results in acute reversible airway distress with no permanent alveoli damage.

5. The narrowing of the airway in either asthma or COPD is ultimately the result of which of the following?
    a. Constriction from inflammation of the airways attributed to different etiologies
    b. Obstruction from thick mucous secretions related to infection
    c. Reaction to medications that reverse the effects on the airways
    d. Impaired gas exchange in the alveoli affecting the bronchial airways

6. Match each of the following pathophysiologic changes with the corresponding type of disease that is associated with CAL. *Answers may be used more than once.*

Characteristics of Diseases of CAL

_____ a. Affects smaller airways

_____ b. Chronic thickening of bronchial walls

_____ c. Decreased surface area of alveoli

_____ d. Destruction of alveolar walls

_____ e. Hypercapnia

_____ f. Impaired mucociliary clearance

_____ g. Increased airway resistance

_____ h. Increased eosinophils

_____ i. Increased secretions

_____ j. Affects work of breathing

_____ k. Intermittent bronchospasm

_____ l. Intermittent mucosal edema

_____ m. Intermittent excess mucus production

_____ n. Loss of elastic recoil

_____ o. Mast cell destabilization

_____ p. Elastin broken down by proteases

_____ q. Stimulation of disease process by allergies

_____ r. Possibly results in respiratory acidosis

_____ s. Narrowed airway lumen due to inflammation

_____ t. Narrowing of airway from smooth muscle constriction

_____ u. Disease triggered by anti-inflammatory drugs used to treat disease

Types of Diseases
1. Asthma
2. Chronic bronchitis
3. Pulmonary emphysema

7. When exercising, a client with asthma should be taught to monitor for which of the following problems? What would the nurse recommend to prevent future episodes of this problem?
   a. Increased peak expiratory flow rates
   b. Wheezing from bronchospasm
   c. Wheezing from atelectasis
   d. Dyspnea from pulmonary hypertension

8. What is the correct statement?
   a. Both emphysema and chronic bronchitis cause a barrel chest.
   b. Emphysema affects the large and small airways, as well as the alveoli; bronchitis affects only the alveoli.
   c. Bronchitis causes the lungs to work hard from hyperventilation of the alveoli.
   d. Emphysema causes hyperventilation of the lung from alveoli damage; bronchitis affects the airways.

9. Which of the following are the classic assessment findings for clients with CAL?
   a. Cyanosis, dyspnea, and wheezing
   b. Cough, dyspnea, and wheezing
   c. Cough, cyanosis, and dyspnea
   d. Cough, dyspnea, and tachypnea

10. For a client who is a nonsmoker, which of the classic assessment findings of CAL is particularly important in diagnosing asthma?
    a. Cough
    b. Dyspnea
    c. Audible wheezing
    d. Tachypnea

11. A client who is allergic to dogs experiences an "asthma attack." In addition to audible wheezing, briefly describe other signs and symptoms that often occur.

12. A client newly diagnosed with asthma has a nursing diagnosis of Deficient Knowledge related to treatment interventions. As a nursing intervention, briefly explain to this client the goals for treating asthma and self-care management.

13. The nurse explains to the client that the rationale for what causes a "barrel chest" is which of the following?
    a. Use of accessory muscles increases the front to back ratio of the chest
    b. Long-term effect of dyspnea as a result of air being trapped in lungs or hyperinflation
    c. Long-term side effect of chronic hypoxia
    d. Collapse of the alveoli, increasing the work of breathing

14. A client with chronic bronchitis often shows signs of hypoxia. The nurse would observe for which of the following clinical manifestations of this problem?
    a. Increased capillary refill
    b. Clubbing of fingers
    c. Pink mucous membranes
    d. Overall pale appearance

15. Match each of the following assessment findings of CAL with the corresponding description.

Assessment Findings

_____ a. Abdominal paradox

_____ b. Asynchronous breathing

_____ c. Barrel chest

_____ d. Blue bloater

_____ e. Pink puffer

_____ f. Respiratory alternans

Descriptions

1. Cachectic emphysemic client
2. Increased anteroposterior-to-lateral chest diameter
3. Diaphragmatic breathing alternating with abdominal breathing
4. Use of intercostal and abdominal muscles to breathe
5. Chronic cyanotic bronchitis client
6. Unorganized chest motion

16. Explain to a client how smoking affects the respiratory tract and why coughing occurs in the morning upon rising.

17. Shortness of breath is often a complaint of clients with chronic pulmonary disease. Which of the following best describes the type of breathing that the client experiences? When does this problem usually occur? What relieves the problem?
    a. Paroxysmal nocturnal dyspnea
    b. Orthopnea
    c. Tachypnea
    d. Cheyne-Stokes

18. In chronic bronchitis, impaired gas exchange occurs as a result of which of the following?
    a. Chronic inflammation, thin secretions, and chronic infection
    b. Respiratory alkalosis, decreased Pa_{CO_2}, and increased Pa_{O_2}
    c. Chronic inflammation and decreased surfactant in the alveoli and atelectasis
    d. Thickening of the bronchial walls, large amounts of thick secretions, and repeated infections

19. The assessment finding related to the chest x-ray of a client with emphysema would be which of the following?
    a. Hypoinflation of the lungs
    b. A flattened diaphragm
    c. A mediastinal shift
    d. No obvious changes

20. What effect does the work of breathing have on the metabolic demands of the client?
    a. Decreases the need for calories and protein requirements since dyspnea causes activity intolerance
    b. Has no effect on caloric protein needs, meal tolerance, satiety, appetite, and weight
    c. Increases metabolism and the need for additional calories and protein supplements
    d. Creates an anabolic state for building body mass, muscle strength, and easier breathing

21. In obtaining a history of a client with CAL, which of the following would not be related to potentially causing/triggering the disease process?
    a. Cigarette smoking
    b. Occupational and air pollution
    c. Genetic tendencies
    d. Smokeless tobacco

22. The nurse explains that smoking cessation affects the disease process of COPD by which of the following?
    a. Completely reversing the damage to the lungs
    b. Slowing the rate of disease progression
    c. Stabilizing the effects on the airways and lungs
    d. Reversing the effects on the airways but not the lungs

23. Which of the following is not a potential complication that can result from COPD?
    a. Respiratory infections
    b. Right-sided heart failure
    c. Left-sided heart failure
    d. Cardiac dysrhythmias

24. When reading a summary of a pulmonary function test, which of the following is the most significant reading to take note of for obstructive pulmonary disease?
    a. FEV_1/FVC ratio
    b. Functional residual capacity
    c. Total lung capacity
    d. Residual volume

25. Over time, a decrease in the FEV_1/FVC ratio indicates to the nurse which of the following?
    a. The disease process is stable.
    b. CAL is progressing.
    c. CAL is improving.
    d. Further testing is needed to determine effects of disease.

26. Match each pulmonary function test with the corresponding test results that can indicate obstructive or restrictive disease. *There may be more than one answer for each test.*

Pulmonary Function Tests

_____ a. Forced vital capacity (FVC)

_____ b. Forced expiratory volume in 1 second (FEV_1)

_____ c. Functional residual capacity (FRC)

_____ d. Total lung capacity (TLC)

_____ e. Residual volume (RV)

_____ f. Diffusion capacity of carbon monoxide

_____ g. Peak expiratory flow (PEF)

Test Results
1. Often reduced in obstructive disease
2. Often reduced/decreased in restrictive disease
3. Increased in obstructive pulmonary disease
4. Increased in obstructive disease
5. Reduced/decreased in certain obstructive or restrictive disorders
6. Normal in restrictive disease
7. Results improve after use of bronchodilators—classic diagnostic test for asthma

27. The purpose of pulmonary function testing for clients with CAL is which of the following?
    a. To determine the oxygen liter flow rates required by the client
    b. To measure arterial and venous blood gas levels before bronchodilators are administered
    c. To evaluate the movement of oxygenated blood from the lung to the heart
    d. To distinguish airway disease from restrictive lung disease

28. An adult client with respiratory difficulty has completed the pulmonary function test before starting any treatment. The peak expiratory flow (PEF) is 18% below what is expected for this client's age, gender, and size. This result is which of the following?
   a. An indication for further diagnostic tests to confirm asthma
   b. A confirmed finding in clients with asthma
   c. High for a client with asthma and COPD
   d. Confirmation of a respiratory disease of unknown type

29. Clients with asthma learn to use the PEF/FVC values for determining interventions. Briefly explain how a client uses this information and what options are available.

30. As the nurse, how would you explain to the client how to determine the FEV_1/peak flow value?

31. As a result of the analysis of assessment findings, what are the common nursing diagnoses for clients with CAL?

32. Clients with asthma are taught self-care activities and treatment modalities according to the "step method." Which of the following relates to step III?
   a. Symptoms occur frequently; increased use of rescue inhalers.
   b. Symptoms occur daily; daily use of anti-inflammatory inhaler with inhaler bronchodilator; no systemic steroids.
   c. Symptoms occur daily; daily use of CSC and long-acting beta agonist; steroids used for rescue.
   d. Frequent exacerbations with limited physical activity; daily CSC; systemic steroids and methylxanthines.

33. A high-liter flow of oxygen is contraindicated in the client with COPD because of which of the following?
   a. The client depends often on a hypercapnic drive to breathe.
   b. The client depends on a hypoxic drive to breathe.
   c. Receiving too much oxygen over a short time results in headache.
   d. Response to high doses needed later will be ineffective.

34. In assisting a client with CAL to relieve dyspnea, which of the following positions would not be of benefit to the client?
   a. Sitting on edge of chair, leaning forward with arms folded and resting on a small table
   b. Leaning back in a low semi-reclining position with the shoulders back and several pillows under the head
   c. Sitting forward in a chair with feet spread apart and elbows placed on the knees
   d. Leaning back against a support with feet spread apart and shoulders slumped forward

35. Which of the following nursing interventions would not be included in the instruction regarding the nursing diagnosis of Deficient Knowledge related to energy conservation measures? Provide a rationale for your answer.
    a. Activities should be at a relaxed pace throughout the day with rest periods.
    b. Avoid working on activities that require using arms at a level higher than the chest.
    c. Eat largest meal when assistance can be provided and eat three large meals a day.
    d. Avoid talking and doing activities at the same time.

36. Identify the main classifications of drugs that are used to treat CAL.

    a. _____

    b. _____

    c. _____

    d. _____

    e. _____

37. Identify and describe the action of the three types of bronchodilators used to treat asthma. Give an example of each type.

    a. _____

    b. _____

    c. _____

38. The lab result for a theophylline level is 18 μ/mL. This would indicate the prescribed dose of theophylline is which of the following?
    a. Within therapeutic range
    b. Too high of a dose
    c. Too low of a dose
    d. Questionable; further information is needed

39. Which of the following information from a client's history would cause a decrease in serum theophylline levels?
    a. Cigarette smoking
    b. Caffeine consumption
    c. Oral contraceptives
    d. Alcohol consumption

40. A client receiving IV theophylline complains of nausea, abdominal pain, headache, and inability to sleep. The nurse would do which of the following?
    a. Administer Compazine for nausea.
    b. Administer an antacid.
    c. Obtain a physician's order for a theophylline level.
    d. Tell the client that these side effects are normal and not to worry.

41. A client with CAL and pneumonia is admitted to the hospital for exacerbation of COPD. Explain why the nurse has a separate IV line for administering aminophylline to this client.

42. A client with asthma has been prescribed a Flovent inhaler. The nurse explains to the client the purpose of this drug is to do what?
    a. Relax the smooth muscles of the airway.
    b. Act as a bronchodilator in severe episodes.
    c. Reduce obstruction of the airway by decreasing the inflammation.
    d. Reduce the histamine effect of the triggering agent.

43. In addition to corticosteroid anti-inflammatory inhalers, indicate other types of anti-inflammatory agents used, and give the action of the drugs. Provide an example of the medication for each category.

    a. _____

    b. _____

    c. _____

44. A client is learning to use an inhaler in the treatment of asthma. Briefly describe how the client should use the inhaler correctly.

45. A client asks about the advantages of using the aerosol route for administering corticosteroids. The nurse replies by saying that this route:
    a. Has less of a bronchodilation effect.
    b. Reduces the risk for fungus infections.
    c. Is easier to use and compliance is better.
    d. Is fast acting with fewer systemic side effects.

46. When teaching a client with CAL, which of the following is the correct sequence for administering aerosol treatments?
    a. Steroid should be given immediately after the bronchodilator.
    b. Steroid should be given 5 to 10 minutes after the bronchodilator.
    c. Bronchodilator should be given immediately after the steroid.
    d. Bronchodilator should be given 5 to 10 minutes after the steroid.

47. Which of the following statements about the use of cromolyn sodium for the treatment of asthma is correct?
    a. It acts by strengthening mast cell membranes to increase histamine release and decrease bronchospasm.
    b. It is useful primarily during acute episodes of asthma attacks.
    c. It is not intended for use during acute episodes of asthma attacks.
    d. It acts by weakening mast cell membranes to decrease histamine releases and bronchospasm.

48. Complete the first chart below to compile a comparison of the classes of medications used in the treatment of CAL.

Drug Name	Usual Route/ Dose	Expected Action	Adverse Actions	Nursing Implications
Sympathomimetics				
Methylxanthines				
Anticholinergics				
Corticosteroids				

49. Complete the second chart below to compare and contrast the classes of respiratory drugs.

Drug Name	Usual Route/ Dose	Expected Action	Adverse Actions	Nursing Implications
Antitussives				
Expectorants				
Mucolytics				

50. The nurse instructs the client with COPD in the proper coughing technique. Which of the following would not be a recommended time to perform this technique and why? What is the purpose of coughing at the recommended times?
   a.   Upon rising in the morning
   b.   Before meals
   c.   After meals
   d.   Bedtime

51. In addition to teaching the client when to perform coughing techniques, the nurse teaches the client how to cough properly to effectively eliminate excessive secretions. Briefly explain the steps for the "controlled coughing" procedure.

52. For a client with CAL, identify at least 10 topics that would be considered for collaborative interventions.

53. Identify appropriate interventions for clients with asthma, including when to seek immediate medical attention.

54. As a result of chronic bronchitis or emphysema, an assessment finding for a client with heart failure, especially cor pulmonale, is which of the following?
    a. Left ventricular hypertrophy
    b. Weak pulse
    c. Fatigue
    d. Dehydration

55. Explain how you would instruct a client with a diagnosis of Ineffective Breathing Pattern to perform the diaphragmatic and pursed-lip breathing techniques.

56. Describe the factors that a nurse should assess for when a client with CAL complains of shortness of breath.

57. Develop a teaching plan that includes home care activities for a newly diagnosed adult client with CAL.

58. Assessment findings of respiratory failure for a client with asthma are which of the following?
    a. Rales, rhonchi, and productive cough of yellowed sputum
    b. Tachypnea, dry cough, and chest pain
    c. Diminished or inaudible breath sounds, wheezing, and use of accessory muscles
    d. Respiratory alkalosis, slow, shallow respiratory rate

59. Develop a concept map relevant to CAL. Consider physiologic, psychosocial, and developmental factors. Identify subjective and objective data.

60. Primary prevention for those employees at high risk for occupational pulmonary disease is which of the following?
   a. Screen all employees by use of chest x-ray films twice a year.
   b. Do not smoke and do use proper masks and ventilation equipment.
   c. Perform pulmonary function tests once a year on all employees.
   d. Perform monthly inspections of areas according to standards.

61. Clients with occupational lung diseases and chronic lung diseases are considered to be at high risk for which of the following?
   a. Tuberculosis
   b. AIDS
   c. Lung cancer
   d. ARDS

62. The most important intervention in the management of dust-related diseases is which of the following?
   a. Using masks and having adequate ventilation for prevention
   b. PFTs to evaluate lung function
   c. Using supplemental oxygen therapy to alleviate hypoxemia
   d. Education about using bronchodilators to relieve dyspnea

63. Match each of the following terms related to occupational lung diseases with the corresponding definition.

Terms

_____ a. Pneumoconiosis

_____ b. Silicosis

_____ c. Asbestosis

_____ d. Talcosis

_____ e. Berylliosis

Definitions
1. Interstitial lung fibrosis related to asbestos exposure
2. Sarcoidosis related to exposure to highly heated or machined metals
3. Pulmonary fibrosis related to long-term talc dust exposure
4. A group of chronic respiratory diseases related to occupational inhaling of dust
5. Chronic fibrosing lung disease related to silica dust inhalation

64. Which of the following statements about lung cancer is correct? Correct the false statements.
   a. The death rate for lung cancer is less than prostate, breast, and colon cancers combined.

   b. The overall 5-year survival rate for all clients with lung cancer is 85%.

   c. Survival can be attributed to early diagnosis and treatment of the lung cancer.

   d. The primary prevention for reducing the risk is to stop smoking and avoid secondhand smoke.

65. *Read the following statements regarding lung cancer and decide whether each is true or false. Write T for true or F for false in the blanks provided. If the statement is false, correct the statement to make it true.*

_____ a. There are two primary classifications of lung cancer—small cell and non–small cell.

_____ b. Non–small cell lung cancer is further divided into three types—squamous, adenocarcinoma, and large cell.

_____ c. Metastasis occurs via three routes—obstruction/direct invasion, blood, and lymph nodes.

_____ d. Common metastasis sites include bone, liver, brain, and adrenal glands.

_____ e. Non–small cell lung cancer is often associated with paraneoplastic syndromes.

_____ f. The risk of lung cancer decreases after 5 years of not smoking.

_____ g. The number of cigarettes and years of smoking do not contribute to the risk; it is the tar and nicotine that contribute to the risk.

_____ h. African-Americans are at less risk for lung cancer than are whites.

_____ i. The death rate for lung cancer is the same for African-Americans and whites.

_____ j. Wearing a specialized mask can decrease the risk of developing occupation-related lung cancer.

_____ k. Female smokers are at a lower risk of developing lung cancer than are men because they have a protective gene.

_____ l. Onset of symptoms is a positive sign of early disease.

_____ m. A chest x-ray film is a good screening tool for lung cancer.

_____ n. Lung cancer is always diagnosed by sputum specimens.

_____ o. Surgical intervention for non–small cell cancer is the goal for curing the client.

_____ p. A wedge resection is a form of surgical intervention that removes a small localized section of the diseased lung.

66. A client with sudden onset of a deep vein thrombosis of unknown origin was diagnosed with lung cancer. This type of paraneoplastic syndrome resulting from lung cancer is a sign of which of the following?
    a. Good prognosis with surgical intervention of diseased lung
    b. A lung cancer that can be treated easily with radiation
    c. The poorest prognosis because of the metastasis
    d. A good prognosis if the client stops smoking

67. Match each of the following features of lung cancer with the corresponding type of lung cancer. More than one answer may apply.

Features of Lung Cancer

_____ a.   Often located in the large bronchi

_____ b.   Slow-growing type of tumor

_____ c.   Often associated with lymph metastasis

_____ d.   Smoking is a high-risk factor

_____ e.   Associated with nonsmokers

_____ f.   Outcome is a poor prognosis

_____ g.   Associated with the classic symptoms of lung cancer

_____ h.   Not a good surgical candidate because of metastasis on diagnosis

_____ i.   Surgical intervention is effective, especially in early stages

_____ j.   Type often found in women

_____ k.   Incidence is about one third of all types

_____ l.   Chemotherapy is used as an adjunct to other treatment

_____ m.   Surgery is treatment of choice for stage I and stage II

Types of Lung Cancer
1. Small cell
2. Squamous
3. Adenocarcinoma
4. Large cell

68. The common signs and symptoms that are often associated with lung cancer are which of the following?
    a. Insidious onset of blood-tinged sputum, cough, hoarseness, shortness of breath
    b. Short onset of cough, shortness of breath, and blood-tinged sputum
    c. Wheezing, coughing, shortness of breath, and palpitations
    d. High-grade fever, chills, and shortness of breath

69. Which is a true statement about radiation therapy?
    a. Radiation treatments are given daily in "cycles" over the course of several months.
    b. Radiation treatments cause hair loss, nausea, and vomiting for the duration of treatment.
    c. Radiation treatments cause dry skin at the radiation site, fatigue, and changes in appetite with nausea.
    d. Radiation is the best method of treatment for systemic metastatic disease.

70. The term used to define the general surgical procedure for lung cancer is which of the following? Define the incorrect answers.
    a. Lobectomy

    b. Thoracotomy

    c. Pneumonectomy

    d. Segmentectomy

71. Which type of surgical intervention for lung cancer does not require a chest tube postoperatively and why?
    a. Segmentectomy
    b. Lobectomy
    c. Wedge resection
    d. Pneumonectomy

72. Immediately after a pneumonectomy, how does the nurse position the client?
    a. Operative side only to allow expansion of the remaining lung
    b. Nonoperative side only to decrease risk of damage to surgical site and improve breathing
    c. Side or back, rotating periodically to prevent stagnation of fluid
    d. Back only, with head elevated to improve breathing

73. Briefly explain the function of each of the chambers/bottles of a three-bottle/chamber water seal drainage system that is used with chest tubes. Indicate key nursing interventions related to each chamber.
    a. Bottle/chamber 1

    b. Bottle/chamber 2

    c. Bottle/chamber 3

74. Which of the following is a correct nursing intervention for clients with chest tubes?
    a. Clients should be encouraged to cough and do deep breathing exercises frequently.
    b. Vigorous "stripping" of the chest tubes should be done routinely to prevent obstruction by blood clots.
    c. Water level in the suction chamber need not be monitored, just the collection chamber.
    d. Drainage containers can be positioned upright or on the side with tubing in no particular position.

75. Upon observation of a chest tube setup, the nurse reports to the physician that there is a leak in the chest tube and system. The nurse assesses this problem by noting which of the following?
    a. Drainage in the collection chamber has decreased.
    b. The bubbling in the suction chamber has suddenly increased.
    c. Fluctuation in the water seal chamber has stopped.
    d. Onset of vigorous bubbling in the water seal chamber.

76. For a client with a chest tube, the physician's orders indicate an increase in the suction to 20 mL. To implement this order, the nurse would perform which of the following interventions?
    a. Increase the wall suction to medium suction to maintain the bubbling in the suction chamber.
    b. Add water to the water seal chamber to the level of 20.
    c. Stop the bubbling in the suction chamber, add sterile water to level of 20, and resume bubbling.
    d. Have client cough and deep breathe, and monitor the level of fluctuation to achieve 20 cm.

77. Discharge teaching considerations for clients with a thoracotomy, especially with a pneumonectomy, is which of the following?
    a. Prevent arm immobility problems by use of range-of-motion exercises and increasing the use of the arm.
    b. Protect the operative site and prevent complications by limiting the motion of the arm/shoulder with a sling.
    c. Resume preoperative activities as soon as possible to promote well-being, independence, and autonomy.
    d. Change pain medication or decrease pain medication to minimize respiratory depression effects of narcotics.

78. Briefly summarize nursing interventions for a client with a thoracotomy.

79. Which of the following is not a factor in the development of lung cancer?
    a. Air pollution
    b. Radon gas exposure
    c. Chronic respiratory disease
    d. Chewing tobacco

80. Identify the nursing diagnoses common to the client with lung cancer.

    a. _____

    b. _____

    c. _____

81. The major complication from treatment with the chemotherapy agent cisplatin is which of the following?
    a. Diarrhea
    b. Nausea
    c. Flatulence
    d. Constipation

82. The most effective intervention for relieving pain resulting from bone metastases caused by lung cancer that still allows for mobility is which of the following?
    a. Radiation therapy
    b. Patient-controlled analgesia
    c. Continuous morphine infusion
    d. Oral meperidine hydrochloride (Demerol)

83. A chest tube system that drains by gravity is functioning correctly when the water seal chamber does which of the following?
    a. Bubbles vigorously and continuously
    b. Bubbles gently and continuously
    c. Fluctuates with the client's respirations
    d. Fluctuates vigorously when the client coughs

84. Interventions to promote comfort in the client with lung cancer include which of the following?
    a. Medicating with analgesics only when requested
    b. Positioning prone with a pillow under abdomen and shins
    c. Ventilating with a high tidal volume and PEEP
    d. Providing supplemental oxygen via cannula or mask

85. A client with small-cell lung cancer is being discharged from the hospital. Which of the following community resources would the nurse potentially discuss with this client?
    a. The local hospice program
    b. A home health care agency
    c. A vendor of durable medical supplies
    d. All of the above

86. A client with repeated pleural effusions, as a result of lung cancer, is injected with a sclerosing agent. The nurse's role is to do which of the following?
    a. Assist in positioning the client so that the affected lung is dependent while the drug is being injected.
    b. Clamp the chest tube securely following the instillation of the drug.
    c. Instruct the client to remain very still for at least 1 hour after the drug has been injected.
    d. Notify the respiratory therapist to administer respiratory therapy treatments.

87. A severe complication of pulmonary hypertension is which of the following problems?
    a. Right side heart enlargement, dilation, and failure
    b. Left side of heart enlargement, dilation, and failure
    c. Decreased cardiac output related to left ventricular failure
    d. Narrowing of the pulse pressure

88. Which of the following is the name of the complication defined in Question 87?
    a. Myocardial infarction
    b. ARDS
    c. Cor pulmonale
    d. Stroke

89. Which of the following is not diagnostic of pulmonary hypertension?
    a. Client complains of fatigue and dyspnea
    b. Normal ventilation-perfusion scans ($\dot{V}/\dot{Q}$ scans)
    c. Changes in pulmonary function test
    d. Cardiac catheterization of right side heart indicates elevated pulmonary pressures

90. A client has developed pulmonary hypertension. Which of the following is not included in the care of this client?
    a. Coumadin
    b. Beta blockers
    c. Oxygen therapy
    d. Diuretics

91. *Decide whether each of the following statements about pulmonary hypertension are true or false. Write T for true or F for false in the blanks provided. Correct the false statements so that they are true.*

    _____ a. Conditions such as COPD, pulmonary fibrosis, and pulmonary emboli can result in pulmonary hypertension.

    _____ b. When treating cor pulmonale, collaborative management is designed around the underlying cause of pulmonary hypertension.

    _____ c. When medical management fails, heart-lung or lung transplantation might be necessary.

92. Which of the following statements about sarcoidosis is correct?
    a. Sarcoidosis is a chronic disorder of the alveoli characterized by granuloma development.
    b. Sarcoidosis is a group of diseases also known as interstitial lung disease.
    c. Sarcoidosis is an acute disorder of the alveoli characterized by granuloma development.
    d. Sarcoidosis is caused by the sarcoid pneumonia bacterium and is highly contagious.

93. Granuloma development in sarcoidosis results from the activation of which of the following?
    a. Lymphocytes
    b. T-lymphocytes
    c. Macrophages
    d. Monocytes

94. Drug treatment of sarcoidosis includes which of the following?
    a. Antibiotics
    b. Bronchodilators
    c. Corticosteroids
    d. Chemotherapeutic agents

95. The similarity between pulmonary fibrosis and sarcoidosis is which of the following?
    a. Both result in death if a lung transplantation is not performed.
    b. Both are treated by steroids.
    c. Both are progressive with a slow onset.
    d. Both are a result of excessive inflammatory response.

96. A client with a history of CAL enters the emergency department with severe dyspnea with noted accessory muscle involvement and neck vein distention, along with severe inspiratory/expiratory wheezing. This respiratory emergency is diagnosed as which of the following life-threatening conditions?
    a. Pulmonary fibrosis
    b. Pulmonary hypertension
    c. Exacerbation of sarcoidosis
    d. Status asthmaticus

97. Status asthmaticus is a potentially life-threatening problem requiring immediate interventions because of which of the following?
    a. Usual interventions are ineffective; it tends to intensify and progress, and IV fluids with medications are required.
    b. The asthma attack causes a pneumothorax resulting in audible wheezing and need of a chest tube.
    c. Neck vein distention is a signal of imminent left-sided heart failure and decreased cardiac output.
    d. Respiratory arrest will occur without the required intubation and mechanical ventilation.

98. Identify specific nursing interventions for an older adult client with respiratory disorders.

Interventions for Clients with Infectious Problems of the Respiratory Tract

LEARNING OUTCOMES

1. Explain the consequences of an untreated streptococcal infection of the upper respiratory tract.
2. Identify adults at highest risk for contracting influenza.
3. Develop a teaching plan to prevent influenza in the older adult.
4. Identify clients at risk for developing community-acquired or hospital-acquired pneumonia.
5. Compare the manifestations of pneumonia in the younger adult with those exhibited by the older adult client with pneumonia.
6. Describe the mechanisms of action, side effects, and nursing implications of drug therapy for pneumonia.
7. Identify adults at risk for tuberculosis (TB).
8. Interpret correctly the TB test results for a person with normal immune function and a person with human immunodeficiency virus/acquired immunodeficiency syndrome (HIV/AIDS).
9. Describe the mechanisms of action, side effects, and nursing implications of drug therapy for TB.
10. Develop a community-based teaching plan for continuing care of the client with active TB.
11. Compare the early and late manifestations of inhalation anthrax with those of other lower respiratory infections.

LEARNING ACTIVITIES

1. Before completing the study guide exercises in this chapter, it is recommended that you review the following:
   - Assessment of the respiratory system
   - Anatomy and physiology of the lower respiratory tract
   - Principles of normal defense mechanisms of the body
   - Principles of infection control and isolation
   - Incentive spirometry technique
   - Collecting sputum specimens
   - Throat culture technique

2. Review the boldfaced terms and their definitions in Chapter 34 to enhance your understanding of the content.

STUDY/REVIEW QUESTIONS

Answers to the Study/Review Questions are provided on the companion Evolve Learning Resources Web site at http://evolve.elsevier.com/Iggy/.

1. Your adult client diagnosed with rhinitis complains of itchy, watery eyes and rhinorrhea every fall season. Which of the following best explains rhinitis?
    a. Allergic rhinitis and coryza are initiated by sensitivity reactions to antigens.
    b. Viral rhinitis and hay fever are initiated by sensitivity reactions to antigens.
    c. Allergic rhinitis and hay fever are initiated by sensitivity reactions to allergens.
    d. Rhinitis medicamentous is relieved with the use of nose drops or sprays.

2. A client's history of which of the following disorders is a contraindication for drug therapy in providing symptomatic treatment of rhinitis?
    a. Sleep apnea
    b. Diverticulitis
    c. Ménière's disease
    d. Urinary retention

3. When prescribing drugs for treatment of rhinitis and sinusitis, which of the following classes of drugs would not be included?
    a. Antihistamines
    b. Antipyretics
    c. Decongestants
    d. Mucolytics

4. An assessment of which of the following would most likely follow or accompany rhinitis?
    a. Pharyngitis
    b. Tonsillitis
    c. Laryngitis
    d. Sinusitis

5. Which of the following statements regarding rhinitis and the older adult is true?
    a. Viral rhinitis is self-limiting and rarely leads to complications in the older adult.
    b. Antihistamines and decongestants should be used with caution.
    c. Antipyretics and antibiotics are not used because of risk of toxicity and allergic reactions.
    d. Complementary and alternative therapies are ineffective in the older adult.

6. A client complains of difficulty breathing, facial pain (especially when head is dependent), sneezing or coughing, green or bloody nasal drainage, productive cough, and low-grade fever. The client will be treated with antibiotics for which of the following diagnoses?
    a. Rhinitis
    b. Tonsillitis
    c. Sinusitis
    d. Pneumonia

7. If the client in Question 6 above had an upper airway infection related to a virus, would this client receive antibiotics? Indicate yes or no and give a reason for your answer.

8. An older adult diagnosed with bacterial pharyngitis may not present with which of the following assessment findings?
    a. Cough and rash
    b. High fever and elevated WBC count
    c. Voice characterized by pain on voicing
    d. Erythema of tonsils with yellow exudate

9. A client is seen in the physician's office for pharyngitis. Which of the following assessment findings is most indicative of a bacteria infection versus a viral infection? Identify other key features of acute viral versus bacterial pharyngitis.
   a. Fever
   b. Erythema of throat
   c. Headache
   d. Positive throat culture

10. A client complains of a "sore throat"/pharyngitis pain, temperature of 101.4° F, scarlatiniform rash, and a positive rapid test throat culture. This client will most likely be treated for which type of bacterial infection?
    a. *Staphylococcus*
    b. *Pneumococcus*
    c. *Streptococcus*
    d. Epstein-Barr virus

11. A client complains of a sore throat that is an indication of "strep throat." To prevent complications such as rheumatic heart disease, this client should receive antibiotic treatment within what time frame?
    a. 24 hours
    b. 48 hours
    c. 1 week
    d. 1 month

12. A priority nursing intervention for the nursing diagnosis of Deficient Knowledge related to the treatment of Group B *Streptococcus* infection would include which of the following?
    a. Administration of penicillin or penicillin-like antibiotics
    b. Gradually resuming activity until there are no physical complaints
    c. Full liquid supplemental diet such as Ensure
    d. Observing for signs and symptoms of glomerulonephritis and rheumatic heart disease

13. A few weeks after having a group A beta-hemolytic streptococcal pharyngitis, a client complains of joint pain, weakness, and a rash of the inner aspects of the upper arm and thigh. These assessment findings are indicative of which complication of group A streptococcal infection?
    a. Acute glomerulonephritis
    b. Arthritis
    c. Rheumatic fever
    d. Scarlet fever

14. A 35-year-old male client with no health problems states that he had a flu shot last year and asks if it is necessary to have a flu shot again this year. Which of the following is the best response by the nurse?
    a. "No, because once you get a flu shot, it lasts for several years and is effective against many different viruses."
    b. "Yes, because the immunity against virus wears off, increasing your chances of getting the flu."
    c. "Yes, because the vaccine guards against a specific virus and reduces your chances of acquiring flu."
    d. "No, flu shots are only for high-risk clients and you are not considered to be at high risk."

15. An active 45-year-old schoolteacher with COPD taking the medication prednisone inquires about getting flu shots. Which of the following is the best response by the nurse?:
    a. "Yes, flu shots are highly recommended for a client with chronic illness and/or receiving immunotherapy."
    b. "No, flu shots are only recommended for clients 50 years old and older."
    c. "Yes, it will help minimize the risk of triggering an exacerbation of COPD."
    d. "No, clients who are active, do not live in a nursing home, and are not health care providers do not need to get flu shots."

16. The body structure primarily affected by pneumonia is which of the following?
    a. Bronchi
    b. Pharynx
    c. Alveoli
    d. Trachea

17. Identify three pathologic results that occur in the lung as a result of pneumonia.

    a. _____

    b. _____

    c. _____

18. Number the following events in sequential order as pertains to the pathophysiologic process of pneumonia.

    _____ a. Atelectasis

    _____ b. Possible septicemia

    _____ c. Decreased surfactant production and compliance

    _____ d. Arterial hypoxemia

    _____ e. Edema formation and inflammation

    _____ f. Tachypnea and tachycardia

    _____ g. Migration of white blood cells (WBCs) to alveoli

    _____ h. Spread of organisms to other alveoli

    _____ i. Shunting of unoxygenated blood

    _____ j. Thickening of alveolar wall and stiffening of lung

    _____ k. Diminished capillary blood flow in alveoli

    _____ l. Invasion of pulmonary tissue by pathogens

19. Decreased lung compliance in pneumonia is the result of which of the following pathologic problems?
    a. Occlusion of the bronchi and alveoli
    b. Inflammatory edema and decreased surfactant production
    c. Inflammatory edema and a ventilation-perfusion defect
    d. Atelectasis and WBC migration to the affected area

20. Which of the following clients are at the highest risk of developing pneumonia?
    a. Any hospitalized client between the ages of 18 and 65 years
    b. A 32-year-old trauma client on a mechanical ventilator
    c. A disabled 54-year-old client living at home with osteoporosis
    d. Any client who has not received the vaccine for pneumonia

21. After being seen at the doctor's office, a client states, "The doctor said I have pneumonia." The nurse gives which of the following explanations for pneumonia?
    a. It is an infection of just the "windpipe" because the lungs are "clear" of any problems.
    b. It is a serious inflammation of the bronchioles from various causes.
    c. It is only an infection of the lungs with mild-to-severe effects on the breathing.
    d. It is an inflammation resulting from lung damage from long-term smoking.

22. For the client in Question 21, which of the following would most likely be the first diagnostic test performed?
    a. Lung scan
    b. Pulmonary function test
    c. Fluorescein bronchoscopy
    d. Sputum Gram stain

23. Which of the following is a common laboratory value finding as a result of pneumonia? What group of clients are exceptions to this finding?
    a. Increased erythrocyte maturation
    b. Increased number of RBCs
    c. Decreased number of WBCs
    d. Increased number of WBCs

24. A client with impaired gas exchange and pneumonia has a primary problem with which of the following? Identify a nursing intervention to correct this problem.
    a. Hypoxemia
    b. Hyperemia
    c. Hypocapnia
    d. Hypercapnia

25. Match each commonly seen organism to the corresponding type of pneumonia. *Answers may be used more than once.*

Organisms

_____ a. *Legionella pneumophila*

_____ b. *Pseudomonas aeruginosa*

_____ c. *Staphylococcus aureus*

_____ d. *Klebsiella pneumoniae*

_____ e. *Mycoplasma pneumoniae*

_____ f. *Streptococcus pneumoniae*

_____ g. *Candida albicans*

_____ h. *Pneumocystis carinii*

Types of Pneumonia
1. Community-acquired pneumonia
2. Nosocomial pneumonia
3. Opportunistic pneumonia

26. A client with acquired immunodeficiency syndrome (AIDS) is diagnosed with *Pneumocystis carinii* pneumonia. Identify the clinical manifestations that a nurse would assess.

27. A history, physical examination, and chest x-ray indicate pneumonia. The physician would suspect community-acquired pneumonia based on what assessment finding?
    a. A dry cough
    b. Slow onset of symptoms
    c. Abrupt onset of fever and chills
    d. Sudden change in mental status

28. Which of the following clients is the least likely to be at risk for developing pneumonia? Explain your answer.
    a. A client with a 5-year history of smoking
    b. A renal transplant client
    c. A postoperative client walking in the halls
    d. A postoperative client with a hip replacement

29. An essential diagnostic test for pneumonia in the older adult is which of the following tests?
    a. Pulse oximetry because of the older adult's normal decreased lung compliance
    b. Sputum specimen for accuracy of antibiotics to decrease risk of renal failure
    c. Elevated white blood cell count confirming findings of pleuritic chest pain, chills, fever, cough, and dyspnea
    d. Chest x-rays because assessment findings can be vague and resemble other problems

30. A client is admitted to the hospital because of pneumonia. The nurse would expect the chest x-ray results to reveal which of following?
    a. Patchy areas of consolidation
    b. Tension pneumothorax
    c. Thick secretions causing airway obstruction
    d. Stenosed pulmonary arteries

31. For most hospitalized clients, prevention of pneumonia is accomplished by which of the following nursing interventions?
    a. Monitoring chest x-rays for early signs of pneumonia
    b. Monitoring lung sounds every shift and forcing fluids
    c. Teaching the client coughing and deep breathing exercises and incentive spirometry
    d. Ensuring respiratory therapy treatments are being performed every 4 hours

32. Education of clients in practices that prevent pneumonia would include which of the following nursing interventions?
    a. Administering vaccines to clients at risk
    b. Implementing strict bedrest for debilitated clients
    c. Restricting food and fluids in immunosuppressed clients
    d. Decontaminating respiratory therapy equipment weekly

33. The rationale for health care providers differentiating between nosocomial versus community-acquired pneumonia is useful because:
    a. Nosocomial infections are more likely to respond to antibiotics.
    b. Nosocomial infections, although common, are caused by organisms that are more resistant to treatment.
    c. The mortality rate is high in individuals with community-acquired pneumonia.
    d. Nosocomial pneumonia often occurs in clients in the fall and winter months after they have had a viral infection.

34. Identify three ways that an individual can develop pneumonia.

    a. _____

    b. _____

    c. _____

35. The key to effective treatment for the nursing diagnosis of Risk for Sepsis is administration of antibiotics. Initial antibiotic therapy is based on which of the following factors?
    a. Gram stains, sputum culture, chest x-ray film
    b. Client's signs and symptoms and type (nosocomial or community-acquired) of pneumonia
    c. Clinical assessment findings with elevated white blood cells
    d. Client's history, physical, and chest x-ray film results

36. A client hospitalized for pneumonia has a nursing diagnosis of Ineffective Airway Clearance related to fatigue, chest pain, excessive secretions, and muscle weakness. The nursing intervention to correct these problems includes which of the following?
    a. Administer oxygen to prevent hypoxemia and atelectasis.
    b. Push fluids to greater than 3000 mL/day to ensure adequate hydration.
    c. Administer respiratory therapy in a timely manner to decrease bronchospasms.
    d. Maintain semi-Fowler's position to facilitate breathing and prevent further fatigue.

37. A client is admitted to the hospital for treatment of pneumonia. Which of the following nursing assessment findings best indicates that the client is responding to the antibiotic?
    a. Wheezing, oxygen at 2 L, respiratory rate 26, no shortness of breath or chills
    b. Temperature 99° F, lung sounds clear, pulse oximetry on 2 L at 98%, cough with yellow sputum
    c. Complains of cough, white sputum, temperature 99° F, pulse oximetry at 96% on room air
    d. Complains of feeling tired, respiratory rate 28 on 2 L of oxygen, loud clear breath sounds

38. Which of the following laboratory values may not be seen in the older adult diagnosed with pneumonia?
    a. RBC 4.0 to 5.0
    b. Hgb 12 to 16
    c. Hct 36 to 48
    d. WBC 12 to 18

39. A client is admitted to the hospital to rule out pneumonia. Regarding isolation technique, the nurse would maintain which of the following nursing interventions?
    a. Strict respiratory isolation and use of a specially designed face mask only
    b. Respiratory isolation and contact isolation for sputum only
    c. Respiratory isolation with the stock surgical mask
    d. Standard precautions and no respiratory isolation

40. Upon admission, a critical concern of a client is often related to impaired gas exchange caused by inadequate ventilation. Which of the following values would indicate to the nurse that oxygen and incentive spirometry need to be administered?
    a. Pao_2 is 64 and clear lung sounds
    b. Pao_2 is 64 with atelectasis
    c. Pco_2 is 38 with crackles
    d. Pco_2 is 38 with atelectasis

41. The client with pneumonia with ineffective airway clearance has developed bronchospasms. The appropriate nursing intervention would be which of the following?
    a. Increase the number of liters of oxygen and deliver humidified oxygen.
    b. Notify the physician of the need for an order for round-the-clock aerosol nebulizer bronchodilator treatments.
    c. Notify the physician of client status and get an order for handheld bronchodilator inhaler as needed.
    d. Notify the physician of the need for prednisone via inhaler or IV to reduce the inflammation causing the spasms.

42. A client is admitted to the hospital because of pneumonia. Which of the following is true regarding administration of antibiotics?
    a. Obtain a sputum culture before starting any antibiotic therapy.
    b. Broad spectrum IV antibiotic therapy should be started without delay to improve client outcomes.
    c. Wait for sputum culture results with specificity before starting antibiotic therapy.
    d. Obtain at least three sputum specimens before starting IV antibiotics to reduce risk of toxicity.

43. An older adult client asks the nurse how often one should receive the pneumococcal vaccine for preventing pneumonia. The nurse's best response would be which of the following?
    a. Every year, when the client is receiving the "flu shot."
    b. The standard of care for clients is every 3 years.
    c. The recommendation is every 5 years; however, older adults may need it more frequently.
    d. There is no standard; it depends on the client's history and risk factors.

44. A client who was hospitalized for pneumonia is being discharged to home. Write a plan of care for the nursing diagnosis of Deficient Knowledge related to prevention of upper respiratory infections.

45. A nurse is providing discharge instructions to a client and family. Which of the following is the correct discharge instruction regarding pneumonia?
    a. Complete antibiotics as prescribed; rest; drink fluids; and minimize contact with crowds.
    b. Take all antibiotics as ordered; resume diet and all activities as before hospitalization.
    c. No restrictions regarding activities, diet, and rest because the client is fully recovered when discharged.
    d. Continue antibiotics only until no further signs of pneumonia are seen.

46. Which of the following medications would be given to the client with Ineffective Airway Clearance related to productive, prolonged coughing?
    a. Guaifenesin with 3.5% alcohol (Robitussin)
    b. Benzonatate (Tessalon)
    c. Oxtriphylline with guaifenesin (Brondecon)
    d. Propylhexedrine (Benzedrex)

47. A client has a nursing diagnosis of Ineffective Airway Clearance. Interventions that help liquefy secretions for expectoration include which of the following measures?
    a. Performing postural drainage twice a day
    b. Using an incentive spirometer every 4 hours
    c. Coughing and deep breathing every 2 hours
    d. Encouraging a minimum fluid intake of 2500 to 3000 mL a day

48. Drug agents used in the management of pneumonia would include which of the following?
    a. Cough suppressants
    b. Antibiotics
    c. Mucolytic agents
    d. Corticosteroids

49. Which of the following instructions should be given to the client with pneumonia who is being discharged to home care?
    a. "You may discontinue the deep breathing exercises after 2 weeks when you stop coughing."
    b. "You will continue to feel tired and will fatigue easily for the next several weeks."
    c. "Try to drink 1 quart of water every day until you have finished all the antibiotics."
    d. "You should be able to return to work full-time in 2 weeks when your energy returns."

50. A complication of pneumonia that creates pain by causing friction between the layers of pleura is which of the following? Identify four other complications and define each of them.
    a. Pleuritic chest pain
    b. Pulmonary emboli
    c. Pleural effusion
    d. Meningitis

    (1) _____

    (2) _____

    (3) _____

    (4) _____

51. Identify clients who are at risk for developing aspiration pneumonia and nursing interventions that can be implemented to prevent aspiration pneumonia.

52. Identify agents that may cause a noninfectious type of pneumonia.

53. A client is admitted to the hospital for pneumonia. What common assessment findings would the nurse expect?

54. A 60-year-old client is admitted to the hospital for treatment of pneumonia. Which of the following antibiotics would be recommended for treatment and why?
    a. Vancomycin
    b. Ampicillin
    c. Levofloxacin
    d. Piperacillin

55. Which of the following clients is at risk for community-acquired pneumonia?
    a. A client on tube feedings
    b. A client with history of tobacco use
    c. A client with poor nutritional status
    d. A client with altered mental status

56. A client with HIV is admitted to the hospital with a temperature of 99.6° F, complaints of bloody sputum, night sweats, feeling of tiredness, and shortness of breath. These assessment findings indicate which of the following diagnoses?
    a. Pneumocystic pneumonia (PCP)
    b. Tuberculosis
    c. Superinfection as a result of a low CD4 count
    d. Bacterial pneumonia

57. Which of the following statements regarding transmission of tuberculosis (TB) is true?
    a. Exposure to a client with TB results in active disease within 2 to 10 weeks.
    b. The causative agent of TB is transmitted via aerosolization (airborne).
    c. It is considered to be an acute disease with no risk for reoccurrence.
    d. The "exposed/infected" client is considered as being the same as having active TB.

58. Number the following steps of type IV delayed hypersensitivity reaction to the infectious microbe *Mycobacterium tuberculosis* in sequential order.
    _____ a. Cavity forms involving connecting bronchi.
    _____ b. T cells become sensitized to the tubercle.
    _____ c. A Ghon tubercle forms.
    _____ d. Tubercles enter the respiratory tract.
    _____ e. Fibrosis and calcification of the lesion occur.
    _____ f. Granuloma becomes necrotic and cheesy in appearance.
    _____ g. Lymphokines are released and activate macrophages.
    _____ h. A multinucleated giant cell (granuloma) forms.

59. Which of the following clients is at the greatest risk for developing TB?
    a. A 22-year-old college woman living in a double room in a dormitory
    b. A 62-year-old retired schoolteacher living in a house with her widowed sister
    c. A 42-year-old alcoholic homeless man who occasionally stays in a shelter
    d. A 53-year-old housewife who does volunteer work in a shelter for the homeless

60. The most substantial impact in incidence of TB is from which of the following high-risk populations?
    a. Older adults, the homeless, minorities
    b. Lower socioeconomic groups
    c. Those in constant frequent contact with untreated individuals
    d. Those with immune dysfunction, particularly HIV

61. After several weeks of "not feeling well," a client is seen in the physician's office for possible TB. The assessment findings include which of the following if TB is present?
    a. Fatigue, night sweats, and low-grade fever
    b. Weight gain, bloody streaked sputum, and night sweats
    c. Hemoptysis, loss of appetite, and high fever
    d. Nonproductive cough, fatigue, and anorexia

62. Which of the following test results indicate the client has clinically active TB?
    a. Induration of 12 mm and positive sputum
    b. Positive chest x-ray for TB only
    c. Positive chest x-ray and clinical symptoms
    d. Client complaints of signs and symptoms

63. After receiving the subcutaneous Mantoux skin test, a client with no risk factors returns to the clinic in the required 48 to 72 hours for a reading of the test. Assessment findings of which of the following would indicate a positive test result?
    a. The test area is red, warm, and tender to touch.
    b. There is induration or a hard nodule of any size at the sight.
    c. The induration/hardened area measures 5 mm or greater.
    d. The induration/hardened area measures 10 mm or greater.

64. A client has a positive skin test result. What explanation does the nurse give to the client?
    a. There is active disease but client is not yet infectious to others.
    b. There is active disease, and client needs immediate treatment.
    c. The client has been infected but that does not mean active disease is present.
    d. A follow-up chest x-ray is necessary because the test could be a false-positive result.

65. A client with TB has been prescribed two or more pharmacologic agents. Explain why this treatment is prescribed.

66. The nurse explains to the client that the minimum treatment time period for TB is which of the following?
    a. 7 to 10 days
    b. 3 weeks
    c. 3 months
    d. 6 months

67. The client is no longer infectious/communicable when which of the following test results is seen?
    a. Negative chest x-ray
    b. No clinical symptoms
    c. Negative skin tests
    d. Three negative sputum cultures

68. In teaching a client about the medication, the best time for a client to take these chemotherapeutic agents for TB is which of the following?
    a. Before breakfast
    b. After breakfast
    c. At midday
    d. At bedtime

69. To prevent TB, clients with HIV infection who have less than 10-mm induration on the TB skin test and no clinical symptoms would receive which of the following medications for a period of 12 months?
    a. Bacille Calmette-Guérin (BCG) vaccine
    b. Isoniazid (INH)
    c. Ethambutol
    d. Streptomycin

70. Describe the initial drug protocol for a client with active TB.

71. Describe the nursing interventions for the nursing diagnosis of Ineffective Health Maintenance related to the client not taking the medication for TB as prescribed.

72. A client diagnosed with TB has been receiving treatment for 3 weeks and has clinically shown improvement. The family asked the nurse if the client is still infectious. The nurse will reply to this question with which of the following statements?
    a. "The client is still infectious until the entire treatment is completed."
    b. "The client is not infectious but needs to continue treatment for at least 6 months."
    c. "The client is infectious until there is negative chest x-ray."
    d. "The client may or may not be infectious. A PPD needs to be done."

73. An older adult client complains of loss of hearing and dizziness after 1 month of taking the medication for TB. The nurse would advise the client to do which of the following?
    a. Continue taking the medication; the symptom will eventually go away.
    b. Consult a physician because this could be a sign of toxicity.
    c. Not be concerned because this symptom is common with all TB medications.
    d. Wait for 3 months, if the symptom continues, consult a physician.

74. Match the following nursing interventions with the medications to treat TB. *Answers may be used more than once.*

Nursing Interventions

_____ a. Assess client's hearing before starting medication.

_____ b. Teach client that urine will be orange in color.

_____ c. Consult physician for dose reduction when the client complains of blurry vision after starting treatment.

_____ d. Teach the client not to take medications such as Maalox with this medication.

_____ e. Obtain baseline and monitor laboratory values: CPK, LDH, SGOT, and uric acid.

_____ f. Monitor creatine and BUN lab values.

_____ g. Teach client to take in morning, preferably before eating unless it causes an "upset stomach."

_____ h. Teach to take with food to decrease GI upset.

_____ i. Closely monitor anticoagulant laboratory values for clients because it may interfere with this medication.

_____ j. Teach clients to identify changes in the ability to differentiate colors.

TB Medications
1. Isoniazid (INH)
2. Rifampin
3. Pyrazinamide
4. Ethambutol
5. Streptomycin
6. Amikacin

75. A client with suspected TB is admitted to the hospital. Which of the following nursing interventions is correct relating to isolation procedure? The nurse would maintain which of the following?
    a. Private room, respiratory isolation, and contact isolation for sputum only
    b. Private room, strict respiratory isolation, and only use specially designed face masks
    c. Private room, respiratory isolation with hospital surgical masks until diagnosis is confirmed
    d. Private room, no respiratory isolation necessary until diagnosis is confirmed

76. A client is admitted to the hospital to "rule-out" TB. What type of mask should the nurse wear when caring for this client?
    a. Surgical face mask
    b. Surgical face mask with eye shield
    c. HEPA respirator
    d. Any type of mask that covers the nose and mouth

77. A client seen in the outpatient clinic is diagnosed with TB. Which of the following nursing interventions is correct related to public health policy?
    a. Only contact the infection control nurse at the hospital.
    b. There are no regulations because the client was seen in the clinic and was not hospitalized.
    c. Contact the public health nurse so that all individuals who have come in contact with client can be screened.
    d. Have the client sign a waiver regarding the hospital's liability for treatment.

78. What interventions can a nurse perform in meeting the Healthy People 2010 objectives for tuberculosis?

79. Which of the following is not a diagnostic test for TB?
    a. Chest radiography
    b. Complete blood count
    c. Mantoux skin test
    d. Sputum culture

80. Identify the subjective data that are relevant to a client with TB.

81. Which of the following is a physical symptom of TB? Identify other physical findings.
    a. Fatigue
    b. Weight gain
    c. High-grade fever
    d. Nonproductive cough

82. The older adult is more susceptible to respiratory infection because of which of the following etiologies?
    a. Inability to force a cough
    b. Weak chest wall muscles
    c. Decreased alveoli surfactant
    d. Macrophages in alveoli are decreased

CASE STUDY: THE OLDER CLIENT WITH TUBERCULOSIS

Answer Guidelines for the Case Study questions are provided on the companion Evolve Learning Resources Web site at http://evolve.elsevier.com/Iggy/.

Your client is a 65-year-old woman who shares a three-room inner-city apartment with two of her daughters and their seven children. She comes into the neighborhood walk-in clinic complaining of extreme fatigue, a 30-pound weight loss, and a cough of 4 months' duration. A Mantoux test, sputum culture, and chest x-ray confirm a diagnosis of tuberculosis. She is to begin a 12-month course of medication therapy with isoniazid (INH) 300 mg PO qd and rifampin (Rifadin) 600 mg PO qd.

1. Discuss why one or more pharmacologic agents are used to treat tuberculosis.

2. When is the best time for this client to take the chemotherapeutic agents to minimize the side effects?

3. Why should rifampin (Rifadin) be taken on an empty stomach?

4. What type of follow-up care should be planned for this client?

5. How long will this client be considered contagious?

6. What measures should be taken with the other family members? Explain your answer.

7. Develop a teaching-learning plan for this client.

Three weeks after diagnosis, the client returns to the clinic stating that she has stopped taking her medications because they make her sick to her stomach. She is unable to eat and has continued to lose weight.

8. Identify the relevant nursing diagnoses for this client based on the above data.

9. Discuss what the nurse should do to assist this client in taking her medications and eating a balanced diet.

CASE STUDY: THE YOUNG CLIENT WITH TUBERCULOSIS

Answer Guidelines for the Case Study questions are provided on the companion Evolve Learning Resources Web site at http://evolve.elsevier.com/Iggy/.

Your client is a 25-year-old inner-city woman with AIDS. She is hospitalized now for active TB. She has four young children who are currently being cared for by her mother, a 42-year-old unemployed woman with diabetes mellitus.

1. What kind of isolation must this client be placed in and why?

2. Sputum cultures for AFB are ordered. When is the best time to collect sputum?

3. Can you send sputum that contains saliva to the laboratory?

4. Before the client is discharged, what interventions need to be done at her home in preparation for her return?

2. What will the nurse probably hear when she auscultates the client's lungs? Explain your answer.

A diagnosis of pneumonia is confirmed by the chest x-ray and sputum cultures. Because the client's blood gases are within normal limits, she will be managed on an outpatient basis.

3. Identify the relevant nursing diagnoses for this client based on above data.

CASE STUDY: THE CLIENT WITH PNEUMONIA

Answer Guidelines for the Case Study questions are provided on the companion Evolve Learning Resources Web site at http://evolve.elsevier.com/Iggy/.

A 75-year-old married woman reports to the outpatient clinic with her husband. She has had a severe cough, says that she has had left-sided chest pain, and holds her left side while coughing. She appears anxious. Her face is flushed. Vital signs are temperature 102.6° F, pulse 118, apical; respirations 32, shallow, and blood pressure 120/80. A diagnosis of pneumonia is suspected. A sputum specimen, chest x-ray, arterial blood gases, and CBC are ordered.

1. What should the nurse teach this client and her husband about the sputum collection and x-ray?

The physician orders cefaclor (Ceclor) 500 mg PO every 8 hours and wants the client to return to the clinic in 1 week. If her condition does not improve within 48 hours or she becomes short of breath, she should call or return to the clinic.

4. Develop teaching-learning and discharge care plans for the client and her husband.

Interventions for Critically Ill Clients with Respiratory Problems

LEARNING OUTCOMES

1. Identify clients at risk for development of pulmonary embolism.
2. Describe the clinical manifestations of pulmonary embolism.
3. Use laboratory data and clinical manifestations to determine the presence of acidosis.
4. Describe the precautions to use for clients receiving heparin or warfarin.
5. Develop a community-based teaching plan for the client who has had a pulmonary embolism.
6. Compare the features of respiratory failure of ventilatory origin with those of respiratory failure of oxygenation origin.
7. Use laboratory data and clinical manifestations to determine the adequacy of ventilatory interventions.
8. Describe the indications for intubation.
9. Prioritize nursing care for the conscious client being mechanically ventilated.
10. Develop interventions to communicate effectively with a client who is unable to talk as a result of intubation.
11. Identify clients at risk for development of pneumothorax.

LEARNING ACTIVITIES

1. Before completing the study guide exercises for this chapter, it is recommended that you review the following:
   - Anatomy and physiology of the lower respiratory tract
   - Process of respiration
   - Principles of diffusion, perfusion, and ventilation
   - Interpretation of blood gas measurements
   - Acid-base balance, acidosis, and alkalosis
   - Hemodynamic monitoring
   - Principles of oxygen therapy
   - Principles of perioperative nursing management
   - Concepts of body image
   - Principles of human sexuality
   - Tracheostomy care and principles of suctioning

2. Review the boldfaced terms and their definitions in Chapter 35 to enhance your understanding of the content.

STUDY/REVIEW QUESTIONS

Answers to the Study/Review Questions are provided on the companion Evolve Learning Resources Web site at http://evolve.elsevier.com/Iggy/.

1. A postoperative client complains of sudden onset of shortness of breath and pleuritic chest pain. Assessment findings include diaphoresis, hypotension, crackles in the left lower lobe, and pulse oximetry of 85%. The nurse interprets these findings as possible:
   a. Bacterial pneumonia
   b. Pneumothorax
   c. Pulmonary embolism
   d. Atelectasis

2. Indicate which of the following clients the nurse would monitor for a pulmonary embolus and provide preventive measures. *Mark Y for yes or N for no, and provide a brief rationale for your answer.*

   _____ a. Client with total hip or knee replacement, postoperative

   _____ b. Client with low protein S or protein C value

   _____ c. First day postoperative client with cervical diskectomy

   _____ d. Client with previous history of deep vein thrombosis

   _____ e. Hospitalized dehydrated older adult client

   _____ f. Client with sickle cell anemia

   _____ g. Pneumonia client, out of bed in chair

   _____ h. 5-foot, 5-inch adult weighing 250 pounds

   _____ i. Pregnant woman

   _____ j. Woman in labor about to deliver

   _____ k. Client with aspiration pneumonia

   _____ l. Client with abdominal surgery, postoperative

   _____ m. Client with atrial fibrillation

   _____ n. Client with spinal cord injury and paralysis

   _____ o. All clients with the nursing diagnosis of Impaired Mobility

3. The most common site of origin for a pulmonary embolism (PE) is which of the following?
   a. Clots in the right side of the heart
   b. Arterial microemboli such as amniotic fluid
   c. Fat particles in venous system
   d. Thrombi in deep veins in the legs or pelvis

4. The most common risk factor for a PE is which of the following?
   a. Hypercoagulability
   b. Heparin therapy
   c. Superficial phlebitis
   d. Minor trauma

5. Which of the following is true regarding the assessment findings (signs and symptoms) of a client with a PE?
   a. Manifestation of a PE is the same for all clients.
   b. Subtle or severe assessment findings depend on the location and type of clot.
   c. In most cases, signs and symptoms are dyspnea, cough, changes in lung sounds, and skin color.
   d. Signs and symptoms are slow in developing over time and insidious in nature.

6. In clients at high-risk for a PE, a unique assessment finding for a small clot in the lung is which of the following?
   a. Respiratory distress
   b. Sudden dry cough, possible chest pain
   c. ECG changes
   d. Changes in lung sounds

7. What assessment findings would indicate to the nurse that the client has developed a PE? List the findings from the most common to the most severe.

8. A nurse suspects a client has a PE and prepares the client for which of the following tests to confirm the diagnosis?
   a. Blood gases, pulse oximetry, CT scan of the chest, echocardiogram
   b. Pulmonary angiography and/or ventilation-perfusion scan
   c. Blood gases, and pulse oximetry, stat 12-lead ECG, and portable chest x-ray
   d. Blood gas, chest x-ray, and cardiopulmonary catheterization

9. Upon diagnosis of a PE in a client, the nurse should expect to perform which of the following therapeutic interventions? Provide a rationale for your answer.
   a. Oral anticoagulant therapy
   b. Bedrest in the supine position and monitor respiratory status as needed
   c. Oxygen therapy via mechanical ventilator
   d. Parenteral anticoagulant therapy

10. The client with a PE asks for an explanation of heparin therapy. Which of the following statements is correct?
    a. "It keeps the clot from getting larger by preventing platelets from sticking together to improve blood flow."
    b. "It will improve your breathing and decrease the chest pain by dissolving the clot in your lung."
    c. "It promotes the absorption of the clot in your leg that originally caused the PE."
    d. "It increases the time it takes for blood to clot, therefore preventing further clotting and improving blood flow."

11. Which of the following nursing interventions pertains to Risk for Injury (bleeding) related to anticoagulation therapy?
    a. Monitor laboratory values for any elevation of PT or PTT value and notify a physician stat.
    b. Monitor PTT values for greater than 2.5 times the control and/or client for bleeding.
    c. Monitor client for a pulmonary infarction by blood in sputum and notify a physician stat.
    d. Monitor PT values for international normalized ratio (INR) for a therapeutic range of 2 to 3 and/or client for bleeding.

12. When PTT values are above the therapeutic range for heparin therapy, the nurse would obtain a physician's order to accomplish which of the following?
    a. Temporarily stop heparin infusion or slow the rate of administration.
    b. Change the concentration of heparin in the IV bag.
    c. Administer the antidote protamine sulfate stat.
    d. Administer a dose of vitamin K by IM injection.

13. Nursing care of a client with a pulmonary embolus would include monitoring for which of the following? *Check all that apply.*

    _____ a. Nausea and vomiting

    _____ b. Symptoms of respiratory failure

    _____ c. Chest pain

    _____ d. Dehydration

14. After receiving heparin anticoagulant therapy, clients should not be discharged from the hospital without a prescription and instructions regarding which of the following drugs?
    a. Dobutamine (Dobutrex)
    b. Antianxiety agents
    c. Coumadin
    d. Vasodilators

15. Nursing responsibilities for a client on Coumadin who has not yet been discharged from the hospital include which of the following?
    a. Having the antidote protamine sulfate available
    b. Administering NSAIDs or aspirin for pain and fever
    c. Teaching the client about foods high in vitamin K
    d. Monitoring platelets for thrombocytopenia

16. The laboratory test used to determine the therapeutic range for Coumadin is which of the following?
    a. PTT level
    b. Platelets
    c. PT and INR
    d. Coumadin peak and trough

17. The INR therapeutic range for a client with a new-onset PE should be which of the following?
    a. 1.0 to 1.5 times the normal
    b. 2.0 to 3.0 times the normal
    c. 3.0 to 4.5 times the normal
    d. 5 times the normal value

18. Develop a discharge teaching plan for a client who has been hospitalized for a pulmonary embolus.

19. Arterial blood gas results from the early stage of a PE would probably indicate which of the following? Provide a rationale for your answer.
    a. Respiratory alkalosis
    b. Respiratory acidosis
    c. Metabolic acidosis
    d. Metabolic alkalosis

20. As a nurse employed on an adult medical-surgical unit, you frequently encounter clients who are at risk for a DVT and PE. Indicate on the chart below the independent and dependent preventive nursing interventions for these clients.

Independent Nursing Functions to Prevent DVT/PE	Dependent Nursing Functions to Prevent DVT/PE

21. Explain the difference between alteplase (tPA), streptokinase, and urokinase in the treatment of a PE.

22. Which of the following clients are at risk for pulmonary contusion?
    a. Client with gunshot wound to the chest
    b. Client with stab wound to the chest
    c. Client with blunt trauma to the chest
    d. Client with rib fracture

23. A client enters the emergency department with a chest injury that resulted from a motor vehicle accident. The client has decreased breath sounds, crackles, wheezing, and blood in the sputum but no open wounds. The nurse would suspect which of the following diagnoses?
    a. Flail chest
    b. Hemothorax
    c. Pneumothorax
    d. Pulmonary contusion

24. Which of the following statements regarding pulmonary contusion is correct? Correct the wrong answers.
    a. It is often a result of a flail chest.

    b. Treatment may require mechanical ventilation with PEEP.

    c. It is treated with aggressive fluids to prevent shock.

    d. Clinical manifestations develop rapidly.

25. Pulmonary contusion is a potentially lethal chest injury because of which of the following?
    a. Broken ribs and flail chest
    b. Laryngospasm
    c. Respiratory failure that can occur over time rather than instantly
    d. High risk of infection from chest tubes

26. A client with a rib fracture is primarily treated with which of the following?
    a. Mechanical ventilation
    b. Tight bandage around chest
    c. Conservative respiratory treatment, e.g., cough and deep breathing
    d. Potent analgesics and muscle relaxants

27. A client can develop a tension pneumothorax when which of the following occurs?
    a. Blood is lost into the thoracic cavity as a result of blunt trauma.
    b. An air leak in the lung or chest wall causes the lung to collapse.
    c. Air accumulates in the pleural space causing a rise in intrathoracic pressure.
    d. There is an infectious process that leads to the accumulation of pus in the pleural space.

28. Which of the following is a significant assessment finding in a client with a tension pneumothorax?
    a. Tracheal deviation to the unaffected side
    b. Inspiratory stridor and respiratory distress
    c. Diminished breath sounds over the affected hemithorax
    d. Hyperresonant percussion note over the affected side

29. During a physical assessment of a client with a hemothorax, percussion of the affected side results in what type of chest sound?
    a. Hypertympanic
    b. Dull
    c. Hyperresonant
    d. Crackles

30. Which of the following is the treatment for a tension pneumothorax?
    a. Inserting a large-bore needle into the intercostal space on the unaffected side
    b. Placement of a chest tube mid sternum to reduce a cardiac tamponade
    c. Attaching the chest to continuous gravity drainage bag
    d. Inserting a large-bore needle into the intercostal space on the affected side

31. A 19-year-old man was seen in the emergency department after a motorcycle accident for multiple rib fractures that resulted in free-floating ribs, paradoxical breathing, and impaired gas exchange. What is this condition called?
    a. Tension pneumothorax
    b. Flail chest
    c. Pulmonary contusion
    d. Subcutaneous emphysema

32. Before suctioning a client with an endotracheal or tracheostomy tube, the nurse preoxygenates the client with what percent oxygen concentration?
    a. 21
    b. 40
    c. 70
    d. 100

33. What is the maximum length of time that suction should be applied to the chest?
    a. 5 to 10 seconds
    b. 10 to 15 seconds
    c. 20 to 30 seconds
    d. 40 to 60 seconds

34. What is the most common cause of ventilatory failure?
    a. Ventilation-perfusion mismatching
    b. Impaired respiratory muscle function
    c. Impaired diffusion at the alveolar level
    d. Abnormal hemoglobin that does not absorb oxygen

35. When does oxygenation failure occur?
    a. When blood shunts from right to left in pulmonary vessels
    b. When the client breathes air that is too concentrated with oxygen
    c. When the respiratory control center in the brain malfunctions
    d. When there is a mechanical abnormality of the chest wall or lungs

36. Match each of the following disorders or events that can cause clients to be at risk for acute respiratory failure with the corresponding type of respiratory failure. *Answers may be used more than once.*

Disorders and Events That Cause Respiratory Failure

_____ a.   Lung tumors

_____ b.   Cerebral edema

_____ c.   Bronchial asthma

_____ d.   Near drowning

_____ e.   Sleep apnea

_____ f.   Multiple sclerosis

_____ g.   Pneumonia

_____ h.   Chronic bronchitis

_____ i.   Atelectasis

_____ j.   Gross obesity

_____ k.   Poliomyelitis

_____ l.   Smoke inhalation

_____ m.   Myasthenia gravis

_____ n.   Meningitis

_____ o.   Pulmonary emphysema

_____ p.   Carbon monoxide poisoning

_____ q.   Opioid overdose

_____ r.   Guillain-Barré syndrome

_____ s.   Liquid aspiration

Types of Respiratory Failure
1. Ventilatory failure
2. Oxygenation failure
3. Combination of ventilatory and oxygenation failure

37. Which of the following conditions is a signal to the nurse of impending acute respiratory failure?
   a.   Orthopnea
   b.   Tachypnea
   c.   Dyspnea on exertion
   d.   Status asthmaticus

38. Indicate the signs and symptoms of respiratory failure for the client with status asthmaticus.

39. Which of the following is not an initial nursing intervention for the client in Question 38 with respiratory failure?
   a.   Administer cromolyn sodium by inhaler.
   b.   Administer bronchodilator treatments.
   c.   Provide energy conservation measures.
   d.   Administer oxygen therapy.

40. What is the major site of injury for ARDS in the respiratory tract?
   a.   Mainstem bronchi
   b.   Respiratory bronchioles
   c.   Alveolar-capillary membrane
   d.   Tracheobronchial tree

41. Which of the following clients is at greatest risk of developing ARDS?
   a.   A 74-year-old client who aspirates a tube feeding
   b.   A 34-year-old client who has nearly drowned
   c.   A 26-year-old client with an electrical burn injury
   d.   An 18-year-old client with a fractured femur

42. Early assessment findings for a client with ARDS include which of the following?
   a.   Adventitious lung sounds
   b.   Hyperthermia and hot, dry skin
   c.   Intercostal and suprasternal retractions
   d.   Increased mental acuity and surveillance

43. Management of ARDS involves which of the following?
   a.   Oxygen therapy via CPAP
   b.   Mechanical ventilation and endotracheal tube
   c.   Antibiotics
   d.   A tracheostomy tube

44. What are four indications for intubation?

    a. _____

    b. _____

    c. _____

    d. _____

45. Match the following parts of an endotracheal tube with their descriptions.

Descriptions

Parts of Endotracheal Tube

_____ a. Device to provide a seal between the trachea and tube

_____ b. Device to allow attachment of ET tube to ventilation source

_____ c. Hollow tube extending from naso-oral cavity to just above the carina

_____ d. Access site for inserting air into the cuff

1. Shaft
2. Cuff
3. Pilot balloon
4. Universal adapter

46. A client in a critical care unit requires an emergency ET intubation. What supplies are needed to perform this procedure?

47. After the insertion of an ET tube, correct placement is conclusively verified when which of the following occurs?
    a. Chest excursion is asymmetrical.
    b. Air emerges from the ET tube on expiration.
    c. Breath sounds are bilaterally equal.
    d. The chest x-ray indicates correct placement.

48. The tape on an endotracheal tube of a client is loose. Describe methods for taping an endotracheal tube and a method to detect tube dislodgment.

49. Which of the following is not a nursing intervention for the care of clients on a ventilator?
    a. Deflating the cuff on the ET tube to check placement
    b. Applying soft wrist restraints as ordered
    c. Suctioning to prevent complications
    d. Maintaining the correct placement of the ET tube

50. Match the following characteristics of ventilators with their types. *Some characteristics may apply to more than one type of ventilator. Indicate all types to which a characteristic applies.*

Characteristics of Ventilators

_____ a. Positive-pressure ventilator

_____ b. Administers consistent volume and gas (oxygen concentration) regardless of the client's lung status until preset tidal volume is reached

_____ c. Preset inspiration and expiration rate with possible variation of tidal volume and pressure

_____ d. Pushes air into the lungs until preset airway pressure is reached

_____ e. Needs an artificial airway such as a tracheostomy or endotracheal tube

_____ f. Tidal volumes and inspiratory time are variable

Types of Ventilators
1. Pressure-cycled
2. Time-cycled
3. Volume-cycled

51. Match the following ventilator terms and settings with their descriptions.

Descriptions

_____ a.   Volumes of air that are 1.5 to 2 times tidal volume

_____ b.   Positive pressure throughout the entire respiratory cycle to prevent alveolar collapse

_____ c.   Number of ventilations delivered per minute

_____ d.   Volume of air the client receives with each breath

_____ e.   Set tidal volume and set rate delivered to the client

_____ f.   Positive pressure exerted during expiration to keep lungs partially inflated

_____ g.   Oxygen concentration delivered to the client

_____ h.   Ventilator takes over the work of breathing for the client and delivers a set tidal volume

_____ i.   Client breathes at own rate, but machine breathes for client as needed

_____ j.   Pressure needed to deliver a set tidal volume

_____ k.   Ventilator delivers mandatory breaths at a preset rate and allows the client to breathe spontaneously between set rate

Terms and Settings

1. Assist-control mode (AC)
2. Breaths per minute (BPM)
3. Continuous positive airway pressure (CPAP)
4. Controlled ventilation
5. Fraction of inspired oxygen (FIO_2)
6. Peak airway inspiratory pressure (PIP)
7. Positive end-expiratory pressure (PEEP)
8. Sighs
9. Synchronized intermittent mandatory ventilation (SIMV)
10. Tidal volume (V1)
11. Intermittent mandatory ventilation (IMV)

52. Identify the acid-base problems and the necessary interventions for each set of ABG data given below.

a.   pH = 7.40, Po_2 = 74 mm Hg, Pco_2 = 40 mEq/L

b.   pH = 7.30, Po_2 = 90 mm Hg, Pco_2 = 40 mEq/L

c.   pH = 7.30, Po_2 = 87 mm Hg, Pco_2 = 50 mEq/L

d.   pH = 7.60, Po_2 = 94 mm Hg, Pco_2 = 21 mEq/L

e.   pH = 7.43, Po_2 = 92 mm Hg, Pco_2 = 40 mEq/L

f.   pH = 7.28, Po_2 = 59 mm Hg, Pco_2 = 40 mEq/L

53. For each of the following body systems, indicate at least one potential complication of mechanical ventilation.

a.   Cardiac: _____

b.   Pulmonary: _____

c.   Gastrointestinal: _____

d.   Immunologic: _____

e.   Muscular: _____

54. A means to determine when a client is ready to be weaned from a ventilator is which of the following assessment findings?
    a. No respiratory infection
    b. Showing signs of becoming ventilator-dependent
    c. Able to maintain blood gases within normal limits
    d. Able to request that the ventilator is not necessary anymore

55. Which of the following findings might delay weaning a client from a ventilator?
    a. Hematocrit = 42%
    b. Arterial Po_2 = 70 mm Hg on a 40% Fio_2
    c. Apical heart rate = 72
    d. Oral temperature = 99° F

56. Which of the following clients might take the longest time to wean from a ventilator?
    a. A 54-year-old man with metastatic colon cancer who has been intubated for 6 days
    b. A 32-year-old woman recovering from a general anesthetic following a tubal ligation
    c. A 25-year-old man intubated for 28 hours following an anaphylactic reaction
    d. A 49-year-old man with a gunshot wound to the chest who was intubated for 8 hours

57. While weaning a client from a ventilator, the nurse should do which of the following?
    a. Assess the monitoring devices regularly from a distance but within the client's sight.
    b. Assess the family member's willingness to stay with the client to provide emotional support.
    c. Plan enough time to stay at the bedside as much as possible to maintain ventilator settings.
    d. Plan to suction the client more frequently as secretions build up.

58. Which of the following is a nursing intervention to implement during extubation?
    a. Ascertain that the cuff is inflated at all times.
    b. Remove the tube during expiration.
    c. Instruct the client not to cough.
    d. Instruct the client to deep breathe and cough.

59. An expected assessment finding in a recently extubated client is which of the following? Why are the other answers incorrect?
    a. Stridor
    b. Dyspnea
    c. Restlessness
    d. Hoarseness

60. Indicate which of the following are nursing interventions related to care of a client on a mechanical ventilator. Why are the other answers incorrect?
    a. Perform mouth care every 2 to 4 hours.
    b. Provide a means of communication.
    c. Administer mandatory muscle-paralyzing agents to ensure ventilation.
    d. Ensure adequate humidity and air temperature.
    e. Empty ventilator tubing back into the cascade.
    f. Perform a respiratory assessment only once a shift.
    g. Include the client and family in care whenever possible.
    h. Monitor for complications such as black tarry stools or constipation.
    i. When setting is PEEP, observe the peak airway pressure dial.

61. A client on a ventilator coughs, gags, and bites on the ET tube. Which of the following is a nursing intervention for this client?
    a. Administer sedation.
    b. Administer a muscle-paralyzing agent.
    c. Insert an oral airway.
    d. Have physician change tube to a tracheostomy.

62. The nurse notices a gradual increase in peak airway pressure over the last several days. Which of the following is the nursing intervention for this client?
    a. Assess for a reason such as ARDS or pneumonia.
    b. Continue to increase peak airway pressure as needed.
    c. Change to another mode such as IMV.
    d. Make arrangements for permanent ventilatory support.

CASE STUDY: CHEST TRAUMA AND ADULT RESPIRATORY DISTRESS SYNDROME (ARDS)

Answer Guidelines for the Case Study questions are provided on the companion Evolve Learning Resources Web site at http://evolve.elsevier.com/Iggy/.

A 72-year-old widow is brought to the hospital following a head-on car accident. She has blunt injury to the chest from hitting the steering wheel. She is having difficulty breathing and shows signs of cyanosis. Initial orders include a stat chest x-ray, arterial blood gases, and oxygen at 4 L/minute per Venturi mask.

1. What other assessments should be made at this time?

2. The chest x-ray reveals a tension pneumothorax. What will an assessment reveal with this diagnosis?

3. What does bubbling in the water seal compartment when the client coughs indicate?

4. Should the nurse "strip" the chest tube? Explain your answer.

5. What should be available at the client's bedside at all times in case the chest tube is accidentally pulled out?

6. Prepare a care plan for the client.

7. Arterial blood gases are drawn. The results are Pao_2 68 mm Hg, $Paco_2$ 32 mm Hg, and pH 7.53. What do these values suggest?

8. What interventions should be implemented based on the laboratory results?

9. The client's oxygen is increased to 6 L/minute. Twenty-four hours later, she develops hemoptysis, crackles, and wheezing. Discuss what may be happening to her. What would contribute to this condition?

A chest x-ray and widening alveolar oxygen gradient confirm a diagnosis of ARDS. A Swan-Ganz catheter is inserted, and the client is intubated and placed on a respirator with PEEP.

11. Why is PEEP necessary?

10. What is the primary laboratory study used to establish the diagnosis of acute respiratory distress syndrome?

12. Explain the rationale for the use of corticosteroids, antibiotics, and colloids in the management of the client with ARDS.

Assessment of the Cardiovascular System

LEARNING OUTCOMES

1. Review the anatomy and physiology of the cardiovascular system.
2. Describe cardiovascular changes associated with aging.
3. Identify factors that place clients at risk for cardiovascular problems.
4. Perform appropriate physical assessment for clients with cardiovascular problems.
5. Interpret laboratory test findings for clients with suspected or actual cardiovascular disease.
6. Explain the pre- and post-test care associated with diagnostic cardiovascular testing.
7. Explain the purpose of hemodynamic monitoring.

LEARNING ACTIVITIES

1. Before completing the study guide exercises for this chapter, it is recommended that you review the following:
   - Anatomy and physiology of the cardiovascular system
   - Techniques for performing a physical assessment
   - Changes in the cardiovascular system of the older adult
   - Pertinent diagnostic tests for the cardiovascular system
   - Basic principles of hemodynamic monitoring

2. Review the boldfaced terms and their definitions in Chapter 36 to enhance your understanding of the content.

STUDY/REVIEW QUESTIONS

Answers to the Study/Review Questions are provided on the companion Evolve Learning Resources Web site at http://evolve.elsevier.com/Iggy/.

1. Match the structures of the heart with their descriptions.

Structures of the Heart

_____ a. Aortic valve

_____ b. Atria

_____ c. Chordae tendineae

_____ d. Coronary arteries

_____ e. Mitral valve

_____ f. Pulmonic valve

_____ g. Septum

_____ h. Tricuspid valve

_____ i. Ventricle

Descriptions

1. Muscular wall dividing the heart into halves
2. Upper heart chamber
3. Lower heart chamber
4. Valve between right atrium and ventricle
5. Valve between right ventricle and pulmonary artery
6. Valve between left atrium and ventricle, bicuspid value
7. Filaments that secure the AV valve leaflets
8. Vessels that supply the heart with oxygenated blood
9. Valve from the left ventricle to the aorta

2. What are the three pacemaker sites in the heart? Name the pacer rate for each site.

   a. _____

   b. _____

   c. _____

3. Increasing the intracellular concentration of which ion causes a chemical interaction within the actin and myosin filaments in the myocardial muscle fibers?
   a. Sodium
   b. Calcium
   c. Potassium
   d. Magnesium

4. Which of the following statements about the cardiac cycle is correct?
   a. Diastole is the shorter of the two phases.
   b. Systole is the longer of the two phases.
   c. S_1 results from tricuspid and mitral valve closure.
   d. S_2 results from the contraction of the ventricles.

5. Identify the two main properties that determine the function of the cardiovascular system.

   a. _____

   b. _____

6. Match the following variables that affect cardiac output with their descriptions.

Descriptions

_____ a. Number of times ventricles contract per minute

_____ b. Degree of myocardial fiber stretch at end of diastole and just before heart contracts

_____ c. Amount of pressure or resistance that the ventricles must overcome to eject blood through the semilunar valves and into the peripheral blood vessels

_____ d. Pressure that ventricle must overcome to open aortic valve

_____ e. Force of contraction independent of preload

Cardiac Output Variables
1. Afterload
2. Contractility
3. Heart rate
4. Impedance
5. Preload

7. Answer the following questions that relate to the mechanical properties of the heart.

   a. How is blood flow from the heart into the systemic arterial circulation measured clinically?

   b. Define cardiac output (CO).

   c. CO is the product of what two variables?

   d. Define the term *stroke volume* and give the variables that impact it and cardiac output.

   e. Define preload.

   f. What is Starling's law of the heart? What happens with excessive filling of the ventricles?

   g. Briefly discuss afterload. What factors affect it?

8. Fill in the blanks:
   a. The ability of all cardiac cells to initiate an impulse spontaneously and repetitively is _____.
   b. Cardiac cells are unable to respond to a stimulus until they have recovered, or repolarized, because of this property: _____

   c. The transmitting of electrical impulses from cardiac cell to cardiac cell is _____.

   d. The ability of a cell to respond to a stimulus by initiating an impulse (depolarization) is _____.

9. Describe the relationship of the left ventricle to maintaining the blood pressure and adequate cardiac output (CO).

10. How is the relationship of the left ventricle to maintenance of blood pressure and adequate CO different in the older adult? Indicate other changes in blood pressure that can occur in the older adult.

11. Briefly explain the three systems/mechanisms and external factors that regulate blood pressure.

12. Identify the three types of sensory receptors in the body that affect the autonomic nervous system in regulating the blood pressure.

   a. _____

   b. _____

   c. _____

13. True or False? Which of the following statements about the various components of blood pressure are true? *Write T for true or F for false in the blanks provided. For those questions that are false, rewrite the statement to make it true.*

_____ a. Systolic blood pressure is the lowest pressure during the relaxation phase of the cardiac cycle.

_____ b. Diastolic blood pressure is the highest pressure during contraction of the ventricles.

_____ c. Diastolic blood pressure is primarily determined by the amount of peripheral vasoconstriction.

_____ d. Pulse pressure is the difference between the systolic and diastolic pressures.

_____ e. Fluid moves from the vascular system into the interstitial spaces when the capillary endothelium is impaired.

14. The chamber of the heart that can generate the greatest amount of blood pressure is the:
    a. Right atrium
    b. Right ventricle
    c. Left atrium
    d. Left ventricle

15. Which of the following statements about the peripheral vascular system is correct?
    a. Veins are equipped with valves that permit one-way flow of blood toward the heart.
    b. The velocity of blood flow varies directly with the diameter of the vessel lumen.
    c. Blood flow decreases and blood tends to clot as the viscosity decreases.
    d. The parasympathetic nervous system has the greatest effect on blood flow to various organs.

16. In the older adult, a common assessment finding is which of the following?
    a. S_4 heart sound
    b. Leg edema
    c. Pericardial friction rubs
    d. Change in point of maximum impulse location

17. For each of the following structures/ functions, identify the changes that occur in the older adult and explain what implications those changes have in regard to nursing care.
    a. Cardiac valves

    b. Conduction system

    c. Left ventricle

    d. Aorta and other large arteries

    e. Baroreceptors

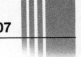

18. On the illustration below, locate and describe the sites for auscultation of the heart sounds and pulse points listed.
    a. Aortic area
    b. Pulmonic area
    c. Erb's point
    d. Right ventricular area
    e. Epigastric area
    f. Mitral area
    g. Tricuspid area

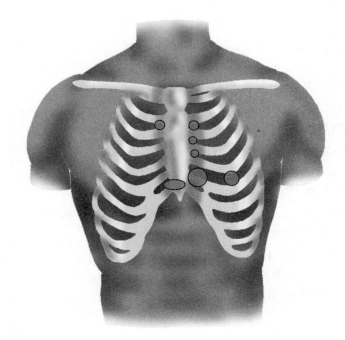

19. The description of S_1 and S_2 refers to which of the following?
    a. First and second heart sounds
    b. Pericardial friction rub
    c. Murmur
    d. Gallop

20. An S_3 or S_4 that is heard on auscultation of the heart refers to which of the following?
    a. Murmur
    b. Pericardial friction rub
    c. Gallop
    d. Normal heart sound

21. Which of the following clients has an abnormal heart sound? *Check all that apply.*
    a. S_1 in a 45-year-old client
    b. S_2 in a 30-year-old client
    c. S_3 in a 15-year-old client
    d. S_3 in a 54-year-old client

22. Which of the following findings from a cardiovascular assessment is abnormal?
    a. Absence of heaves, lifts, or thrills
    b. Splitting of S_2; decreases with expiration
    c. Jugular venous distention to level of the mandible
    d. Point of maximal impulse (PMI) in fifth intercostal space at midclavicular line

23. Describe clubbing, how it is assessed, and the indication for a positive result.

24. Which of the following statements about symptoms of heart disease in women are true? *Check all that apply.*

_____ a. Pain typically occurs with activity or stress.

_____ b. Symptoms are subtle or atypical.

_____ c. Pain is often relieved by rest.

_____ d. Woman may not respond to rest or medication.

_____ e. Antacids, rather than nitroglycerin, may relieve pain.

_____ f. Pain responds to nitroglycerin.

_____ g. Other symptoms, such as back pain, indigestion, nausea, vomiting, and anorexia are common.

25. Match each source of chest pain with assessment findings. Each source of chest pain may be used more than once.

Assessment Findings

_____ a. Sudden onset

_____ b. Moderate ache, worse on inspiration

_____ c. Substernal, may spread to shoulders or abdomen

_____ d. Intermittent, relieved with sitting upright

_____ e. Substernal, may spread across chest, back, arms

_____ f. Usually lasts less than 15 minutes

_____ g. Continuous until underlying condition is treated

_____ h. Intense stabbing, vice-like pain

_____ i. Dull ache to sharp stabbing, may have numbness of fingers

_____ j. Sudden onset, often in early morning

_____ k. Usually on left side of chest without radiation

_____ l. Sharp stabbing, moderate to severe

_____ m. Squeezing, heartburn, variable in severity

Sources of Chest Pain
1. Angina
2. Myocardial infarction
3. Pericarditis
4. Esophageal-gastric
5. Anxiety
6. Pleuroplumonary

26. A 50-year-old man with a history of recent cardiac surgery enters the emergency department very anxious and complaining of sudden, sharp, stabbing chest pain that spreads to the left side. He states that he is having a "heart attack." His skin is pink, warm to the touch, and diaphoretic. Capillary refill is within normal limits. He has no signs of clubbing. HR is 110; BP is 122/82. How would you analyze these assessment findings? Is he experiencing a "heart attack"?

27. A client in the emergency department with chest pain has a possible myocardial infarction (MI). Which of the following laboratory tests would be performed to determine this diagnosis?
   a. CK-MB
   b. Serum potassium
   c. Homocysteine
   d. Lactate dehydrogenase

28. Which of the following laboratory tests are used to predict a client's risk for coronary artery disease? *Check all that apply.*

    _____ a. Cholesterol level

    _____ b. Triglyceride level

    _____ c. Prothrombin time

    _____ d. Low-density lipoprotein level

    _____ e. Albumin level

29. Which of the following tests would be performed to determine the location and extent of coronary artery disease?
    a. Electrocardiogram (ECG)
    b. Echocardiogram
    c. Cardiac catheterization
    d. Chest x-ray

30. Use Gordon's functional health patterns to identify questions a nurse would ask a client in assessing that client's cardiovascular status.

31. Identify subjective data that would be included in assessment findings related to cardiovascular disease.

32. Identify objective data that would be included in assessment findings related to cardiovascular disease.

33. One of the most modifiable, controllable risk factors for cardiovascular disease is which of the following?
    a. Obesity.
    b. Diabetes mellitus.
    c. Ethnic background.
    d. Family history of cardiovascular disease.

34. Calculate the number of pack-years for the client who has smoked half a pack of cigarettes per day for 2 years, one pack per day for 4 years, and 2 packs per day for 20 years. Discuss the significance of the number of pack-years and how those data can be used to predict a client's risk for cardiovascular disease.

35. The following is a partial client history. Discuss the significance of these data as they relate to the cardiovascular system.

    White male client, 45 years old. Married with three children. Works as an investment banker. Reports that he feels a lot of pressure to perform his job well. Began to have syncope episodes 3 months ago; feeling light-headed and sometimes dizzy. Denies loss of consciousness. States that he often skips lunch to continue working through the lunch hour. Entertains clients several times per week by taking them out to lunch or dinner. Commutes to and from work via his own automobile and often gets upset and angry with traffic snarls. Tends to have late dinners with wife at home, consuming several cocktails with meals. Admits to having a "weight problem" off and on. Denies hypertension. His father has had a cerebrovascular accident (CVA).

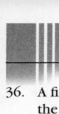

36. A finding of pallor is indicative of which of the following?
    a. Anemia
    b. Thrombocytosis
    c. Dehydration
    d. Chest pain

37. Which of the following terms describes the difference between the systolic and diastolic values?
    a. Paradoxical blood pressure
    b. Pulse pressure
    c. Ankle-brachial index
    d. Normal blood pressure

38. An ankle-brachial index of 0.7 is an indication of which of the following?
    a. Normal arterial circulation to the lower extremities
    b. Moderate arterial disease of the lower extremities
    c. Severe arterial disease of the lower extremities
    d. Inconclusive test results

39. True or False? Decide whether each of the following statements is true or false. *Write T for true or F for false in the blanks provided.*

    _____ a. Dyspnea can occur with both cardiac disease and pulmonary disease.

    _____ b. A cardinal symptom of heart disease is dyspnea.

    _____ c. Paroxysmal nocturnal dyspnea occurs when the client has been lying down for several hours.

    _____ d. Orthopnea is defined as dyspnea on exertion.

    _____ e. Dyspnea on exertion may be the only sign of early heart failure in women.

40. True or False? Read the following statements regarding performing a pericardium assessment and decide whether each is true or false. *Write T for true or F for false in the blanks provided. If the statement is false, correct the statement to make it true.*

    _____ a. The assessment begins with auscultation.

    _____ b. The client is in a supine position with the head of bed elevated for comfort and ease of breathing.

    _____ c. Inspect for point of maximal impulse or pulsations at the apex of the heart.

    _____ d. Heaves and lifts are associated with inspection and with valve disease.

    _____ e. The nurse palpates with fingers and the most sensitive part of the palm of the hand.

    _____ f. When palpating, turn the client to the right side to bring the heart closer to the surface of the chest.

    _____ g. When auscultating, use the diaphragm to listen for low-frequency sounds.

    _____ h. The skill of accurately auscultating sounds requires a good stethoscope and lots of practice.

41. Which of the following procedures requires informed consent from the client? *Check all that apply.*

    _____ a. Electrocardiogram

    _____ b. Use of a Holter monitor

    _____ c. Stress test

    _____ d. Echocardiography

    _____ e. Cardiac catheterization

    _____ f. Electrophysiologic study

42. Preparation for an electrocardiogram (ECG) includes which of the following?
    a. Asking the client to lie on his or her left side
    b. Applying leads over the client's gown
    c. Cleaning the client's skin with soap and water
    d. Placing the leads on as flat an area as possible

43. Which of the following assessment findings in a client who has had a cardiac catheterization should the nurse report immediately to the physician?
    a. Pain at the catheter insertion site
    b. Catheterized extremity dusky with decreased peripheral pulses
    c. Small hematoma at the catheter insertion site
    d. Pulse pressure of 40 mm Hg with slow, bounding pulse

44. Match each of the following serum lipid values with the serum lipid laboratory test used to determine the value in an adult male.

Name of Lipid Test

    _____ a. Cholesterol

    _____ b. Triglycerides

    _____ c. Plasma high-density lipoproteins (HDLs)

    _____ d. Plasma low-density lipoproteins (LDLs)

    _____ e. HDL:LDL ratio

Normal Laboratory Value

1. 60 to 180 mg/dL; older than 65 years of age is 92 to 221 mg/dL
2. Females 35 to 135; males 40 to 160; and older adults is 55 to 260 mg/dL
3. 122 to 200 mg/dL; older adults is 144 to 280 mg/dL
4. 3:1
5. Females 55 to 60; males 45 to 50; range increases with age

45. From the list of lipid tests in Question 44, identify the laboratory values that increase the risk for coronary artery disease when the values are elevated.

46. From the list of lipid tests in Question 44, which one is considered to protect against coronary artery disease when the values are elevated?

47. Define each hemodynamic monitoring term and cite the normal values:
    a. Right atrial pressure

    b. Pulmonary artery pressure (PAP)

    c. Pulmonary artery wedge pressure (PAWP)

    d. Pulmonary artery occlusion pressure (PAOP)

48. A right atrial pressure (RAP) reading of less than 3 cm H_2O indicates which of the following?
    a. Right-sided heart failure
    b. Left-sided heart failure
    c. Cardiac tamponade
    d. Hypovolemia

49. A client's Svo$_2$ (mixed venous oxygen saturation) is 70%. What is your interpretation of this finding?
    a. The client's oxygen demand is balanced by the oxygen supply.
    b. The client's oxygen demand exceeds the available oxygen supply.
    c. The client's available oxygen supply exceeds the current oxygen demand.
    d. The client's venous oxygen saturation is equal to the arterial oxygen saturation.

50. A client develops complications from a cardiac catheterization and is admitted to the critical care unit where hemodynamic monitoring (HM) is initiated.
    a. Explain the purpose of HM.

    b. Describe the client position for accurate hemodynamic monitoring.

51. Which type of hemodynamic monitoring technique directly measures the mean arterial pressure in the critically ill client?

52. How is impedance cardiography different than what was previously discussed regarding conventional HM?

53. What is essential for the nurse to monitor when a client has an invasive arterial line?

54. A client is scheduled for an angiography. What is the purpose of this invasive test?
    a. Determine the size, silhouette, and position of the heart.
    b. Identify abnormal structures, calcifications, and tumors of the heart by fluoroscopy.
    c. Assess cardiovascular response to an increased workload.
    d. Determine arterial obstruction, narrowing, or aneurysm in specific locations.

55. The most definitive, yet invasive test for studying the right or left side of the heart and the coronary arteries is a

    _____.

56. It important for the nurse to ask the client who is scheduled for any type of angiography with dye about an allergy to _____

    _____

    _____.

57. Explain what you would tell a client about the sensations that may be felt during a cardiac catheterization.

58. Explain the nursing responsibilities involved in preparing a client for a scheduled cardiac catheterization.

59. The alternative to injecting dye into the coronary arteries is to use a test called

    _____ _____,

    which uses a flexible catheter with a miniature transducer at the distal tip to visualize the coronary arteries.

60. Postprocedural care of a client following a cardiac catheterization includes which of the following? *Check all that apply.*

    _____ a. Client is to remain on bedrest for 12 to 24 hours.

    _____ b. Client is to lie flat at all times.

    _____ c. Assess dressing for bloody drainage or hematoma.

    _____ d. Peripheral pulses in the affected extremity, as well as skin temperature and color, are monitored with every vital sign check.

    _____ e. Assess pain at insertion site.

    _____ f. Report to physician any chest pain, nausea, or feelings of light-headedness.

    _____ g. Provide adequate oral and IV fluids for hydration.

    _____ h. Monitor intake and output because the dye is an osmotic diuretic.

    _____ i. Monitor vital signs every hour for 24 hours.

61. To determine valve disease of the mitral valve, left atrium, or aortic arch, the client would be scheduled for which of the following?
    a. Transesophageal echocardiogram
    b. Electrocardiogram (ECG)
    c. Myocardial nuclear perfusion imaging
    d. Phonocardiography

62. Briefly discuss the purpose, client preparation, and procedure for a Holter monitor.

63. True or False? Decide whether each of the following statements is true or false. *Write T for true or F for false in the blanks provided. If the statement is false, correct it to make it true.*

    _____ a. There is no follow-up care for clients who undergo echocardiograms.

    _____ b. Echocardiograms require an informed consent.

    _____ c. MNPI is a radioactive technique used to view cardiovascular abnormalities.

    _____ d. Technetium scanning is effective for diagnosing old infarctions.

    _____ e. After an MNPI, the client is placed in isolation because of radioactive isotopes.

    _____ f. Thallium imaging can be done with the client at rest or during exercise.

    _____ g. For clients who cannot perform a treadmill stress test, thallium imaging can be used.

    _____ h. Clients should be aware that thallium can cause flushing, headache, dyspnea, and chest tightness a few moments after the injection.

    _____ i. An echocardiogram is a risk-free, pain-free test that uses sound waves to assess cardiac structure and mobility, particularly that of the valves.

_____ j.   A PET scan takes 2 to 3 hours and a client may be asked to use a treadmill.

_____ k.   During multigated blood pool scanning, several blood samples are taken for measurement of oxygen saturation.

_____ l.   Electronic beam computed tomography (EBCT) can look for calcifications within the arteries.

64. Identify reasons a client would be scheduled for a thallium imaging.

65. Which of the following statements about the coronary arteries of the heart is correct?
   a.   There are three main coronary arteries: left coronary artery (LCA), right coronary artery (RCA), and circumflex.
   b.   In most individuals, the left coronary artery supplies both the sinoatrial (SA) and atrioventricular (AV) nodes.
   c.   To maintain adequate blood flow through the coronary arteries, diastolic blood pressure must be at least 60 mm Hg.
   d.   Coronary artery blood flow to the myocardium occurs primarily during systole when coronary vascular resistance is minimal.

CASE STUDY: ASSESSMENT OF THE CARDIOVASCULAR SYSTEM

Answer Guidelines for the Case Study questions are provided on the companion Evolve Learning Resources Web site at http://evolve.elsevier.com/Iggy/.

Your client is a 72-year-old man who had an extensive left ventricular myocardial infarction (MI) at 36 years of age. At the time of his MI, he was overweight by 50 pounds and smoked two packs of unfiltered cigarettes per day. He had smoked for 20 years. Alcohol consumption was part of his ethnic background; it was customary for him to drink one or two beers per day and several mixed drinks per week. His father had also suffered an MI, at the age of 48, and was a chain smoker. Your client slowly recovered from his MI, gave up smoking, and lost weight. His weight stabilized within 15 pounds of the upper limit of his ideal weight. His wife became an active participant in his recovery by changing her style of cooking and virtually eliminating saturated fats from their diets. He no longer drank beer, but he continued to consume an average of two mixed drinks per day. He began a moderate exercise program that included walking several miles a day at least three times a week. He has had stable angina for many years and has annual physical checkups and ECGs at the cardiologist's office. He took up the hobby of downhill skiing at the age of 66, with his cardiologist's approval. He is a retired accountant with a type A personality. Over the past 6 months, he has experienced infrequent periods of light-headedness. He has "blacked out" on at least one occasion and was unable to remember any details of what happened. A second episode of loss of consciousness occurred on a clear, cold winter day while he was skiing. He revived spontaneously. The next day, he scheduled an appointment with his physician.

1.   Which lifestyle changes decreased his risk status after his MI? Which habits increased his risk status?

2.   Compare and contrast the risk factors of CV disease for a 36-year-old man and a 72-year-old man.

3. The cardiologist performs an ECG and orders blood work drawn for AST, CK and CK-MB, LDH and isoenzymes, and serum potassium. What are the purposes for these tests?

4. The ECG and blood work are inconclusive, but the physician is concerned about his symptoms. Discuss why there is reason for concern.

5. He is scheduled for an inpatient cardiac catheterization. The physician tells him that, based on the findings at the time of the catheterization, he may go ahead and perform an angioplasty. Develop a teaching-learning plan for this client.

The cardiac catheterization is completed, and a 95% blockage of the left anterior descending (LAD) artery is seen along with an 80% blockage of the circumflex artery. A balloon angioplasty is performed in the catheterization laboratory. After the procedure, the LAD has a 40% blockage, and the circumflex has a 25% blockage. The physician counsels the client to resume activity gradually. A stress test will be scheduled in several weeks for further evaluation of his exercise tolerance and cardiac status.

6. Develop a teaching-learning plan for this client to prepare him for the upcoming tests.

Interventions for Clients with Dysrhythmias

LEARNING OUTCOMES

1. Correlate the components of the electrocardiogram (ECG) with the cardiac conduction system.
2. Analyze a rhythm strip or ECG tracing to identify common cardiac dysrhythmias.
3. Identify typical physical assessment findings associated with common dysrhythmias.
4. Prioritize nursing diagnoses for clients experiencing dysrhythmias.
5. Plan care for clients experiencing common dysrhythmias.
6. Implement appropriate treatment modalities, including antidysrhythmic drugs, for common and lethal dysrhythmias.
7. Develop a teaching plan for clients experiencing common dysrhythmias.
8. Explain the purpose and types of pacing used as interventions for clients with dysrhythmias.
9. Differentiate between defibrillation and cardioversion, identifying the indications for the use of each.
10. Plan community-based care for a client after pacemaker or implantable cardioverter/defibrillator insertion.

LEARNING ACTIVITIES

1. Before completing the study guide exercises for this chapter, it is recommended that you review the following:
   - Anatomy and physiology of the heart and vascular system
   - Principles of fluid and electrolyte balance
   - Assessment of the cardiovascular system including changes in the older adult
   - Conduction system of the heart
   - Principles of acid-base balance
   - Principles related to cardiac output
   - Anatomy and physiology of respiratory system
   - Assessment of the respiratory system
   - Principles of cardiac output
   - Examples of ECG rhythm strips from various basic ECG interpretation textbooks

2. Review the boldfaced terms and their definitions in Chapter 37 to enhance your understanding of the content.

STUDY/REVIEW QUESTIONS

Answers to the Study/Review Questions are provided on the companion Evolve Learning Resources Web site at http://evolve.elsevier.com/Iggy/.

1. The primary pacemaker of the heart is

   _____.

2. Match each of the electrophysiologic properties or specialized cells of the cardiac conduction system with its definition.

Electrophysiologic Properties/Specialized Cells

_____ a. Contractility

_____ b. Conductivity

_____ c. Excitability

_____ d. Action potential

_____ e. Automaticity

_____ f. SA node (sinoatrial node)

_____ g. Depolarization

_____ h. Sarcolemma

_____ i. Atrial kick

_____ j. Purkinje fibers

_____ k. AV node (atrioventricular node)

Definitions
1. Ability of a cell to respond to an electrical impulse
2. Extra amount of blood added to ventricles
3. Heart's primary pacemaker
4. Ability of the heart to circulate blood; the mechanical response to an impulse
5. Changing a cell membrane from negatively charged to positively charged
6. Ability to spontaneously and repeatedly generate a cardiac impulse
7. Specialized cells in the ventricles
8. Cell permeability that creates an electrical imbalance
9. Cardiac cell membrane
10. Cell-to-cell transmission of impulse
11. Slows down impulses to the ventricles

3. The SA node fires at the rate of which of the following times per minute?
   a. Less than 60
   b. 60 to 100
   c. 80 to 100
   d. Greater than 100

4. The electrical impulse of the heart moves through the ventricles from the _____ to
   _____ _____ to
   _____.

5. Identify the sequential order of the cardiac tissues that assume the cardiac pacemaker's role if the sinoatrial (SA) node fails to function.

   a. _____

   b. _____

   c. _____

6. Briefly describe the difference between the terms *arrhythmia* and *dysrhythmia*.

7. True or False? Read the following statements regarding characteristics of an ECG complex and decide whether each is true or false. *Write T for true or F for false in the blanks provided. If the statement is false, correct the statement to make it true.*

   _____ a. The P wave represents atrial depolarization followed by atrial contraction.

   _____ b. The P-R interval is the period of time from the firing of the SA node to just before ventricular depolarization.

_____ c. When depolarization occurs in the ventricles, the T wave is formed on the ECG.

_____ d. The period between ventricular depolarization and the beginning of ventricular repolarization is the S-T segment.

_____ e. The T wave represents ventricular repolarization.

_____ f. Q-T interval is the total time it takes the depolarization and repolarization of atrial and ventricles to occur.

8. ECG signal transmission is enhanced by which of the following?
   a. Cleaning the skin with povidone-iodine solution before applying the electrodes
   b. Ensuring that the area for electrode placement is dry and nonhairy
   c. Applying tincture of benzoin to the electrode sites and waiting for it to become "tacky"
   d. Abrading the skin by rubbing the electrode sites briskly with a rough surface such as a washcloth

9. Match the following placements with the limb leads for ECG monitoring.

Placement

_____ a. Right arm (+)

_____ b. Right arm (-), left arm (+)

_____ c. Left arm (-), left leg (+)

_____ d. Left leg (+)

_____ e. Left arm (+)

_____ f. Right arm (-), left leg (+)

Limb Lead

1. Lead I
2. Lead II
3. Lead III
4. aVr
5. aVL
6. aVF

10. List in sequence the six recommended steps for analyzing ECG rhythms.

   1. _____

   2. _____

   3. _____

   4. _____

   5. _____

   6. _____

11. Which of the following statements about ECG waves is *correct*?
   a. The amplitude of the wave reflects the muscular strength of the contraction.
   b. If the rhythm is regular, heart rate can be estimated by counting the number of QRS complexes within a given time.
   c. If the rhythm is irregular, heart rate is estimated by counting the number of QRS complexes within a given time.
   d. Assessment of a rapid rhythm is best done by decreasing the recorder speed.

12. Identify the components of a normal electrocardiogram.

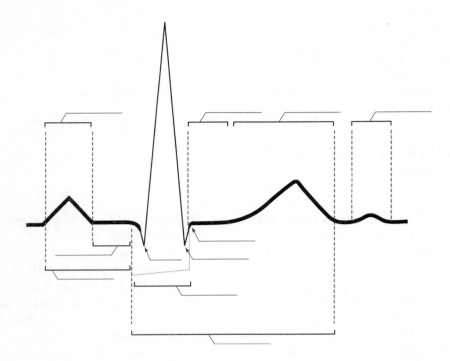

13. With the speed set for 25 mm/second, the segment between the dark lines on a monitor ECG strip represents how many seconds?
    a. 3 seconds
    b. 6 seconds
    c. 10 seconds
    d. 20 seconds

14. ECG waveforms are measured in which of the following?
    a. Pressure and cardiac output
    b. Seconds and minutes
    c. Beats per minute
    d. Amplitude (voltage) and duration (time)

15. Calculate the heart rate from an ECG strip when there are 25 small blocks from one R wave to the next R wave.

16. Calculate the heart rate shown on a 6-second ECG strip when the number of R-R intervals is 5. What is this rhythm?

17. How does a nurse interpret the measurement of the P-R interval when it is six small boxes on the ECG strip?
    a. Atrium is taking longer to repolarize.
    b. Longer than normal impulse time from the SA node to the ventricles is shown.
    c. There is a problem with the length of time the ventricles are depolarizing.
    d. This is the normal length of time for the P-R interval, and there is no cause for concern.

18. A wide distorted QRS complex of 0.14 second followed by a p wave is an indication of which of the following?
    a. Wide but normal complex and no cause for concern
    b. A premature ventricular contraction
    c. A problem with the speed set on the ECG machine
    d. A delayed time of the electrical impulse through the ventricles

19. The monitor technician notifies the nurse that the client's rhythm is showing artifact. What should the nurse do?
    a. Document the artifact.
    b. Monitor the rhythm until the artifact disappears.
    c. Check the client.
    d. Notify the physician.

20. A client in a cardiac critical care unit has a sustained bradydysrhythmia. Identify key clinical manifestations of this problem.

21. Identify treatment modalities for the following common dysrhythmias:
    a. Atrial fibrillation

    b. Ventricular tachycardia (sustained)

    c. Ventricular fibrillation

    d. Premature ventricular contractions (PVCs)

    e. Sinus bradycardia

    f. Sinus tachycardia

    g. Atrial flutter

    h. Supraventricular rhythms

22. True or False? Read the following statements regarding heart block and decide whether each is true or false. *Write T for true or F for false in the blanks provided. If the statement is false, correct the statement to make it true.*

    _____ a. Mobitz type II second degree is a constant block in one of the bundle branches.

    _____ b. First-degree heart block is the complete blockage of impulses from the SA node.

    _____ c. Third-degree AV block results in ventricular rhythm.

    _____ d. Wenckebach is characterized by a progressive prolonged PR interval followed by a dropped beat.

    _____ e. A characteristic feature of third-degree block is that the P-R interval is not constant.

    _____ f. All heart blocks require interventions.

    _____ g. Clients with first-degree and type I blocks may be asymptomatic, whereas type II blocks may have symptoms.

23. Match each type of dysrhythmia with its description. *Answers may be used more than once.*

Descriptions

_____ a. A straight line on the cardiac monitor

_____ b. Results in the atria and the ventricles contracting independently of one another

_____ c. A ventricular rhythm that in most cases results in loss of consciousness

_____ d. Rapidly fatal if not corrected in 3 to 5 minutes

_____ e. Results in a QRS complex width that exceeds 0.12 second

_____ f. Results in uncoordination of atrial contraction and decreased cardiac output

_____ g. May result from sympathetic nervous system stimulation of the heart or vagal inhibition

_____ h. Characterized by rapid atrial depolarization occurring at a rate of 250 to 350 times per minute

_____ i. Causes the ventricles to quiver, resulting in absence of cardiac output

Types of Dysrhythmias
1. Sinus tachycardia
2. Atrial flutter
3. Atrial fibrillation
4. Atrioventricular dissociation
5. Ventricular tachycardia
6. Ventricular fibrillation
7. Asystole
8. Bundle branch blocks

24. Identify common causes of ectopic foci for cardiac contraction.

25. A client in a critical care unit on telemetry develops the following rhythm: normal P waves at a regular rate of 88 beats per minute. There is a separate ventricular regular rate of 55 with a normal QRS complex. An AV dissociation exists because the atria and ventricles are independent of each other.

a. Based on this ECG, what assessment findings might the nurse identify with this dysrhythmia?

b. What would make a difference in the physical findings?

c. What type of heart block has been identified?
   (1) First degree
   (2) Mobitz type I
   (3) Mobitz type II
   (4) Third degree

d. What interventions are necessary for this client?

e. Would the client have a temporary or permanent pacemaker? Provide a rationale for your answer.

f. Indicate nursing interventions including discharge teaching for this client.

26. An adult client with ventricular fibrillation or pulseless ventricular tachycardia will receive which of the following medications? What is the usual dose for this drug and its side effects? What are the nursing interventions?
    a. Propranolol (Inderal)
    b. Adenosine (Adenocard)
    c. Diltiazem hydrochloride (Cardizem)
    d. Lidocaine

27. Differentiate between invasive and noninvasive temporary pacing. Describe the two types of invasive temporary pacing.

28. Identify the three complications that can occur with noninvasive pacemaker therapy.

    a. _____

    b. _____

    c. _____

29. Briefly describe what the synchronous, or demand, mode means regarding pacemaker therapy.

30. Defibrillation for cardioversion is synchronized with which part of the ECG complex?
    a. T wave
    b. Q-T interval
    c. S-T segment
    d. QRS complex

31. All clients who have a dysrhythmia should be instructed to do which of the following?
    a. Stay at least 4 feet away from a microwave oven that is operating.
    b. Avoid going through any electronic metal detectors, such as those at airports.
    c. Learn the procedure for assessing their apical pulses and have a family member learn the procedure as well.
    d. Purchase an automatic external defibrillator for home use.

32. A nurse observes changes in mental status and orientation and notes client complaints of chest pain while ambulating a client. The nursing diagnosis for this patient would be which of the following?
    a. Activity Intolerance
    b. Decreased Cardiac Output
    c. Acute Confusion
    d. Impaired Gas Exchange

33. When performing external defibrillation, which of the following is a vital step in the procedure?
    a. The gel pads are placed anterior over the apex and posterior for better conduction.
    b. A second shock cannot be administered for 1 minute to allow for recharging.
    c. No one is to be touching the client at the time shock is delivered.
    d. Continue to ventilate the client via endotracheal tube during the procedure.

34. Which of the following is the most life-threatening consequence of cardiac dysrhythmias?
    a. Severe hypotension
    b. Sinus bradycardia
    c. Stroke
    d. Sudden death

35. On a separate sheet of paper, develop a concept map relevant to dysrhythmias. Consider factors that put clients at risk for atrial and for ventricular dysrhythmias. Identify subjective and objective data.

36. Based on assessment findings, what are the two most common nursing diagnoses for clients with dysrhythmia?

    a. _____

    b. _____

37. Discuss the four factors that are considered when interventions for dysrhythmias are planned.

    a. _____

    b. _____

    c. _____

    d. _____

38. Which of the following statements about antidysrhythmic agents is *correct*?
    a. Class I agents stabilize phase 4 to decrease automaticity.
    b. Class II agents control dysrhythmias associated with too much parasympathetic stimulation.
    c. Class III agents decrease the absolute refractory time and help to increase cardiac rate.
    d. Class IV agents impede the flow of sodium into the cell during depolarization and decrease cardiac rate.

39. Which of the following procedures should be avoided on the client who has a dysrhythmia?
    a. Giving an intramuscular injection
    b. Monitoring temperature rectally
    c. Cleaning the mouth using a Water Pik
    d. Assisting transfer to a bedside commode for bowel movement

40. Which of the following statements about sinus dysrhythmias is *correct*?
    a. A too-rapid rate lengthens diastolic filling time and leads to increased cardiac output.
    b. The body attempts to compensate for a decreased stroke volume by decreasing the heart rate.
    c. Sinus bradycardia occurs in trained athletes because the stroke volume is adequate without a higher rate.
    d. Sinus tachycardia is uncommon in the general population and causes symptoms of coronary insufficiency.

41. A client is found pulseless; the cardiac monitor shows a rhythm that has no recognizable deflections, but instead has coarse "waves" of varying amplitudes. What is the priority ACLS intervention for this rhythm?
    a. Immediate defibrillation
    b. Administration of magnesium IVP
    c. Administration of lidocaine IVP
    d. Noninvasive temporary pacing

42. Which of the following drugs would a nurse prepare to administer to a client during a cardiac arrest? *Check all that apply.*

    _____ a. Lidocaine

    _____ b. Epinephrine

    _____ c. Calcium chloride

    _____ d. Sodium bicarbonate

    _____ e. Dopamine hydrochloride (Intropin)

    _____ f. Verapamil (Calan)

    _____ g. Amiodarone (Cordarone)

    _____ h. Adenosine (Adenocard)

43. Which of the following is the correct placement for defibrillator paddles?
    a. The anterior paddle is placed on the client's upper left chest, below the clavicle and to the left of the sternum; the apex paddle is placed on the lower right chest in a mid-axillary line.
    b. The anterior paddle is placed on the client's upper left chest below the clavicle and to the right of the sternum; the apex paddle is placed on the lower right chest in a mid-axillary line.
    c. The anterior paddle is placed on the client's upper right chest below the clavicle and to the right of the sternum; the apex paddle is placed on the client's lower left chest in a mid-axillary line.

44. A client is in ventricular fibrillation. Which of the following actions is *correct* in regard to defibrillation?
    a. Defibrillate at 360 joules
    b. Defibrillate at 200 joules
    c. Defibrillate at 50 joules
    d. Defibrillate at 100 joules

45. True or False? Write T for true or F for false in the blanks provided. *If the statement is false, correct it to make it true.*

    _____ a. The implantable cardioverter defibrillator (ICD) treats bradyarrhythmia.

    _____ b. Dobutamine is a beta-adrenergic agent used to improve contractility.

    _____ c. Ventricular aneurysms are a complication of myocardial infarction.

    _____ d. A cardioversion shock is synchronized with the T wave.

    _____ e. Class III antidysrhythmics lengthen the absolute refractory period and prolong repolarization.

    _____ f. Confusion, drowsiness, and slurring of speech are signs of lidocaine toxicity.

46. A 45-year-old client is being treated with ibutilide fumarate (Covert) for an atrial fibrillation. The nurse should closely observe the client for which of the following? *Check all that apply.*

    _____ a. Heart failure

    _____ b. Orthostatic hypotension

    _____ c. Conversion to a sinus rhythm

    _____ d. Hypokalemia

    _____ e. Prolonged QT intervals

    _____ f. Acute ventricular dysrhythmias.

47. Which of the following is the drug of choice for symptomatic bradycardia?
    a. Epinephrine
    b. Atropine
    c. Calcium
    d. Lidocaine

48. Which of the following drugs controls dysrhythmias associated with excessive beta-adrenergic stimulation?
    a. Amiodarone hydrochloride (Cordarone)
    b. Propranolol hydrochloride (Inderal)
    c. Diltiazem (Cardizem)
    d. Verapamil hydrochloride (Calan)

49. Identify three important topics to review with clients who have premature beats and ectopic rhythms.

    a. _____

    b. _____

    c. _____

50. Develop a teaching plan for a client with a pacemaker.

51. Develop a teaching plan for clients with implantable cardioverters/defibrillators.

52. The older adult is at risk for dysrhythmias because of changes in the cardiac conduction system. Identify at least three nursing interventions that are specific for the older adult.

    a. _____

    b. _____

    c. _____

53. The P wave represents which of the following?
    a. Atrial depolarization
    b. Atrial repolarization
    c. Ventricular depolarization
    d. Ventricular repolarization

54. Which of the following is the normal measurement of the PR interval?
    a. Less than 0.11 second
    b. 0.06 to 0.10 second
    c. 0.12 to 0.20 second
    d. 0.16 to 0.26 second

55. The QRS complex normally measures which of the following?
    a. Less than 0.12 second
    b. 0.10 to 0.16 second
    c. 0.12 to 0.20 second
    d. 0.16 to 0.24 second

56. The ST segment is normally which of the following?
    a. Isoelectric
    b. Elevated
    c. Depressed
    d. Biphasic

57. The total time required for ventricular depolarization and repolarization is represented on the ECG by which of the following?
    a. PR interval
    b. QRS complex
    c. ST segment
    d. QT interval

58. When the myocardium is refractory, it is which of the following?
    a. Able to accept another impulse
    b. Fibrillatory
    c. Unable to accept another impulse
    d. Prone to re-entry mechanism

59. Stimulation of the sympathetic nervous system produces which of the following effects?
    a. Decreased heart rate and decreased force of contraction
    b. Increased heart rate, increased contractility, and dilation of coronary vessels
    c. Has virtually no effect on the ventricles of the heart
    d. Slows the heart rate and slows AV conduction time

60. Which of the following is responsible for the major pumping action of the heart?
    a. Endocardium
    b. Myocardium
    c. Epicardium
    d. Pericardium

61. What is the function of the AV node?
    a. Increase the automaticity of the SA node.
    b. Pace the heart at 60 to 100 beats per minute.
    c. Provide structural support for the tricuspid valve.
    d. Delay impulses between the atria and ventricles.

Interpret the following ECG strips. Write your answers in the blanks provided.

62. _____

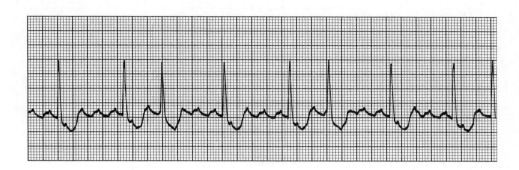

RATE _____ RHYTHM _____ P WAVES _____
PR INTERVAL _____ QRS DURATION _____ INTERPRETATION _____

63. _____

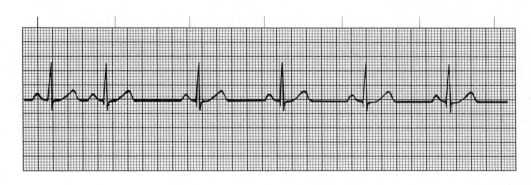

RATE _____ RHYTHM _____ P WAVES _____
PR INTERVAL _____ QRS DURATION _____ INTERPRETATION _____

64. _____

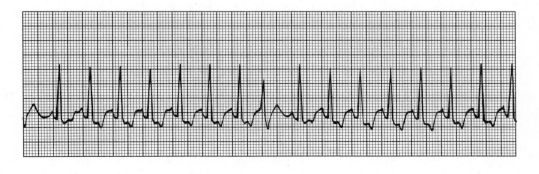

RATE _____ RHYTHM _____ P WAVES _____
PR INTERVAL _____ QRS DURATION _____ INTERPRETATION _____

65. _____

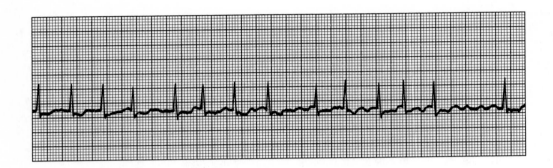

RATE _____ RHYTHM _____ P WAVES _____
PR INTERVAL _____ QRS DURATION _____ INTERPRETATION _____

66. _____

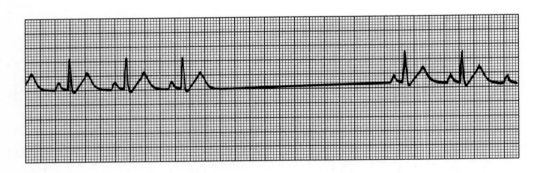

RATE _____ RHYTHM _____ P WAVES _____
PR INTERVAL _____ QRS DURATION _____ INTERPRETATION _____

67. _____

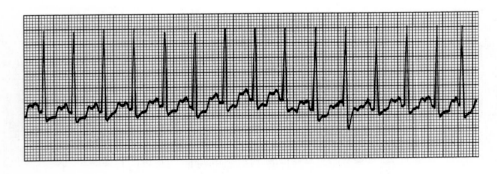

RATE _____ RHYTHM _____ P WAVES _____
PR INTERVAL _____ QRS DURATION _____ INTERPRETATION _____

68. _____

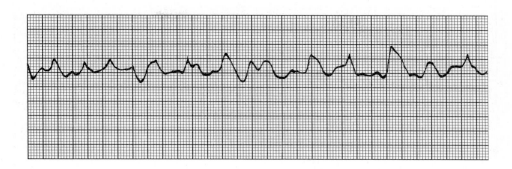

RATE _____ RHYTHM _____ P WAVES _____
PR INTERVAL _____ QRS DURATION _____ INTERPRETATION _____

69. _____

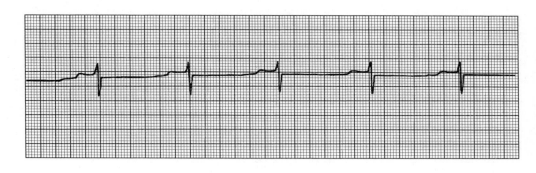

RATE _____ RHYTHM _____ P WAVES _____
PR INTERVAL _____ QRS DURATION _____ INTERPRETATION _____

70. _____

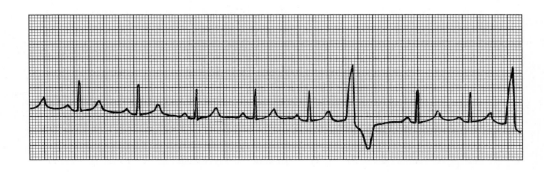

RATE _____ RHYTHM _____ P WAVES _____
PR INTERVAL _____ QRS DURATION _____ INTERPRETATION _____

71. _____

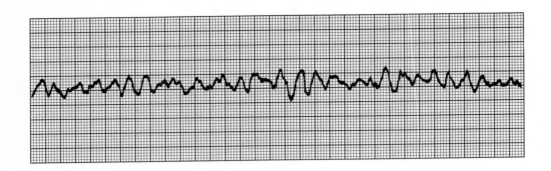

RATE _____ RHYTHM _____ P WAVES _____
PR INTERVAL _____ QRS DURATION _____ INTERPRETATION _____

72. _____

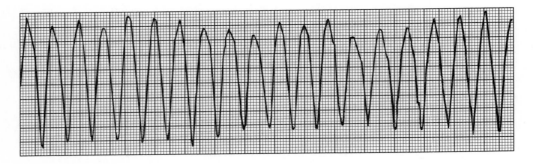

RATE _____ RHYTHM _____ P WAVES _____
PR INTERVAL _____ QRS DURATION _____ INTERPRETATION _____

73. _____

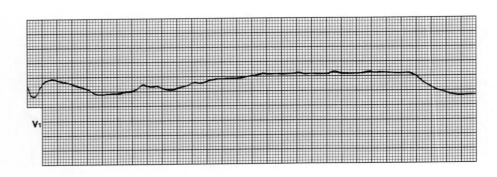

RATE _____ RHYTHM _____ P WAVES _____
PR INTERVAL _____ QRS DURATION _____ INTERPRETATION _____

74. _____

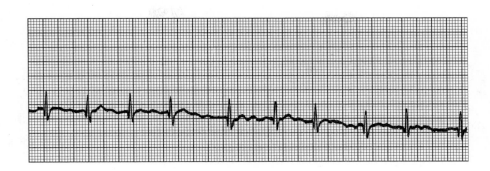

RATE _____ RHYTHM _____ P WAVES _____
PR INTERVAL _____ QRS DURATION _____ INTERPRETATION _____

75. _____

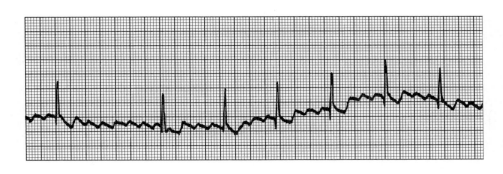

RATE _____ RHYTHM _____ P WAVES _____
PR INTERVAL _____ QRS DURATION _____ INTERPRETATION _____

76. _____

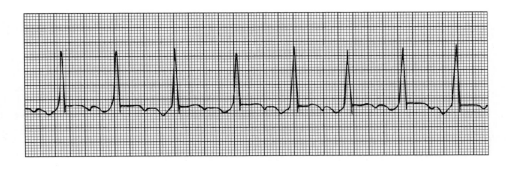

RATE _____ RHYTHM _____ P WAVES _____
PR INTERVAL _____ QRS DURATION _____ INTERPRETATION _____

77. _____

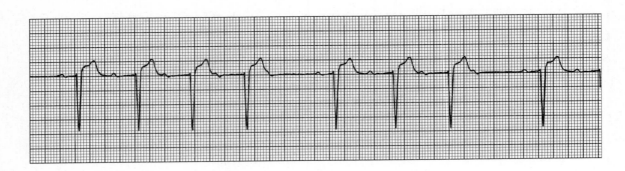

RATE _____ RHYTHM _____ P WAVES _____
PR INTERVAL _____ QRS DURATION _____ INTERPRETATION _____

78. _____

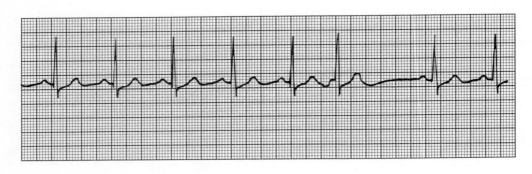

RATE _____ RHYTHM _____ P WAVES _____
PR INTERVAL _____ QRS DURATION _____ INTERPRETATION _____

79. _____

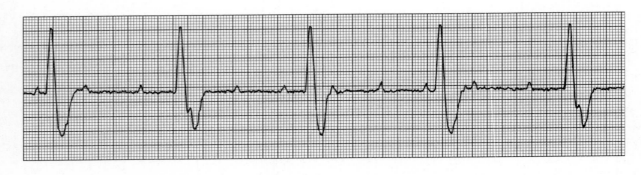

RATE _____ RHYTHM _____ P WAVES _____
PR INTERVAL _____ QRS DURATION _____ INTERPRETATION _____

80. _____

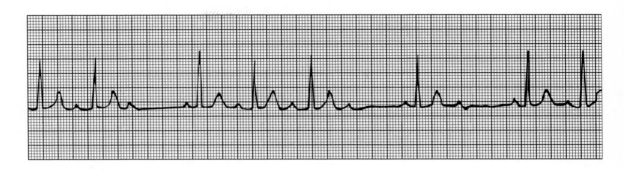

RATE _____ RHYTHM _____ P WAVES _____
PR INTERVAL _____ QRS DURATION _____ INTERPRETATION _____

81. _____

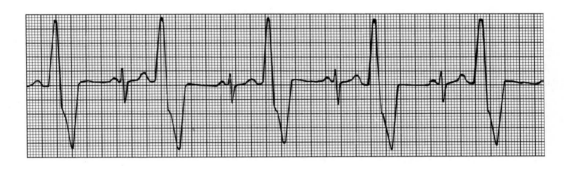

RATE _____ RHYTHM _____ P WAVES _____
PR INTERVAL _____ QRS DURATION _____ INTERPRETATION _____

CASE STUDY: THE CLIENT WITH A DYSRHYTHMIA

Answer Guidelines for the Case Study questions are provided on the companion Evolve Learning Resources Web site at http://evolve.elsevier.com/Iggy/.

A 78-year-old woman is admitted to a telemetry unit directly from her physician's office for evaluation and management of congestive heart failure. She has a history of systemic hypertension and chronic moderate mitral regurgitation. Her medication orders include furosemide (Lasix) 80 mg PO four times a day, digoxin 0.125 mg PO daily, and diltiazem (Cardizem) 60 mg PO three times a day. Your initial assessment of the client reveals a pulse rate that is rapid and very irregular. The client is restless, her skin is pale and cool, she states she is dizzy when she stands up, and she is slightly short of breath. Her blood pressure is 106/88. She is short of breath and anxious. Her ECG monitor pattern shows uncontrolled atrial fibrillation, with a rate ranging from 150 to 170 beats per minute. Her oxygen saturation level is 90%.

1. Given the assessment findings, what should you do first?

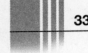

2. What additional physical assessment techniques would you perform?

3. Because the length of time the client has been in atrial fibrillation is unknown, what potential complication may occur?

4. Based on your answer for number 3, what should be done before elective cardioversion is attempted?

5. What other medical therapy might this client receive before elective cardioversion is done?

6. Later that evening, the client calls the nurse because she feels "like something terrible is going to happen." She complains of chest pain, has increased shortness of breath, and has coughed up blood-tinged sputum. What do you suspect? What is the first thing the nurse should do, and what further assessments should be performed at this time?

Interventions for Clients with Cardiac Problems

LEARNING OUTCOMES

1. Explain the pathophysiology of heart failure.
2. Compare and contrast left-sided and right-sided heart failure.
3. Perform a comprehensive assessment of clients experiencing heart failure.
4. Identify common nursing diagnoses and collaborative problems for clients with heart failure.
5. Evaluate the effects of interventions for reducing preload and afterload.
6. Identify common drug therapies to improve cardiac output.
7. Describe special considerations for older adults with heart failure.
8. Discuss the prevention of complications for clients with heart failure.
9. Prioritize nursing care for clients experiencing heart failure.
10. Identify essential focused assessments used by the home care nurse for clients with heart failure.
11. Compare and contrast common valvular disorders.
12. Discuss surgical management for clients with valvular disease.
13. Develop a teaching-learning plan for clients with valvular disease.
14. Differentiate between common cardiac inflammations and infections—endocarditis, pericarditis, and rheumatic carditis.
15. Discuss the legal/ethical aspects related to heart transplantation, including resource management.

LEARNING ACTIVITIES

1. Before completing the study guide exercises for this chapter, review the following:
   - Anatomy and physiology of the cardiovascular system
   - Principles of fluid and electrolyte balance
   - Principles of acid-base balance including blood gas values
   - Regulation of blood pressure
   - Cardiovascular assessment
   - Respiratory assessment
   - Conduction system of the heart
   - Principles related to cardiac output
   - Principles of infection

2. Visit your local organ donation service or its Web site.

3. Review the boldfaced terms and their definitions in Chapter 38 to enhance your understanding of the content.

STUDY/REVIEW QUESTIONS

Answers to the Study/Review Questions are provided on the companion Evolve Learning Resources Web site at http://evolve.elsevier.com/Iggy/.

1. Indicate which of the following clients are at greatest risk of developing infective endocarditis. *Check all that apply.*

   _____ a. An intravenous drug user

   _____ b. A client with pancreatitis

   _____ c. A client with a myocardial infarction

   _____ d. A client with a prosthetic mitral valve replacement, postoperative

   _____ e. A client with mitral stenosis who recently had an abscessed tooth removed

   _____ f. An older adult client with urinary tract infection and valve damage

   _____ g. A client with cardiac arrhythmias

2. On a separate sheet of paper, develop a concept map relevant to infective endocarditis. Consider physiologic, psychological, and developmental factors. Identify subjective and objective data.

3. A client with aortic valve endocarditis complains of fatigue and shortness of breath. Crackles are heard on lung auscultation. These assessment findings may indicate which of the following?
   a. Emboli to the lung
   b. Valve incompetence resulting in heart failure
   c. Valve stenosis, resulting in increased chamber size
   d. Coronary artery disease

4. A client has an admitting diagnosis of infective endocarditis. The nurse would anticipate which of the following tests to be performed to confirm a positive diagnosis?
   a. CT scan
   b. MRI
   c. Blood cultures
   d. Echocardiogram

5. Self-care measures for the client who has had infective endocarditis include teaching the client to do which of the following?
   a. Take an oral temperature reading daily for the remainder of his or her life.
   b. Begin a moderate exercise program to strengthen the myocardium.
   c. Administer prophylactic antibiotics for every invasive procedure including dental care.
   d. Weigh daily to monitor for weight gain, which is then reported to the physician.

6. Which of the following procedures is the client with infective endocarditis most likely to report having had recently?
   a. Teeth cleaning
   b. Urinary bladder catheterization
   c. Chest radiography
   d. Colonoscopy

7. Arterial embolization to the brain resulting from infective endocarditis may cause which of the following symptoms?
   a. Dysarthria
   b. Dysphagia
   c. Atelectasis
   d. Electrolyte imbalances

8. Treatment interventions for a client with infective endocarditis would include which of the following?
   a. Administration of oral penicillin for 6 weeks or more
   b. Hospitalization for initial intravenous antibiotics, possibly with a central line
   c. Complete bedrest for the duration of treatment
   d. Long-term anticoagulation therapy with heparin

9. Which of the following clients could be at risk for developing viral pericarditis?
   a. 35-year-old woman with tuberculosis
   b. 45-year-old man who has had radiation therapy for lung cancer
   c. 30-year-old man with a respiratory infection
   d. 50-year-old woman with chest trauma

10. True or False? Read the following statements regarding assessment findings of pericarditis and decide whether each is true or false. *Write T for true or F for false in the blanks provided. If the statement is false, correct the statement to make it true.*

   _____ a. A common assessment finding is a grating substernal pain, mainly on inspiration when in supine position.

   _____ b. Initially, pain is best relieved by sitting up and leaning forward.

   _____ c. Acute pericarditis is usually short-term, lasting approximately 2 to 6 weeks.

   _____ d. Pericardial friction rub is best heard using the diaphragm at the right upper sternal border.

   _____ e. ECG changes are insidious.

   _____ f. Pericardiocentesis is a treatment for pericardial effusion.

   _____ g. Tuberculosis can be a cause of chronic constrictive pericarditis.

   _____ h. Interventions for the client with pericarditis include preparing for a paracentesis if cardiac tamponade develops.

11. A client has been admitted with acute pericarditis. Assessment findings indicate neck vein distention, clear lungs, muffled heart sounds, tachycardia, tachypnea, and a greater than 10 mm Hg difference in systolic pressure on inspiration than on expiration. Which of the following would be the nurse's response to these assessment findings?
   a. Continue to monitor client; these are normal signs of pericarditis.
   b. Immediately report findings to the physician, because these are signs of cardiac tamponade.
   c. Administer oxygen, monitor oxygen saturation, and seek pain medication order to control symptoms.
   d. Check ECG, administer morphine for pain to slow respiratory rate, and administer diuretic as ordered.

12. Summarize the nursing interventions for a client with pericarditis.

13. A client with rheumatic heart disease needs to understand that signs of rheumatic carditis must be recognized immediately so that the client receives prompt treatment with which of the following?
   a. Pericardiocentesis
   b. Antibiotics for 10 days
   c. Pain medication for substernal pain control
   d. Rest with observation for further necessary treatment

14. The nurse should anticipate the client receiving which medication of choice for treatment of rheumatic carditis?
    a. Antibiotic (penicillin)
    b. NSAIDs
    c. Pain medications (opioids)
    d. Steroids

15. Match each description to the corresponding key feature/finding.

Key Features/Findings

_____ a. Percardial friction rub

_____ b. Splinter hemorrhages

_____ c. Petechiae

_____ d. Systemic emboli

_____ e. Pulsus paradoxus

_____ f. Aschoff's bodies

_____ g   Cardiac tamponade

Descriptions
1. Vegetation fragments in circulation resulting in a CVA or TIA
2. Red, flat pinpoint spots/lesions in mucous membrane and conjunctive
3. Small red streaks or black longitudinal lines of nail beds
4. Having a systolic blood pressure higher on expiration than on inspiration
5. Scratchy, high-pitched sound heard at left lower sternal border
6. Small nodules on myocardium replaced by scar tissue
7. Excess fluid in the pericardial cavity

16. True or False? Which of the following is true regarding cardiac tamponade? *Write T for true or F for false in the blanks provided.*

    _____ a. Cardiac tamponade may occur with as little as 20 to 50 mL fluid.

    _____ b. If fluid accumulates slowly, the pericardium accommodates the fluid by stretching.

    _____ c. This condition is not a medical emergency.

_____ d. Chest x-ray and echocardiogram can confirm the diagnosis, but hemodynamic monitoring may be necessary.

_____ e. A pericardiocentesis is performed to remove the fluid.

17. What is the nurse's role before, during, and after a pericardiocentesis?

18. Match each assessment finding with the corresponding inflammatory cardiac disease. *Answers may be used more than once.*

Assessment Finding

_____ a. Grating pain that is aggravated by breathing

_____ b. A new, regurgitant murmur

_____ c. Janeway's lesions

_____ d. Streptococcal infection

_____ e. Osler's nodes

_____ f. Scratchy, high-pitched sound heard on auscultation over left lower sternal border

_____ g. Petechiae

_____ h. Aschoff's bodies

Inflammatory Cardiac Disease
1. Endocarditis
2. Pericarditis
3. Rheumatic carditis

19. True or False? For the following statements about cardiomyopathies, determine whether they are true or false. *Write T for true or F for false in the blanks provided.*

    _____ a. Dilated cardiomyopathy results in symptoms of left ventricular failure.

_____ b. Most clients with hypertrophic cardiomyopathy are asymptomatic until early adulthood.

_____ c. Sudden death may be the first manifestation of hypertrophic cardiomyopathy.

_____ d. The earliest sign of restrictive cardiomyopathy is edema.

_____ f. Dilated cardiomyopathy and restricted cardiomyopathy are initially managed the same as heart failure.

_____ g. Heart transplantation is the treatment of choice for severe hypertrophic cardiomyopathy.

20. The client with a heart transplantation will do which of the following?
    a. Have an increased risk for developing coronary artery disease.
    b. Respond to carotid sinus pressure and vagal stimulation.
    c. Experience numerous episodes of acute organ rejection.
    d. Report episodes of angina with increased activity.

21. A client has decreased cardiac output related to dilated cardiomyopathy and is being considered for heart transplantation. Review the section on cardiomyopathy, including criteria for selection for transplantation, along with the legal/ethical issues in health care to formulate your own personal thoughts as a nurse health care provider. Write your answer on a separate sheet of paper. Be able to discuss and defend your position on the subject with other health care providers.

22. Where is the most common site of valvular disease?
    a. The aortic valve
    b. The pulmonary valve
    c. The tricuspid valve
    d. The mitral valve

23. True or False? Read the following statements regarding valvular disease and decide whether each is true or false. _Write T for true or F for false in the blanks provided. If the statement is false, correct the statement to make it true._

_____ a. Stenosis is a term referring to the narrowing of the heart valve opening.

_____ b. Regurgitation is a term referring to the heart valves no longer being able to close completely.

_____ c. The right side of the heart is more often affected.

_____ d. The aortic valve is the most common valve affected.

_____ e. The most common valve disorder is mitral stenosis.

_____ f. The most common cause of mitral stenosis is rheumatic carditis.

_____ g. The tricuspid valve is not affected often unless damage occurs after endocarditis resulting from intravenous drug abuse.

_____ h. Women are diagnosed with mitral regurgitation of nonrheumatic origin more often than are men.

_____ i. Nitrates can cause decreased preload and dizziness with aortic stenosis.

_____ j. Nonsurgical treatment modality is most concerned with maintaining right-side heart function.

24. Which of the following is the most common preventable cause of valvular heart disease?
    a. Congenital disease or malformation
    b. Calcium deposits and thrombus formation
    c. Beta-hemolytic streptococcal infection
    d. Hypertension or Marfan syndrome

25. Pitting edema is a sign for which type of valvular disease?
    a. Mitral valve stenosis and insufficiency
    b. Aortic valve stenosis and insufficiency
    c. Both aortic and mitral valve insufficiency
    d. Mitral valve prolapse

26. Which of the following is the diagnostic test most often performed to assess valvular heart disease?
    a. Echocardiography
    b. Electrocardiography
    c. Exercise testing
    d. Thallium scanning

27. Long-term anticoagulant therapy for the client with valvular heart disease includes which drug?
    a. Heparin sodium
    b. Warfarin sodium (Coumadin)
    c. Tubocurarine chloride
    d. Protamine sulfate

28. The most common invasive procedure for a client with valvular heart disease that requires prophylactic antibiotic therapy is which of the following?
    a. Intravenous therapy
    b. Colonoscopy
    c. Dental cleaning
    d. Gastroscopy

29. Match the types of valvular disease with their characteristics. *Answers may be used more than once.*

Characteristics

_____ a. Fatigue and chronic weakness are first signs, followed by dyspnea

_____ b. Classic signs of dyspnea, angina, and syncope

_____ c. A first sign is dyspnea and dry cough

_____ d. Blowing type of murmur; "bounding" arterial pulse

_____ e. Irregular rhythm; atrial fibrillation can cause emboli

_____ f. Most clients are asymptomatic

_____ g. Right-side heart failure; later cardiac output fails

_____ h. The client may experience palpitations while lying on left side

_____ i. Symptom-free for decades, later related to left ventricle failure

_____ j. Rumbling apical diastolic murmur

_____ k. Right-sided failure results in neck vein distention

_____ l. Leaflets enlarge and fall back into left atrium during systole

_____ m. Normal heart rate and blood pressure

_____ n. Becoming a disorder of aging populations

_____ o. Murmur, systolic crescendo-decrescendo

_____ p. S_3 often present due to severe regurgitation

Types of Valvular Disease
1. Mitral valve stenosis
2. Mitral valve insufficiency
3. Mitral valve prolapse
4. Aortic stenosis
5. Aortic insufficiency

30. Compare and contrast the pathophysiology and clinical manifestations of each of the following valve disorders.

Valve Disorder	Pathophysiology	Clinical Manifestations
Mitral stenosis		
Mitral insufficiency		
Mitral valve prolapse		
Aortic stenosis		
Aortic insufficiency		

31. The surgical noninvasive intervention of a balloon valvuloplasty is often used for which type of client?
    a. Young adults with a genetic valve defect
    b. Adults who are nonsurgical candidates
    c. Adults whose open heart surgery failed
    d. Older adults needing replacement valves

32. Which of the following is a complication of postvalvuloplasty?
    a. Myocardial infarction
    b. Angina
    c. Bleeding and emboli
    d. Infection

33. A client with a prosthetic valve replacement should understand that postoperative care will include lifelong therapy with which of the following?
    a. Antibiotics
    b. Anticoagulant therapy
    c. No exercise program
    d. Aspirin therapy

34. A client with a xenograft valve must realize that this type of valve does not require anticoagulant therapy but will require which of the following?
    a. Replacement in about 7 to 10 years
    b. An exercise program to develop collateral circulation
    c. Daily temperature check to watch for signs of rejection
    d. Frequent monitoring for pulmonary edema

35. Summarize items that are covered when educating clients and their families about mitral valve disease.

36. What is the most common nursing diagnosis for a client with valvular heart disease?
    a. Decreased Cardiac Output
    b. Ineffective Coping
    c. Ineffective Breathing Pattern
    d. Disturbed Body Image

37. The client undergoing heart valve surgery is instructed to do which of the following?
   a. Continue taking oral anticoagulants until the time of admission for surgery.
   b. Prepare for a cardiac catheterization, at which time the defective valve will be replaced.
   c. Expect to have open heart surgery and be admitted to an intensive care unit postoperatively.
   d. Refill the prescription for oral anticoagulants because it will be resumed postoperatively.

38. Home care of the client following heart valve surgery includes which of the following?
   a. Using an electric toothbrush for regular dental hygiene
   b. Flossing of teeth daily to prevent plaque formation
   c. Starting a rehabilitation regimen using weight training
   d. Taking measures to prevent bleeding due to anticoagulant therapy

39. Impaired cardiac function from heart failure results in which of the following?
   a. Low ventricular end-diastolic blood pressure
   b. Reduced systemic diastolic blood pressure
   c. Decreased pulmonary venous pressure
   d. Decreased cardiac output

40. What is the initial compensatory mechanism of the heart that maintains cardiac output?
   a. Increased parasympathetic stimulation
   b. Increased sympathetic stimulation
   c. The Starling mechanism
   d. Myocardial hypertrophy

41. In the table below, describe how each of the following compensatory mechanisms increases cardiac output (CO) as a result of heart failure. Indicate the long-term effect of each mechanism.

Compensatory Mechanism	Action to Increase CO with Long-Term Damaging Effect
SNS—adrenergic receptors	
Cardiac hypertrophy	
Hormonal response	

42. Complete the table below to compare and contrast the two subtypes of left heart failure.

Heart Failure Classification	Definition	Effect on System
Systolic dysfunction (systolic ventricular dysfunction)		
Diastolic dysfunction		

43. Which of the following statements about the classification of heart failure is correct?
    a. Most heart failure begins with failure of the left ventricle and progresses to failure of both ventricles.
    b. Left ventricular failure is usually caused by right ventricular failure.
    c. High-output failure occurs when the body's metabolic needs are met with an increased cardiac output.
    d. Chronic heart failure develops over time and is caused by a sudden myocardial infarction.

44. The main cause of heart failure is related to which of the following conditions?
    a. Renal failure
    b. Myocardial infarction/coronary artery disease
    c. High-fat diet
    d. Hypertension

45. The client with left ventricular failure is most likely to report which of the following?
    a. Nocturia
    b. Weight gain
    c. Swollen legs
    d. Nocturnal coughing

46. Assessment findings of the client with left-sided heart failure may include which of the following? *Check all that apply.*
    _____ a. S_2 splitting
    _____ b. S_3 heart sound
    _____ c. Paroxysmal nocturnal dyspnea
    _____ d. Jugular venous distention
    _____ e. Splenomegaly
    _____ f. Wheezes or crackles

47. Assessment findings of a client with right-sided heart failure may include which of the following? *Check all that apply.*
    _____ a. Dependent edema
    _____ b. Weight loss
    _____ c. Polyuria at night
    _____ d. Hypotension
    _____ e. Hepatomegaly
    _____ f. Angina

48. A client with congestive heart failure develops pulmonary edema. Identify the nursing interventions for this client.

49. Which of the following correctly describes drug therapy for heart failure?
   a. Inotropic agents to increase the heart rate
   b. Sympathomimetics to decrease contractility
   c. Diuretics to increase the cardiac preload
   d. Vasodilators to decrease systemic resistance

50. Clients may receive any of the following medications for the treatment of heart failure. Complete the following chart.

Drug	Action	Nursing Interventions
Angiotensin-converting enzyme (ACE) inhibitors, such as enalapril (Vasotec)		
Human B-type natriuretic peptides, such as nesiritide (Natrecor)		
Various diuretics, such as furosemide (Lasix), bumetanide (Bumex), metolazone (Zaroxolyn)		
Nitrates (nitroglycerin)		
Digoxin (Lanoxin)		
Beta-adrenergic blockers, such as carvedilol (Coreg), metoprolol (Lopressor)		

51. A client taking digoxin therapy would be educated to have which of the following laboratory tests to monitor for potential cardiac problems and digoxin toxicity?
    a. Complete blood counts
    b. BUN and creatinine levels
    c. Serum potassium levels
    d. Prothrombin time and INR

52. Which of the following is an outcome for the collaborative problem Potential for Pulmonary Edema?
    a. No dysrhythmias
    b. Clear lung sounds
    c. Less fatigue
    d. No disorientation

53. In addition to oxygen and a diuretic, which of the following drugs is commonly administered to relieve dyspnea resulting from pulmonary edema?
    a. Beta blockers
    b. Dopamine
    c. Morphine sulfate
    d. Digoxin

54. Chronic heart failure results in which of the following problems?
    a. Xanthelasma
    b. Leg edema
    c. Hemangioma
    d. Palpitations

55. The best way for a nurse to assess for orthopnea is to ask the client about which of the following?
    a. Number of times the client voids at night
    b. Dry hacking coughs
    c. The use of two or more pillows to sleep
    d. Sudden awakening with a feeling of breathlessness at night

56. Identify preventive measures for delaying heart failure in clients with pre-existing heart disease.

    a. _____

    b. _____

    c. _____

    d. _____

    e. _____

57. Indicate which of the following medications are used to reduce afterload. *Check all that apply.*
    _____ a. Digoxin
    _____ b. Human B-type natriuretic peptides
    _____ c. ACE inhibitors
    _____ d. Beta blockers

58. The client is at risk for developing significant hypotension after the first dose of which of the following medications?
    a. Furosemide (Lasix)
    b. Captopril (Capoten)
    c. Digoxin
    d. Nesiritide (Natrecor)

59. Discharge planning for the client with heart failure includes which of the following?
    a. Teaching the client to take diuretics at bedtime to enhance the effect on increased renal perfusion
    b. Demonstrating to the client how to monitor an apical pulse and what symptoms to report to the physician
    c. Determining whether the client has a bathroom scale to monitor weight to facilitate reporting a gain of more than 5 pounds
    d. Providing the client with dietary exchange list of foods allowed on a low-potassium diet.

60. Correct the *italicized word* in each of the following assessment findings that indicate that heart failure is worsening
    a. Weight gain of *5 pounds* in a week
    b. Complaints of not being able to perform activities of daily living for *1 week*
    c. Dry cough for *2 days*
    d. Getting up *one time* during the night to urinate
    e. Shortness of breath on *exertion*

61. Which of the following statements is an indication that the client needs more teaching regarding a treatment regimen for heart failure?
    a. "I should only weigh myself once a month and watch for fluid retention."
    b. "If my heart feels like it is racing, I should call the doctor."
    c. "I need to consider my activities for the day and take rests as needed."
    d. "I need to have periods of rest and activity and need to avoid activity after meals."

62. Home care for the client with heart failure is a focus for Healthy People 2010. Summarize areas that the home health nurse assesses in clients with heart failure.

CASE STUDY: THE CLIENT WITH HEART FAILURE

Answer Guidelines for the Case Study questions are provided on the companion Evolve Learning Resources Web site at http://evolve.elsevier.com/Iggy/.

A 74-year-old woman is admitted to the hospital with heart failure. She had been growing progressively weaker and had ankle edema, dyspnea on exertion, and three-pillow orthopnea. On admission, she is severely dyspneic and can answer questions only with one-word phrases. She is diaphoretic, with a heart rate of 132 beats/min, and blood pressure 98/70. She is extremely anxious.

1. Because this client cannot breathe or talk easily, prioritize the immediate nursing assessments upon admission.

2. Considering the process of congestive heart failure, explain the symptoms she is having.

3. Based on assessment, identify nursing diagnoses for this client.

4. The physician orders the following items for this client. Explain the rationale for these medications and treatments.

- Start an IV, then give dobutamine 3 mg/kg/hr IV

- Furosemide (Lasix) 40 mg IV stat

- Digoxin 0.5 mg PO stat, then 0.125 every 6 hours for three doses, with ECG before doses 3 and 4

- Morphine 2 mg IV stat and then 2 mg IV every 1 to 2 hours prn

- Oxygen 4 L/min per nasal cannula

- Schedule for an echocardiogram

- No added salt diet

- Weigh daily and monitor input and output

Interventions for Clients with Vascular Problems

CHAPTER

39

LEARNING OUTCOMES

1. Explain the pathophysiology of arteriosclerosis and atherosclerosis, including the factors that cause arterial injury.
2. Interpret essential laboratory data related to risk for atherosclerosis.
3. Discuss the role of diet therapy in the management of clients with arteriosclerosis.
4. Describe the differences between essential and secondary hypertension.
5. Develop a collaborative plan of care for a client with essential hypertension.
6. Explain the purpose, action, and nursing implications of drugs used to manage hypertension.
7. Identify cultural considerations that impact care for clients with hypertension.
8. Evaluate the effectiveness of interdisciplinary interventions to improve hypertension.
9. Compare and contrast assessment findings typically present in clients with peripheral arterial and peripheral venous disease.
10. Prioritize postoperative care for clients who have undergone peripheral bypass surgery.
11. Assess clients at risk for venous thromboembolism (VTE) and identify when VTE occurs.
12. Describe nursing interventions used to help prevent venous thromboembolism (VTE).
13. Describe the nurse's role in monitoring clients who are receiving anticoagulants.
14. Develop a continuing care plan for a client who has undergone an abdominal aortic aneurysm repair.
15. Compare and contrast Raynaud's and Buerger's disease.
16. Identify evidence-based practice for care of clients with venous leg ulcers.

LEARNING ACTIVITIES

1. Before completing the study guide exercises for this chapter, it is recommended that you review the following:
    • Anatomy and physiology of the cardiovascular system
    • Cardiovascular assessment
    • Regulation of blood pressure
    • Coagulation cascade
    • Cultural diversity
    • Low-fat diet

2. Review the boldfaced terms and their definitions in Chapter 39 to enhance your understanding of the content.

STUDY/REVIEW QUESTIONS

Answers to the Study/Review Questions are provided on the companion Evolve Learning Resources Web site at http://evolve.elsevier.com/Iggy/.

1. Differentiate between the terms *arteriosclerosis* and *atherosclerosis*.

2. Number in sequence the development of atherosclerosis.

    _____ a.   Fibrous plaque develops.

    _____ b.   Intimal layer of artery is injured.

    _____ c.   Calcification, thrombosis, ulceration of fibrous lesions occur.

    _____ d.   Fatty streak is deposited on intimal layer.

3. Describe each of the following as it relates to the development of atherosclerosis.

    a.   The characteristics of plaque

    b.   Causes of injury to the inner layer of the arterial wall

    c.   The rate of progression and factors that influence it

    d.   The characteristics of a fatty streak

4. Which of the following has a high incidence and primary risk factor related to atherosclerosis and cardiac and vascular diseases?
    a.   Smoking
    b.   Stress
    c.   Hypertension
    d.   Sedentary lifestyle

5. Noted as a result of cholesterol screening, the HDL value for an adult client is greater than 40 with no other cardiac or vascular risk factors. The total serum cholesterol level is 188. The nurse would advise the client to do what?
    a.   Complete a full-fasting lipoprotein analysis.
    b.   Repeat total and HDL cholesterol testing.
    c.   Repeat total and HDL cholesterol testing in 6 to 12 weeks.
    d.   Repeat total and HDL cholesterol testing in 5 years or with physical examination.

6. Which of the following is a nonmodifiable factor that can be a major factor attributing to injury to the intimal layer?
    a.   Smoking
    b.   High-fat diet
    c.   Hypertension
    d.   Aging

7. Which of the following are indicators of metabolic syndrome, thus indicating an increased risk for coronary heart disease? *Check all that apply.*

    _____ a.   Triglyceride level 170 mg/dL

    _____ b.   HDL cholesterol 45 mg/dL in a male

    _____ c.   HDL cholesterol 45 mg/dL in a female

    _____ d.   Blood pressure 130/86

    _____ e.   Fasting blood sugar 100 mg/dL

8.   True or False? Read the following statements regarding atherosclerosis and decide whether each is true or false. *Write T for true or F for false in the blanks provided. If the statement is false, correct the statement to make it true.*

_____ a.   The exact cause of atherosclerosis is unknown; however, there are theories and risk factors.

_____ b.   Atherosclerosis progresses for years before clinical manifestations are evident.

_____ c.   An example of a step one diet is 630 calories a day of fat in a 2100 calorie/day diet.

_____ d.   Meats and eggs contain the lowest amount of saturated fats.

_____ e.   Clients with LDL values of 130 to 159 are advised to follow a fat-modified diet.

_____ f.   Cigarette smoking increases the risk by raising the levels of HDLs.

_____ g.   Routine exercises can promote optimal lipid levels, prevent atherosclerosis, and lead to regression of plaque.

_____ h.   An NIC intervention for smoking cessation is to encourage the client to "listen to relaxation tapes."

_____ i.   Generally, medications for hyperlipidemia should be taken with meals.

9.   On a separate sheet of paper, develop a concept map relevant to atherosclerosis. Consider physiologic, psychosocial, and developmental factors. Identify data that are subjective and data that are objective.

10.   Develop a teaching plan to minimize the risk of atherosclerosis for a 62-year-old client with a total cholesterol laboratory value of 260 mg/dL, triglyceride laboratory value of 210 mg/dL, and normal blood pressure.

11.   Which of the following blood pressure findings for an adult client with no other medical problems should be evaluated further for hypertension? *Check all that apply.*

_____ a.   118/78

_____ b.   124/86

_____ c.   138/78

_____ d.   140/96

12. Complete the following table to compare antihypertensive medications.

ANTIHYPERTENSIVE DRUGS COMPARISON			
Category and Action	**Common Drugs**	**Unique Side Effects**	**Nursing Implications***
Diuretics	Thiazide (low ceiling)		
	Loop (high ceiling)		
	Potassium-sparing		
Calcium channel blockers			
Angiotensin-converting enzyme (ACE) inhibitors			
Angiotensin II receptor antagonists			
Aldosterone receptor antagonists			
Beta-adrenergic blockers			

*Nursing implications in addition to checking blood pressure before administering the medication.

13. Identify reasons why a client being treated with antihypertensive medications may not be compliant with the prescribed regimen.

14. Which of the following organs are affected by complications of hypertension? *Check all that apply.*

_____ a. Kidneys

_____ b. Heart

_____ c. Brain

_____ d. Stomach

_____ e. Eyes

15. Which of the following items should the client with hypertension have available for home use?
    a. Ambulatory blood pressure monitoring device
    b. Exercise bicycle
    c. Blood glucose monitor scale
    d. Food scale

16. At a mall health fair, a client's blood pressure reading is 128/80. Two weeks later, he is seen by his health care provider, and his blood pressure is 130/84. One month later, the reading is unchanged. This client's blood pressure would be classified as which of the following?
    a. Normal
    b. Prehypertension
    c. Stage 1 hypertension
    d. Stage 2 hypertension

17. Initial therapy for uncomplicated hypertension would include which of the following drugs?
    a. Alpha adrenergic blockers
    b. Aldosterone receptor antagonists
    c. ACE inhibitors
    d. Thiazide-like diuretics

18. A client with hypertension also has renal disease and type 2 diabetes mellitus. The goal blood pressure for this client would be which of the following?
    a. 120/80
    b. 130/80
    c. 135/90
    d. 140/90

19. Tissue damage as a result of peripheral arterial disease (PAD) is related to which of the following? *Check all that apply.*

_____ a. Extent of the arterial blockage

_____ b. Length of time there is decreased blood flow

_____ c. Location of the arterial blockage

_____ d. Venous circulation

20. A client who complains of numbness or burning pain that is severe enough to awaken the client at night with dependent rubor is in which of the following stages of PAD? What can the client do to temporarily relieve this pain? What is the implication of these findings?
    a. Stage I
    b. Stage II
    c. Stage III
    d. Stage IV

21. A client with peripheral vascular disease is admitted to the hospital. Which of the following assessment findings are indicative of peripheral arterial disease (PAD) and which are indicative of peripheral vascular disease (PVD)? *Write A for arterial and V for venous.*

_____ a. Decreased peripheral pulses

_____ b. Reproducible leg pain when walking that is relieved by rest

_____ c. Neurologic assessment intact in legs

_____ d. Edema around ankles

_____ e. Paresthesia

_____ f. Loss of hair

_____ g. Skin is cool-to-cold to touch

_____ h. Skin color is pale, dusky, mottled

_____ i. Brown pigmentation of the legs

_____ j. Dependent rubor

_____ k. Thickened toenails

_____ l. Pain in distal portion of extremity

_____ m. Aching pain

_____ n. Pain relieved in dependent position

_____ o. Discomfort relieved with elevation

22. The result of a vascular study related to claudication in the legs indicates a brachial systolic blood pressure of 135 mm Hg with an ankle systolic blood pressure of 105 mm Hg. The ankle-brachial index (ABI) is _____. Evaluate this finding.

23. A client with a history of vascular disease as a result of diabetes has developed a peripheral neuropathy. This client is at risk for which of the following nursing diagnoses?
    a. Fatigue
    b. Acute Pain
    c. Risk for Injury
    d. Disturbed Sensory Perception

24. Which of the following assessment findings indicates arterial ulcers rather than diabetic or venous ulcers?
    a. Ulcer located over the pressure points of the feet.
    b. Ulcer has deep, pale color with even edges and little granulation tissue.
    c. Severe pain or discomfort occurs at the ulcer site.
    d. Ankle discoloration and edema are associated.

25. A complication that can result from severe PAD includes which of the following? *Check all that apply.*

    _____ a. Gangrene

    _____ b. Varicose veins

    _____ c. Septicemia

    _____ d. Amputation

26. A walking program to build collateral arterial circulation in the legs is advised only for clients with which of the following?
    a. Severe pain at rest
    b. Venous ulcers
    c. Gangrene
    d. Intermittent claudication

27. Develop a teaching plan for a client with PAD.

28. Which of the following drugs may be used to promote circulation in the client with chronic PAD? *Check all that apply.*

    _____ a. Pentoxifylline (Trental)

    _____ b. Propranolol hydrochloride (Inderal)

    _____ c. Aspirin

    _____ d. Clopidogrel (Plavix)

29. True or False? A client with PAD is scheduled for a percutaneous transluminal balloon angioplasty. Which of the following statements are true regarding this procedure? *Write T for true or F for false in the blanks provided. For false answers, rewrite to make the statement true.*

_____ a.   A laser probe is advanced through a cannula into the stenosed/occluded artery to open the vessel lumen by heat from the laser vaporization.

_____ b.   This procedure is for the purpose of curing the client of any atherosclerosis of the artery.

_____ c.   Preparation for this procedure is similar to that for a diagnostic angiography.

_____ d.   The nurse monitors for the primary complication of bleeding at the puncture site.

_____ e.   After the procedure, the client is usually on bedrest with the limb straight for 6 to 8 hours.

_____ f.   The occurrence of reocclusion is rare in most clients.

30. A 77-year-old woman has just had femoral-popliteal bypass surgery to treat severe arterial disease.

a.   What are the six Ps that are assessed for after femoral-popliteal bypass surgery in relation to arterial flow and lack of oxygenation to the tissues? Indicate techniques, equipment, and principles that are used by the nurse to assess these findings.

b.   Which of the six Ps written above is often the first indicator of a graft site occlusion and requires immediate attention from the physician? Give an explanation for your answer.

c.   What is the procedure to be followed if a graft occlusion occurs?

31. Which of the following is a postoperative nursing intervention for a client with arterial revascularization?
a.   Promote graft patency by maintaining hypotension and hypovolemic state.
b.   Have the client avoid bending at the hip or knee.
c.   Diet is resumed immediately after surgery for all clients regardless of type of surgery.
d.   Cough and deep breathing exercises are contraindicated because of high risk of ruptured grafts.

32. After arterial revascularization, the extremity becomes edematous with tenseness, pain, decreased sensation, and pulses. The physician is immediately notified regarding a possible _____.

33. What is the most common cause of an acute arterial occlusion related to an emboli?
    a.   Diabetes
    b.   Atherosclerosis
    c.   Atrial fibrillation
    d.   Hypertension

34. A client is seen in the physician's office with a recurrence of a superficial ankle ulcer that is pink in color. Pulses are present. There is edema and discoloration of the leg. The client complains of "discomfort" in the leg but no claudication pain.
    a.   What type of ulcer does this client have? Compare its characteristics with other types of leg ulcers.

    b.   How would the teaching for a client with chronic venous insufficiency differ from teaching for clients with arterial disease?

35. True or False? A client with a venous stasis ulcer has been prescribed an "Unna boot" as a form of treatment. Which of the following statements regarding an Unna boot are true? *Write T for true or F for false in the blanks provided, and rewrite false statements to make them true.*

    _____ a.   It is a type of dressing applied by a health care provider and changed daily.

    _____ b.   It consists of a gauze dressing and is moistened with Betadine or soaked in hydrogen peroxide.

    _____ c.   The Unna boot is covered with elastic wrap that hardens like a cast to promote venous circulation.

    _____ d.   The boot promotes healing by forming a sterile environment for the ulcer.

    _____ e.   The boot is applied around the ankle.

    _____ f.   The ulcer is cleaned with normal saline only before application of dressing.

    _____ g.   Instruct client to assess for signs and symptoms of arterial occlusion if boot is too tight.

36. Indicate whether the following are related to Buerger's disease (B) or Raynaud's disease (R). *Write B or R in the blanks provided.*

    _____ a.   Occurs in smokers and often in young males

    _____ b.   Occurs in both sexes, predominately female

    _____ c.   Episodic, causing white then blue fingers

    _____ d.   Triggered by exposure to cold or tobacco

    _____ e.   Occurs in medium and small arteries and veins

    _____ f.   Severe episodes may lead to gangrene

37. Match the following physical findings with their related arterial disorders.

Physical Findings

_____ a. Blood pressure different in each arm

_____ b. Intermittent claudication in one or both legs

_____ c. Intermittent neck and shoulder pain

Arterial Disorders
1. Popliteal entrapment
2. Subclavian steal
3. Thoracic outlet syndrome

38. Name two common phenomena that can occur as a result of damage to veins.

  a. _____

  b. _____

39. The greatest risk for a pulmonary embolus is a result of which venous disorder?
   a. Bilateral varicose veins
   b. Phlebitis of superficial vein
   c. Thrombophlebitis in deep vein of lower extremity
   d. Venous insufficiency throughout the leg

40. Identify the classic signs and symptoms of a deep vein thrombosis (DVT).

41. A client is admitted to the hospital with a deep vein thrombosis. The physician would order which of the following? Give a rationale for your answer.
   a. Heparin 5000 units SQ twice a day
   b. Loading high dose of Coumadin, then smaller doses on following days
   c. Alternate heparin and Coumadin depending on the laboratory values
   d. Heparin via IV infusion, and starting Coumadin therapy at the same time

42. What is the medication regimen and nursing intervention for a client receiving LMW heparin (Enoxaparin)?

43. The antidote for heparin is _____ and for Coumadin is _____.

44. Which of the following is the most definitively preferred noninvasive test to diagnose a DVT?
   a. Venogram
   b. Duplex ultrasonography
   c. X-ray films
   d. CT scan

45. True or False? Read the following statements regarding venous disorders and decide whether each is true or false. _Write T for true or F for false in the blanks provided. If the statement is false, correct the statement to make it true._

_____ a. Classic signs and symptoms of a DVT are always present.

_____ b. Checking for Homans' sign should be done to assess for a DVT.

_____ c. The focus of treatment for a DVT is to prevent complications and increase in size of the thrombus.

_____ d. DVTs are often treated medically with rest, anticoagulants, and elevation of leg and compression stockings.

_____ e. Thrombolytic agents are only effective if administered within the first 24 hours.

_____ f. To prevent leg edema, elevate legs when in bed or in a chair.

_____ g. To minimize risk of venous insufficiency after a DVT, clients should wear prescribed compression stockings.

46. Which of the following symptoms in the client with DVT who is receiving heparin therapy should the nurse report to the physician immediately?
    a. Pruritus
    b. Rash
    c. Hematuria
    d. Tinnitus

47. Which of the following is the recommended therapeutic range for the INR that is done along with prothrombin time in the client receiving warfarin sodium (Coumadin)?
    a. 0.5 to 1.0
    b. 1.0 to 1.5
    c. 1.5 to 2.0
    d. 2.0 to 2.5

48. A client who is prescribed warfarin sodium (Coumadin) should be instructed that which of the following foods decrease the effect of Coumadin, and therefore, if those foods are eaten, consistency in amount consumed each day is important?
    a. Fresh fruits
    b. Chicken and fish
    c. Green leafy vegetables and cabbage
    d. Milk and cheese

49. In addition to diet and desired laboratory values, indicate additional information a client receiving Coumadin should receive.

50. Which of the following is included in health teaching for the client with chronic venous stasis? *Check all that apply.*

    _____ a. Elevate the legs when sitting.

    _____ b. Avoid crossing legs.

    _____ c. Wear antiembolic stockings at night during sleep

    _____ d. Avoid standing still for any length of time.

51. Which of the following clients are at greatest risk for developing varicose veins?
    a. A 37-year-old mail carrier
    b. A 19-year-old retail store clerk
    c. A 40-year-old operating room scrub technician
    d. A 25-year-old pregnant woman in the first trimester

52. Which of the following is the preferred treatment for phlebitis?
    a. Dry heat
    b. Ice packs
    c. Warm, moist packs
    d. Massage and elevation

53. Identify three common types of vascular injury.

    a. _____

    b. _____

    c. _____

54. Which of the following is the type of vascular injury most likely to result from blunt trauma?
    a. Arteriovenous fistula
    b. Hematoma
    c. Dissection
    d. Incompetent valves

55. Which of the following clients with vascular trauma is a candidate for immediate surgery?
    a. A 54-year-old with fractured humerus
    b. A 36-year-old with a ruptured renal artery
    c. An 18-year-old with a contusion of the leg
    d. A 67-year-old with a chronic subdural hematoma

56. Identify, in order of priority, the three top principles of management of vascular trauma.

    a. _____

    b. _____

    c. _____

57. An aneurysm is a permanent localized dilation of an artery. Match the following types of aneurysms with their descriptions.

Descriptions

_____ a. Involves the entire circumference of artery

_____ b. Involves a distinct portion of the artery

_____ c. Is caused by blood in wall of the artery

Types of Aneurysms
1. Dissecting aneurysm
2. Saccular
3. Fusiform

58. What is the most common location for an aneurysm?
    a. Abdominal aorta
    b. Thoracic aorta
    c. Femoral arteries
    d. Popliteal arteries

59. What is the most common cause of an aneurysm?
    a. Emboli
    b. Trauma
    c. Atherosclerosis
    d. Thrombus formation

60. A 75-year-old man with a history of atherosclerosis enters the emergency department with pain in his abdomen. What finding would indicate a possible abdominal aortic aneurysm? *Check all that apply.*

    _____ a. Chest pain

    _____ b. Steady, gnawing pain for the past 3 days

    _____ c. Visible pulsation on the upper abdominal wall

    _____ d. Decreased blood pressure

61. The client in Question 60 is admitted to the hospital. The physician would order which of the following tests to confirm an accurate diagnosis as well as to determine the size and location of the AAA? *Check all that apply.*

    _____ a. Abdominal x-rays

    _____ b. Ultrasound

    _____ c. Electrocardiogram

    _____ d. MRI

62. Which of the following is the best nonsurgical intervention to use to decrease the risk of rupture of an aneurysm and to slow the rate of enlargement?
    a. Maintenance of normal blood pressure and avoidance of hypertension
    b. Bedrest until there is shrinkage of the aneurysm
    c. Heparin and Coumadin therapy to increase blood flow
    d. Intra-arterial thrombolytic therapy

63. The client with a ruptured aneurysm may exhibit which of the following symptoms? *Check all that apply.*

    _____ a. Decreased heart rate

    _____ b. Increased heart rate

    _____ c. Increased blood pressure

    _____ d. Decreased blood pressure

    _____ e. Severe pain

    _____ f. Diaphoresis

    _____ g. Dilated pupils

    _____ h. Decreased level of consciousness

64. Which of the following actions should the nurse take first if a client has a suspected aneurysm rupture?
    a. Start an intravenous infusion with a large-bore needle.
    b. Assess baseline measurements of blood pressure and pulse rate.
    c. Palpate the pulsating abdominal mass to determine its size.
    d. Assess all peripheral pulses to use as a baseline for comparison.

65. Why is the client with a repair of an abdominal aneurysm being monitored postoperatively for urinary output and renal function studies (creatinine and BUN)?
    a. The client was probably in shock preoperatively and there may be glomerular damage.
    b. The client is usually in a critical care nursing unit where this is done routinely.
    c. The aorta was clamped during the surgery and the kidneys may have been inadvertently damaged.
    d. Repair of the aneurysm improves renal perfusion and the urinary output should increase.

66. Before surgery to repair an aneurysm, monitoring of which of the following is most important?
    a. Peripheral pulses
    b. Temperature
    c. Blood pressure
    d. Color of extremity

67. Following an aortic aneurysm repair, the nurse would monitor which of the following for several days after surgery? What is the complication that may result?
    a. ECG
    b. Blood pressure
    c. Bowel sounds
    d. Pulse oximetry

68. Following repair of a thoracic aneurysm, the nurse monitors for and immediately reports which of the following?
    a. Shallow respirations and poor coughing
    b. Increased drainage from the chest tubes
    c. Sternal pain with coughing and deep breathing
    d. Increased urinary output from the indwelling catheter

69. In addition to hemorrhage, clients with repair of thoracic aneurysm are monitored for which of the following complications? *Check all that apply.*
    _____ a. Cardiac dysrhythmias
    _____ b. Paraplegia
    _____ c. Respiratory distress
    _____ d. Hemorrhage

70. Which of the following activities is allowed after discharge of the client who has had an aneurysm repair?
    a. Playing golf
    b. Washing dishes
    c. Raking leaves
    d. Driving a car

71. Summarize the discharge teaching for a client with an abdominal aortic aneurysm (AAA) repair.

72. Which statement regarding aortic dissection is true?
    a. It is relatively uncommon in the United States.
    b. It occurs primarily in adults in their 50s and 60s.
    c. There is a high survival rate.
    d. Hypotension and atherosclerosis are the primary causes.

CASE STUDY: THE CLIENT WITH HYPERTENSION

Answer Guidelines for the Case Study questions are provided on the companion Evolve Learning Resources Web site at http://evolve.elsevier.com/Iggy/.

Your client is a 64-year-old African-American man who is diagnosed with hypertension. He is 6 feet tall and weighs 300 pounds. He smokes two packs of cigarettes per day. He works as a salesman and has two to three drinks a week. He admits that he does not get as much exercise as he used to when he was 40 years old. His mother and brother have high blood pressure, and his father died of a heart attack at age 68.

1. Does he have essential or secondary hypertension? Can you tell at this point? Give a rationale for your answer.

2. What diseases would have made this client at risk for developing secondary hypertension?

3. What cultural aspects need to be considered in controlling his hypertension?

4. How does this client's age impact the diagnosis and treatment of hypertension?

5. During the initial workup for hypertension, what laboratory testing would you expect to be ordered? Explain.

6. An interdisciplinary team consult was completed. What assessment findings would indicate successful outcomes have been met?

This client was later seen in the emergency department with severe headache, extremely high blood pressure, dizziness, blurred vision, and disorientation.

7. His diagnosis is _____. Describe the medical interventions for this problem.

CASE STUDY: THE CLIENT WITH DEEP VEIN THROMBOSIS

Answer Guidelines for the Case Study questions are provided on the companion Evolve Learning Resources Web site at http://evolve.elsevier.com/Iggy/.

A 58-year-old woman was discharged from the hospital 4 days ago after lower abdominal surgery. She has been readmitted for pain and edema in her right calf. She has a tentative diagnosis of thrombophlebitis.

1. Discuss the probable etiology of this client's thrombophlebitis.

2. The physician prescribes heparin sodium 1000 units per hour intravenously for this client, and also begins therapy with warfarin (Coumadin). Discuss the purpose of these medications, the nursing precautions, and laboratory tests to monitor their effectiveness.

3. The client asks you, "Which medication dissolves the clot? The IV or the pill?" What do you say to her? How does heparin differ from warfarin in the treatment of thrombophlebitis?

4. This client is placed on strict bedrest with her legs elevated, and a warm, moist pack is to be applied. What are the purposes of these interventions?

5. The following morning, the client complains of leg cramps and asks the nurse to massage her calf because it is "cramping." Should the nurse comply with this request? Why or why not?

6. The client's activated partial thromboplastin time is 70 seconds (the hospital's control range is 22.1 to 34.1 seconds) and the INR is 1. Discuss the significance of these test results.

7. The client's laboratory values are now within therapeutic range, and the client is being discharged from the hospital on Coumadin. Develop a teaching-learning plan for this client.

Interventions for Clients with Shock

LEARNING OUTCOMES

1. Describe the clinical manifestations associated with the compensatory mechanisms for shock.
2. Identify clients at risk for hypovolemic shock.
3. Use laboratory data and clinical manifestations to determine the effectiveness of therapy for shock.
4. Explain the basis for intravenous therapy for shock.
5. Describe the mechanisms of action, side effects, and nursing implications for pharmacologic management of shock.
6. Prioritize nursing care for the client experiencing the nonprogressive stage of hypovolemic shock.
7. Compare the pathophysiology and clinical manifestations of the hyperdynamic and hypodynamic phases of septic shock.
8. Identify clients at risk for septic shock.
9. Identify nursing practices to reduce infection risk in an immunocompromised client.
10. Explain the rationale for the drug therapy for septic shock.
11. Prioritize nursing care for the client experiencing the hyperdynamic stage of septic shock.
12. Prioritize nursing care for the client experiencing the hypodynamic stage of septic shock.
13. Develop a community-based teaching plan for the client at risk for septic shock.

LEARNING ACTIVITIES

1. Before completing the study guide exercises for this chapter, it is recommended that you review the following:
    *   General adaptation syndrome
    *   Fluid and electrolytes
    *   Acid-base balance
    *   Anatomy and physiology of respiratory, cardiovascular, and renal systems
    *   Principles of cardiac output
    *   Respiratory and cardiac assessment, including peripheral vascular assessment

2. Review the boldfaced terms and their definitions in Chapter 40 to enhance your understanding of the content.

STUDY/REVIEW QUESTIONS

Answers to the Study/Review Questions are provided on the companion Evolve Learning Resources Web site at http://evolve.elsevier.com/Iggy/.

1. As the foundation for understanding the mechanism of shock, complete the following statement related to human physiology. The ability of the circulatory system to deliver oxygen to the tissues is related to the _____.

2. Which factors listed below affect mean arterial pressure? *Check all that apply.*
   - _____ a. Size of the capillary bed
   - _____ b. Total blood volume
   - _____ c. Cardiac output
   - _____ d. Heart size

3. Which factors identified in Question 2 directly correlate with the MAP when it increases or decreases?

4. Which factor in Question 2 is inversely related to the MAP?

5. Which of the following statements about the control of blood flow is correct?
   a. The most influential factor is the regional control.
   b. The brain can independently control its own blood flow.
   c. Blood vessels contain nerves from the sympathetic nervous system.
   d. Blood flow in all organs is increased at the same rate.

6. Which of the following best describes shock?
   a. A disease state involving the heart, blood vessels, or blood
   b. Abnormal cellular metabolism caused by inadequate delivery of oxygen
   c. Physiologic changes in cardiac output
   d. Lack of oxygenation related to an increase in mean arterial pressure

7. Which hormones are released in response to decreased MAP? *Check all that apply.*
   - _____ a. Insulin
   - _____ b. Renin
   - _____ c. ADH
   - _____ d. Epinephrine
   - _____ e. Aldosterone
   - _____ f. Serotonin

8. True or False? Read the following statements regarding shock and decide whether each is true or false. *Write T for true or F for false in the blanks provided. If the statement is false, correct the statement to make it true.*

   - _____ a. Regardless of the cause, the pathophysiologic cellular response is the same for all types of shock.

   - _____ b. When shock occurs, the body fails and death is the inevitable result.

   - _____ c. The older adult and immunosuppressed clients are the only clients who are at risk for shock.

   - _____ d. The most reliable indicator that would cause a nurse to suspect shock in a client is changes in the systolic blood pressure.

   - _____ e. Anaphylactic shock is a result of an antigen-antibody reaction.

   - _____ f. Oxygen administration is appropriate therapy for any type of shock.

_____ g. Most clinical manifestations of shock are related to the body's compensatory response to shock and not the cause of shock.

_____ h. Changes in systolic blood pressure are a reliable indicator of the early stage of shock.

9. The body's ability to initiate the compensatory response for the anaerobic metabolism and decreased MAP is stimulated by which of the following?
    a. Coronary arteries
    b. Carotid and aortic baroreceptors
    c. Respiratory center in the brain
    d. Parasympathetic nervous system

10. Identify clinical manifestations of shock as they relate to the various body systems.
    a. Cardiovascular manifestations:

    b. Respiratory manifestations:

    c. Neuromuscular manifestations:

    d. Renal manifestations:

    e. Integumentary manifestations:

    f. Gastrointestinal manifestations:

11. In the table below, summarize stages of shock according to the general MAP response, the related compensatory mechanism, and specific clinical manifestations.

Stage of Shock	General Body Response, Compensatory Mechanism, and Clinical Manifestations
Initial/early stage	
Nonprogressive/ compensatory stage	
Progressive/ intermediate stage	
Refractory stage of shock/irreversible	

12. The major pathophysiologic event in the refractory or irreversible stage is which of the following?
    a. Renal failure
    b. Cardiac failure
    c. Sympathetic nervous system failure
    d. Hormone failure

13. Which of the following is an early sign of shock?
    a. Cool, clammy skin
    b. Decreased urinary output
    c. Restlessness
    d. Hypotension

14. Match the overall pathophysiology response that occurs with various types of shock.

Types of Shock	**General Pathophysiology Responses**
_____ a. Hypovolemic	1. Indirect pump failure
_____ b. Cardiogenic	2. Vascular tone/volume decreased
_____ c. Distributive	3. Intravascular volume depleted
_____ d. Obstructive	4. Direct pump failure

15. Match each of the following types of clients who may be at risk with the corresponding type of shock. *Answers may be used more than once.*

Types of Clients

_____ a. Client with cardiac tamponade

_____ b. Older adult with urinary tract infection

_____ c. Client who recently received a vaccine

_____ d. Client who had a myocardial infarction

_____ e. Client who had a ruptured aortic aneurysm

_____ f. Client with a bowel obstruction

_____ g. Client with insect bites

_____ h. Client with ruptured spleen resulting from trauma

_____ i. Client receiving chemotherapy

_____ j. Client with pulmonary emboli

_____ k. Client receiving heparin therapy

_____ l. Older adult who has a spinal cord reunion

_____ m. Client with electrolyte imbalance and dehydration

_____ n. Client with diabetes insipidus

_____ o. Older adult with sacral pressure ulcers

_____ p. Client who has cancer of the head and neck, with a nasogastric tube

_____ q. Client with VRE or MRSA

_____ r. Client with heart failure, receiving diuretic therapy

Types of Shock
1. Hypovolemic
2. Cardiogenic
3. Distributive-neurogenic
4. Obstructive
5. Distributive-chemical
6. Distributive-septic

16. Which of the following assessment findings is most indicative of the early phase of sepsis-induced distributive shock?
    a. Crackles in lung bases
    b. Weak, rapid peripheral pulses
    c. Cool, clammy, and cyanotic skin
    d. Increased cardiac output with warm, pink skin

17. A client has cardiac dysrhythmias and pulmonary problems as a result of receiving an IV antibiotic. What type of shock would this represent?
    a. Hypovolemic
    b. Cardiogenic
    c. Anaphylactic
    d. Septic

18. What is the most common cause of distributive (septic) shock?
    a. Gram-negative bacteremia
    b. Gram-positive bacteremia
    c. Viral sepsis
    d. Fungal sepsis

19. What is the most common cause of hypovolemic shock?
    a. Traumatic limb amputation
    b. Ruptured esophageal varices
    c. Wound dehiscence and evisceration
    d. Deep lacerations and blunt trauma

20. What is the most common cause of anaphylaxis?
    a. Poisonous snake bites
    b. Food reaction
    c. A drug reaction
    d. Human bites

21. What is the most common cause of cardiogenic shock?
    a. Heart failure
    b. Myocardial infarction (MI)
    c. Valvular disease
    d. Cardiac tamponade

22. Which of the following is an assessment finding that is consistent with hypovolemic shock?
    a. Pulse pressure of 40 mm Hg
    b. A rapid, weak, and thready pulse
    c. Cyanotic, cool extremities
    d. Increased muscle strength

23. Which of the following is a life-threatening pulmonary complication of shock?
    a. Adult respiratory distress syndrome
    b. Oxygen toxicity
    c. Status asthmaticus with bronchospasm
    d. Alveolar collapse and altered perfusion

24. What is the priority for managing a client with cardiogenic shock?
    a. Open heart surgery
    b. Insertion of intra-aortic balloon pump
    c. Administration of thromboembolic agents
    d. Determination and treatment of the cause of the shock state

25. Match either the colloid or crystalloid solution with each of the indications. *Answers will be used more than once.*

Indications

_____ a. Hemorrhagic shock

_____ b. Fluid replacement

_____ c. Restore osmotic pressure

_____ d. Carries oxygen to peripheral tissues

_____ e. Does not cause allergic reactions

_____ f. Substitute for blood

Solutions

1. Colloid
2. Crystalloid

26. Indicate which solutions are colloids and which are crystalloids. Mark colloids as 1 and crystalloids as 2.
    a. Normal saline
    b. Hetastarch
    c. Packed red cells
    d. Ringer's lactate
    e. Fresh frozen plasma (FFP)

27. Which intravenous fluid solution would result in the greatest increase in oxygen-carrying capacity for a person with hypovolemic shock?
    a. Lactated Ringer's solution
    b. Hetastarch
    c. Fresh frozen plasma
    d. Packed red cells

28. Which of the following data indicate that a client is responding to treatment for shock?
    a. Blood pH of 7.28
    b. Arterial Po_2 of 65 mm Hg
    c. Distended neck veins
    d. Increased urinary output

29. Which of the following statements about drug therapy for hypovolemic shock is correct?
    a. Vasoconstricting agents stimulate venous return by increasing venous pooling of blood.
    b. Atropine increases the contractile response of cardiac muscle cells.
    c. Digoxin (Lanoxin) prolongs ventricular filling time and stimulates the ventricle to contract.
    d. Sodium nitroprusside (Nitropress) dilates coronary blood vessels and causes systemic vasoconstriction.

30. The nurse's role includes prevention of shock by which of the following interventions?
    a. Assessing arterial blood gas values
    b. Monitoring all clients at risk for shock
    c. Instructing clients in lifestyle changes
    d. Performing blood cultures

31. Which of the following would be part of a deficient knowledge teaching plan related to prevention of septic shock in at-risk clients? *Check all that apply.*

    _____ a. Wash hands frequently using antimicrobial soap.

    _____ b. Avoid aspirin and aspirin-containing products.

    _____ c. Avoid large crowds or gatherings where people might be ill.

    _____ d. Do not share utensils; wash toothbrush in dishwasher.

    _____ e. Take temperature once a week.

    _____ f. Do not change pet litter boxes.

32. A 70-year-old man is admitted to the hospital with an infected finger of several days' duration. He is lethargic, confused, and has a temperature of 101.3° F. Other assessment findings are BP of 94/50, HR 105, RR 40, and shallow breathing. Pulmonary arterial wedge pressure (PAWP) was 4 mm Hg. These assessment findings indicate what type of shock?
    a. Hypovolemic
    b. Cardiogenic
    c. Anaphylactic
    d. Septic shock

33. A postsurgical hospitalized client has a falling blood pressure; elevated, thready pulse; shallow respirations of 26; and pale skin. The client is in what phase of shock?
    a. Compensatory/nonprogressive
    b. Progressive
    c. Refractory
    d. Multiple organ dysfunction

34. Assessment findings of a client with trauma injuries reveals cool, pale skin; complaints of thirst, urine output 100 mL/8 hr, BP 122/78, HR 102, RR 24 with decreased breath sounds. This client is in what phase of shock?
    a. Compensatory/nonprogressive
    b. Progressive
    c. Refractory
    d. Multiple organ dysfunction

35. Drug therapy specific to distributive (septic) shock management includes which of the following?
    a. Inotropics
    b. Antibiotics
    c. Vasoconstrictors
    d. Antidysrhythmics

36. List four treatment modalities for a client with hypovolemic shock.

    a. _____

    b. _____

    c. _____

    d. _____

37. List four treatment modalities for a client with septic shock.

    a. _____

    b. _____

    c. _____

    d. _____

38. When dopamine is administered 20 mcg/kg/min IV in the treatment of shock, the nurse will assess for which of the following?
    a. Decreased urine output and decreased blood pressure
    b. Increased respiratory rate and increased urine output
    c. Chest pain and hypertension
    d. Bradycardia and headache

39. When administering Levophed, the nurse needs to monitor for which of the following?
    a. Decreased tissue perfusion
    b. Profuse sweating
    c. High output renal failure
    d. Chest pain

40. Which of the following is the best indicator of progressing shock?
    a. Elevated body temperature
    b. Absent peristalsis
    c. Decreasing urine output
    d. Vasodilation

41. A hospitalized client received an antibiotic and developed anaphylactic shock. Which of the following assessment findings indicates this type of shock?
    a. Cool skin, rapid heart rate, and changes in mental status
    b. Decreased heart rate, cyanosis, and bronchospasm
    c. Hypertension, distended neck veins, and bounding pulses
    d. Bronchospasm, dysrhythmias, massive vasodilation

42. A head injury client was treated for a cerebral hematoma. After surgery, this client is at risk for what type of shock?
    a. Obstructive
    b. Cardiogenic
    c. Distributive-chemical
    d. Distributive-neural

43. After discharge from the hospital, which of the following is a common psychosocial problem faced by the client who has suffered from hypovolemic shock?
    a. Confusion related to loss of fluids
    b. Anxiety regarding recurrence of shock or fear of dying
    c. Inability to perform activities of daily living
    d. Acceptance of resulting self-care limitations

44. Identify three common nursing diagnoses associated with hypovolemic shock.

    a. _____

    b. _____

    c. _____

45. Which of the following is a factor that increases the older adult's risk for distributive (septic) shock?
    a. Reduced skin integrity
    b. Diuretic therapy
    c. Cardiomyopathy
    d. Musculoskeletal weakness

46. The clinical manifestations in the first phase of sepsis-induced distributive shock results from the body's reaction to which of the following?
    a. Leukocytes
    b. Endotoxins
    c. Hemorrhage
    d. Hypovolemia

47. Identify nursing interventions for a client with hypovolemic shock.

48. Which of the following is typically given intravenously in the treatment of hypovolemic shock due to hemorrhage?
    a. Ringer's lactate
    b. Blood and blood products
    c. Normal saline
    d. Fresh frozen plasma

49. The nurse would expect which of the following when a client with sepsis is in phase 2 of shock?
    a. Drop in blood pressure
    b. Dyspnea
    c. Tachycardia with a bounding pulse
    d. Increased urine output

50. True or False? Read the following statements regarding shock and decide whether each is true or false. *Write T for true or F for false in the blanks provided. If the statement is false, correct the statement to make it true.*

    _____ a. Hypovolemic shock occurs when there is a decrease in blood volume that causes the MAP to decrease, resulting in lack of tissue oxygenation.

    _____ b. Examples of external causes of hypovolemic shock are trauma, wounds, and surgery.

    _____ c. Dehydration, as a result of decreased fluid intake or increased fluid loss, can cause hypovolemic shock.

    _____ d. Distributive shock is a result of a decrease in the MAP caused by a loss of sympathetic tone, blood vessel dilation, pooling of blood in venous and capillary beds, and increased blood vessel permeability (leak).

    _____ e. Sepsis leading to distributive shock occurs when antibiotic therapy causes an allergic reaction.

    _____ f. Anaphylactic shock results from large amounts of histamines and other inflammatory substances being rapidly released throughout the circulatory system, causing massive blood vessel dilation and increased capillary permeability.

    _____ g. Age is not a risk factor in the development of sepsis.

    _____ h. During the hyperdynamic phase of septic shock, the endotoxins cause a decrease in cardiac output.

    _____ i. The clinical manifestations of the first phase of septic shock are unique, often opposite to other types of shock, and therefore can be misinterpreted by the health care provider as a shock state.

51. Septic shock is the result of:

52. Unlike other types of shock, septic shock has the following two phases:

    a. _____

    b. _____

53. The assessment findings of a client suspected of septic shock reveals lethargy, disorientation, tachycardia, changes in white blood cell count, and normal temperature. This client is in which phase of septic shock? Give a rationale for your answer.
    a.   Hyperdynamic
    b.   Hypodynamic

54. Which of the following is appropriate for the care of a client in septic shock? *Choose all that apply.*

    _____   a.   Elevate feet, with the head flat or elevated 30 degrees

    _____   b.   Monitor vital signs every 5 minutes until they are stable

    _____   c.   Administer clotting factors or plasma in phase 1

    _____   d.   Administer heparin in phase 2

    _____   e.   Provide oxygen therapy

55. Can shock be prevented? Discuss this question with your classmates and instructor.

CASE STUDY: THE CLIENT WITH HYPOVOLEMIC SHOCK

Answer Guidelines for the Case Study questions are provided on the companion Evolve Learning Resources Web site at http://evolve.elsevier.com/Iggy/.

A 38-year-old female client returned to the post-anesthesia recovery area 2 hours ago after undergoing a tubal ligation by colposcopy (through the back wall of the vagina behind the cervix). Her last documented vital signs, taken 30 minutes ago, were BP = 102/80, pulse = 88, and respirations = 22. You now note that her face is pale, and the skin around her lips has a bluish cast. Her vital signs are now BP = 90/76, pulse = 98, and respirations = 28.

1. What additional assessment techniques would you perform?

2. Where would you look for the hemorrhage?

3. What other data would you gather?

4. When you reassess her in 15 minutes, you find the following vital signs: BP = 88/70, pulse = 102, and respirations = 30. She awakens when you shake her arm and complains of back pain and thirst. Given these findings, what are your priority actions?

5. What expected outcomes would be specific to this situation?

Interventions for Critically Ill Clients with Acute Coronary Syndromes

CHAPTER 41

LEARNING OUTCOMES

1. Describe the relationship between coronary artery disease (CAD) and acute coronary syndromes (ACS).
2. Explain the pathophysiology of ACS.
3. Compare and contrast stable angina, unstable angina, and myocardial infarction (MI).
4. Identify modifiable and nonmodifiable risk factors for ACS.
5. Interpret physical and diagnostic assessment findings in clients who have ACS.
6. Describe the psychosocial aspects of ACS.
7. Prioritize nursing care for clients who have ACS.
8. Identify the life-threatening complications of ACS.
9. Explain the advantages of thrombolysis for a client experiencing an MI.
10. Compare and contrast the drug classifications used to treat ACS.
11. Describe the appropriate nursing interventions for monitoring clients receiving drug therapy for ACS.
12. Develop a plan of care for the client who has undergone a percutaneous transluminal coronary angioplasty.
13. Manage care for the client who has undergone coronary artery bypass graft (CABG) surgery.
14. Discuss the differences between CABG surgery, minimally invasive direct coronary artery bypass, off-pump CABG, and transmyocardial laser revascularization.
15. Develop a discharge plan for the client with ACS.

LEARNING ACTIVITIES

1. Before completing the study guide exercises for this chapter, it is recommended that you review the following:
   - Anatomy and physiology of the cardiovascular system
   - Atherosclerosis
   - Arteriosclerosis
   - Diabetes
   - Hypertension
   - Myocardial infarction
   - Cardiovascular and respiratory assessment

- Postoperative care
- Principles of cardiac output
- Shock, cardiogenic shock

2. Review the boldfaced terms and their definitions in Chapter 41 to enhance your understanding of the content.

STUDY/REVIEW QUESTIONS

Answers to the Study/Review Questions are provided on the companion Evolve Learning Resources Web site at http://evolve.elsevier.com/Iggy/.

1. What is the leading cause of coronary artery disease (CAD)?
   a. Aging
   b. Atherosclerosis
   c. Diabetes
   d. Hypertension

2. Which of the following statements best describes the pathophysiology regarding the leading cause of CAD as indicated in the previous question?
   a. There is a blockage of blood that supplies oxygen and nutrients to the cardiac cells.
   b. There is an accumulation of lipids in the intimal layer of the arteries that blocks the flow of blood.
   c. CAD is the result of ischemia and infarction of the myocardium.
   d. CAD occurs when there is an increase in demand of arterial blood flow with activity.

3. Differentiate stable and unstable angina pectoris.

4. Which of the following assessment findings is associated with calcium channel blocker therapy?
   a. Wheezes
   b. Hypotension
   c. Bradycardia
   d. Forgetfulness

5. In addition to atherosclerosis, indicate other common causes of a myocardial infarction.

6. Denial is a common reaction of clients with cardiovascular disease. What other psychosocial reactions should a nurse assess for?

7. Which of the following statements about the heart's physiologic response to an infarction is correct?
   a. The infarcted area shows signs of inflammation after 24 hours.
   b. Neutrophils invade the areas to remove necrotic cells within 6 hours.
   c. Granulation tissue begins to form 8 to 10 days after infarction.
   d. Scar tissue remodeling resembles the original tissue in size and shape.

8. The location of a myocardial infarction (MI) associated with the highest mortality rate is which of the following, and why?
   a. Anterior wall
   b. Lateral wall
   c. Inferior wall
   d. Posterior wall

9. The ECG reading may indicate which of the following as a result of an anterior wall MI?
   a. Bradycardia
   b. PVCs
   c. Atrial fibrillation
   d. Second-degree heart block

10. What complication of an anterior wall MI may result in an insertion of a pacemaker?
    a. Third-degree heart block
    b. PVCs
    c. Bradycardia
    d. Second-degree AV block

11. Which of the following clients is at greatest risk for having a fatal MI?
    a. A 36-year-old athletic man who smokes
    b. A 72-year-old woman who smokes and is obese
    c. A 24-year-old man with a family history of hypertension
    d. A 32-year-old woman with elevated serum cholesterol levels

12. Which of the following tests is diagnostic for myocardial damage caused by an MI?
    a. Positive chest x-ray
    b. Creatine kinase (CK) elevation
    c. ECG: ST depression, T-wave inversion, wide Q
    d. CK-MB isoenzymes elevation

13. An assessment finding that may indicate heart failure as a result of an MI is which of the following heart sounds?
    a. Murmur
    b. S_3 gallop
    c. Split S_1 and S_2
    d. Pericardial friction rub

14. Which of the following regarding thrombolytic therapy is correct?
    a. Streptokinase is the drug of choice for all clients.
    b. Monitor for bleeding—laboratory values, stool, urine, CVA, epistaxis.
    c. Wait until 12 hours after onset of chest pain to administer medication.
    d. Therapy is quick and easy to use with few allergic reactions.

15. A client who has been admitted for surgery with a history of angina reports to you, the nurse, symptoms of tightness or pressure in the chest radiating to the left arm. Your assessment also includes cool, clammy skin, BP 150/90, P 100, R 32.
    a. What is the priority nursing diagnosis?

    b. Based on the assessment findings, summarize the priority nursing interventions for this client.

16. Which of the following are examples of acute coronary syndromes? *Choose all that apply.*
    _____ a. Variant angina
    _____ b. New-onset angina
    _____ c. Stable angina
    _____ d. Crescendo angina
    _____ e. Myocardial infarction

17. Which of the following diagnostic tests is used to identify the client who may benefit from further invasive management after acute angina or an MI?
    a. Exercise tolerance test
    b. Cardiac catheterization
    c. Thallium scan
    d. Multigated angiogram (MUGA) scan

18. Which of the following statements indicates correct understanding regarding the effects of angina on sexual activity?
    a. "I will not be able to resume the same level of physical exertion as I did before I had chest pain."
    b. "I will discuss alternative methods with my partner since I will no longer be able to have sexual intercourse."
    c. "I should stress myself to see if sexual activity is a problem."
    d. "I should engage in sexual activity after a rest period."

19. Identify subjective data that would be included in the nursing assessment of a client with CAD.

20. Identify objective data that would be included in the nursing assessment of a client with CAD.

21. What complication can occur as a result of necrosis of more than 40% of left ventricle failure?
    a. Hypovolemic shock
    b. Cardiogenic shock
    c. Valve regurgitation
    d. PVCs

22. Indicate your assessment findings for the complication indicated in Question 21.

23. What treatment modality would you expect for the complication in Question 21, and why?

24. Interventions for the clients with heart failure following an MI include which of the following?
    a. Administering digoxin (Lanoxin), 1.0 mg, as a loading dose and then daily
    b. Infusing IV fluids to maintain a urinary output of 60 mL/hr
    c. Titrating vasoactive drugs to maintain a sufficient cardiac output
    d. Observing for such complications as hypertension, flushed hot skin, and agitation

25. A client with angina who is scheduled for PTCA should also sign a consent for which of the following?
    a. Intra-aortic balloon pump
    b. Coronary artery bypass graft (CABG)
    c. Cardiac catheterization
    d. Carotid endarterectomy

26. Identify the primary indications for CABG and give examples of clients who would be candidates for this surgery.

27. A client is not responding to drug therapy to improve tissue perfusion from cardiogenic shock and requires an intra-aortic balloon pump (IABP). Briefly describe IABP and when it is designed to inflate and deflate during systole and diastole.

_____ e. Premenopausal women have a lower incidence of MI than men do.

_____ f. Postmenopausal women in their 70s have a higher incidence of MI than men.

_____ g. More women than men die within 1 year of initial recognition of an MI.

28. A client with an inferior MI has a 30% chance of developing which of the following?
    a. Valve damage
    b. Atrial fibrillation
    c. Right ventricular infarction and failure
    d. Left ventricular infarction and failure

_____ h. For women, impaired glucose tolerance (e.g., diabetes) seriously increases the risk of CAD.

29. True or False? Read the following statements and decide whether each is true or false. _Write T for true or F for false in the blanks provided. If the statement is false, correct the statement to make it true._

_____ a. More men than women have angina.

_____ b. Some women may experience atypical angina as indigestion or a choking sensation.

_____ c. Angina in women has often been misdiagnosed.

_____ d. Cardiac disease is the leading cause of death for men in the most prevalent ethnic groups, but not for women.

30. A post-MI client in phase 1 cardiac rehabilitation would perform which of the following activities?
    a. Range-of-motion exercises
    b. Modified weight training
    c. Brisk walking
    d. Jogging

31. An MI client has advanced to phase 3 cardiac rehabilitation. Which activity is indicated for this phase?
    a. Biking in the mountains
    b. Playing doubles in tennis
    c. Working out with weights at a fitness center
    d. Walking several miles three times a week

32. Identify at least three reasons for treating dysrhythmias.

    a. _____

    b. _____

    c. _____

33. Which of the following statements regarding nitroglycerin are true? *Check all that apply.*

    _____ a. Reduces venous return to the heart

    _____ b. Increases coronary artery blood flow

    _____ c. Reduces coronary artery spasm

    _____ d. Increases heart rate and contractility

34. A client is prescribed nitroglycerin tablets. Which of the following should be included in the client education? *Check all that apply. Give a rationale as to why the other choices are wrong.*

    _____ a. If one tablet does not relieve the angina after 5 minutes, take two pills.

    _____ b. You can tell the pills are active when your tongue feels a tingling sensation.

    _____ c. Keep your nitroglycerin in your pocket with your other pills at all times.

    _____ d. The prescription should last you about 6 months before having it refilled.

    _____ e. If the pain doesn't go away, sit down and wait; the medication takes a while to take effect.

    _____ f. The medication causes the blood vessels to dilate or widen in order to let more blood flow to the heart.

    _____ g. It can cause a temporary headache or a flushed face.

35. Interventions for the hospitalized client who is being treated initially with intravenous nitroglycerin include which of the following?

    a. Increasing dose rapidly to achieve pain relief
    b. Assisting the client to bathroom as needed
    c. Monitoring blood pressure continuously
    d. Elevating the head of the bed to 45 degrees

36. A client complains of chest pain that is unrelieved with nitroglycerin. The nurse should prepare to administer which of the following?

    a. Valium IM
    b. Morphine sulfate IV
    c. Haldol IV push
    d. Chewable aspirin

37. Indicate whether the characteristics listed below are angina (A) or myocardial infarction (MI).

    _____ a. Pain is precipitated by exertion or stress.

    _____ b. Pain occurs without cause, usually in the morning.

    _____ c. Pain is relieved only by opioids.

    _____ d. Pain is relieved by nitroglycerin or rest.

    _____ e. Nausea, diaphoresis, feelings of fear, and dyspnea may occur.

    _____ f. There are few associated symptoms.

    _____ g. Pain lasts less than 15 minutes.

    _____ h. Pain lasts 30 minutes or more.

    _____ i. Pain radiates to left arm, back, or jaw.

38. Which drug is given within 24 hours of a myocardial infarction to help the heart to perform 25% to 30% more work without ischemia?
    a. Opioid analgesic, such as morphine sulfate
    b. Beta-adrenergic blocking agents, such as metoprolol (Lopressor)
    c. Antiplatelet agents, such as aspirin
    d. Calcium channel blockers, such as diltiazem (Cardizem)

39. A client is being evaluated for thrombolytic therapy. Contraindications for this procedure include which of the following? *Check all that apply*.

    _____ a. CVA within the last 6 months

    _____ b. Pregnancy

    _____ c. Surgery within the last 10 days

    _____ d. Major trauma in the last 3 months

    _____ e. Endocarditis

    _____ f. Pericarditis

    _____ g. DVT

40. Before having a CABG, a client is taking a beta blocker, digitalis, and a diuretic. What teaching should be given to the client regarding these drugs before this surgery?

41. Identify the complications for which the nurse should monitor in a postoperative client with CABG.

42. Which of the following is a problem that may result in the collapse of a vein graft?
    a. Cardiac tamponade
    b. Hypotension
    c. Hypertension
    d. Hypothermia

43. Which electrolytes are closely monitored in a postoperative client with a CABG ? *Check all that apply*.

    _____ a. Sodium

    _____ b. Potassium

    _____ c. Calcium

    _____ d. Magnesium

    _____ e. Phosphorus

44. Identify how the fluids are regulated in the postoperative client with a CABG to avoid complications.

45. A postoperative client suddenly has a decrease in mediastinal drainage, jugular vein distention with clear lung sounds, pulsus paradoxus, and equalizing PAWP and right atrial pressure. These are signs of which of the following? Indicate the nursing interventions for this problem.
    a. Severe postoperative pain
    b. Occlusion of the venous graft
    c. Cardiac tamponade
    d. Anxiety reaction

46. True or False? Read the following statements and decide whether each is true or false. *Write T for true or F for false in the blanks provided. If the statement is false, correct the statement to make it true.*

    _____ a. One third of all clients with CABG develop dysrhythmias.

    _____ b. Sternal wound infections develop within 24 hours of surgery.

    _____ c. Signs and symptoms of mediastinitis are fever, bogginess of wound, and increased WBCs.

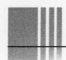

47. Identify special considerations for the older adult with a CABG.

48. A client is being discharged from the hospital after a CABG. Indicate topics that would be covered in the discharge teaching for home care and provide an example of what is included for each topic.

49. Which of the following is the most significant risk factor for coronary artery disease (CAD)?
    a. Smoking
    b. High-calorie diet
    c. Inactivity
    d. Stress

50. Develop a teaching plan for preventing CAD.

51. Which of the following is an over-the-counter product that is often used by clients on a daily basis as a preventive measure for CAD?
    a. Ibuprofen
    b. Aspirin
    c. Acetaminophen
    d. Caffeine

52. A hospitalized client with a history of angina complains of chest pain. Summarize the nursing interventions for this client.

53. The client in the previous question is being discharged from the hospital. Tell what information you, as the nurse, would reinforce for this client with CAD regarding activity.

54. True or False? A client is scheduled to receive a thrombolytic agent to dissolve thrombi in the coronary arteries. Which of the following statements are true regarding this intervention? *Write T for true or F for false in the blanks provided, and correct statements that are false.*

_____ a.   Examples of agents are t-PA and streptokinase.

_____ b.   These agents are most effective when administered within the first 6 hours of the coronary event.

_____ c.   Streptokinase is the most commonly used thrombolytic agent.

_____ d.   It is indicated when a client has chest pain of duration greater than 1 hour and that is unrelieved by other medication.

_____ e.   The nurse must monitor for bleeding by assessing IV site, laboratory values, and neurologic status, and by observation.

55. A client has arrived at the open-heart surgical intensive care unit after surgery for a triple bypass graft. Indicate what your responsibilities as nurse would be for this client at this time.

56. Which of the following diagnostic tests is performed after angina or MI to determine ECG changes that are consistent with ischemia, to evaluate medical interventions, and to determine whether invasive intervention is necessary?
    a.   Stress test
    b.   ECG
    c.   Cardiac catheterization
    d.   Chest x-ray

57. Identify the common nursing diagnoses for clients with CAD.

    a.   _____

    b.   _____

    c.   _____

    d.   _____

58. What is the purpose of administering morphine sulfate IV to relieve chest pain?

59. What are signs of morphine toxicity? What is used to treat this?

60. After an MI, which of the following drugs is prescribed within 48 hours to prevent the development of heart failure?
    a.   Calcium channel blockers
    b.   ACE inhibitors
    c.   Beta blockers
    d.   Digoxin

61. For patients who are hypertensive and continue to have angina despite therapy with beta blockers, which drug is indicated?
    a. Calcium channel blocker
    b. Digoxin
    c. ACE inhibitor
    d. Dopamine

62. After an inferior MI, the client is at risk for developing which of the following dysrhythmias?
    a. Bradycardia and second-degree heart block
    b. PVCs
    c. Third-degree heart block
    d. Bundle branch block

63. A relatively common complication after an MI is _____, and the most severe form is _____.

64. When a client is hemodynamically stable, the client should show evidence of this by:

    a. _____

    b. _____

    c. _____

    d. _____

    e. _____

65. Clients with class I heart failure respond best to which of the following medications?
    a. Digoxin
    b. Beta blockers
    c. Calcium channel blockers
    d. Diuretics

66. A client with discrete, proximal, noncalcified lesions of only one or two vessels is more than likely to benefit from which of the following procedures?
    a. PTCA
    b. Stress test
    c. IABP
    d. Thrombolytic therapy

67. Identify the postprocedure care of a client receiving PTCA.

68. Treatment of hypothermia, a common problem after CABG surgery, with warming blankets is necessary because this condition can cause the client to be at risk for which of the following?
    a. Hypotension
    b. Hypertension
    c. Heart failure
    d. Loss of consciousness

69. True or False? Which of the following statements are true regarding the level of consciousness for a client with CABG? *Write T for true or F for false in the blanks provided, and correct false statements to make them true.*

    _____ a. It can be transient or permanent.

    _____ b. Permanent deficits may be associated with CVA.

    _____ c. Return to baseline usually occurs within 4 to 8 hours.

    _____ d. Seventy-five percent of clients experience some form of transient mental status changes.

    _____ e. Signs and symptoms can include slowness of arousal, memory loss, and confusion.

70. Following a CABG, the nurse must be knowledgeable to monitor what areas in order to provide safe quality client care?

4. What instructions should this client have received regarding managing her chest pain at home?

CASE STUDY: THE CLIENT WITH ANGINA

Answer Guidelines for the Case Study questions are provided on the companion Evolve Learning Resources Web site at http://evolve.elsevier.com/Iggy/.

A 68-year-old woman arrives in the emergency department stating, "I think I had a heart attack." She states that she had an episode of chest pain that lasted a couple of minutes during her daily 3-mile walk; the pain was relieved by rest. ECG rhythm is normal sinus rhythm. She has no abnormal heart sounds or laboratory values. VS are stable. PO_2 by pulse oximetry is 97% on room air. She is diagnosed with angina.

1. How would this client's clinical manifestations be different if she had had an MI?

2. How would you explain to the client the diagnosis of angina?

3. What teaching would you provide for this client regarding her diagnosis of angina?

The client is seen by a cardiologist who prescribes nitroglycerin tablets, nifedipine, and one baby aspirin per day. After 6 months, the client returns to the cardiologist with additional complaints regarding her chest pain. A cardiac catheterization reveals the following results: 50% blockage of the circumflex artery, 60% blockage of the anterior descending (LAD), and 90% blockage of the right coronary artery.

5. On this client's return appointment, what assessment findings indicate to the cardiologist that her angina is now unstable?

6. This client is a 68-year-old woman. Describe the relationship between older adults, particularly older women, and heart disease.

7. Procardia was prescribed for this client. Identify the drug classification of this medication and the pertinent information that a client needs to know about it.

2. What client education would you provide for this client?

CASE STUDY: THE CLIENT WITH CORONARY ARTERY DISEASE

Answer Guidelines for the Case Study questions are provided on the companion Evolve Learning Resources Web site at http://evolve.elsevier.com/Iggy/.

3. Explain to this client his risk factors for developing CAD.

Your client is a 40-year-old African-American man with a history of hypertension. He is being seen for an annual physical and admits that he has experienced chest pain "a time or two" when he takes the stairs at work, so lately he has avoided the stairs. The chest pain subsided once he rested for a few minutes in his office. He smokes one pack of cigarettes per day. He is 5 feet, 8 inches tall and weighs 250 pounds. He takes hydrochlorothiazide and Procardia for his hypertension. His last serum cholesterol level was 220 mg/dL, with the HDL 35 mg/dL and LDL 105 mg/dL. His father died of an MI at age 54 and his mother has hypertension. He works 50 hours a week as a lawyer and takes occasional walks on weekends.

1. What are this client's modifiable risks for CAD? What are his nonmodifiable risks for CAD?

Assessment of the Hematologic System

LEARNING OUTCOMES

1. Describe the hematologic changes associated with aging.
2. Explain the process of erythrocyte maturation.
3. Describe the role of platelets in hemostasis.
4. Compare the structure and function of platelet plugs and fibrin clots.
5. Interpret blood cell counts and clotting tests to assess the client's hematologic status.
6. Compare the actions and uses of anticoagulants, fibrinolytics, and inhibitors of platelet activity.
7. Develop a community-based teaching plan for the client on anticoagulant therapy at home.
8. Prioritize nursing care for the client after bone marrow aspiration.

LEARNING ACTIVITIES

1. Before completing the study guide exercises in this chapter, it is recommended that you review the anatomy and physiology of the blood and blood components.

2. Review the boldfaced terms and their definitions in Chapter 42 to enhance your understanding of the content.

STUDY/REVIEW QUESTIONS

Answers to the Study/Review Questions are provided on the companion Evolve Learning Resources Web site at http://evolve.elsevier.com/Iggy/.

1. The hematologic system is concerned with blood formation and storage. Identify the parts that compose the system.

2. Define the following terms and abbreviations:
   Hematopoietic

   RBC

   Erythrocytes

   WBC

   Leukocytes

   Stem cells

   Erythropoietin

   Oxygen dissociation

   Hypoxia

   Aggregation

   Macrocytic

   Microcytic

   Hypochromic

3. Identify the hematopoietic organ that is also involved in the immune response.

4. Identify the types of cells produced by the bone marrow.

5. Describe the formation of blood components from fetus to adulthood.

6. Explain how the bone marrow produces blood cells. Refer to Figure 42-1 in the textbook.

7. Plasma is the extracellular fluid of the body and carries three to four times the amount of protein in interstitial fluid. Identify the three types of plasma protein and their functions.

   a. _____

   b. _____

   c. _____

8. Describe the RBC and its special features; give the normal range for RBCs.

9. Describe the formation of RBCs. Use Figures 42-1 and 42-2 in the textbook.

10. An RBC life span is 120 days; destruction is done by a cooperative effort of which of the following?
     a.   Bone marrow and the spleen
     b.   Macrophages, spleen, and liver
     c.   Platelets, spleen, and liver
     d.   RBCs, spleen, and liver

11. Identify the parts that must be present in the RBC to transport oxygen.

12. Identify the functions of RBCs.

13. Identify the body organ that controls RBC production and destruction. Describe how it determines the need for production or destruction of RBCs.

14. Identify the seven substances needed to form RBCs and hemoglobin.

15. If any of the above substances are missing from your client's diet, what might the client develop?

16. In the formation of platelets, what is the role of the megakaryocyte?
     a.   It is a part of the formation of any cell type.
     b.   It breaks into pieces called platelets.
     c.   It is necessary for RBC formation.
     d.   It does not release platelets.

17. Describe the functions of a platelet in the body.

18. What stimulates platelet production?

19. Describe the life activities of a platelet.

20. Describe the three tissues of the spleen and their functions.
     a.   _____
     b.   _____
     c.   _____

21. Identify the four functions of the spleen.
     a.   _____
     b.   _____
     c.   _____
     d.   _____

22. The liver plays an important part in the hematologic process. Identify its functions and its relationship to vitamin K.

23. Describe homeostasis of blood clotting and anticlotting.

24. Identify the three-step process of blood clotting.

25. Explain why platelets normally do not stick together.

26. What is formed when the platelets are stimulated to aggregate?

27. Compare and contrast a platelet plug and a blood clot.

28. Explain the cascade reaction that begins when a platelet plug is formed.

29. Identify the intrinsic events that stimulate platelet aggregation.

30. Review Table 42-2 in the textbook, and identify the clotting factors and cofactors for forming fibrin.

31. Platelets aggregate in response to extrinsic factors, such as which of the following?
    a. Trauma
    b. Bacteria
    c. WBCs
    d. Antibody-antigen reactions

32. Identify the two specific substances on which the formation of a platelet plug is dependent.

    a. _____

    b. _____

33. Describe the sequence in which clotting factor and inactive proteins result in activating fibrinogen into fibrin. Use Table 42-2 in the textbook.

34. Using Figure 42-5 in the textbook, describe fibrin and its role in clot formation.

35. Which of the following describes the formation of fibrin mesh?
    a. More platelets and cells stick to the mesh, clotting factor XIII stabilizes it, and serum is extruded.
    b. Clotting factor XIII stabilizes it; more platelets, blood cells, and protein form a clot; and serum is extruded.
    c. Serum seals it with clotting factor XIII to stabilize it and more platelets and blood cells and protein form a clot.
    d. Heparin is mobilized, clotting factor XIII encircles it, and protein binds to the mesh.

36. Compare and contrast the roles of the spleen and the liver in hematopoiesis.

37. Explain the importance of anticoagulation forces in maintaining the control of blood flow in the body during formation of clots.

38. Describe the breakdown of plasminogen into plasmin, and identify what the enzyme digests to break down a fibrin clot. See Figure 42-6 in the textbook.

39. Identify eight changes in the hematologic system of older adults. Review Chart 42-1 in the textbook to learn how to identify some of these changes upon physical assessment of an older adult.

   a. _____

   b. _____

   c. _____

   d. _____

   e. _____

   f. _____

   g. _____

   h. _____

40. Describe how anticoagulants exert their effect on the blood-clotting cascade and identify the categories.

41. Describe the action of thrombolytic agents and identify the four agents used most commonly.

42. Identify the four conditions for which thrombolytic therapy is used.

   a. _____

   b. _____

   c. _____

   d. _____

43. Clots older than 6 hours are not recommended for thrombolytic therapy because of which of the following?
   a. Cost
   b. Anoxic tissue
   c. Large size of clot
   d. Too many clots

44. Thrombolytic therapy is not used for deep vein thrombosis or massive pulmonary emboli because of which of the following?
   a. The clots are easily accessed and can be treated with other methods.
   b. Tissue that has been anoxic for some time is not worthwhile to preserve.
   c. The amount of drug and the duration of therapy needed are cost-prohibitive and risky.
   d. The clots are too small to be affected by the drug.

45. List and discuss four areas the nurse should investigate when taking a history from a client with a clot.

46. Assessment for anemia should include a detailed list of what client behaviors for a period of at least one week?

47. Identify the major way that alcohol consumption can affect the hematologic system.

48. A person subsisting on a low income may have a diet deficient in what dietary nutrients?

49. When performing a physical assessment, the nurse should question women about their menorrhagia. What questions would the nurse ask to get an estimate and pattern of menorrhagia?

50. Which symptom of anemia is the client most likely to report?

51. Identify five additional symptoms of anemia.

    a. _____

    b. _____

    c. _____

    d. _____

    e. _____

52. Identify sites the nurse would check to assess for pallor and jaundice.

53. Describe the differences between petechiae and ecchymoses.

54. Describe the different looks of the tongue in pernicious anemia, iron deficiency anemia, and nutritional deficiencies.

55. In performing a client examination, the nurse requests a urine specimen. The client asks why this specimen is being collected. What would the nurse explain to answer this question?

56. Describe abdominal organs the nurse would assess, and explain why this is important in determining a diagnosis of a hematologic disorder.

57. Identify the types of neurologic impairment that can occur with vitamin B_{12} deficiency.

58. Identify the parts of a complete blood count.

59. Describe the difference in mean corpuscular volume being elevated and being decreased, and the effect these changes have on the body.

60. What is indicated by an elevated neutrophil count without an accompanying elevation in leukocyte alkaline phosphate?

61. Demonstrate on a classmate a capillary fragility test. Count the petechiae.

62. Identify the drugs monitored by PT levels and identify their therapeutic levels.

63. State the therapeutic range of INR when used to monitor warfarin therapy.

64. What test is used to monitor heparin therapy and what is the desirable range?

65. State the missing factors that are produced in the liver that can extend a PTT.

66. von Willebrand's disease is characterized by what phenomenon?

67. What procedure can be used to evaluate iron storage sites in bone marrow?

68. Describe the difference between a bone marrow biopsy and bone marrow aspiration.

69. What sensations should the nurse tell the client to expect during a bone marrow biopsy or aspiration procedure?

CASE STUDY: HEMATOLOGY ASSESSMENT

Answer Guidelines for the Case Study questions are provided on the companion Evolve Learning Resources Web site at http://evolve.elsevier.com/Iggy/.

The client is a 45-year-old woman who is married to a career military officer. Her father was a miner, leading an itinerant life as he worked in uranium mines. She grew up in a western state and remembers playing with other children on slag heaps from the mines. She recalls being ill often as a child and attributes this to being chronically undernourished. The family was often cold during the winter months when there was no money to buy warm clothing or fuel for heat.

Over the past 6 months, the client has had episodes of epistaxis and prolonged bleeding after having her teeth cleaned by a dental hygienist. She has also noticed that she seems to bruise easily: There are multiple ecchymotic areas on her legs and arms. She reported to the military hospital for a checkup and was referred to a regional civilian hospital for further evaluation. During the admission history, she tells the nurse that she tires easily and often has little energy. Her husband and children are worried about her.

1. What additional data should the nurse elicit from the client at this time?

2. Based on the above data, formulate relevant nursing diagnoses for the client.

As part of the diagnostic workup, the client is scheduled to have blood work drawn for CBC with differential, platelets, electrolytes, bleeding time, PT, PTT, iron, TIBC, and albumin.

3. What are the purposes of these laboratory studies?

4. The results of the laboratory tests and bone scan indicate that the client has depressed bone marrow function. The hematologist discusses plans to perform a bone marrow aspiration with her. What is the purpose of this procedure?

5. Develop a teaching-learning plan for the bone marrow aspiration procedure.

6. Just before the hematologist is expected to arrive to perform the aspiration, the client asks the nurse if she is going to die. She says she is scared and begins to cry. How should the nurse respond?

Interventions for Clients with Hematologic Problems

CHAPTER 43

LEARNING OUTCOMES

1. Identify three clinical manifestations common to clients who have any type of anemia.
2. Explain the pattern of inheritance for sickle cell disease.
3. Prioritize nursing care for the client who has sickle cell disease.
4. Plan a diet for a client who has iron deficiency anemia or vitamin B_{12} deficiency anemia.
5. Explain the mechanism of action and potential side effects of epoetin alpha therapy.
6. Compare the pathologic mechanisms of hemolytic anemia versus aplastic anemia.
7. Compare leukemia and lymphoma for etiology, pathophysiology, and clinical manifestations.
8. List four risk factors for the development of leukemia.
9. Analyze laboratory data and clinical manifestations to determine the presence of infection in a client who has neutropenia.
10. Compare the purposes and scheduling of induction therapy, consolidation therapy, and maintenance therapy for leukemia.
11. Prioritize nursing interventions for the client with neutropenia.
12. Prioritize nursing interventions for the client with thrombocytopenia.
13. Develop a community-based teaching plan for a client with thrombocytopenia.
14. Prioritize nursing responsibilities during transfusion therapy.
15. Identify clients at risk for complications of transfusion therapy.

LEARNING ACTIVITIES

1. Before completing the study guide exercises in this chapter, it is recommended that you review the following:
   - Anatomy and physiology of the blood and blood products
   - Normal laboratory values for red and white cells
   - Principles of inflammation and infection
   - Function of vitamins
   - Principles of good nutrition

2. Review the boldfaced terms and their definitions in Chapter 43 to enhance your understanding of the content.

STUDY/REVIEW QUESTIONS

Answers to the Study/Review Questions are provided on the companion Evolve Learning Resources Web site at http://evolve.elsevier.com/Iggy/.

1. Discuss the origins of problems with erythrocytes.

2. Describe two types of anemias based on reduction in components of the hematologic system.

   a. _____

   b. _____

3. Identify and briefly describe four types of anemia caused by deficiencies.

   a. _____

   b. _____

   c. _____

   d. _____

4. Identify which of the following descriptors relate to RBCs and which relate to sickle cells. *Write R for RBCs or S for sickle cells in the blanks provided.*

   _____ a. 20-day life span

   _____ b. 120-day life span

   _____ c. Destroyed in spleen

   _____ d. Chronically stimulated bone marrow

   _____ e. HbS

   _____ f. Clumps with hypoxia

   _____ g. May not be able to return to proper shape

   _____ h. Biconcave disk

   _____ i. HbA

   _____ j. Sickle-shaped and twisted

5. Describe the difference between sickle cell disease and sickle cell trait.

6. When counseling a client with sickle cell disease, what should the nurse say about an offspring's chance of having the disease?

7. The client with the sickle cell trait asks the nurse about problems that might occur with the disease. What should teaching include when replying to the client?

8. Identify six causes of a sickle cell crisis.

   a. _____

   b. _____

   c. _____

   d. _____

   e. _____

   f. _____

9. State the major problem of sickle cell disease crisis and describe how it is treated.

10. For each body system listed, identify an assessment finding in a client with sickle cell disease.
    a. Cardiovascular

    b. Integumentary

    c. Abdominal

    d. Musculoskeletal

    e. Psychosocial

11. Identify four therapies that can be used for sickle cell disease in conjunction with opioids.

    a. _____

    b. _____

    c. _____

    d. _____

12. Clients with sickle cell disease are more susceptible to infections, specifically *Streptococcus pneumoniae* and *Haemophilus influenzae*, which can be prevented with which of the following? *Check all that apply.*
    _____ a. Consistent good handwashing technique
    _____ b. Yearly vaccination
    _____ c. Twice daily oral penicillin
    _____ d. NSAIDs

13. Indicate which of the following the nurse would administer to a client with multiple organ dysfunction and explain why. *Choose all that apply.*
    _____ a. IV fluid up to 500 mL/hr
    _____ b. Oxygen with nebulization
    _____ c. Transfusions
    _____ d. Albumin

14. Transfusions of RBCs are therapeutic because of which of the following? *Choose all that apply.*
    a. HbA levels are sustained as HbS levels are diluted.
    b. It suppresses erythropoiesis.
    c. It decreases menstrual flow in women.
    d. It decreases incidence of organ dysfunction and stroke.

15. What would the nurse emphasize in teaching the teenage female client with sickle cell disease with respect to contraception?

16. Identify three clinical manifestations common to clients who have any type of anemia.

    a. _____

    b. _____

    c. _____

17. Plan a diet for a client with an iron deficiency anemia or vitamin B_{12} deficiency anemia.

18. Which of the following relates to polycythemia vera?
    a. Has the symptom of hypocellularity
    b. Causes plethoric appearance of the face
    c. Causes hypotension and thrombosis
    d. Can be cured with anticoagulants

19. Explain the rationale for periodic phlebotomy for the client with polycythemia vera.

20. Polycythemia vera has many negative effects on the body. List and describe four of them

    a. _____

    b. _____

    c. _____

    d. _____

21. Identify the more intensive therapies for polycythemia vera.

22. Identify and define the two categories of leukemia with respect to cell types.

    a. _____

    b. _____

23. Describe the pathophysiology of leukemia.

24. Several categories of leukemia are listed in the textbook. Review these and identify a condition or substance that may be a risk factor for each category.

25. Indicate which type of leukemia is most common in adults, in children, and in older adults.

26. Which of the following types of leukemia is the least common?
    a. Chronic myelogenous leukemia
    b. Acute myelogenous leukemia
    c. Acute lymphocytic leukemia
    d. Chronic lymphocytic leukemia

27. List three areas that are important to assess when doing a hematologic assessment and interviewing a client.

    a. _____

    b. _____

    c. _____

28. Explain what it means when bone marrow is full of blast phase cells.

29. Identify the common nursing diagnoses for an adult client with leukemia.

30. Define autocontamination and cross-contamination.

31. Match the types of therapy with their descriptions. *Answers may be used more than once.*

Descriptions

_____ a. Aimed at achieving a rapid, complete remission

_____ b. Prescribed orally, 3 to 5 years

_____ c. Intent to cure; repeat of previous treatment therapy

_____ d. Has many side effects, including immunosuppression

Types of Therapy
1. Maintenance therapy
2. Induction therapy
3. Consolidation therapy

32. What are the disadvantages of treatment with granulocyte transfusions?

33. Drugs used for prophylaxis in the client with leukopenia include which of the following? *Check all that apply.*

_____ a. Antibiotics

_____ b. Antifungal vaginal creams

_____ c. Antiviral agents

_____ d. Analgesics

34. Describe each of the following types of protection that can be provided to a client with leukopenia.
    a. Protective (reverse) isolation

    b. Cross-contamination prevention

    c. Minimal bacteria diet

    d. HEPA filtration system

35. Bone marrow transplants are most ideally done during which stage of therapy? *Check all that apply.*

_____ a. Induction therapy

_____ b. Consolidation therapy

_____ c. Maintenance therapy

_____ d. Radiation therapy

36. What is the goal of bone marrow or stem cell transplantation?

37. Along with chemotherapy, the client with leukemia is routinely given which of the following?
    a. Hormone therapy
    b. Radiation therapy
    c. Psychotherapy
    d. Heat shock therapy

38. Match each type of transplant to the source of transplant tissue.

Source		Type of Transplant
_____ a.	From a sibling or HLA match	1. Allogeneic
		2. Autologous
		3. Syngeneic
_____ b.	From an identical twin	
_____ c.	From own stem cells	

39. Identify the five phases of transplant procedures.

    a. _____

    b. _____

    c. _____

    d. _____

    e. _____

40. What should the nurse tell the client in describing the bone marrow transplant procedure?

41. In addition to having the aspiration sites monitored, what else do bone marrow donors need and why? *Choose all that apply.*

    _____ a. Fluid for hydration

    _____ b. Pain management

    _____ c. Possible RBC infusion

    _____ d. Antibiotic therapy

42. Peripheral blood stems are obtained by pheresis during which stage?
    a. Collection
    b. Reinfusion
    c. Mobilization
    d. Suppression

43. Define *mobilization*.

44. Identify the common complications of pheresis.

45. How long after a bone marrow transplant might a client have effects of conditioning for the procedure?

46. How is the bone marrow transplant administered?

47. Which of the following symptoms should the nurse observe for and treat in a bone marrow transplant recipient? *Choose all that apply.*

    _____ a. Fever

    _____ b. Hypertension

    _____ c. Chills

    _____ d. Red urine

48. Engraftment is the settling in of stem cells and the beginning of producing new cells. Indicate when success of this procedure is known and explain.
    a. 8 to 12 hours after infusion
    b. 8 to 12 days after infusion
    c. 12 to 28 days after infusion
    d. b or c

49. Identify the reasons for possible failure of an engraftment.

50. Describe graft-versus-host disease (GVHD) and common areas of damage.

51. GVHD occurs most frequently in which clients?

52. Describe the kind of treatment for a client with veno-occlusive disease (VOD) and explain the choice.

53. Early detection enhances the chance of survival for a patient with veno-occlusive disease (VOD). How would the nurse monitor this client?
    a. The same as any other client
    b. The same as a client with hepatic problems
    c. While he or she is in isolation
    d. While he or she is on bedrest

54. Explain nadir.

55. Referring to Charts 43-10 and 43-11 in the textbook, describe the interventions for bleeding precautions.

56. When should the nurse start to administer a thrombopoietic agent?

57. How do leukemic cells compare with normal white blood cells in terms of metabolism and oxygen consumption?

58. Explain the mechanism of action and the potential side effects of epoetin alpha therapy.

59. Identify the needs of a marrow transplant recipient being discharged home after transplantation.

60. Compare and contrast leukemia and lymphoma in regard to etiology, pathophysiology, and clinical manifestations.

61. Match each descriptor, symptom, or treatment with the corresponding disease.

Descriptor, Symptom, or Treatment

_____ a.   White men older than 50

_____ b.   Sixth most common cause of cancer death

_____ c.   Mid-to-late 20s; men older than 50 years

_____ d.   Viral infections and exposure to alkylating chemical agents

_____ e.   Twelve subtypes

_____ f.   Reed-Sternberg cell

_____ g.   Enlarged painless lymph node or nodes

_____ h.   Prognosis best in women

_____ i.   Stages I and II: treat with radiation; add chemotherapy for more extensive disease

Disease
1. Non-Hodgkin's lymphoma
2. Hodgkin's lymphoma

62. Prioritize nursing care for the client with thrombocytopenia.

63. Develop a teaching plan for a client who is at home and has thrombocytopenia.

64. Identify which of the following applies to autoimmune thrombolytic purpura (ATP) and which applies to thrombotic thrombocytopenic purpura (TTP). Write ATP for autoimmune thrombolytic purpura or TTP for thrombotic thrombocytopenic purpura in the blanks provided.

    _____ a. Was idiopathic

    _____ b. Platelets clump

    _____ c. Antibodies directed against own platelets

    _____ d. Inappropriate aggregation of platelets

    _____ e. Women 20 to 40 years of age

    _____ f. Pre-existing autoimmune condition

    _____ g. Plasmapheresis

    _____ h. Immunosuppressive therapy to reduce intensity

    _____ i. Corticosteroids and azathioprine

65. Describe three ways that coagulation disorders or bleeding disorders can develop.

    a. _____

    b. _____

    c. _____

66. List three common congenital disorders that result in defects of the clotting factor.

    a. _____

    b. _____

    c. _____

67. Disseminated intravascular coagulation (DIC) is an acquired clotting disorder closely related to which of the following?
    a. Hemophilia
    b. Septic shock
    c. von Willebrand's disease
    d. Leukemia

68. Christmas disease is also known as which of the following?
    a. Hemophilia A
    b. Hemophilia B
    c. Thrombocytopenia
    d. Sickle cell disease

69. Describe how the X-linked recessive trait for hemophilia is transmitted by the mother.

70. Distinguish the clinical characteristics of hemophilia A and hemophilia B.

71. Explain why clients with hemophilia have bleeding problems when injured.

72. Clients with hemophilia have which of the following problems in comparison with healthy clients?
    a. Bleeding more often
    b. Bleeding more rapidly
    c. Bleeding for a longer period
    d. Bleeding internally more often

73. Common history of the client with hemophilia is which of the following? *Check all that apply.*

_____ a. Excessive hemorrhage from minor cuts

_____ b. Joint and muscle hemorrhages

_____ c. Easily bruised

_____ d. Potential for postoperative hemorrhage

74. The laboratory tests for a client with hemophilia include all but which of the following?
    a. INR in the normal range
    b. Prolonged partial thromboplastin
    c. Normal prothrombin time
    d. Normal bleeding time

75. What therapy is used for the client with hemophilia A to control bleeding?

76. What is the most common health problem of the client with hemophilia?

77. List nursing actions performed during transfusion of a client receiving a blood transfusion.

78. What are the necessary components of a physician's order for transfusion therapy?

79. What document may require signing before administration of a blood transfusion?

80. Explain the reason for typing and cross-matching blood.

81. What size intravenous needle is appropriate for administering a blood transfusion?
    a. 22-gauge needle
    b. 20-gauge needle
    c. 19-gauge needle or larger
    d. Butterfly needle

82. What special administration equipment is necessary for a blood transfusion?

83. The protocol for giving blood calls for the use of what solution with the blood?
    a. Ringer's lactate
    b. Normal saline
    c. Dextrose in water
    d. Dextrose in saline

84. Why is D_5W contraindicated when giving blood?
    a. It causes hemolysis of blood cells.
    b. It dilutes the cells.
    c. It shrinks the blood cells.
    d. It causes blood cells to coagulate.

85. What infusions are acceptable to add to blood products?

86. What precaution with respect to the physician's order for transfusion is taken before administration?

87. Any severe reactions from a blood transfusion usually occur within the first:
    a. 15 minutes.
    b. 50 mL of blood.
    c. Hour.
    d. 100 mL of blood.

88. How often should vital signs be checked for the client receiving a transfusion?
    a. Every 15 minutes throughout the transfusion
    b. Every 15 minutes times 2, and then every hour throughout the infusion
    c. Every 15 minutes times 4, and then every hour throughout the infusion
    d. Every 15 minutes times 2, and then every 2 hours throughout the infusion

89. Describe the protocols for administration of other blood components without RBCs.

90. What would the nurse explain to the client who asks why so many precautions are needed for a blood transfusion?

91. Identify the blood types and list the associated antigens.

92. Explain the mechanism of the Rh antigen system and state the significance of this with respect to blood transfusions.

93. What is given to treat possible sensitization to Rh+ during a pregnancy and delivery?

94. Explain why platelets are given quickly with a special filter and short tubing.

95. The client receiving a platelet transfusion may be premedicated with which of the following to prevent a reaction?
    a. Demerol and Vistaril
    b. Valium and aspirin
    c. Benadryl and Tylenol
    d. Hydrocortisone and Demerol

96. A client is receiving an infusion of amphotericin B. Before starting administration of blood products, the nurse should do which of the following?
    a. Premedicate the client to reduce the risk of reaction.
    b. Stop the infusion of the antifungal agent.
    c. Set up piggyback administration so that the infusions can run in together.
    d. Start another IV line to run the blood products in so the amphotericin can run uninterrupted.

97. Describe how fresh frozen plasma is infused and give rationale for the answer.

98. Identify different reactions a client can have to a blood transfusion; identify the clinical signs of hemolytic transfusion reaction.

99. What symptoms commonly signal a transfusion reaction, and how long after the transfusion might they occur?

100. Identify the symptoms of a febrile reaction to a transfusion and describe the appropriate care for the client.

101. A client experiencing bacterial transfusion reaction needs to be treated for which of the following?
    a. Allergic reaction
    b. Anaphylaxis
    c. Septic shock
    d. Infection only

102. Identify the symptoms of circulatory overload and indicate who is most at risk.

103. Describe transfusion-associated graft-versus-host disease.

104. List three characteristics of TA-GVHD.

    a. _____

    b. _____

    c. _____

105. How may TA-GVHD be prevented?

106. (a) Identify the advantages of autologous blood transfusion. (b) Identify the types of autologous blood transfusion. (c) Explain intraoperative and postoperative autologous infusions and when they are used.

Assessment of the Nervous System

LEARNING OUTCOMES

1. Compare the functions of the major divisions of the nervous system.
2. Describe the mechanisms of nerve impulse transmission.
3. Identify the structure and function of different areas of the central and peripheral nervous system.
4. Identify common physiologic changes associated with aging that affect the nervous system.
5. Perform a neurologic history.
6. Perform a comprehensive neurologic physical assessment.
7. Perform a rapid neurologic assessment and interpret findings.
8. Interpret results of cerebrospinal fluid analysis.
9. Plan and implement pretest and follow-up care for clients undergoing common neurologic diagnostic tests.

LEARNING ACTIVITIES

1. Before completing the study guide exercises for this chapter, it is recommended that you review the following:
    *   The anatomy and physiology of the neurologic system (central and peripheral)
    *   The process of nerve conduction
    *   The principles of acid-base balance

2. Review the boldfaced terms and their definitions in Chapter 44 to enhance your understanding of the content.

STUDY/REVIEW QUESTIONS

Answers to the Study/Review Questions are provided on the companion Evolve Learning Resources Web site at http://evolve.elsevier.com/Iggy/.

1. Which of the following statements is true about the neuron?
    a. Axons, the efferent pathway, may travel great distances from the cell body.
    b. All axons are covered with a myelin sheath that enhances nerve conduction.
    c. Dendrite processes send information out of the cell body.
    d. Synaptic knobs are responsible for storing and releasing transmitter substances.

2. List and describe the three areas that constitute a synapse.

    a. _____

    b. _____

    c. _____

3. Identify factors that influence transmission of impulses between neurons.

4. The speed of neural transmission depends on which of the following?
    a. Number and intensity of stimuli
    b. Myelination of the axon
    c. Diameter of the nerve fibers
    d. Width of the synaptic cleft

5. Which factors inhibit and which enhance transmission? *Answers may be used more than once.*

Factors

_____ a. Acetylcholine

_____ b. Anoxia

_____ c. Distance from the cell body

_____ d. Aspartic acid

_____ e. GABA

_____ f. CSF alkalosis

_____ g. Tea or coffee

Actions

1. Inhibit
2. Enhance
3. May do either

6. Match each cell type with the role it plays.

Cell Type

_____ a. Microglia cells

_____ b. Astroglia cells

_____ c. Ependymal cells

_____ d. Oligodendrocytes

Role

1. Physical support
2. Part of blood-brain barrier
3. Scavengers
4. Form myelin sheath

7. Identify the two components of the central nervous system.

    a. _____

    b. _____

8. Which of the following statements about the meninges is correct?
    a. The dura mater is thin and delicate and adheres to the brain.
    b. Cerebrospinal fluid (CSF) fills the subarachnoid layer.
    c. The dura mater is a single tough membrane that protects the pia mater.
    d. The epidural space only extends down to the cervical vertebrae.

9. The dura mater dips down between the cerebral hemispheres and the cerebrum and the cerebellum. Which of the following statements is true?
   a. The dura between the hemispheres is called the tentorium.
   b. The dura between the cerebellum and the cerebrum is called the falx.
   c. The falx enhances transmission of forces between the cerebral hemispheres.
   d. The falx and the tentorium protect the lower brainstem.

10. Match the following cerebral areas with their functions.

Cerebral Areas

_____ a. Motor cortex of the frontal lobe
_____ b. Broca's area
_____ c. Occipital lobe
_____ d. Parietal lobe
_____ e. Limbic lobe
_____ f. Wernicke's area
_____ g. Temporal lobe

Functions
1. Speech center
2. Visual center
3. Initiate voluntary movement
4. Process language
5. Spatial perception
6. Complicated memory patterns
7. Emotional and visceral patterns

11. Match each area of the diencephalon with its function.

Areas of the Diencephalon
_____ a. Thalamus
_____ b. Hypothalamus
_____ c. Epithalamus
_____ d. Subthalamus

Functions
1. Point of reference in x-rays
2. Connects to basal ganglion
3. Crudely perceives all sensations except smell
4. Regulates water metabolism

12. Which of the following is true of the hypophysis?
    a. Is also called the pineal gland
    b. Regulates the hypothalamus
    c. Is called the "master gland"
    d. Has four lobes that secrete specific hormones

13. The corticospinal tracts, also called the pyramidal tracts, cross over in the medulla. What does this mean?
    a. The RAS (reticular activating system) controls only right-sided functions.
    b. Reflexes are ipsilateral.
    c. Motor function is contralateral.
    d. Sensation is interpreted in the medulla.

14. What is the cerebellar function?
    a. Controls alertness
    b. Is ipsilateral
    c. Is contralateral
    d. Initiates voluntary movement

15. An interruption of the blood supply in the area served by the middle cerebral artery does which of the following?
    a. Causes loss of vision
    b. Affects upper body movement
    c. Causes increased intracranial pressure
    d. Interferes with temperature regulation

16. Which of the following pass through the blood-brain barrier and which are blocked by the barrier?

Substance
_____ a. Oxygen
_____ b. Albumin
_____ c. Most bacteria
_____ d. Alcohol
_____ e. Water
_____ f. Anesthetics
_____ g. Many antibiotics
_____ h. Carbon dioxide

Blood-Brain Barrier Access
1. Passes through
2. Is blocked

17. Match the spinal tract with the function of the tract.

Spinal Tract

_____ a. Spinothalamic

_____ b. Spinocerebellar

_____ c. Fasciculus gracilis or cuneatus

_____ d. Corticospinal

Function

1. Proprioception
2. Voluntary movement
3. Carry sensations of pain, temperature, pressure
4. Vibratory sense

18. Identify the parts of the peripheral nervous system (PNS).

a. _____

b. _____

c. _____

19. Which of the following statements about spinal nerves is correct?

_____ a. Loss of sensation and motor function can be caused by a problem with one particular spinal nerve.

_____ b. The anterior tract transmits impulses of proprioception.

_____ c. The posterior branch transmits impulses to the muscles.

_____ d. Sensory receptors do not transmit information on special senses.

20. Reflexes:
    a. Are mediated by the cerebellum.
    b. Are under direct control of the motor cortex and are therefore contralateral.
    c. Require sensory input from muscles, tendons, skins organs, and special senses.
    d. Involve only the sensory neuron and the motor neuron.

21. Name the components of the autonomic nervous system.

a. _____

b. _____

22. Match each statement below to the corresponding part of the autonomic nervous system.

Statement

_____ a. Has cell bodies in the gray matter of the spinal cord from S2 to S4

_____ b. Lies beside the spinal cord in a chain

_____ c. Has some sensory function

_____ d. Is part of cranial nerves III, VII, IX, and X

_____ e. Causes the heart to pump faster

_____ f. Constricts pupils

Component of the Autonomic Nervous System

1. Parasympathetic nervous system (PNS)
2. Sympathetic nervous system (SNS)

23. Which of the following changes occurs in the older adult?
    a. Sense of smell is heightened.
    b. Intellect declines.
    c. Long-term memory seems better than recall.
    d. Touch sensation increases.

24. Identify the components of a neurologic assessment.

25. Which of the following chronic conditions can impact neurologic function?
    a. Hypertension
    b. Obesity
    c. Crohn's disease
    d. Coronary artery disease

26. A baseline physical assessment is used to do which of the following?
    a. Determine a level of function for later comparison.
    b. Show the family what problems the older adult has.
    c. Gain information on past sensory changes.
    d. Determine rehabilitation potential.

27. Match each question that the nurse would pose with the type of information sought.

Questions

_____ a. Ask client to repeat three unrelated words.

_____ b. "What is your birth date?"

_____ c. Ask client to follow simple instructions.

_____ d. "What health care providers have you seen during the last year?"

_____ e. Ask client to repeat a series of numbers.

_____ f. "Tell me about your hobbies."

Information Sought
1. Attention span
2. Recent memory
3. Remote memory
4. New memory
5. Language comprehension
6. Cognitive skills

28. Assessment of sensory function:
    a. Is limited to light touch and pain.
    b. Is done routinely every 4 hours.
    c. Is reserved for clients with problems affecting the spinal cord.
    d. Includes assessment of the hypoglossal nerve.

29. If temperature sensation is intact, which of the following can be omitted from an assessment of nerve function?
    a. Vibration
    b. Pain
    c. Light touch
    d. Pressure

30. Match the component of motor testing with the corresponding test performed.

Test Performed

_____ a. Walk across room, and return.

_____ b. Client stands, eyes open, feet close together.

_____ c. Client holds arms perpendicular to body, eyes closed.

_____ d. Client grasps and squeezes nurse's fingers.

_____ e. With arms out to side, client touches nose two to three times.

Test Component
1. Brainstem integrity
2. Coordination
3. Muscle strength
4. Gait
5. Equilibrium

31. Which of the following is not a deep tendon reflex?
    a. Achilles tendon
    b. Plantar
    c. Biceps
    d. Brachioradialis

32. Which of the following statements regarding the Glasgow coma scale is true?
    a. It is a thorough neurologic assessment tool.
    b. It establishes a baseline for eye opening, motor response, and verbal response.
    c. It establishes a baseline cognitive function.
    d. A score of 15 indicates serious neurologic impairment.

33. It would be inappropriate to use contrast medium in which of the following tests?
    a. MRI
    b. Computed tomography
    c. X-rays of skull or spine
    d. Cerebral angiography

34. Which of the following statements about lumbar punctures is true? *Check all that apply.*

    _____ a. They are indicated for clients with infections at or near the puncture site.

    _____ b. They are done at the T1 to T3 spinal level.

    _____ c. They require the client to lie flat for 24 to 48 hours after the procedure.

    _____ d. They are done with the client in the "fetal" position.

35. Which of the following findings in CSF is normal?
    a. Protein 15 to 45 mg/100 mL
    b. Pressure 70 to 180 mm H_2O
    c. Color straw yellow
    d. Glucose 80 to 120 mg/100 mL

36. Preparing a client for an EEG would include which of the following?
    a. Giving a sedative before bedtime
    b. Having the client drink coffee or tea before the test
    c. Keeping the client NPO after midnight
    d. Keeping the client awake from 2 AM to the scheduled test time

CASE STUDY: NEUROLOGIC ASSESSMENT

Answer Guidelines for the Case Study questions are provided on the companion Evolve Learning Resources Web site at http://evolve.elsevier.com/Iggy/.

The client is a 48-year-old male client, married, and the father of three children. He works as a draftsman, designing decorative iron and other metal products. He is scheduled for a neurologic diagnostic workup. Over the past month, he has noticed that he has had difficulty drawing figures accurately. At times, he has been unable to hold a pencil with sufficient strength to mark the drawing paper. He denies visual changes; however, at times he has difficulty walking without tripping. A lumbar puncture is scheduled following x-rays of the skull and spine.

1. What additional data should the nurse collect initially?

2. Describe the preparation of the client for the x-ray studies.

3. Develop a teaching-learning plan for the client about the lumbar puncture.

4. The hospital requires that a consent form be signed by the client before the lumbar puncture. What is the purpose of this document?

5. The client asks about complications from the procedure. He asks "Will the test make my symptoms worse? I don't need anymore problems right now." What should the nurse reply?

6. The lumbar puncture is performed and five tubes of cerebrospinal fluid (CSF) are collected. The CSF pressure is 165 mm Hg. What is the significance of this finding?

The physician orders that the specimens be analyzed for cells, protein, and glucose. The laboratory results are color = straw; cells = 7 lymphocytes/mm3; RBCs = absent; protein = 60 mg/100 mL; glucose = 68 mg/100 mL.

7. Which of the laboratory findings are normal? Which are abnormal?

Following the lumbar puncture, the client is to be kept on bedrest for 24 hours with the head of the bed flat. A regular diet may be resumed and fluids encouraged.

8. What is the purpose of these postprocedure interventions?

9. What assessments should the nurse make following the procedure?

10. The client calls the nurse and says that he has a throbbing headache. What should the nurse do? What is the most likely explanation for his headache? What interventions are indicated to help make the client more comfortable?

Interventions for Clients with Problems of the Central Nervous System: The Brain

LEARNING OUTCOMES

1. Compare the assessment findings of migraine, cluster, and tension headaches.
2. Develop a teaching plan for a client diagnosed with migraine headaches.
3. Differentiate the common types of seizures, including presenting clinical manifestations.
4. Identify collaborative management options for treating clients diagnosed with epilepsy.
5. Explain the nursing interventions required when providing care for a client having a seizure.
6. Outline the priorities for care of clients with meningitis and encephalitis.
7. Describe the pathophysiology of Parkinson disease.
8. Develop a community-based plan of care for a client with Parkinson disease.
9. Identify nursing implications related to giving medications for Parkinson disease.
10. Identify the roles of the interdisciplinary health care team and family in developing a comprehensive individualized treatment plan for the client with Alzheimer's disease.
11. Explain the use of drug therapy for clients with Alzheimer's disease.
12. Prioritize care for clients with Alzheimer's disease.
13. Develop a teaching plan for caregivers of clients with Alzheimer's disease.
14. Analyze legal/ethical concerns related to genetic counseling of clients with Huntington disease.

LEARNING ACTIVITIES

1. Before completing the study guide exercises for this chapter, it is recommended that you review the following:
   - Anatomy and physiology of the neurologic system (central and peripheral)
   - Process of nerve conduction
   - Principles of acid-base balance
   - Principles of fluid and electrolytes
   - Normal function of the musculoskeletal system, including joint range of motion
   - Process of rehabilitation and related interventions

2. Review the boldfaced terms and their definitions in Chapter 45 to enhance your understanding of the content.

STUDY/REVIEW QUESTIONS

Answers to the Study/Review Questions are provided on the companion Evolve Learning Resources Web site at http://evolve.elsevier.com/Iggy/.

1. Match each characteristic with the corresponding type of headache.

Characteristics

_____ a.   Familial disorder

_____ b.   Occurs more often in men

_____ c.   Associated with runny nose and ptosis

_____ d.   Has no known cause

_____ e.   May be caused by hyperexcitability of nerves

_____ f.   Client may walk or rock

_____ g.   May last for several days

_____ h.   Duration limited to 15 to 45 minutes

_____ i.   Occurs at regular intervals with long remission periods

_____ j.   Occurs more often in women

Type of Headache

1.   Migraine
2.   Cluster headache

2. The assessment of migraine headaches includes asking about which of the following?
    a.   Abuse of drugs
    b.   History of smoking
    c.   Presence of aura prior to onset of headaches
    d.   Stuffy or runny nose associated with headaches

3. A teaching plan for a client with a migraine would include which of the following?
    a.   Management of urinary incontinence
    b.   Psychotherapy
    c.   Forcing fluids to maintain hydration
    d.   Information on preventive drug therapy

4. Which of the following is an intervention for cluster headaches?
    a.   Modification of diet: eliminating caffeine and chocolate
    b.   Providing preventive medication
    c.   Administering oxygen
    d.   Psychotropic medications

5. Match the type of generalized seizure with the correct definition.

Definitions

_____ a.   Brief jerking of extremities, singly or in groups

_____ b.   Brief period of staring or loss of consciousness

_____ c.   Rigidity followed by rhythmic jerking

_____ d.   Sudden loss of body tone

Types of Generalized Seizures

1.   Tonic-clonic
2.   Absence
3.   Myoclonic
4.   Atonic

6. Which of the following statements about partial seizures is true?
    a.   They are also called absence seizures.
    b.   Automatisms may occur.
    c.   They involve both cerebral hemispheres.
    d.   Medical treatment tends to be more effective for partial seizures than for generalized seizures.

7. Identify the subjective data needed for assessment of seizures.

8. Which of the following statements is true for the older adult?
    a.   Seizures are unlikely to be associated with metabolic changes.
    b.   Drug monitoring is very important because of changes in metabolism and elimination.
    c.   Seizure medication produces fewer adverse reactions.
    d.   Drug interactions are uncommon and usually mild.

9. List interventions the nurse would initiate for seizure precautions.

10. List interventions for the client with a seizure.

11. Which of the following statements is true about status epilepticus?
    a. It is hereditary.
    b. It is characterized by a rapid succession of seizures.
    c. It is a potential complication of atonic seizures only.
    d. IV diazepam is contraindicated for treatment.

12. List four topics for education of the client and family regarding status epilepticus.

    a. _____

    b. _____

    c. _____

    d. _____

13. Organisms enter the nervous system through which routes?

    a. _____

    b. _____

    c. _____

14. Match each factor with its associated type of meningitis.

Factors

_____ a. Condition is usually self-limiting; full recovery is expected.

_____ b. Manifestations vary according to the state of the immune system.

_____ c. Cerebrospinal fluid (CSF) is hazy.

_____ d. No organisms grow from the CSF.

_____ e. Outbreaks occur in crowded conditions such as dormitories.

Types of Meningitis
1. Bacterial meningitis
2. Viral meningitis
3. Fungal meningitis

15. Describe and explain the advantages of a PET scan in comparison with other diagnostic procedures.

16. The nurse can anticipate that which of the following tests will be performed on the client suspected of having meningitis?
    a. X-rays of the mastoid area
    b. Lumbar puncture
    c. Myelography
    d. Cerebral angiogram

17. Which of the following symptoms in a client with meningitis would need to be communicated to the physician?
    a. Capillary refill of 3 seconds
    b. Urinary incontinence
    c. Inability to visually follow a moving object from side to side
    d. Temperature of 100.6° F orally

18. Briefly describe TCD and compare it to other diagnostic procedures.

19. What structure must be intact to prevent the risk of CNS infections such as encephalitis?

20. Compare and contrast decerebrate and decorticate posturing.

21. What should the nurse explain to the client who is apprehensive about having a CT scan done?

22. Which of the following interventions should be implemented before a cerebral blood flow evaluation?
    a. Withhold medications that affect the CNS for 24 hours.
    b. Shave the client's scalp in the area where the examination is focused.
    c. Instruct the client that bedrest is required for 24 hours after the examination.
    d. Make the client NPO for at least 12 hours before the examination.

23. Other staff on the unit are concerned about a client's elimination of radioisotopic matter following a PET scan. What should the nurse explain to them about this?

24. What points should the nurse include when teaching a client before undergoing an MRI scan?

25. Follow-up care for a client who has had contrast media injected should include what assessments?

26. Briefly describe a reflex arc.

27. List the cranial nerves and give their related functions.

28. Compare and contrast the sympathetic and the parasympathetic nervous systems.

29. Circadian rhythm changes in the older adult may lead to which common problem?

30. What method of learning may help the older adult acquire and retain new information?

31. What is being assessed when the nurse asks the client to explain statements such as "A stitch in time saves nine?"

32. Briefly describe proprioception and explain why assessment of it is important.

33. Describe the type of abnormal findings associated with motor cortex lesions.

36. Describe ways to assess for pain perception.

34. In the older adult, what might be the cause of confusion other than a nervous system problem?

37. Describe the extinction phenomenon and how to assess for it.

35. List at least five questions that could be used in an interview to test the client's recall or recent memory.

Interventions for Clients with Problems of the Central Nervous System: The Spinal Cord

LEARNING OUTCOMES

1. Identify risk factors that contribute to back pain.
2. Explain health promotion measures to prevent back pain.
3. Plan care for the client having a diskectomy, laminectomy, or spinal fusion.
4. Analyze the common nursing diagnoses and collaborative problems for the client with an acute spinal cord injury (SCI).
5. Describe the role of the health care team in the recognition and treatment of typical medical complications that are experienced by clients with an SCI.
6. Prioritize the nursing care of the client with an SCI.
7. Evaluate the expected outcomes for the client with an SCI.
8. Identify the clinical manifestations and treatment options associated with spinal cord tumors.
9. Explain the pathophysiology of multiple sclerosis (MS), including the six basic types.
10. Discuss the role of medications in managing clients with MS.
11. Develop a community-based teaching plan for the client with MS.
12. Compare and contrast the clinical manifestations of MS and amyotrophic lateral sclerosis.

LEARNING ACTIVITIES

1. Before completing the study guide exercises for this chapter, it is recommended that you review the following:
   - Anatomy and physiology of the neurologic system (central and peripheral)
   - Process of nerve conduction
   - Principles of acid-base balance
   - Principles of fluid and electrolytes
   - Normal function of the musculoskeletal system, including joint range of motion
   - Process of rehabilitation and related interventions
   - Concepts of body image and self-esteem
   - Concepts of loss, death, and grieving
   - Pain and pain management, coping, and stress management
   - Principles of perioperative nursing management

2. Review the boldfaced terms and their definitions in Chapter 46 to enhance your understanding of the content.

STUDY/REVIEW QUESTIONS

Answers to the Study/Review Questions are provided on the companion Evolve Learning Resources Web site at http://evolve.elsevier.com/Iggy/.

1. Acute back pain usually results from trauma. Identify other factors that contribute to the occurrence of back pain.

2. Identify what additional factors contributing to back pain in the older adult.

3. Which of the following statements is true about back pain?
   a. The pain follows the dermatome of the affected nerve.
   b. Opiates are more effective in relieving pain than NSAID medications.
   c. Sensation is often heightened in the extremity affected by the pain.
   d. Straight-leg raising alleviates pain.

4. Identify the nonsurgical interventions used for back pain.

5. Which of the following surgical procedures is used when the spine is unstable?
   a. Laparoscopic discectomy
   b. Spinal fusion
   c. Laminectomy
   d. Traditional discectomy

6. Which of the following postoperative findings should be reported to the surgeon immediately?
   a. Minimal drainage in the surgical drain after 8 hours
   b. Pain at the operative site
   c. Swelling or bulging at the operative site
   d. Altered sensation in the affected limb

7. Identify the intervention done postoperatively for a client with a spinal fusion but not a laminectomy.
   a. Log roll the client every 2 hours.
   b. Have client dangle legs on the evening of surgery.
   c. Have client wear a brace when out of bed.
   d. Do a neurologic assessment and check vital signs.

8. Which of the following statements indicates that the client does not understand the postoperative instructions he or she was given?
   a. "I use ice on my back for pain."
   b. "I put a piece of plywood under my mattress."
   c. "Dieting is difficult but important."
   d. "I have a new ergonomic chair at work."

9. Match each of the following symptoms with its corresponding complication.

Symptoms

_____ a. Hypertension

_____ b. Flaccid paralysis

_____ c. Hypotension

_____ d. Severe headache

_____ e. Loss of reflexes below the injury

_____ f. Blurred vision

Complications
1. Spinal shock
2. Autonomic dysreflexia

10. Describe the four major mechanisms of spinal cord injury and their causes.

   a. _____

   b. _____

   c. _____

   d. _____

11. Match each type of partial cervical spinal cord lesion with the corresponding physical findings.

Physical Findings

_____ a. Motor function is lost on the same side of the body as the injury.

_____ b. Motor function is lost below the injury.

_____ c. Motor function remains intact; sensory function is lost.

Types of Spinal Cord Lesions
1. Anterior cord injury
2. Posterior cord injury
3. Brown-Séquard's syndrome

12. List three important questions in completing an assessment of a client with a cervical SCI.

a. _____

b. _____

c. _____

13. Which of the following is an important nursing intervention for the client at risk for autonomic dysreflexia?
   a. Careful monitoring of urinary output
   b. Keeping the room warm
   c. Using an elastic corset to raise blood pressure
   d. Frequently ambulating client

14. Autonomic dysreflexia can lead to which of the following?
   a. Heat stroke resulting from loss of thermoregulation
   b. Paralytic ileus
   c. Hypertensive stroke
   d. Aspiration and pneumonia

15. Match each of the following medications with the corresponding indication/effect.

Medication

_____ a. Methylprednisolone

_____ b. Dextran

_____ c. Atropine

_____ d. Dopamine

_____ e. Dantrolene

Indication/Effect
1. Increases heart rate
2. Relieves spasticity
3. Increases capillary blood flow
4. Reduces inflammation
5. Regulates blood pressure

16. List nursing interventions to maintain a patent airway.

17. Identify the major complications of prolonged immobility.

18. When implementing bowel and bladder retraining, the nurse should do all the following except what?
   a. Ensure that the client gets a sufficient quantity of fluid each day.
   b. Assist the client in developing a schedule.
   c. Teach the client about high-fiber foods.
   d. Teach the client that regaining continence is dependent upon how well the spinal cord heals.

19. Identify the major area of education for the client with a spinal cord injury.

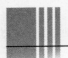

20. The nurse assists the client with psychosocial adaptation to successful rehabilitation of a client with spinal cord injury by doing what kinds of interventions?

21. Which of the following statements about spinal cord tumors is correct?
    a. The majority are malignant.
    b. They occur mostly in the lumbar area.
    c. More men than women develop spinal cord tumors.
    d. The symptoms vary by location of the tumor and its rate of growth.

22. Which of the following is the major pathologic feature of multiple sclerosis (MS)?
    a. Destruction of the dendrite processes on nerve cells
    b. Destruction of the myelin sheath
    c. Destruction of the axon
    d. Destruction of the cell body

23. Which of the following statements about MS is true?
    a. It is a chronic progressive disease.
    b. It has a defined genetic cause.
    c. It is more prevalent in the 40- to 60-year age group.
    d. Life expectancy is prolonged if the client moves to an area of low prevalence.

24. Which of the following tests may aid in diagnosing MS?
    a. EMG and PET scan
    b. EEG and EMG
    c. MRI and CT scan
    d. CT scan and ultrasound

25. Identify educational topics for a client with MS.

26. Which of the following statements about amyotrophic lateral sclerosis is true?
    a. It is a progressive disease involving the motor system.
    b. It has a specific known cause.
    c. It affects mental ability first.
    d. There is specific treatment.

27. Early symptoms of amyotrophic lateral sclerosis include which of the following?
    a. Bowel and bladder incontinence
    b. Tongue atrophy
    c. Blurred vision
    d. Headaches

Interventions for Clients with Problems of the Peripheral Nervous System

LEARNING OUTCOMES

1.   Compare and contrast the pathophysiology and etiology of Guillain-Barré syndrome (GBS) and myasthenia gravis (MG).

2.   Analyze assessment data for a client with GBS or MG to determine common nursing diagnoses.

3.   Prioritize nursing care for the client with GBS or MG.

4.   Evaluate nursing care for the client with GBS or MG based on expected outcomes.

5.   Differentiate between a myasthenic crisis and a cholinergic crisis.

6.   Identify specific nursing actions regarding medication administration for the client with MG.

7.   Develop a teaching plan for the client with peripheral neuropathy.

8.   Prioritize postoperative care for the client undergoing peripheral nerve repair.

9.   Compare and contrast trigeminal neuralgia and facial paralysis.

10. Discuss the role of drug therapy in managing the client with trigeminal neuralgia and facial paralysis.

11. Explain the purpose of surgery for clients with trigeminal neuralgia.

LEARNING ACTIVITIES

1.   Before completing the study guide exercises for this chapter, review the following:
     *   Anatomy and physiology of the neurologic system (central and peripheral)
     *   Process of nerve conduction
     *   Principles of acid-base balance
     *   Principles of fluid and electrolytes
     *   Normal function of the musculoskeletal system, including joint range of motion
     *   Process of rehabilitation and related interventions
     *   Concepts of body image and self-esteem
     *   Concepts of loss, death, and grieving
     *   Pain and pain management, coping, and stress management
     *   Principles of perioperative nursing management

2.   Review the boldfaced terms and their definitions in Chapter 47 to enhance your understanding of the content.

STUDY/REVIEW QUESTIONS

Answers to the Study/Review Questions are provided on the companion Evolve Learning Resources Web site at http://evolve.elsevier.com/Iggy/.

1. Which statement about Guillain-Barré syndrome (GBS) is correct?
   a. Clients with GBS usually present with an acute respiratory illness or injury.
   b. Males are affected twice as often as females.
   c. Most evidence points to a cell-mediated immunologic reaction as the cause.
   d. The major problem in GBS is the destruction of the muscle receptor site.

2. Identify the subjective information sought by the nurse from the client in assessing for GBS.

3. Identify symptoms associated with GBS.

4. What tests would you expect to be performed on a client with GBS?

5. Which of the following would the nurse report to the physician immediately for a client with GBS?
   a. Increasing loss of motor function
   b. Ineffective cough
   c. Dyspnea and confusion
   d. Analgesia following administration of opioids

6. Explain each intervention for the client with GBS who has respiratory compromise.
   a. Provision of appropriate pain medication to enhance breathing
   b. Auscultation of breath sounds every 2 hours
   c. Checking the vital capacity every 4 hours
   d. Suction as needed using sterile technique

7. Which of the following statements about treatment for GBS is correct?
   a. Immunoglobulins are curative.
   b. Second treatments with plasmapheresis have increased risk of side effects.
   c. Treatment is supportive because this disease is usually self-limiting.
   d. Immunoglobulins have no major side effects.

8. Discuss the goals and intervention for impaired mobility for the client with GBS.

9. What should be included in health care teaching for the GBS client?
   a. Always include a family member or significant other.
   b. Instructions given in oral form only.
   c. Always include information on range-of-motion exercises.
   d. Include information on the need for continued plasmapheresis.

10. Which of the following statements about myasthenia gravis (MG) is correct?
    a. It is a progressive disease marked by a steep decline in function.
    b. Increased activity delays onset of symptoms.
    c. It is a genetically inherited disease.
    d. It is highly correlated with hyperplasia of the thymus gland.

11. Outline the subjective information gathered by the nurse as part of the client history when assessing for MG.

12. Which of the following statements about Tensilon testing is correct?
    a. A false-positive test may occur if the muscle is extremely weak.
    b. The drug has a long duration of action.
    c. The test can be used to distinguish between a cholinergic crisis and a myasthenic crisis.
    d. A false-negative test can result from increased effort by the client.

13. The client with MG is deficient in which of the following transmitters:
    a. Serotonin
    b. Acetylcholine
    c. Dopamine
    d. GABA

14. Which of the following symptoms of an MG client should the nurse report to the physician immediately? Why?
    a. Diarrhea
    b. Blurry vision
    c. Inability to swallow
    d. Tinnitus

15. In planning activities for the client with MG, the nurse should use which of the following parameters? Why?
    a. Time of day
    b. Severity of symptoms
    c. Medication times
    d. Sleep schedule

16. MG is associated with which of the following diseases?
    a. Diabetes
    b. Peripheral vascular disease
    c. Hyperthyroidism
    d. Hypothyroidism

17. Identify the objective data gathered by the nurse from the client with MG.

18. Which of the following is important information about MG drug therapy?
    a. If a dose of cholinesterase is missed, a double dose is taken the next day.
    b. Antibiotics such as neomycin and kanamycin have a synergistic effect with cholinesterase inhibitors.
    c. Medications must be taken on an empty stomach.
    d. Drugs containing morphine or sedatives can increase muscle weakness.

19. List and explain three common causes of respiratory compromise in the client with MG.

20. Postoperative care for the client with MG consists of which of the following?

    _____ a. Use of an incentive spirometer every 8 hours

    _____ b. Assessing for onset of chest pain, dyspnea, hypotension

    _____ c. Turning, coughing, and deep breathing once every 8 hours

    _____ d. Ambulating client hourly

21. Identify the most common causes of polyneuritis.

22. Which of the following statements regarding polyneuritis is true?
    a. All forms of polyneuritis have an inflammatory component.
    b. Polyneuritis usually begins in the hands (glove neuropathy) before going to the legs.
    c. Vitamins in excess of dietary allowances have been found useful in treating polyneuropathies.
    d. Rapid recovery may follow if the toxin causing the polyneuropathy is removed.

23. Which of the following diseases is associated with polyneuropathy?
    a. Raynaud's syndrome
    b. Diabetes
    c. Leukemia
    d. Hyperthyroidism

24. Discuss why each of the following would or would not be suited for the client with polyneuropathy.
    a. Checking feet for cuts and reddened areas
    b. Checking bath water for proper temperature
    c. Using a heating pad to keep feet warm
    d. Proper shoe selection

25. Identify the four major ways peripheral nerves can be injured.

    a. _____

    b. _____

    c. _____

    d. _____

26. Which of the following statements about peripheral nerve damage is true?
    a. Successfully remyelinated nerves conduct impulses at 80% of original velocity.
    b. Nerves regenerate at the rate of 10 to 40 mm/day.
    c. After injury, the proximal nerve degenerates within 24 hours.
    d. Some motor function may return before regeneration is complete.

27. Discuss the subjective data that may be given by the client with peripheral nerve damage.

28. Postoperative care for the client with peripheral nerve damage includes which of the following?
    a. ROM exercises for the affected limb to maintain mobility
    b. Joint extension to keep the nerve properly aligned
    c. Joint flexion to keep tension off the suture site
    d. Making sure the skin around the edge of the splint is blanched

29. Match each statement to the corresponding condition. *Answers can be used more than once.*

Statements

_____ a. Pain provoked by stimulation of trigger zone

_____ b. More common in women

_____ c. Incidence may be higher in diabetic clients

_____ d. Thought to be related to brainstem activity

_____ e. Inflammatory in nature

_____ f. Taste impaired

_____ g. Requires protection of the cornea

_____ h. Arterial compression removed by surgery

_____ i. Prednisone prescribed

_____ j. Soft diet and frequent small meals encouraged

Conditions
1. Trigeminal neuralgia
2. Facial paralysis

Interventions for Critically Ill Clients with Neurologic Problems

LEARNING OUTCOMES

1. Identify the common types of strokes.
2. Discuss risk factors that increase the likelihood of strokes.
3. Describe typical clinical manifestations associated with stroke.
4. Analyze assessment data to determine common nursing diagnoses that are pertinent to clients with strokes.
5. Identify the purpose of intracranial pressure (ICP) monitoring and signs of increasing ICP.
6. Explain the role of drug therapy in managing clients with strokes.
7. Prioritize nursing care for a client who has experienced a stroke.
8. Discuss the purpose of rehabilitation for the client who has had a stroke.
9. Develop a teaching plan for the client who has experienced a stroke.
10. Differentiate the common types of traumatic brain injury (TBI).
11. Explain the pathophysiologic changes that can result from moderate or severe TBI.
12. Describe the psychosocial and behavioral manifestations associated with TBI.
13. Prioritize nursing care for the client with TBI.
15. Explain the role of sedation and analgesia in managing the client with intracranial hypertension.
16. Describe common complications of brain tumors.
17. Develop a postoperative plan of care for a client having a craniotomy.

LEARNING ACTIVITIES

1. Before completing the study guide exercises for this chapter, it is recommended that you review the following:
   - Anatomy and physiology of the neurologic system (central and peripheral)
   - Process of nerve conduction
   - Principles of acid-base balance
   - Principles of fluids and electrolytes
   - Normal function of the musculoskeletal system, including joint range of motion
   - Process of rehabilitation and related interventions
   - Concepts of body image and self-esteem
   - Concepts of loss, death, and grieving

- Pain and pain management, coping, and stress management
- Principles of perioperative nursing management

2. Review the boldfaced terms and their definitions in Chapter 48 to enhance your understanding of the content.

STUDY/REVIEW QUESTIONS

Answers to the Study/Review Questions are provided on the companion Evolve Learning Resources Web site at http://evolve.elsevier.com/Iggy/.

1. A stroke is caused by which of the following?
   a. Pressure on central neurons caused by swelling
   b. Interruption of blood flow to the brain
   c. Severing of pyramidal tracts in the brain
   d. Increased pressure due to increased CSF

2. Which of the following statements about stroke is true?
   a. Incidence of stroke has been increasing in recent years.
   b. Strokes are the tenth leading cause of death in the United States.
   c. Strokes have a variety of causes.
   d. Costs of strokes are now at $10 billion per year.

3. When do strokes cause damage?
   a. Within minutes of occurring
   b. When the stored oxygen in the brain is depleted
   c. When too much glucose is delivered to the brain
   d. When the glia cells constrict

4. Fill in the following table with the distinguishing features of each type of stroke. Copy to a separate sheet of paper if necessary.

	TYPE OF STROKE		
Feature	Thrombotic	Embolic	Hemorrhagic
Onset			
Evolution			
Contributing Factors			
Duration			

5. Which of the following statements about stroke is true?
   a. Thrombotic strokes account for one tenth of all strokes.
   b. Collateral circulation may develop and decrease the effects of an embolic stroke.
   c. The lack of elasticity of the artery is an important feature of a thrombotic stroke.
   d. Bifurcations are protected from thrombus formation because of increased blood flow.

6. What is a lacunar stroke?
   a. It is a type of thrombotic stroke.
   b. It is a type of embolic stroke.
   c. It causes cavities to develop in the white matter of the brain only.
   d. It always causes severe damage.

7. In embolic stroke, the middle cerebral artery is involved most often. Which of the following deficits are associated with middle cerebral artery occlusion?
   a. Contralateral hemiparesis: arm greater than leg
   b. Contralateral hemiparesis: leg greater than arm
   c. Unilateral neglect
   d. Dysconjugate gaze

8. Which of the following statements about the causes of stroke is correct?
   a. Hypertension is the leading cause of embolic stroke.
   b. Rupture of an arteriovenous malformation is the most common cause of hemorrhagic stroke.
   c. Embolic stroke is associated with myocardial infarction.
   d. Transient ischemic attacks last longer than 24 hours and often precede ischemic strokes.

9. Which of the following clients are at increased risk for stroke? *Check all that apply.*
   _____ a. A 66-year-old man with well controlled diabetes
   _____ b. A 35-year-old healthy pregnant woman
   _____ c. A 77-year-old woman who exercises regularly
   _____ d. A 17-year-old male smoker

10. Identify three factors that are thought to contribute to the "stroke belt" in the southern United States.

    a. _____

    b. _____

    c. _____

11. Match each symptom of stroke with the hemisphere most often affected by that symptom. *Answers can be used more than once.*

Symptom

_____ a. Loss of depth perception

_____ b. Aphasia

_____ c. Loss of hearing

_____ d. Cannot recognize faces

_____ e. Impaired sense of humor

_____ f. Depression

_____ g. Denies illness

_____ h. Frustration and anger

_____ i. Disoriented to person, place, and time

_____ j. Poor judgment

Affected Hemisphere
1. Left hemisphere
2. Right hemisphere

12. When assessing motor changes in a client who has had a stroke, which of the following is important to remember?
    a. Motor deficit is ipsilateral to the hemisphere affected.
    b. Motor deficit is contralateral to the hemisphere affected.
    c. Bowel and bladder function remain intact.
    d. Flaccid paralysis is not an expected finding and should be reported promptly.

13. Match each deficit with its corresponding definition.

Definitions

_____ a. Inability to comprehend language

_____ b. Sensitivity to light

_____ c. Difficulty writing

_____ d. Blindness in half of the visual field

_____ e. Blindness in one eye

_____ f. Difficulty reading

_____ g. Drooping eyelid

Deficits
1. Ptosis
2. Hemianopsia
3. Amaurosis fugax
4. Receptive aphasia
5. Agraphia
6. Alexia
7. Photophobia

14. Identify laboratory tests after a stroke that may show changes and explain why.

15. Identify radiology tests that may be used to establish a diagnosis of stroke and determine the type.

16. Which of the following is not an indication of intracranial pressure?
    a. Nonreactive pupils
    b. Nausea and vomiting
    c. Hypotension
    d. Seizures

17. List nursing interventions for the client with any type of stroke and give rationales.

18. Which of the following drugs can a nurse expect to give to a client who has had a hemorrhagic stroke?
    a. Enteric-coated aspirin
    b. Warfarin sodium (Coumadin)
    c. Sodium heparin
    d. Docusate (Colace)

19. Which of the following drugs is used to control cerebral vasospasm?
    a. Nimodipine
    b. Phenytoin
    c. Dipyridamole (Persantine)
    d. Clopidogrel (Plavix)

20. Identify the nursing interventions for a client with a hemorrhagic stroke.

21. Which of the following surgical procedures may be used to treat an ischemic stroke?
    a. Craniotomy to remove clots
    b. Inserting a detachable silicone balloon into the affected artery
    c. Carotid endarterectomy
    d. Craniotomy to clip the artery

22. The expected outcomes for the diagnosis of Impaired Physical Mobility are to increase the client's exercise intolerance, to prevent the client from experiencing the consequences of immobility, and to teach the client to become independent in ADLs. Which of the following would be contraindicated in the client with a stroke?

_____ a.   Position the client with a pillow under the knees to decrease spasticity.

_____ b.   Teach the client how to do active and passive ROM exercises.

_____ c.   Splint the arm to prevent contractures.

_____ d.   Apply sequential compression stockings.

23. Match each of the following interventions for a client who has had a stroke to the hemisphere most commonly affected. *Answers may be used more than once.*

Intervention

_____ a.   Scan side-to-side.

_____ b.   Place pictures and familiar objects around client.

_____ c.   Approach client from unaffected side.

_____ d.   Reorient client frequently.

_____ e.   Place objects within the client's field of vision.

_____ f.   Establish a structured routine for the client.

_____ g.   Teach client to wash both sides of body.

_____ h.   Repeat names of objects commonly used.

Affected Hemisphere
1. Right hemisphere
2. Left hemisphere

24. If the client has impaired swallowing, the nurse should do which of the following?
   a. Limit the diet to clear liquids so if aspiration occurs the client still will be able to breathe.
   b. Make sure the client is in semi-Fowler's position for all meals.
   c. Monitor the client's weight.
   d. Make meals more enjoyable by making sure the family is present.

25. To re-establish urinary continence, the nurse should do which of the following?
   a. Request a Foley catheter.
   b. Offer the urinal to a male client every 4 hours.
   c. Restrict fluid intake to 1500 mL/day.
   d. Determine barriers to continence and correct them.

26. Identify the areas of education that need to be addressed with the client who has had a stroke.

27. Which of the following statements does not reflect the home management of the client who has had a stroke?
   a. Home caregivers need to plan for respite care.
   b. The home should be evaluated for potential safety risks such as throw rugs.
   c. Teach the family to give the medications used to treat emotional lability.
   d. Have family members give a return demonstration on transfer techniques.

28. Which of the following statements about traumatic brain injury (TBI) is correct?
   a. TBIs are the leading cause of death of persons between 50 and 64 years of age.
   b. TBIs are most often caused by falls.
   c. The incidence of injury is higher in older women.
   d. Only serious brain injury can lead to permanent disability.

29. Match each type of trauma with the corresponding definition.

Definitions

_____ a.   The head hits a stationary object.

_____ b.   There is a simple, clean break in the skull.

_____ c.   Cortical surface is torn.

_____ d.   The head is in motion.

_____ e.   Bone presses inward into brain tissue.

_____ f.   CSF leaks from nose or ears.

_____ g.   There is a direct opening to brain tissue.

_____ h.   Fragments of bone are in brain tissue.

_____ i.   There is a brief loss of consciousness.

Types of Trauma
1.   Laceration
2.   Acceleration
3.   Concussion
4.   Linear fracture
5.   Basilar skull fracture
6.   Comminuted fracture
7.   Depressed fracture
8.   Deceleration
9.   Open fracture

30. Explain how each of the following causes cerebral edema.
   a.   Vasogenic edema

   b.   Cytotoxic edema

   c.   Interstitial edema

31. Match each type of hematoma with the corresponding description.

Descriptions

_____ a.   Caused by tearing of small vessels within brain tissue

_____ b.   Occurs between the skull and the dura

_____ c.   May present as acute, subacute, or chronic

Types of Hematomas
1.   Epidural hematoma
2.   Subdural hematoma
3.   Intracranial hemorrhage

32. Blood flow to the brain remains fairly constant as a result of which of the following processes?
   a.   Autostasis
   b.   Automobilization
   c.   Hemodynamic stasis
   d.   Autoregulation

33. Identify and discuss three factors in the development of hydrocephalus.

   a.   _____

   b.   _____

   c.   _____

34. In light of the common causes of traumatic brain injury, identify factors that make it difficult to obtain a history.

35. List questions that are important to ask when obtaining an initial history from the client with traumatic brain injury or from the family of the client, and explain why they are important.

36. Match each type of breathing to the area of the brain that is affected by such breathing.

Types of Breathing

_____ a.   Cheyne-Stokes

_____ b.   Central neurogenic hyperventilation

_____ c.   Apneustic breathing

_____ d.   Cluster breathing

_____ e.   Ataxic breathing

Affected Areas of the Brain

1. Low midbrain, upper pons
2. Medulla
3. Cerebral hemispheres, cerebellar
4. Low pons, high medulla
5. Mid pons, low pons

37. The first priority in assessment of the client with traumatic brain injury is to determine which of the following?
    a. Whether spinal injury is present
    b. Whether the client is hypotensive
    c. Whether a patent airway is present
    d. The level of consciousness using the Glasgow scale

38. Identify the indications of intracranial pressure (ICP).

39. Which of the following statements is correct in regard to a client with a traumatic brain injury?
    a. The appearance of abnormal posturing occurs only when the client is not positioned for comfort.
    b. Cushing reflex, an early sign of ICP, consists of severe hypertension, widening pulse pressure, and bradycardia.
    c. Papilledema, edema, and hyperemia of the optic disk are always signs of ICP.
    d. Areas of tenderness over the scalp indicate the presence of contrecoup injuries.

40. Nursing interventions for the client with traumatic brain injury include which of the following?
    a. Assessment of vital signs every 8 hours
    b. Positioning to avoid extreme flexion
    c. Encouraging fluid intake over the first 48 hours to compensate for diabetes insipidus
    d. Administration of glucocorticosteroids to prevent ICP

41. Which of the following nursing interventions applies to clients with sensory functions?
    a. Play tapes for at least 30 minutes to make sure the comatose client has heard them.
    b. Teach the client to test the water temperature used for bathing.
    c. Position the client reclining in bed or in a chair for meals.
    d. Teach the client to place food on the unaffected side of the mouth.

42. Identify the types of ICP monitoring devices and their major advantages and disadvantages.

43. Identify the most common sites of primary tumors that metastasize to the brain.

    a. _____

    b. _____

    c. _____

    d. _____

44. Which of the following does not result in increased ICP in clients with brain tumors?
    a. Vasogenic edema
    b. Hemorrhage into the brain
    c. Obstruction of CSF flow
    d. Pituitary dysfunction

45. Which of the following statements is correct?
    a. Hands-free cellular phones prevent brain tumors.
    b. The exact cause of brain tumors is not known.
    c. Genetics and heredity are important risk factors for brain tumors.
    d. A high-fat diet has been linked to brain tumor development.

46. Match each key feature of brain tumors with the most likely site of the tumor. *Answers may be used more than once.*

Features of Brain Tumors

_____ a. Vomiting unrelated to food intake

_____ b. Hemiparesis

_____ c. Facial pain or weakness

_____ d. Nystagmus

_____ e. Seizures

_____ f. Headache

_____ g. Hoarseness

_____ h. Aphasia

_____ i. Ataxia

_____ j. Hearing loss

Site of Tumor
1. Cerebral tumor
2. Brainstem tumor

47. Drug therapy for the client with a brain tumor includes which of the following?
    a. Glucocorticosteroids for edema
    b. NSAIDs for pain
    c. Insulin for diabetes insipidus
    d. Antihistamines to prevent stress ulcers

48. Which of the following is true of gamma knife therapy?
    a. It is used for easily reached tumors.
    b. It is noninvasive and has few complications.
    c. It requires general anesthesia.
    d. It replaces conventional radiation therapy.

49. Education for the client and family concerning craniotomy would include which of these statements?
    a. Your head will not need to be shaved at the surgical site.
    b. The client may be in a coma for up to several days after surgery.
    c. Drainage of CSF after surgery is normal; blood drainage is not.
    d. The family should remind the client of their names and relationships.

50. Which of the following positions is preferred for a client who has had an infratentorial craniotomy?
    a. High-Fowler's position, turned to the operative side
    b. Head of bed at 30 degrees, turned to the nonoperative side
    c. Flat in bed, turned to the operative side
    d. Flat in bed, may turn to either side

51. Which statements about increased ICP in the surgical client is correct?
    a. It is a minor postoperative complication.
    b. Diuretics such as furosemide may be given to decrease it.
    c. Cerebral edema usually subsides within 72 hours.
    d. If not contraindicated, the head of the bed should be at 30 degrees.

52. In regard to respiratory problems, the nurse should remember which of the following points?
    a. Atelectasis and pneumonia can be prevented by proper pulmonary hygiene.
    b. Suctioning and chest physiotherapy should be avoided because they increase ICP.
    c. Neurologic pulmonary edema occurs frequently.
    d. The client should be discouraged from breathing deeply to avoid increasing ICP.

53. Health care teaching for a client with brain tumors includes which of the following?
    a. Instructing the client on avoiding physical activity
    b. Teaching the client and family to avoid over-the-counter medications
    c. Teaching the client and family that seizures may occur in the immediate postoperative period
    d. Instructing the client on dietary changes needed to prevent recurrence of the tumor

54. Organisms that cause brain abscesses most often originate from:

    a. _____

    b. _____

    c. _____

55. Septic emboli often originate from:

    a. _____

    b. _____

    c. _____

    d. _____

56. Which of following could be found in the history of a client with a brain abscess?
    a. A family history of Huntington disease
    b. Recent chemotherapy treatment for cancer
    c. A history of osteoarthritis
    d. Vaccination against influenza

57. Which of the following organisms is found mostly in AIDS clients?
    a. *Streptococcus* species
    b. *Enterobacter* species
    c. *Haemophilus influenzae*
    d. Toxoplasmosis

58. Which of the following statements about diagnostic testing is correct?
    a. The WBC may be normal, even in the presence of infection.
    b. Blood cultures are the only cultures likely to grow the causative organism.
    c. MRI is useful late in the course of the disease to identify permanent lesions.
    d. The first test performed is a lumbar puncture to determine whether the CSF is cloudy.

59. If a client has an abscess that was caused by anaerobic bacteria, the nurse would expect to give the client which of the following medications?
    a. Nafcillin sodium (Nafcil)
    b. Clindamycin (Cleocin)
    c. Metronidazole (Flagyl)
    d. Penicillin G benzathine (Bicillin)

Assessment of the Eye and Vision

LEARNING OUTCOMES

1. Explain the concept of refraction in relation to how the cornea, lens, aqueous humor, and vitreous humor contribute to vision.
2. Describe age-related changes in the eye, eyelids, and vision.
3. List five systemic disorders that have an impact on the eye and vision.
4. Discuss which elements of a client's history might predict visual impairment later in life.
5. Interpret the findings of visual acuity by the Snellen chart.
6. Describe two methods of assessing extraocular muscle function.
7. Describe the proper technique for examining the client's eyes with an ophthalmoscope.
8. Discuss the educational needs of a client undergoing fluorescein angiography.
9. Explain the relationship between intraocular pressure and eye health.
10. Use proper technique to instill eyedrops.

LEARNING ACTIVITIES

1. Before completing the study guide exercises for this chapter, it is recommended that you review the following:
   - Anatomy and physiology of the eye
   - Instillation of eyedrops

2. Review the boldfaced terms and their definitions in Chapter 49 to enhance your understanding of the content.

STUDY/REVIEW QUESTIONS

Answers to the Study/Review Questions are provided on the companion Evolve Learning Resources Web site at http://evolve.elsevier.com/Iggy/.

1. Which of the following statements about the optic disk is true?
    a. Nerve fibers and photoreceptor cells are contained in this depressed area on the retina.
    b. It is the clear layer that forms the external coat on the front of the eye.
    c. It is sometimes called the blind spot.
    d. It forms a circular, convex structure behind the iris.

2. Light waves pass through each of the eye structures listed below to reach the retina. Place them in sequence, with the first one being the outermost structure, ending at the retina.

    _____ a. Vitreous humor

    _____ b. Aqueous humor

    _____ c. Lens

    _____ d. Cornea

    _____ e. Retina

3. Match each characteristic or function of the eye with its associated structure.

Characteristic/Function of the Eye

_____ a. Maintains the form of the eyeball

_____ b. Is responsible for light refraction

_____ c. The external layer of the eye

_____ d. Pigmented, vascular coating of the eye

_____ e. Transparent layer over the anterior eye

_____ f. Responsible for peripheral vision

_____ g. Secretes aqueous humor

_____ h. Central circular opening

_____ i. Center of the macula

_____ j. Point where optic nerve enters the eyeball

Structure of the Eye
1. Rods
2. Lens
3. Ciliary body
4. Vitreous humor
5. Uvea
6. Pupil
7. Cornea
8. Fovea centralis
9. Optic disk
10. Sclera

4. Which of the following muscles is responsible for pulling the eye upward?
    a. Inferior oblique
    b. Lateral rectus
    c. Medial rectus
    d. Superior oblique

5. Match each cranial nerve with its function.

Nerve		Function
_____ a.	Cranial nerve II (optic)	1. Corneal reflex
_____ b.	Cranial nerve III (oculomotor)	2. Visual acuity
		3. Eyelid closure
_____ c.	Cranial nerve V (trigeminal)	4. Eyelid muscle movements
_____ d.	Cranial nerve VII (facial)	

6. Name the term used to identify each of the vision problems described below.
    a. A refractive error caused by an irregular curvature

    b. Refraction power is too strong, or nearsightedness

    c. Loss of accommodation resulting from aging

    d. Insufficient refracting power, or farsightedness

    e. Perfect refraction of the eye

7. Match each description with the corresponding name for the eye change associated with aging.

Descriptions

_____ a. Accumulation of fatty deposits

_____ b. Decreased ability of iris to dilate

_____ c. Loss of subcutaneous fat, skin elasticity, and muscle tone

_____ d. Flattened cornea, resulting in irregular curvature

_____ e. Loss of lens elasticity

Eye Changes Associated with Aging
1. Sunken eyes
2. Decreased ability to accommodate
3. Astigmatism
4. Yellowed sclerae
5. Loss of night vision

8. Identify at least five ocular signs and symptoms that may be the result of a reaction to a systemic medication.

a. _____

b. _____

c. _____

d. _____

e. _____

9. Write a brief answer for why it is important to address each of the following areas of health history with your client when assessing the eyes.

Health History	Reason for Obtaining Information
Family history and genetic risk	
Current medical systemic diseases	
Types of sports activities in which client participates	
All medications	

10. Which of the following statements is true?
    a. A client with myopia has smaller pupils.
    b. Normal pupil size is between 1 and 3 mm.
    c. Pupils are larger in older adults.
    d. Anisocoria is normal in 5% of the population.

11. a. Your client complains of not seeing objects in his peripheral vision. Which test would you perform to evaluate this complaint?

    b. Your findings indicate that he has blindness in one half of his field of vision. What is this condition called?

12. Your client, who works in a machine shop, has presented with a suspected foreign body in his eye. What diagnostic test would be done?

13. Match each of the following physical findings with the corresponding related technique.

Physical Finding

_____ a. Alignment of anteroposterior axes

_____ b. Visual acuity

_____ c. Peripheral vision

_____ d. Eye muscle strength

_____ e. Eye drifting

_____ f. Color blindness

Related Technique
1. Ishihara chart
2. Cover-uncover test
3. Corneal light reflex
4. A Snellen chart
5. Confrontation
6. Cardinal gaze position

14. Your client is scheduled for a computed tomography (CT) scan. Which of the following statements are true? *Check all that apply.*

_____ a. CT can be used to detect tumors in the orbital space.

_____ b. The client will need to be positioned in a confined space.

_____ c. A cross-section image is formed using beams of high-intensity x-rays.

_____ d. Contrast dye is used if trauma is suspected.

_____ e. Metal in the eye is an absolute contraindication.

15. When preparing your client for a fluorescein angiography, which of the following statements would be included in your teaching? *Check all that apply.*

_____ a. An intravenous access is necessary.

_____ b. Client must avoid sunlight for 2 days.

_____ c. Urine voided after the test will be bright orange.

_____ d. Fluids are limited for the first 24 hours after the procedure.

_____ e. The skin may temporarily have a yellow or green hue for a few hours after the procedure.

_____ f. Mydriatic drops will be instilled one hour before the procedure.

16. When instilling ophthalmic drops in a client's eyes, which of the following procedures are correct? *Check all that apply.*

_____ a. Check the name, strength, and expiration date of the solution.

_____ b. Have the client tilt head backward and look down.

_____ c. Release drops into the conjunctival pocket.

_____ d. Avoid contaminating the tip of the bottle.

_____ e. After instilling the drop, have the client close eyes tightly.

17. Which of the following statements about tonometry are correct? *Check all that apply.*

_____ a. Tonometer readings are indicated for all clients older than 50 years of age.

_____ b. Tonometry is used to measure intraocular pressure.

_____ c. Adults with a family history of glaucoma should be checked once or twice a year.

_____ d. Intraocular pressure stays constant throughout the day.

18. When using the ophthalmoscope, which of the following procedures are correct? *Check all that apply.*

_____ a. The nurse comes toward the client's eye from 6 inches away.

_____ b. The nurse comes toward the client to the side of the client's line of vision.

_____ c. When examining the right eye, the nurse holds the ophthalmoscope in the left hand.

_____ d. The nurse stands on the same side as the eye being examined.

_____ e. The test should be done in a brightly lit room to enhance visibility.

_____ f. The nurse should observe for the presence of the red reflex, which should be seen in the pupil.

19. Which structures or reflexes should be assessed by direct ophthalmoscopy?

a. _____

b. _____

c. _____

d. _____

e. _____

20. Match the assessment findings listed below to the structures observed by ophthalmoscopy. *Answers may be used more than once.*

Assessment Finding

_____ a. Bleeding

_____ b. Nicking at arteriovenous crossings

_____ c. Presence or absence

_____ d. Tears or holes

_____ e. Margins

_____ f. Presence of blood vessels

_____ g. Light reflection

_____ h. Lesions

_____ i. Kinks or tangles

Structure
1. Red reflex
2. Optic disk
3. Optic blood vessels
4. Fundus
5. Macula

True or False? *Write T for true or F for false in the blanks provided. For those questions that are false, rewrite the statement to make it true.*

_____ 21. Presence of the arcus senilis is a change of aging that affects vision.

_____ 22. The fovea centralis is the point in the macula where the vision is the most acute.

_____ 23. The lacrimal gland is located in the inner canthus and secretes tears over the eye surface.

_____ 24. Exophthalmos is the sunken appearance of the eye.

_____ 25. A vision acuity of 20/70 means that the client is able to see at 70 feet what a "healthy eye" can see at 20 feet.

26. Which of the following assessment findings are normal? *Check all that apply.*

_____ a. Presbyopia in a 45-year-old woman

_____ b. Ptosis of the eyelids

_____ c. Yellow sclera with small pigmented dots in a dark-skinned person

_____ d. Pupil constriction in response to accommodation

_____ e. Pupil constriction within two seconds in response to light

_____ f. Nystagmus in the far lateral gaze

_____ g. Consensual pupil response

For the following questions, describe the purpose of each diagnostic test or procedure.

27. Corneal staining

28. Slit-lamp examination

29. Jaeger card

30. Radioisotope scanning

Interventions for Clients with Eye and Vision Problems

LEARNING OUTCOMES

1. Describe how to correctly instill ophthalmic drops and ointment into the eye.
2. Explain the consequences of increased intraocular pressure (IOP).
3. Identify common actions, conditions, and positions that increase IOP.
4. Prioritize educational needs for the client after cataract surgery with and without lens replacement.
5. Compare myopia with hyperopia for pathophysiology and the correction needed for each.
6. Describe the pathologic bases, manifestations, and nursing care priorities for primary open-angle glaucoma and acute angle-closure glaucoma.
7. Identify the nursing care priorities for the donor when corneal donation is planned.
8. Explain how diabetes mellitus and hypertension affect vision.
9. Develop a community-based teaching plan for the client after corneal transplantation.
10. Describe the common visual deficits for the client with dry macular degeneration.
11. Identify nursing interventions to promote home safety for the client with reduced vision.

LEARNING ACTIVITIES

1. Before completing the study guide exercises for this chapter, it is recommended that you review the following:
   - Anatomy and physiology of the eye
   - Instillation of eyedrops and ointments
   - Assessment of the eye and vision
   - Concept of body image and self-esteem
   - Concept of loss and grief
   - Principles of perioperative management

2. Review the boldfaced terms and their definitions in Chapter 50 to enhance your understanding of the content.

STUDY/REVIEW QUESTIONS

Answers to the Study/Review Questions are provided on the companion Evolve Learning Resources Web site at http://evolve.elsevier.com/Iggy/.

1. Match each of the following eyelid disorders with the corresponding description.

Disorder

_____ a. Ectropion

_____ b. Blepharitis

_____ c. Hordeolum

_____ d. Chalazion

_____ e. Entropion

Description
1. Eyelid margin inflammation
2. Sweat gland infection at the lash/lid margin
3. Inflammation of a sebaceous gland of the eyelid
4. The turning inward of the eyelid
5. The turning outward and sagging of the eyelid

2. Which of the following statements about an entropion are true? *Check all that apply.*

_____ a. Pain and tearing may be present.

_____ b. The orbicular muscle can be surgically tightened for correction.

_____ c. Entropion can be caused by eyelid spasms.

_____ d. The client lacks sufficient tears to wash adequately over the eye.

3. Identify four important safety points to emphasize with clients who will be instilling an ophthalmic ointment.

   a. _____

   b. _____

   c. _____

   d. _____

4. Your client presents with a red swollen area on one eyelid; it is painful and is on the conjunctival side of the eyelid-eyelash margin.
   a. What is the problem?

   b. What would facilitate healing?

5. Which of the following statements about keratoconjunctivitis sicca and its management is true?
   a. Use of antihistamines can stimulate tear production.
   b. Warm, moist compresses help restore moisture to the eye.
   c. Artificial tears can be used as often as necessary.
   d. Care must be taken to avoid transferring contamination from one eye to the other.

6. Your client has been diagnosed with trachoma. What is the main focus of your nursing interventions?

7. When examining a client with bacterial conjunctivitis, the nurse remembers that this eye disorder is associated with which of the following? *Check all that apply.*

   _____ a. Significant ocular discharge

   _____ b. Tearing

   _____ c. Itching

   _____ d. Blurred vision

   _____ e. Mild conjunctival edema

   _____ f. Formation of scales and granulations on the eyelids

8. Identify three nursing care priorities for the donor when a corneal donation is planned.

   a. _____

   b. _____

   c. _____

9. Your client is scheduled for a keratoplasty. What are four possible complications of this surgery?

    a. _____

    b. _____

    c. _____

    d. _____

10. Which of the following statements is correct about the postoperative care for a client who has had a keratoplasty?
    a. The client should lie on the operative side to reduce intraocular pressure.
    b. The client's eye will be covered for 1 week with the initial dressing and shield.
    c. The client should wear the patch at night for the first month after surgery.
    d. The head of the bed must be elevated 15 degrees.

11. On a separate sheet of paper, develop a concept map relevant to corneal disorders. Consider physiologic, psychosocial, and developmental factors. Identify data that are subjective and objective and include significant diagnostic studies.

12. True or False? Which of the following statements about cataracts are true? *Write T for true or F for false in the blanks provided. For those questions that are false, rewrite the statement to make it true.*

    _____ a. Age-related cataract formation is associated with pain and eye redness.

    _____ b. Early manifestations include slightly blurred vision and decreased color perception.

    _____ c. A cataract is an opacity of the lens that distorts the image projected onto the retina.

    _____ d. Cataracts develop in both eyes at the same rate.

    _____ e. Cataracts may be present at birth.

13. Your client has had cataract surgery and she is ready to go home. What activities should she avoid?

14. The client who has had cataract surgery should know the signs and symptoms of complications. Which signs and symptoms should the client report to her physician?

15. Which of the following statements about glaucoma are true? *Check all that apply.*

    _____ a. Glaucoma is actually a group of diseases resulting in increased intraocular pressure.

    _____ b. Warning signs of glaucoma include gradual loss of central vision.

    _____ c. The most common form is acute glaucoma, which has a sudden onset.

    _____ d. Blindness may result from reduced blood flow to the optic nerve and retina.

16. Compare and contrast primary open-angle glaucoma and angle-closure glaucoma.

	Primary Open-Angle Glaucoma	**Angle-Closure Glaucoma**
Prevalence		
Symptoms		
Onset		
Physical examination		
Tonometry reading		

17. Drug therapy for glaucoma focuses on reducing increased ocular pressure through what two mechanisms?

    a. _____

    b. _____

18. Compare the following medications used for glaucoma by completing the chart below.

Drug	**Classification**	**Action**	**Nursing Implication**
Timolol	1a	1b	1c
Pilocarpine	2a	2b	2c
Latanoprost	3a	3b	3c

19. Identify three causes of blood leakage into the vitreous.

    a. _____

    b. _____

    c. _____

20. Which of the following statements about uveitis is correct?
    a. Anterior uveitis is also known as retinitis.
    b. Posterior uveitis is an inflammation of the iris.
    c. Symptoms include seeing a red haze or series of floaters.
    d. Steroid drops are given hourly to prevent adhesion of the iris to the cornea and lens.

21. Which of the following conditions are associated with posterior uveitis? *Check all that apply*.

    _____ a. Tuberculosis

    _____ b. Syphilis

    _____ c. Herpes zoster

    _____ d. Rheumatoid arthritis

    _____ e. Toxoplasmosis

    _____ f. Allergies

22. Nursing interventions for a client with uveitis include which of the following?
    a. Patching the affected eye
    b. Offering aspirin and opioids for increased pain
    c. Darkening the room
    d. Instructing the client to drive only when necessary

23. Identify the retinal changes that occur in hypertensive retinopathy.

24. What are the two types of diabetic retinopathy?

    a. _____

    b. _____

25. Which of the following statements about retinal detachment is true?
    a. Onset is usually sudden and painful.
    b. Clients may notice loss of peripheral vision.
    c. Clients may suddenly see bright flashes of light.
    d. Hyperopia is directly associated with its occurrence.

26. A client is told by his ophthalmologist that he has a retinal tear and that it should be closed or sealed. What are the three mechanisms for doing this?

    a. _____

    b. _____

    c. _____

27. Following a sclera buckling procedure involving a gas bubble insertion, the client should be placed in what position?
    a. High Fowler's
    b. Supine with head to nonoperative side
    c. Prone with head turned so that the operative eye is facing up
    d. Trendelenburg position

28. Which of the following is the most common early clinical manifestation of retinitis pigmentosa?
    a. Cataracts
    b. Night blindness
    c. Headache
    d. Vitamin A deficiency

29. A client states that he has developed problems seeing the exit signs on the highway when he is driving. What should he be checked for?

30. Match the following refractive errors with their definitions.

Definitions

_____ a.   Short eye length causes images to be focused behind the retina.

_____ b.   Curve of the cornea is not even.

_____ c.   Images are bent and fall in front of the retina.

_____ d.   This condition usually appears in people in their 30s and 40s.

Refractive Errors
1. Myopia
2. Astigmatism
3. Presbyopia
4. Hyperopia

31. Complete the following chart comparing the surgical management for the treatment of the following refractive errors: radial keratotomy, photorefractive keratectomy (PRK), and laser-in-situ keratomileusis (LASIK).

	Radial Keratotomy (RK)	Photorefractive Keratotomy (PRK)	Laser-in-situ Keratomileusis (LASIK)
Indication			
Procedure			
Postoperative recovery			

32. A 10-year-old client was hit in his left eye with a baseball. He has a "black eye," but his vision is not affected and he is applying ice. He wants to know how long the discoloration will last. What would you tell him about the discoloration?

33. What is the most common intraocular malignant tumor in adults?

34. Clients are classified as blind if their best visual acuity with corrective lenses is which of the following?
    a.   20/50
    b.   20/100
    c.   20/150
    d.   20/200

35. Clients who have lost their sight may experience which of the following? *Check all that apply.*

    _____ a. Hopelessness

    _____ b. Grieving

    _____ c. Anger

    _____ d. Immobility

36. A client with impaired vision has been found to be making errors on her medications. What suggestions would help her manage her medicines yet remain independent?

37. When teaching a client about self-medication with eyedrops, the nurse teaches the client to apply pressure to the nasal punctal area after instilling the drop. Explain the rationale for this action.

38. If more than one ophthalmic drug is prescribed, what should the nurse teach the client regarding the timing of the drops?

39. Are gloves required when the nurse is preparing to administer eye drops? Explain.

40. What are two important nursing measures to take before giving ophthalmic drops for conjunctivitis?

    a. _____

    b. _____

41. A client is taking an ocular NSAID, flurbiprofen (Ocufen), for an inflammatory disorder. The client calls the clinic to ask about wearing contact lenses while taking these eye drops. What instructions should the client receive?

CASE STUDY: THE CLIENT WITH EYE AND VISION PROBLEMS

Answer Guidelines for the Case Study questions are provided on the companion Evolve Learning Resources Web site at http://evolve.elsevier.com/Iggy/.

A 45-year-old woman comes into the ophthalmology office for an annual eye examination. She has had progressive myopia and astigmatism since age 11 years. In addition to her job as a high school PE teacher, she also plays in local recreation league volleyball teams and plays tennis with friends. She wears eyeglasses that now also correct for beginning presbyopia and has satisfactory correction. This year, the physician notes that she has a very small hole in the retina of her left eye, but no treatment is indicated for now. However, the physician does recommend that she stop playing tennis and volleyball at this time.

1. What is the probable cause of this retinal hole? Why did the physician recommend that she stop these activities?

Later, the client works in her yard trimming hedges with an electric clipper. Despite wearing her eyeglasses, a branch whips backward and strikes her in the left eye. She immediately sees bright flashes of light, and at first notes that it seems as if a curtain or shadow is pulled over her eye.

2. What should the client do?

3. Upon ophthalmoscopic examination, the physician sees gray bulges in the retina that quiver. A tear is seen at the lateral edge of retina. What is the probable diagnosis? Be specific.

4. The client is scheduled for immediate surgery. Describe the type and purpose of the surgery needed for this condition.

5. Postoperatively, the client has an eye patch and shield over her left eye. She is now fully awake and wants to use the bathroom. She also is complaining of severe nausea. What should the nurse do?

6. The client tells the nurse that she is looking forward to going home because she wants to be able to work outside in her garden for relaxation. What instructions should the nurse give to the client about her activity, diet, and postoperative care?

Assessment of the Ear and Hearing

LEARNING OUTCOMES

1. Describe the key elements to inspect when performing assessment of the external ear.
2. Describe age-related changes in the structure of the ear and hearing.
3. Identify 10 common drugs that affect hearing.
4. Demonstrate the correct use of an otoscope.
5. Describe the landmarks of the tympanic membrane (eardrum).
6. Compare air conduction of sound with bone conduction of sound.
7. Demonstrate the correct use of a tuning fork in performing the Weber and Rinne tests for hearing.
8. Prioritize educational needs for the client about to undergo pure-tone audiometry and electro-nystagmography.

LEARNING ACTIVITIES

1. Before completing the study guide exercises for this chapter, it is recommended that you review the anatomy and physiology of the ear.

2. Review the boldfaced terms and their definitions in Chapter 51 to enhance your understanding of the content.

STUDY/REVIEW QUESTIONS

Answers to the Study/Review Questions are provided on the companion Evolve Learning Resources Web site at http://evolve.elsevier.com/Iggy/.

1. Which of the following is the spiral organ of hearing?
   a. Cochlea
   b. Semicircular canal
   c. Pinna
   d. Stapes

2. The two critical functions of the ear are _____ and maintaining _____.

3. Match each ear structure with the corresponding locations. Answers may be used more than once.

Structure

_____ a. Mastoid process

_____ b. Incus

_____ c. Stapes

_____ d. Cochlea

_____ e. Tympanic membrane

_____ f. Organ of Corti

_____ g. Malleus

Location

1. External ear
2. Middle ear
3. Inner ear

4. Identify the events, in sequential order, that lead to the sense of hearing.

   _____ a. Sound waves are transferred to the malleus.

   _____ b. Sound waves are transferred to the incus and the stapes.

   _____ c. Vibrations are transmitted to the cochlea.

   _____ d. Neural impulses are conducted by the auditory nerve.

   _____ e. Sound waves strike the mastoid and the movable tympanic membrane.

   _____ f. Sound is processed and interpreted by the brain.

5. Which of the following is a change in the ear that is related to aging? *Check all that apply.*

   _____ a. The tympanic membrane may appear dull and retracted.

   _____ b. The pinna becomes shorter and thickened.

   _____ c. Cerumen-producing glands decrease in number and function.

   _____ d. Bony ossicles have decreased movement.

   _____ e. Hearing for high-frequency sound increases.

6. Match the following terms with their definitions.

Term

_____ a. Decibel

_____ b. Masking

_____ c. Vestibular hearing loss

_____ d. Otosclerosis

_____ e. Sensorineural

Definition

1. Relating to the functions of the ear needed for the sense of balance and position
2. A unit of sound for expressing loudness
3. Formation of spongy bone around structures of the middle and inner ear
4. The process of hiding a specific sound from one ear while the other ear is tested
5. Hearing loss resulting from neural defects

7. A sensorineural hearing loss results from impairment of which of the following?
   a. Fused bony ossicles
   b. The first cranial nerve
   c. The seventh cranial nerve
   d. The eighth cranial nerve

8. Your adult client is having problems with his hearing. Below are his medications. Which of his medications are ototoxic? *Check all that apply.*

   _____ a. Ibuprofen (Motrin)

   _____ b. Digoxin (Lanoxin)

   _____ c. Furosemide (Lasix)

   _____ d. Levothyroxine (Synthroid)

   _____ e. Aspirin

   _____ f. Gentamicin (Garamycin)

9. Which of the following statements about an otoscopic assessment is true?
   a. The client's head should be tilted slightly toward the nurse for support.
   b. The nurse holds the otoscope upside down, like a large pen.
   c. The pinna is pulled down and back.
   d. The internal canal is visualized while the speculum is slowly inserted.

10. Upon otoscopic assessment, which of the following findings indicate a normal tympanic membrane? *Check all that apply.*

    _____ a. The membrane is slightly convex in nature.

    _____ b. The membrane is a pink to deep-red color.

    _____ c. The membrane has a mobile pars tensa.

    _____ d. The membrane is opaque or pearly gray.

    _____ e. The membrane is always intact.

11. Which structures are seen through the normal tympanic membrane?

12. What is the main difference between air conduction and bone conduction of sound?

13. Fill in the blanks regarding hearing intensity.

    a. The lowest intensity at which a young, normal ear can detect sound is _____ dB.
    b. Conversational speech is generally around _____ dB.
    c. A soft whisper is around _____ dB.
    d. Sound at _____ dB is so intense that it is painful for most people with normal hearing.
    e. A person with a hearing loss of _____ dB may not be able to hear speech even with a hearing aid.
    f. A person with a hearing loss of _____ to _____ dB will be unable to hear speech without a hearing aid.

14. Match the following hearing test terms with their correct definitions.

Hearing Test

    _____ a. Voice test

    _____ b. Electronystagmography

    _____ c. Dix-Hallpike test

    _____ d. Audiometry

    _____ e. Watch test

    _____ f. Weber tuning fork test

Definition
1. Measurement of hearing acuity
2. Test for high-frequency sounds
3. Used to differentiate between conductive and sensorineural hearing losses
4. Test for detecting central and peripheral disease of vestibular system
5. Tests for vertigo
6. A simple acuity test

15. When conducting a Weber tuning fork test:
    a. The preferred site for testing is above the upper lip over the teeth.
    b. Ask the client in which ear the sound is louder.
    c. Proper handling of the fork includes grasping the upper part of the fork for stability.
    d. Lateralization is a normal result.

16. Which of the following statements are true regarding the Rinne tuning fork test? *Check all that apply*.

_____ a. The test assists in differentiating hearing by air conduction and bone conduction.

_____ b. The test involves timed responses.

_____ c. The vibrating fork stem is placed on the client's mastoid process.

_____ d. Sound is normally heard longer by bone conduction than by air conduction.

17. It is important for the nurse to understand the terminology of pure tone audiometry. Match each of the following terms with the corresponding definition.

Definition

_____ a. Lowest level of intensity heard by client (50% of the time)

_____ b. Expressed in decibels

_____ c. Highness or lowness of tones

_____ d. Results of pure tone audiometry testing

Term
1. Frequency (time)
2. Threshold
3. Audiogram
4. Intensity

18. A client is scheduled for an electronystagmography (ENG). What should the nurse tell this client to prepare him for this test?

19. Which clients should not have electronystagmography?

20. The ability to understand speech is the most important aspect of human auditory function. What does speech discrimination testing determine?

21. Tympanometry is helpful in distinguishing which of the following?
    a. Middle ear infections
    b. Outer ear infections
    c. Furuncles
    d. Indurated lesions on the pinna

22. What is the normal response to caloric testing?

23. In bone conduction testing, which ear is tested first?

24. What is the purpose of using a gentle puff of air when examining the external ear canal with an otoscope?

25. Match the type of hearing loss with its definition.

Definition

_____ a. Profound hearing loss

_____ b. Results from a defect in the cochlea, eighth cranial nerve, or the brain

_____ c. Results from any physical obstruction of sound wave transmission

Type of Loss
1. Sensorineural hearing loss
2. Conductive hearing loss
3. Mixed conductive-sensorineural hearing loss

Interventions for Clients with Ear and Hearing Problems

LEARNING OUTCOMES

1. Compare the clinical manifestations and interventions for external otitis with those of otitis media.
2. Describe how to correctly instill medications into the ear.
3. Describe the mechanisms of action, side effects, and nursing interventions of drug therapy for ear infections.
4. Explain the procedures to safely remove impacted cerumen from the ear canal of an older client.
5. Prioritize educational needs for the client with Ménière's disease.
6. Describe the mechanisms of action, side effects, and nursing implications of drug therapy for Ménière's disease.
7. Compare the causes and interventions for conductive hearing loss with those for sensorineural hearing loss.
8. Prioritize nursing care needs for the client after tympanoplasty.
9. Prioritize educational needs for the client after stapedectomy.
10. Identify an appropriate method for communicating with a client who has recently become hearing impaired.
11. Develop a community-based teaching plan for a client who is learning to use a hearing aid.

LEARNING ACTIVITIES

1. Before completing the study guide exercises for this chapter, it is recommended that you review the following:
   - Anatomy and physiology of the ear
   - Assessment of the ear and hearing
   - Maintenance of hearing aids
   - Concepts of body image and self-esteem

2. Review the boldfaced terms and their definitions in Chapter 52 to enhance your understanding of the content.

STUDY/REVIEW QUESTIONS

Answers to the Study/Review Questions are provided on the companion Evolve Learning Resources Web site at http://evolve.elsevier.com/Iggy/.

1. Which of the following treatments are used for external otitis? *Check all that apply.*

    _____ a. Application of heat

    _____ b. Oral analgesics

    _____ c. Topical antibiotics

    _____ d. Myringotomy

2. What are the most common organisms associated with external otitis? *Check all that apply.*

    _____ a. *E. coli*

    _____ b. *Aspergillus*

    _____ c. *Pseudomonas aeruginosa*

    _____ d. *Staphylococcus aureus*

3. Identify at least four conditions affecting the external ear.

    a. _____

    b. _____

    c. _____

    d. _____

4. Which of the following statements about necrotizing or malignant external otitis are true? *Check all that apply.*

    _____ a. It is the most virulent form of external otitis.

    _____ b. There is a low mortality rate related to complicating disorders.

    _____ c. It can destroy cranial nerves, especially the facial nerve.

    _____ d. It is a very common problem among younger adults.

5. Your adult client has external otitis. After the inflammation resolves, which of the following actions should the client avoid?
    a. Use earplugs while swimming.
    b. Drop diluted alcohol in the ear to prevent recurrence.
    c. Use cotton-tipped applicators to dry the ears thoroughly after bathing.
    d. Use analgesics for pain relief.

6. Describe the clinical manifestations of a furuncle.

7. Ear irrigation fluid would be least likely to stimulate the vestibular sense at what temperature?
    a. 78° F
    b. 98° F
    c. 110° F
    d. 120° F

8. An adult client has otitis media. The nurse would expect the client's chief complaint to be which of the following?
    a. Ear pain
    b. Rhinitis
    c. Drainage from the ear canal
    d. Itchiness in the ear canal

9. Your adult client has a history of otitis media. He states that his left ear pain is better, but he has noticed some pus with some blood in that ear.
    a. What does the nurse suspect has happened?

    b. What would reveal an infecting agent?

10. As part of the procedure for instilling ear drops, a nurse would do which of the following? *Check all that apply.*

    _____ a. Irrigate the ear if the membrane is not intact.

    _____ b. Place the bottle of eardrops in a bowl of warm water for 5 minutes.

    _____ c. Tilt the client's head in the opposite direction of the affected ear.

    _____ d. Use sterile gloves during the procedure.

11. Your adult client has wax in his left ear. When irrigating his ear, you would use no more than _____ mL of solution.
    a. 50 to 70
    b. 90 to 120
    c. 125 to 140
    b. 150 to 170

12. The nurse would stop irrigating the ear if the client complained of which of the following?
    a. Headache
    b. Nausea
    c. Tingling sensation
    d. Fatigue

13. What would the nurse's instructions to the client include after a myringotomy? *Check all that apply.*

    _____ a. Report an excessive drainage to your physician.

    _____ b. Restrict hair washing for 1 week.

    _____ c. Use a straw for drinking liquids.

    _____ d. Do not change the ear dressing until the next office visit.

14. Mastoiditis is an inflammation of which of the following?
    a. Bones in the middle ear
    b. Temporal bone behind the ear
    c. Sixth and seventh cranial nerves
    d. Labyrinth structure

15. Which of the following statements about tinnitus are true? *Check all that apply.*

    _____ a. It is one of the most common complaints of clients with hearing disorders.

    _____ b. Diagnostic tests cannot confirm the disorder.

    _____ c. This disorder does not have observable characteristics.

    _____ d. Tinnitus can lead to particularly disturbing emotional consequences.

16. Identify at least four causes of tinnitus.

    a. _____

    b. _____

    c. _____

    d. _____

17. What is the difference, if any, between vertigo and dizziness?

18. Ménière's disease is associated with which of the following? *Check all that apply.*

    _____ a. Viral or bacterial infection

    _____ b. Allergic reactions

    _____ c. Biochemical disturbances

    _____ d. Genetic and familiar traits

19. Identify the three distinct characteristics of Ménière's disease and give the pathologic changes associated with the disease.

20. An adult client has been diagnosed with Ménière's disease. Which of the following would the nurse include in teaching for this client? *Check all that apply.*

_____ a. Make slow head movements.

_____ b. Reduce the intake of salt.

_____ c. Stop smoking.

_____ d. Take aspirin every 4 hours.

21. Which of the following defines an acoustic neuroma?
    a. Tumor that is benign and rarely causes a problem
    b. Malignant tumor that metastasizes quickly
    c. Benign tumor that can be neurologically damaging
    d. Benign tumor of cranial nerve VI

22. Identify the causes of conductive hearing loss.

23. Identify the causes of sensorineural hearing loss.

24. Presbycusis is a common cause of sensorineural hearing loss associated with aging. What are some physiologic changes associated with this loss?

25. What percentage of the population of clients 65 to 75 years of age suffers hearing loss?
    a. 10%
    b. 25%
    c. 35%
    d. 50%

26. Which of the following actions could prevent ear trauma?
    a. Holding your nose when sneezing to reduce pressure.
    b. Not using small objects to clean your external ear canal.
    c. Occluding one nostril when blowing your nose.
    d. Avoiding washing your external ear and canal.

27. A client has just started to wear a hearing aid. Identify what special tips the nurse should offer to help this client adapt more easily to its use.

28. Which of the following is proper care of a hearing aid?
    a. Cleaning the entire hearing aid with mild soap and water
    b. Storing the device with the battery in place
    c. Adjusting the volume at the highest setting to maximize hearing
    d. Cleaning the debris from the hole in the middle with a pipe cleaner

29. Which of the following statements are true regarding a tympanoplasty reconstruction of the middle ear? *Check all that apply.*

    _____ a. The goal of a tympanoplasty is to improve hearing caused by conductive hearing loss.

    _____ b. Hearing loss after surgery is usually normal but temporary.

    _____ c. Local anesthesia is preferred over general anesthesia.

    _____ d. Activity is permitted after 6 hours of bedrest.

30. A client is recovering from ear surgery. Identify the instructions the nurse should incorporate in the discharge teaching.

31. The client who has had a stapedectomy should be told which of the following? *Check all that apply.*

    _____ a. Hearing is initially worse after surgery.

    _____ b. Success rate is high.

    _____ c. There is a risk of total hearing loss on the affected side.

    _____ d. Hearing is improved immediately after surgery.

32. Briefly discuss some strategies for communicating with a hearing-impaired client.

33. Match each term with its definition.

Definition

    _____ a. Calcification and hardening of the auricle that occurs as a result of trauma and subsequent hematoma

    _____ b. Swimmer's ear

    _____ c. Complete absence of the auditory canal

    _____ d. Damage to the middle ear due to extreme pressure changes

    _____ e. Has three forms: acute, chronic, and serous

    _____ f. Disturbed sense of a person's proper relationship in space

    _____ g. A sensation of whirling or turning in space

    _____ h. Hearing loss that occurs with aging

    _____ i. Term that describes drugs that damage inner-ear structures

Term
1. Ototoxic
2. Vertigo
3. Cauliflower or boxer's ear
4. Atresia
5. External otitis
6. Dizziness
7. Presbycusis
8. Otitis media
9. Barotrauma

34. Which statement about hearing loss is true? *Check all that apply.*

    _____ a. Hearing loss is always gradual.

    _____ b. The ability to hear high-frequency, soft consonants (such as *s, sh, f, th, ch*) sounds is lost first.

    _____ c. Tinnitus rarely accompanies hearing loss.

    _____ d. Vertigo may be present with hearing loss.

    _____ e. Clients often state that they cannot understand specific words.

35. True or False? Which of the following statements about otitis are true? *Write T for true or F for false in the blanks provided. For those questions that are false, rewrite the statement to make it true.*

_____ a. For external otitis, topical antibiotics and steroid therapies are most effective in decreasing inflammation and pain.

_____ b. Cerumen is the most common cause of an impacted ear canal.

_____ c. Irrigation is indicated for eardrum perforation or otitis media.

_____ d. Insects in the ear canal are best removed while still alive, if possible.

_____ e. Anyone can easily remove earwax using a small curette or cerumen spoon.

_____ f. Topical antibiotics are not used to treat otitis media.

_____ g. A myringotomy may be used to drain fluids and ease inner-ear pain.

_____ h. Tinnitus, or ringing in the ears, is a common problem that rarely causes problems.

CASE STUDY: OTOSCLEROSIS

Answer Guidelines for the Case Study questions are provided on the companion Evolve Learning Resources Web site at http://evolve.elsevier.com/Iggy/.

A 53-year-old client is visiting the ENT clinic today. She has had progressive hearing loss since her late 20s. Her ability to hear is better with her right ear, and she has been using bilateral hearing aids for the past 5 years. After being evaluated, it is determined that she has otosclerosis. She discusses options with her physician and the decision is made for her to have a stapedectomy of the left ear.

1. Why is the procedure done on the left ear rather than the right ear?

2. Develop a preoperative teaching-learning plan for the client. What should the nurse discuss about the hearing aids?

3. Discuss alternative ways for the client to cope with her reduced hearing ability until the surgery is performed.

Postoperatively, the client is nauseated and states that "things are spinning" when she tries to sit up. Her postoperative orders include meclizine (Antivert) and droperidol (Inapsine).

4. What interventions are implemented for client safety? What side effects should the nurse monitor for while the client is receiving these medications?

Following removal of the external dressing, the client becomes upset and begins to cry. She states, "I don't notice any difference; in fact, I think it's worse! Now I can't hear anything with my right ear!"

5. What is the probable cause of her hearing loss? What can the nurse say to the client to assist her at this time?

Assessment of the Musculoskeletal System

LEARNING OUTCOMES

1. Recall the anatomy and physiology of the musculoskeletal system.
2. Explain how physiologic aging changes of the musculoskeletal system affect care of older adults.
3. Conduct a musculoskeletal history using Gordon's Functional Health Patterns.
4. Evaluate important assessment findings in a client with a musculoskeletal health problem.
5. Explain the use of laboratory testing for a client with a musculoskeletal health problem.
6. Identify the use of radiography in diagnosing musculoskeletal health problems.
7. Plan follow-up care for clients undergoing musculoskeletal diagnostic testing.
8. Develop a teaching plan for clients undergoing arthroscopic procedures.

LEARNING ACTIVITIES

1. Before completing the study guide exercises for this chapter, it is recommended that you review the following:
   - Anatomy and physiology of the musculoskeletal system (muscles, bones, and joints)
   - Physiology of muscle contraction
   - Active and passive range-of-motion (ROM) exercises for each joint
   - Assessment of the musculoskeletal system
   - Normal ROM for each joint
   - Effect of immobility on the musculoskeletal system

2. Review the boldfaced terms and their definitions in Chapter 53 to enhance your understanding of the content.

STUDY/REVIEW QUESTIONS

Answers to the Study/Review Questions are provided on the companion Evolve Learning Resources Web site at http://evolve.elsevier.com/Iggy/.

1. Identify five types of bones and give an example of each.

    a. _____

    b. _____

    c. _____

    d. _____

    e. _____

2. Match each of the following musculo-skeletal terms with the corresponding description.

Term

_____ a. Cancellous

_____ b. Cortex

_____ c. Diaphysis

_____ d. Epiphysis

_____ e. Haversian system

_____ f. Osteoblast

_____ g. Osteoclast

_____ h. Osteocyte

_____ i. Periosteum

_____ j. Trabeculae

_____ k. Volkmann's canal

Description
1. Living bone cells
2. Shaft of a long bone
3. Outer layer of bone tissue
4. Longitudinal canal network containing microscopic blood vessels
5. End of a long bone
6. Spongy inner layer of bone
7. Network connecting bone marrow vessels to outer bone covering
8. Bone-forming cells
9. Bone tissue containing marrow
10. Highly vascular bone covering
11. Bone-destroying cells

3. Identify the six major functions of the skeletal system.

    a. _____

    b. _____

    c. _____

    d. _____

    e. _____

    f. _____

Describe each of the following types of joints and give an example of each.

4. Synarthrodial joints

5. Amphiarthrodial joints

6. Diarthrodial joints

True or False? *Write T for true or F for false in the blanks provided. If a statement is false, correct it to make it true.*

_____ 7. The knee is considered to be a "ball-and-socket" joint.

_____ 8. The elbow is considered to be a "hinge" joint.

_____ 9. Pivot joints allow for flexion and extension only.

_____ 10. Biaxial joints allow for gliding movement such as that done with the wrist.

_____ 11. Condylar joints allow for flexion and extension only.

Describe each of the following types of muscle tissue and identify their functions.

12. Smooth muscle

13. Cardiac muscle

14. Skeletal muscle

15. Match each of the following musculoskeletal terms with the corresponding definition.

Term

_____ a. Atrophy

_____ b. Bursa

_____ c. Cartilage

_____ d. Fascia

_____ e. Fasciculi

_____ f. Ligament

_____ g. Synovium

_____ h. Synovial fluid

_____ i. Tendon

Definition
1. Membrane that secretes a lubricating fluid
2. Decrease in size and number of muscle fibers
3. Small sacs lined with synovial membrane.
4. Band of tough, fibrous tissue attaching muscle to bone
5. Bundles of muscle fibers
6. Lubricates joints
7. Band of tough, fibrous tissue attaching bone to bone
8. Fibrous tissue surrounding muscle
9. Collagen fibers at bone ends

True or False? Write T for true or F for false in the blanks provided. If a statement is false, correct it to make it true.

_____ 16. As one ages, bone density often increases.

_____ 17. As one ages, synovial joint cartilage regenerates.

_____ 18. Degenerative joint disease, muscle atrophy, slowed movement, and decreased strength are common changes in the musculoskeletal system of the older adult.

For each of the categories of assessment listed below, identify one finding that would indicate a risk factor for an actual or potential problem of the musculoskeletal system.

Category of Assessment	Potential Risk Factor for Problem
19. Demographic data	
20. Personal and family history	
21. Diet history	
22. Socioeconomic status	
23. Psychosocial	

24. While observing a client performing range-of-motion (ROM) exercises, the nurse notes that the client can move his leg outward from the side of the body. The nurse would document this movement as which of the following?
    a. Flexion
    b. Extension
    c. Adduction
    d. Abduction

25. Which instrument is used to assess joint range of motion?
    a. An odometer
    b. An ergometer
    c. A goniometer
    d. A spectrometer

26. Which of the following is an abnormal finding in the physical assessment of the musculoskeletal system?
    a. Upper extremities symmetric, equal muscle mass
    b. Gait balanced, stride smooth and regular
    c. Flexion, extension, and rotation of the neck
    d. Opposition of three of four fingers to the thumb

27. Which of the following is primarily responsible for regulating serum calcium levels?
    a. Calcitonin
    b. Vitamin D
    c. Glucocorticoids
    d. Growth hormone

28. Which of the following is present in bone and serum in inverse proportion to calcium?
    a. Estrogen
    b. Phosphorus
    c. Thyroxine
    d. Insulin

29. Which of the following laboratory results may indicate bone or liver damage, such as metastatic cancer of the bone?
    a. Serum calcium 9.5 mg/dL
    b. Serum calcium 8.2 mg/dL
    c. Lactate dehydrogenase (LDH) 185 units/L
    d. Alkaline phosphatase 140 U/L

30. Read the following scenario, then complete the chart using the PQRST model to assess the client's pain with the data provided in the scenario.

A client with a 5-year history of osteoarthritis comes to the clinic with severe intermittent left knee pain. She describes the pain as starting yesterday in her foot and moving up her shin to her knee. At the time, she was gardening in her yard and was walking to the curb to put out the trash when the pain suddenly stopped her. She says that the pain is a burning pain, "like nothing I've ever had before," and rates it as between an 8 and 9 on a 10-point scale. She says that she hobbled up to her house, put an ice pack on her knee, and rested for the rest of the evening after taking a pain pill. The ice helped at first, but her knee throbbed all night and this morning the pain has resumed even though she has tried to stay off of her leg.

	Assessment Findings
P	
Q	
R	
S	
T	

31. Match the following substances related to the musculoskeletal system with its function.

Function

_____ a.   Promotes absorption of calcium and phosphorus from the small intestine

_____ b.   Responsible for increasing bone length

_____ c.   If serum calcium levels are increased above normal, this hormone decreases serum calcium levels by inhibiting bone resorption and increasing renal excretion of calcium and phosphorus

_____ d.   Regulate protein metabolism

_____ e.   If serum calcium levels are lowered, this hormone stimulates bone to promote osteoclastic activity and release calcium to the blood, thus raising serum calcium levels

Substance
1. Glucocorticoids
2. Calcitonin
3. Vitamin D
4. Parathyroid hormone
5. Growth hormone

True or False? *Write T for true or F for false in the blanks provided. If a statement is false, correct it to make it true.*

_____ 32.   African-American women have denser bones than African-American men.

_____ 33.   Caucasian women are more likely, out of all groups, to have osteoporosis and fractures.

_____ 34.   Lactose intolerant individuals need to obtain calcium from other sources, such as yogurt and cheeses.

35. Complete the puzzle by answering the questions related to physical assessment of the musculo-skeletal system.

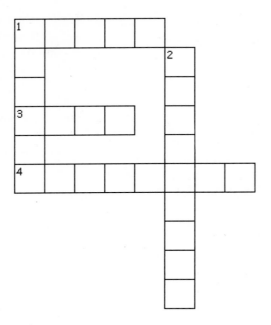

Across

1. Genu _____, also called bowlegged.
3. Assess the stance phase and the swing phase.
4. Assess by asking the client to perform activities of daily living.

Down

1. Genu _____, also called knocked-knee.
2. A lateral curve in the spine found upon inspection when the client flexes forward from the hips.

36. Match each of the following radiographic examinations and diagnostic tests with the corresponding definition.

Radiographic Examination

_____ a. Tomography

_____ b. Xeroradiography

_____ c. Myelography

_____ d. Arthrography

_____ e. Computed tomography (CT)

_____ f. Bone biopsy

_____ g. Muscle biopsy

_____ h. Electromyography (EMG)

_____ i. Arthroscopy

_____ j. Bone scan

_____ k. Gallium/thallium scan

_____ l. Magnetic resonance imaging (MRI)

_____ m. Ultrasonography

Definition

1. A more sensitive and specific isotope scan used to detect bone problems. Can be used to examine the brain, liver, and breast tissue when disease is suspected.
2. Used to detect musculoskeletal problems, particularly in the vertebral column. Can produce three-dimensional images. Can be done with or without contrast.
3. Helpful in detailing the musculoskeletal system because it produces planes, or slices, for focus and blurs the images of other structures.
4. Invasive test that may confirm the presence of infection or neoplasm of the bone.
5. Margins and edges are clearly seen because this test highlights the contrast between structures.
6. A contrast medium or dye is injected into the subarachnoid space of the spine. The vertebral column, intervertebral disks, spinal nerve roots, and blood vessels all can be visualized.
7. Used for the diagnosis of atrophy (as in muscular dystrophy) and inflammation (as in polymyositis).
8. A fiberoptic tube is inserted into a joint (usually the knee or shoulder) for direct visualization. Procedures such as synovial biopsy or repair of traumatic injury may also be done.
9. Radioactive material is injected for visualization of the entire skeletal system. This test is used to detect tumors, arthritis, osteomyelitis, vertebral compression fractures, osteoporosis, and unexplained bone pain.
10. A test that uses sound waves to produce an image of the tissue. This test may be used to visualize osteomyelitis, soft-tissue disorders (such as masses and fluid accumulation), and traumatic injuries.
11. An image is produced through the interaction of magnetic fields, radio waves, and atomic nuclei showing hydrogen density. This test is particularly useful in identifying problems with muscles, tendons, and ligaments.
12. An x-ray study of a joint after contrast medium (air or solution) is injected to enhance visualization. Most commonly done on the knee and shoulder joints.
13. Used to determine the electrical potential of an individual muscle, and usually accompanied by nerve conduction studies. Used to diagnosis neuromuscular, lower motor neuron, and peripheral nerve disorders.

Interventions for Clients with Musculoskeletal Problems

LEARNING OUTCOMES

1. Explain the risk factors for primary and secondary osteoporosis.
2. Implement interventions to decrease the risk for developing osteoporosis.
3. Develop a teaching plan for all age-groups concerning osteoporosis.
4. Describe the role of drug therapy in the prevention and management of osteoporosis.
5. Compare and contrast osteoporosis and osteomalacia.
6. Identify common assessment findings in clients with Paget's disease of the bone.
7. Differentiate acute and chronic osteomyelitis.
8. Prioritize care for clients with osteomyelitis.
9. Analyze assessment data to determine common nursing diagnoses and collaborative problems for the client with a malignant bone tumor.
10. Discuss the psychosocial aspects associated with a diagnosis of bone cancer.
11. Evaluate the nursing care of a client with a bone tumor using expected outcome criteria.
12. Explain the pathophysiology and risk factors for carpal tunnel syndrome.
13. Identify treatment options for the client diagnosed with carpal tunnel syndrome.
14. Describe common disorders of the foot, including hallux valgus and plantar fasciitis.
15. Explain the role of the nurse when caring for an adult client with muscular dystrophy.

LEARNING ACTIVITIES

1. Before completing the study guide exercises for this chapter, it is recommended that you review the following:
   - Anatomy and physiology of the musculoskeletal system (muscles, bones, and joints)
   - Perioperative nursing management
   - Postoperative nursing management
   - Wound and skin isolation, contact isolation, and drainage precautions
   - Metabolism of calcium and vitamin D
   - Parameters of a complete musculoskeletal and neurologic assessment
   - Principles of IV therapy
   - Concepts of growth and development
   - Concept of body image and self-esteem
   - Concepts of grief, loss, death, and dying

2. Review the boldfaced terms and their definitions in Chapter 54 to enhance your understanding of the content.

STUDY/REVIEW QUESTIONS

Answers to the Study/Review Questions are provided on the companion Evolve Learning Resources Web site at http://evolve.elsevier.com/Iggy/.

1. Briefly describe each of the following metabolic bone diseases.
   a. Osteoporosis

   b. Primary osteoporosis

   c. Secondary osteoporosis

   d. Osteomalacia

   e. Paget's disease

2. Match each of the following musculoskeletal disorders with the corresponding risk factors.

Musculoskeletal Disorder

_____ a. Osteoporosis

_____ b. Osteomalacia

_____ c. Paget's disease

Risk Factor

1. Older adults; vitamin D deficiency; insufficient exposure to sunlight
2. Possibly a result of latent viral infection
3. Female; white; menopause; thin; lean; immobilization

3. Describe three ways a person could reduce his or her risk for osteoporosis.

   a. _____

   b. _____

   c. _____

4. Match the following subjective client data with the musculoskeletal disorders they are primarily associated with. *Answers may be used more than once.*

Subjective Client Data

_____ a. Headache

_____ b. Loss of height

_____ c. Muscle cramps

_____ d. Smokes two packs of cigarettes per day

_____ e. Back pain relieved by rest

_____ f. Deep pain worsened by pressure and weight bearing

_____ g. Milk intolerance

_____ h. Sedentary lifestyle

_____ i. Pelvic bone pain, worse at night

_____ j. Drinks eight cups of coffee per day

_____ k. Dizziness or loss of balance

_____ l. Muscle weakness in legs

_____ m. Loss of height

Musculoskeletal Disorder
1. Osteoporosis
2. Osteomalacia
3. Paget's disease

5. Match the following objective client data with the musculoskeletal disorders they are primarily associated with. *Answers may be used more than once.*

Objective Client Data

_____ a. Unsteady gait

_____ b. Hip flexion contractures

_____ c. Flushed warm skin

_____ d. Vertebral fracture

_____ e. Bone tenderness over rib cage

_____ f. Kyphosis

_____ g. Long bone bowing

_____ h. Discomfort on vertebral palpation

_____ i. Soft skull

Musculoskeletal Disorder
1. Osteoporosis
2. Osteomalacia
3. Paget's disease

Explain briefly why each of the following drug therapies would benefit the client in the prevention of and/or management of osteoporosis.

6. Hormone replacement therapy (HRT)

7. Parathyroid hormone

8. Calcium

9. Vitamin D

10. Biphosphonates (BPs)

11. Selective estrogen receptor modulators (SERMs)

12. Calcitonin

13. Match each of the following precautions and/or side effects to the appropriate drug therapy.

Precaution/Side Effect

_____ a. Esophagitis and esophageal ulcers

_____ b. Hypercalcemia; can cause serious damage to the urinary system

_____ c. Low doses prescribed due to potentially serious side effects, such as endometrial or breast cancer

_____ d. May cause nasal mucosal irritation when given intranasally

_____ e. Should not be given to women with a history of venous thromboembolism

_____ f. Hypercalcemia and hyperphosphatemia

Drug Therapy
1. Calcitonin
2. Vitamin D
3. Estrogen
4. Calcium
5. Selective estrogen receptor modulators (SERMs)
6. Bisphosphonates (BPs)

14. Osteomalacia can be a complication of the intake of certain drugs. Identify the three drugs commonly associated with this circumstance.

a. _____

b. _____

c. _____

Briefly describe the two major types of osteomyelitis to differentiate between them.

15. Acute osteomyelitis

16. Chronic osteomyelitis

17. Your adult client is a carpenter. One day he was building a house and using an automatic nailing gun for his work. As he reached up to nail a piece of wood in place, he missed the wood and the nail fired into his hand. This would be an example of which of the following routes that could lead to osteomyelitis?
    a. Acute hematogenous spread
    b. Contiguous spread
    c. Direct inoculation
    d. Indirect inoculation

18. Which of the following is an assessment finding that the nurse would note for the client with acute osteomyelitis? *Check all that apply.*

    _____ a. Fever; temperature usually above 101° F

    _____ b. Sinus tract formation

    _____ c. Erythema of the affected area

    _____ d. Swelling around the affected area

19. Which of the following statements is correct regarding antibiotic therapy for the client with osteomyelitis?
    a. Single-agent therapy is the most effective treatment for acute infections.
    b. Chronic osteomyelitis may require 1 month of antibiotic therapy.
    c. Clients usually remain hospitalized to complete the full course of antibiotic therapy.
    d. The infected wound may be irrigated with one or more types of antibiotic solutions.

20. Match each of the following terms related to bone tumors with its corresponding definition.

Bone Tumor

_____ a. Chondrogenic

_____ b. Fibrogenic

_____ c. Osteogenic

_____ d. Sarcoma

_____ f. Secondary tumor

Definition
1. Tumor arising from bone
2. Malignant tumor metastasizing to bone
3. Tumor arising from cartilage
4. Tumor arising from fibrous tissue
5. Malignant bone tumor arising from underlying tissue

21. Match each type of benign tumor with its most common location.

Types of Benign Tumors

_____ a. Chondroma

_____ b. Giant cell tumor

_____ c. Osteoblastoma

_____ d. Osteoid osteoma

Most Common Location
1. Vertebra
2. Femur and tibia
3. Often spreads to lungs
4. Hands and feet

22. Match each of the following types of malignant bone tumors with the associated signs and symptoms.

Types of Malignant Bone Tumors

_____ a.   Chondrosarcoma

_____ b.   Ewing's sarcoma

_____ c.   Fibrosarcoma

_____ d.   Osteosarcoma

Signs and Symptoms

1.   Local tenderness in lower extremity long bones
2.   Short-term pain and swelling in distal femur
3.   Long-term dull pain near proximal femur
4.   Pain and swelling in lower pelvis

23. a.   Differentiate primary and secondary bone tumors.

 b.   Identify five common sites of formation of primary tumors that metastasize to the bone.

   (1) _____

   (2) _____

   (3) _____

   (4) _____

   (5) _____

 c.   Explain the term "bone seeking" regarding tumors.

24. Identify four common sites for bone tumor metastases.

 a. _____

 b. _____

 c. _____

 d. _____

True or False? *Write T for true or F for false in the blanks provided. For those questions that are false, rewrite the statement to make it true.*

_____ 25.   Osteosarcoma is the most common type of primary malignant bone tumor.

_____ 26.   Ewing's sarcoma is the most malignant of all the bone tumors.

_____ 27.   Ewing's sarcoma rarely extends into the soft tissue.

_____ 28.   Clients with chondrosarcoma typically verbalize complaints of swelling and constant, severe, throbbing pain.

_____ 29.   Fibrosarcoma clinically presents slowly and without specific symptoms.

Identify the pertinent data in each of the following categories that the nurse would collect in an assessment of the client with suspected metastatic bone disease.

30.   History

31.   Clinical manifestations

32.   Psychosocial

33. Identify two nursing diagnoses and one collaborative problem based on your assessment findings relevant to the client with suspected metastatic bone disease.

34. Match the following radiographic findings with their associated types of bone tumor growths. *Answers may be used more than once.*

Radiographic Finding

_____ a.   Poor margination

_____ b.   Intact cortices

_____ c.   Bone destruction

_____ d.   Cortical breakthrough

_____ e.   Smooth uniform periosteal bone

_____ f.   Irregular new periosteal bone

_____ g.   Sharp margins

Type of Bone Tumor
1. Benign
2. Malignant

35. Identify six interventions for pain management relevant to the client with bone tumors.

a.   _____

b.   _____

c.   _____

d.   _____

e.   _____

f.   _____

36. Which of the following assessment findings in the client who has undergone a bone graft for a tumor should the nurse report to the physician immediately?
   a.   Extremity distal to operative site warm and pink
   b.   Cast over operative site cool
   c.   Capillary refill in digits distal to operative site lasting longer than 5 seconds
   d.   Pain in operative extremity

37. Interventions to assist the client with a bone tumor who is grieving and anxious include which of the following? *Check all that apply.*

   _____ a.   Allowing the client to verbalize feelings

   _____ b.   Offering to call the client's clergy person or religious leader

   _____ c.   Preparing the client for death

   _____ d.   Listening attentively while the client talks

38. Identify six expected outcomes for the client with a malignant bone tumor, based on identified nursing diagnoses and collaborative problems.

a.   _____

b.   _____

c.   _____

d.   _____

e.   _____

f.   _____

39. Briefly describe the pathophysiology and related risk factors for carpal tunnel syndrome.
   a.   Pathophysiology

   b.   Risk factors

40. Briefly describe Phalen's maneuver.

41. What is Tinel's sign?

42. Identify the two common conservative measures the health care provider may use before surgical intervention as a treatment option for the client with carpal tunnel syndrome. Give an example of each.

    a. _____

    b. _____

43. Identify and briefly describe the two common surgical procedures for carpal tunnel syndrome.

    a. _____

    b. _____

44. Match the following characteristics to the hand disorders they are primarily associated with. *Answers may be used more than once.*

Characteristic

_____ a.   Pain worse at night

_____ b.   Round, cyst-like lesion

_____ c.   First three digits affected

_____ d.   Progressive palmar flexion deformity

_____ e.   Joint discomfort after strain

_____ f.   Median nerve compression

_____ g.   Fourth and fifth digits affected

_____ h.   Swollen synovium

_____ i.   Familial tendency common

_____ j.   Colles' fracture or hand burns

_____ k.   Occupational hazard

Hand Disorder

1. Carpal tunnel syndrome
2. Dupuytren's contracture
3. Ganglion

45. Match each of the following characteristics to the foot disorder it is primarily associated with. *Answers may be used more than once.*

Characteristic

_____ a.   Dorsiflexion of any MTP joint with plantar flexion of the adjacent PIP joint

_____ b.   A small tumor in a digital nerve of the foot

_____ c.   Often referred to as a bunion

_____ d.   Acute pain; burning sensation in the web space

_____ e.   Compressed posterior tibial nerve in ankle

_____ f.   Pain in the arch of the foot, especially when getting out of bed

_____ g.   Can occur as a result of poorly fitted shoes

_____ h.   Corns may develop on the dorsal side of the toe

_____ i.   Surgical procedure involves removal of the bony overgrowth and bursa

_____ j.   Diagnosis and treatment similar to those for carpal tunnel syndrome

_____ k.   May be seen in athletes, especially runners

_____ l.   Inflammation of the plantar fascia

_____ m.   Insertion of wires or screws for fixation

Foot Disorder

1. Hallux valgus
2. Hammertoe
3. Morton's neuroma
4. Tarsal tunnel syndrome
5. Plantar fasciitis

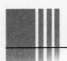

Read the following statements regarding scoliosis and decide whether each is true or false. Write T for true or F for false in the blanks provided. If a statement is false, correct it to make it true.

_____ 46. Scoliosis is a C- or S-shaped lateral curvature of the vertebral spine.

_____ 47. The abnormal curvature can cause low back pain.

_____ 48. Males are affected more than females.

_____ 49. Children are typically screened for scoliosis before starting school.

_____ 50. Surgical intervention is the least common treatment for adults.

_____ 51. Methods of treatment for adults are the same as for children.

52. Match each of the following characteristics and physical findings with the associated musculoskeletal disorder. *Answers may be used more than once.*

Characteristic/Physical Finding

_____ a. Muscle atrophy and weakness

_____ b. Fragile and deformed bones

_____ c. Cardiac involvement

_____ d. Hearing loss

_____ e. Poor skeletal development

Musculoskeletal Disorder
1. Osteogenesis imperfecta
2. Muscular dystrophy

CASE STUDY: THE CLIENT WITH OSTEOPOROSIS

Answer Guidelines for the Case Study questions are provided on the companion Evolve Learning Resources Web site at http://evolve.elsevier.com/Iggy/.

A 67-year-old postmenopausal woman has come to your clinic complaining of lower backache. She states that this pain is interfering with her sleep. She gets together weekly with her friends to play cards, and lately she has had to cancel. She says she is afraid her back will give out on her and she will fall. She states that the pain is interfering with her social life and other daily activities and that the episodes are becoming unbearable, so she has decided to seek treatment.

1. You suspect she may have osteoporosis. Identify six questions that you would ask her while performing her assessment.

2. During your assessment you discover that she does not take estrogen. What main question would you ask the client that would be important in determining any contraindications or precautions if the physician decides to place her on estrogen replacement therapy?

3. This client tells you that she does not like milk and rarely drinks it. How could you get her to increase her calcium intake?

4. The physician suspects osteoporosis as well and has ordered x-ray studies of her spine. When the films come back, they appear normal. The client asks you, "How can this be?" How would you respond to her?

5. The client is given a prescription for alendronate (Fosamax). What should you tell her before she begins therapy with this drug?

6. Determine appropriate measures to relieve this client's back pain.

7. The client states that she does not exercise. She tells you that the most exercise she gets is going up and down a few stairs to get to and from her car. What advice could you give her in regard to exercise?

Interventions for Clients with Musculoskeletal Trauma

LEARNING OUTCOMES

1. Compare and contrast common types of fractures.
2. Discuss the usual healing process for bone.
3. Identify common complications of fractures.
4. Explain the typical clinical manifestations that are seen in clients with fractures.
5. Analyze common nursing diagnoses for the client with a fracture.
6. Describe the nursing care of the client with a cast, including client education.
7. Describe the nursing care of the client in traction.
8. Discuss pain management for the client with a fracture.
9. Prioritize nursing care for the postoperative client who has undergone open reduction with internal fixation of the hip.
10. Evaluate the nursing care of a client with a fracture.
11. Identify common types of amputations.
12. Explain the psychosocial aspects related to amputations.
13. Develop a community-based teaching plan for a client who has undergone an elective amputation.
14. Describe the collaborative management for the client with complex regional pain syndrome.
15. Identify the common types of sports-related injuries and their management.

LEARNING ACTIVITIES

1. Before completing the study guide exercises for this chapter, it is recommended that you review the following:
   - Anatomy and physiology of the musculoskeletal system
   - Principles of body mechanics
   - Normal ROM for joints
   - Parameters for a complete musculoskeletal and neurologic assessment
   - Principles of perioperative and postoperative nursing management
   - Principles of traction
   - Concept of body image
   - Principles of hot and cold therapy
   - Concepts of grief and loss

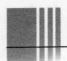

• Gaits for crutch and cane walking: use of a walker
• Principles of rehabilitation

2. Review the boldfaced terms and their definitions in Chapter 55 to enhance your understanding of the content.

STUDY/REVIEW QUESTIONS

Answers to the Study/Review Questions are provided on the companion Evolve Learning Resources Web site at http://evolve.elsevier.com/Iggy/.

1. Compare and contrast the following pairs of fracture types.
   a. Complete versus incomplete

   b. Open versus closed

   c. Pathologic versus fatigue

   d. Impacted versus spiral

2. Match each of the following descriptions to the corresponding type of fracture.

Description

_____ a. An adult client was riding his four-wheeler on a country road late one evening. Off in the distance he saw several cows in the middle of the road. He turned sharply to avoid hitting them and spun out of control. His four-wheeler landed on top of him. His lower leg is obviously broken. It is bleeding and bone fragments are protruding from the skin.

_____ b. One afternoon in her classroom, a schoolteacher slipped on some chalk that had fallen from the blackboard. She did not fall far and seemed to be all right. With the help of a student she was able to walk to the office. The secretary drove her to the emergency department.

_____ c. Your adult female client has osteoporosis. She plays cards often with her friends. One morning she was opening her car door while on her way to play cards when she fell suddenly. She said it was as though her "leg gave way" and caused her to fall.

Type of Fracture
1. Pathologic (spontaneous) fracture
2. Incomplete fracture
3. Open (compound) fracture

3. Match each of the following terms related to the fracture healing process with its definition.

Term

_____ a. Callus

_____ b. Granulation

_____ c. Hematoma

_____ d. Remodeling

Definition

1. Mass of clotted blood at fracture site
2. Process of bone building and resorption
3. Vascular and cellular proliferation
4. Nonbony union at fracture site

4. Indicate the numeric sequence of bone healing from the beginning.

_____ a. Callus formation

_____ b. Bone remodeling

_____ c. Hematoma formation

_____ d. Osteoblastic proliferation

_____ e. Hematoma to granulation tissue

5. Identify at least six complications associated with fractures.

a. _____

b. _____

c. _____

d. _____

e. _____

f. _____

6. Briefly explain why acute compartment syndrome is a medical emergency.

7. Identify eight signs and symptoms associated with acute compartment syndrome.

a. _____

b. _____

c. _____

d. _____

e. _____

f. _____

g. _____

h. _____

8. Identify four possible complications resulting from acute compartment syndrome.

a. _____

b. _____

c. _____

d. _____

9. Briefly describe a fasciotomy.

10. Identify the type of shock that is a possible complication of fractures.

11. Identify the four types of fractures that are primarily associated with fat embolism syndrome.

a. _____

b. _____

c. _____

d. _____

12. What is the single, earliest manifestation of fat embolism syndrome?

13. Identify the signs and symptoms the client would exhibit in response to low arterial oxygen levels.

14. Identify the types of clients with fractures who are at an increased risk for developing deep vein thrombosis.

15. Match each of the following fracture complications with its corresponding definition.

Fracture Complication

_____ a.   Disrupted blood supply to the bone, resulting in the death of bone tissue

_____ b.   Incorrect fracture healing

_____ c.   Fat globules released from the yellow bone marrow into the bloodstream

_____ d.   Incomplete fracture healing

_____ e.   Extensive tissue edema allowing fluid to move into the weakened space between the epidermis and the dermis

_____ f.   Lack of fracture healing

Definition

1. Delayed union
2. Fat embolism
3. Fracture blisters
4. Malunion
5. Avascular necrosis
6. Nonunion

16. Briefly define crepitation (crepitus).

17. Identify five common nursing diagnoses for clients with fractures.

18. Briefly describe the emergency measures taken in an acute trauma situation to assist a client who may have suffered a fracture.

19. Identify five methods used to immobilize fractures.

   a.   _____

   b.   _____

   c.   _____

   d.   _____

   e.   _____

20. The nurse's primary responsibility is to assess the area distal to an immobilization device. Briefly describe what the nurse would be evaluating.

21. Describe nursing interventions used to preserve cast integrity from the time of application to removal.

22. Explain why a nurse may cut a "window" into a cast.

23. Identify complications that may result from cast application.

24. Match each of the following definitions to the corresponding type of traction.

Definition

_____ a. Involves the use of a fabric fastener boot (Bucks), belt, or halter, which is secured around a body part

_____ b. Pins, wires, tongs, or screws surgically inserted directly into bone

_____ c. Combines skeletal traction and a plaster cast

_____ d. Exerts a pull for correction of alignment deformities

_____ e. Uses a belt around the body

Type of Traction
1. Plaster traction
2. Brace traction
3. Skin traction
4. Circumferential traction
5. Skeletal traction

25. Describe the nurse's role in caring for the client in traction.

26. Define the major disadvantage of skin traction.

27. Define the major disadvantages of skeletal traction.

28. Identify the three most common types of medications prescribed for the client with a fracture.

a. _____

b. _____

c. _____

29. Identify complementary/alternative (nondrug) nursing interventions that may be used to relieve pain in the client with a fracture.

30. Explain why open reduction with internal fixation (ORIF) is often the preferred surgical method for older adults.

31. Briefly describe four advantages and one disadvantage of external fixation.

32. Identify the nursing diagnoses appropriate for the client who has undergone ORIF of the hip.

33. Identify at least five potential complications related to impaired physical mobility in the client with a fracture.

    a. _____

    b. _____

    c. _____

    d. _____

    e. _____

34. Which of the following mobilization devices is usually preferred for the older client?
    a. Crutches
    b. Cane
    c. Walker
    d. Wheelchair

35. Briefly describe an open (guillotine) method amputation.

36. Briefly describe a closed (flap) method amputation.

37. Briefly describe a traumatic amputation and provide examples of such.

38. Identify at least four complications that may result from an amputation.

    a. _____

    b. _____

    c. _____

    d. _____

39. Describe the two groups of clients most likely to experience an amputation.

40. Identify two psychosocial manifestations exhibited by the client who experiences an amputation.

41. Describe the three stages of complex regional pain syndrome (CRPS).

42. Identify the first priority of management in the client with CRPS.

43. Identify three members of the health care team with whom the nurse would collaborate for management of the client with CRPS.

    a. _____

    b. _____

    c. _____

44. Identify the most common injuries to the knee.

45. Briefly define and describe the McMurray test.

Read the following statements and decide whether each is true or false. Write T for true or F for false in the blanks provided. If a statement is false, correct it to make it true.

_____ 46. The lateral meniscus is more likely to tear than the medial meniscus.

_____ 47. When the anterior cruciate ligament (ACL) is torn, the person may feel a "snap."

_____ 48. Complete healing of knee ligaments after surgery only takes 3 to 4 weeks.

_____ 49. Rupture of the Achilles tendon is common in older adults.

_____ 50. Dislocation is most common in the hip, shoulder, knee, and fingers.

_____ 51. A strain is excessive stretching of a ligament.

_____ 52. Management of a strain usually involves cold and heat applications.

_____ 53. Sprains are usually precipitated by twisting motions from a fall or sports injury.

_____ 54. Clients with a torn rotator cuff have shoulder pain and cannot initiate or maintain adduction of the arm at the shoulder (drop arm test).

55. Match each of the following terms related to musculoskeletal injuries with the corresponding definition.

Definition

_____ a. Partial joint surface separation

_____ b. Injury to ligament

_____ c. Joint surfaces not approximated

_____ d. Excessive stretching of muscle or tendon

Type of Musculoskeletal Injury
1. Dislocation
2. Sprain
3. Strain
4. Subluxation

Provide the answers for the following questions regarding fractures.

56. What is the major concern with rib and sternal fractures?

57. After head injuries, which type of fracture is the most common cause of death from trauma? Why?

58. What type of fracture is associated with osteoporosis rather than acute spinal injury?

59. What is the major complication associated with a femoral fracture?

60. What types of fractures are associated with ankle or foot fractures?

CASE STUDY: THE CLIENT WITH TRAUMATIC AMPUTATION

Answer Guidelines for the Case Study questions are provided on the companion Evolve Learning Resources Web site at http://evolve.elsevier.com/Iggy/.

A 25-year-old carpenter comes running into the emergency department where you are working with a blood-soaked rag over his right hand. He states that while working on a house he was building, he sawed off his right index finger. He has the finger in his pocket. You put on gloves and apply pressure with sterile gauze to the amputated area. You find out during your assessment that he has a history of depression and takes medication for it. You have identified during your assessment that he has no significant medical history other than depression.

1. Identify the type of amputation that would be considered for this client.

2. Identify the top nursing priority in dealing with the client's amputated finger.

3. What would you do with the client's finger?

4. Identify two appropriate nursing diagnoses for this client.

5. Identify the type of shock for which this client is at risk.

6. Considering this client's history, what recommendations would you make?

CASE STUDY: THE CLIENT WITH FRACTURE

Answer Guidelines for the Case Study questions are provided on the companion Evolve Learning Resources Web site at http://evolve.elsevier.com/Iggy/.

A 20-year-old client was admitted with fractures of the right tibia and fibula after a fall. She has a long leg cast that was applied this morning. The physician has ordered bedrest for now until her condition stabilizes.

1.   What is the priority for assessment during this time?

2.   Later that evening, as the nurse performs an assessment, the client states that the cast seems "too tight." It was difficult, but not impossible, for the nurse to insert one finger between the top of the cast and the client's skin. Is this a concern, and what actions, if any, should the nurse take at this time?

3.   A few days later, the client is allowed to get out of bed with crutches. The crutches have been delivered, but the physical therapist has not yet been in to see the client. The client states, "I can't wait any longer. Let me try walking with those crutches—I'm sure I can do it because I've played with my brother's crutches before." Should you let her walk with the crutches? Why or why not?

4.   What type of gait will she be taught to use while crutch-walking?

5.   The client has been discharged, and has received instructions for cast care. One week later, she calls the office and asks, "Can I get a new cast? This one smells moldy or musty! And it's getting uncomfortable." What do you suspect? When she comes to the office to have it checked, what further assessments should be done?

6.   The physician decides to remove the cast. The client is fearful when she sees the cast cutter. What should you tell her?

Assessment of the Gastrointestinal System

LEARNING OUTCOMES

1. Recall the anatomy and physiology of the gastrointestinal (GI) system.
2. Identify GI system changes associated with aging.
3. Perform a GI history using Gordon's Functional Health Patterns.
4. Evaluate important physical assessment findings in a client with digestion, nutrition, and elimination (GI) health problems.
5. Explain the use of laboratory testing for a client with a GI health problem.
6. Describe the use of radiography in diagnosing GI health problems.
7. Explain follow-up care for clients who have invasive radiographic examinations.
8. Plan preprocedure and follow-up care for clients having endoscopic procedures.

LEARNING ACTIVITIES

1. Before completing the study guide exercises in this chapter, it is recommended that you review the following:
   - Anatomy and physiology of the gastrointestinal system
   - Effect of the central and autonomic nervous systems on the gastrointestinal organs
   - Normal nutrition, including the essential vitamins, minerals, and foods in the recommended food groups
   - Special diets (such as low-salt, high- or low-protein, high-carbohydrate, high- or low-fiber, low-fat, bland, liquid, and pureed) for clients with gastrointestinal organ disorders
   - Parameters of a complete gastrointestinal assessment
   - Principles of enema administration
   - Normal fluid and electrolyte values

2. Review the boldfaced terms and their definitions in Chapter 56 to enhance your understanding of the content.

STUDY/REVIEW QUESTIONS

Answers to the Study/Review Questions are provided on the companion Evolve Learning Resources Web site at http://evolve.elsevier.com/Iggy/.

1. Identify the layers of the gastrointestinal (GI) tract and describe the composition of each.

2. Identify the four major functions of the GI tract.

   a. _____

   b. _____

   c. _____

   d. _____

3. Briefly describe the process of digestion.

4. Innervation of the GI tract occurs in two ways. Identify them and briefly describe their purpose.

   a. _____

   b. _____

5. Where does the blood supply to the GI tract originate?

6. The venous system that carries absorbed nutrients away from the lumen of the GI tract drains into what structure?

7. Describe the circulation of blood beginning with the portal vein to general systemic circulation.

8. Identify the components of the oral cavity.

9. What term refers to the process of chewing food in preparation for swallowing and digestion?

10. Identify the three major salivary glands and describe their purpose.

    a. _____

    b. _____

    c. _____

11. Match the following terms associated with the GI system with their corresponding definitions.

Definition

_____ a. Organ with both exocrine and endocrine functions

_____ b. Last 8 to 12 feet of the small intestine

_____ c. Finger-like projections into the small intestine

_____ d. Oral secretion that softens food

_____ e. Thick, liquid mass of partially digested food

_____ f. Temporary reservoir for food

_____ g. Intestinal hormone that inhibits acid secretion and decreases gastric motility

_____ h. Epithelial cell layer lining GI tract

_____ i. Process of expelling feces

_____ j. Central part of small intestine

_____ k. Organ where water absorption occurs

_____ l. Conduit for food from mouth to stomach

_____ m. First 10 inches of small intestine

_____ n. Connective tissue layer of GI lumen

_____ o. Functional unit of liver

_____ p. Liver secretion essential to fat emulsification

_____ q. Largest abdominal organ with numerous functions

_____ r. Organ that concentrates and stores bile

_____ s. Circular folds of mucosa projecting into the GI lumen

_____ t. Beginning pathway for digestion

Term

1. Bile
2. Chyme
3. Duodenum
4. Elimination
5. Esophagus
6. Gallbladder
7. Ileum
8. Jejunum
9. Large intestine
10. Liver
11. Lobule
12. Mouth
13. Mucosa
14. Pancreas
15. Plicae circulates
16. Saliva
17. Secretin
18. Stomach
19. Submucosa
20. Villi

12. List the assessment data (both subjective and objective) you would include when performing a GI assessment on your client.

13. What is the correct sequence of examination procedures for abdominal assessment? Briefly explain why the sequence used for assessing the abdomen is different than the sequence that is used to examine other body systems.

Explain the significance of each of the following assessment findings.

14. Fruity breath smell

15. Asymmetry in the upper quadrants of the abdomen

16. Asymmetry in the lower quadrants of the abdomen

17. The presence of ecchymosis around the umbilicus (Cullen's sign)

18. A bruit heard over the abdominal aorta

19. Diminished or absent bowel sounds

20. Loud, gurgling bowel sounds

21. Laboratory values for the client with liver disease would show which of the following?
    a. Decreased prothrombin time
    b. Increased AST and ALT
    c. Increased albumin values
    d. Decreased ammonia levels

22. Laboratory values for the client with acute pancreatitis may show decreased levels of which of the following?
    a. Calcium
    b. Serum amylase
    c. Serum lipase
    d. Urine amylase

23. State what the fecal occult blood test (FOBT) measures and identify a common finding associated with it.

24. Match the diagnostic studies on the following page with the corresponding descriptions.

Description

_____ a. Useful in evaluating hepatocellular disease; IV injection of radioactive colloid is used.

_____ b. X-ray study of the gallbladder and biliary ducts. IV injection of contrast material is given and films are taken at 20-minute intervals for 1 hour (or until the biliary ducts are visualized).

_____ c. Visualizes organs in the abdomen. May reveal masses, tumors, strictures or obstructions. Patterns of bowel gas appear light on the film. Jewelry and belts should be removed before the test.

_____ d. Cross-sectional x-ray that detects tissue densities and abnormalities in the abdomen, liver, spleen, pancreas, and biliary tract. Clients are instructed to lie still and hold their breath when asked; clients are confined in a rather enclosed space inside the machine.

_____ e. A radiographic visualization of the large intestine; usually ordered for the client with blood or mucus in the stool or a change in bowel habits.

_____ f. Visualization of the gallbladder after oral ingestion of radiopaque, iodine-based contrast medium. The day before the test, the client eats a fat-free or low-fat meal and takes six radiopaque iodine tablets approximately 2 hours after the meal. Client is NPO from midnight on the night before the test.

_____ g. X-ray study of the biliary duct system using instillation of an iodinated dye into the liver.

_____ h. Visualization from the oral part of the pharynx to the duodenojejunal junction. Used to detect disorders of structure or function of the esophagus, stomach, or duodenum.

_____ i. An extension of the upper GI series; this test continues to trace the barium through the small intestine, up to and including the ileocecal junction, to detect disorders of the jejunum or ileum.

Diagnostic Study

1. Flat plate film of the abdomen
2. Upper GI radiographic series
3. Small bowel series (SBFT)
4. Barium enema
5. Percutaneous transhepatic cholangiography
6. Gallbladder radiographic series
7. Intravenous cholangiography
8. Computed tomography
9. Liver-spleen scan

25. Match the following endoscopic procedures to the appropriate follow-up care.

Follow-up Care

_____ a. The client is informed that mild gas pain and flatulence may be experienced as a result of air instilled into the rectum during the examination. If a biopsy specimen is obtained, a small amount of bleeding may be observed.

_____ b. Vital signs must be checked every 15 minutes until the client is stable. Side rails are kept up until sedation wears off. Observe for signs of perforation or hemorrhage. The nurse instructs the client that a feeling of "fullness," cramping, and passage of flatus can be expected for several hours after the test. A small amount of blood may be in the first stool after the test if a biopsy specimen is taken or a polypectomy is performed. Excessive bleeding should be reported immediately.

_____ c. Vital signs are assessed frequently until the client is stable. Observe for cholangitis, perforation, sepsis, and pancreatitis (these problems may not occur immediately after the procedure and may take several hours to 2 days to develop). The client is instructed to report abdominal pain, fever, nausea, or vomiting that fails to resolve. The client is on NPO status until the gag reflex returns.

_____ d. Vitals checked frequently (usually every 30 minutes) and side rails are up until sedation wears off. Client remains NPO until the gag reflex returns. Monitor for signs of perforation, such as pain, bleeding, or fever. Client is instructed not to drive for 12 hours after the test. A hoarse voice and sore throat may persist for several days; throat lozenges may be used to relieve the discomfort.

Endoscopic Procedure

1. Esophagogastroduodenoscopy (EGD)
2. Endoscopic retrograde cholangiopancreatography (ERCP)
3. Colonoscopy
4. Proctosigmoidoscopy

CASE STUDY: UPPER GI PAIN

Answer Guidelines for the Case Study questions are provided on the companion Evolve Learning Resources Web site at http://evolve.elsevier.com/Iggy/.

The client is an 87-year-old woman who is admitted to a medical nursing unit from a local nursing home. She had surgery for abdominal adhesions 4 weeks ago and is now passing blood-streaked stools. She also reports that her stomach hurts, especially during the night. "It feels like someone is burning a hole inside me." The client states that she lives alone in an apartment building for retirees. Last week, a close friend and neighbor visited her at the nursing home and reported news of deaths of two mutual friends who were residents of the apartment building.

1. What additional data should the nurse collect for a thorough GI system assessment of the client?

2. The client is scheduled to have an upper GI and small bowel series the next day. What does the nurse do to prepare her for these diagnostic studies? Devise a teaching-learning plan for the client.

3. The client is unable to tolerate the barium solution, becomes nauseated, and vomits. Her physician orders that an esophagogastroduodenoscopy (EGD) be done. What additional preparation is needed before this procedure can be performed on the client?

4. Following the EGD, the client is returned to her room by stretcher. The nurse assists her to transfer to bed. What position should the client be assisted to assume? What assessments should the nurse initially perform? Why?

5. While the nurse is assessing her, the client asks for some water to drink because "my mouth is so dry that my tongue is sticky." What should the nurse do?

Interventions for Clients with Oral Cavity Problems

57

LEARNING OUTCOMES

1. Develop a teaching plan for clients who have stomatitis.
2. Explain the common causes of malignant oral tumors.
3. Describe health promotion strategies to prevent oral cancer.
4. Identify common nursing diagnoses for clients with oral cancer.
5. Prioritize postoperative care for clients undergoing surgery for oral cancer.
6. Develop a teaching plan for community-based care of clients with oral cancer.
7. Plan care for clients who have disorders of the salivary glands.

LEARNING ACTIVITIES

1. Before completing the study guide exercises in this chapter, it is recommended that you review the following:
   - Anatomy and physiology of the oral cavity
   - Special diets (such as bland, liquid, and pureed) for clients with oral cavity disorders
   - Parameters of a complete oral assessment
   - Principles of oral hygiene
   - Care of nasogastric tubes
   - Normal fluid and electrolyte values
   - Principles of perioperative and postoperative nursing management
   - Concepts of body image and self-esteem
   - Concepts of grief, loss, death, and dying

2. Review the boldfaced terms and their definitions in Chapter 57 to enhance your understanding of the content.

497

STUDY/REVIEW QUESTIONS

Answers to the Study/Review Questions are provided on the companion Evolve Learning Resources Web site at http://evolve.elsevier.com/Iggy/.

1. Identify five etiologic factors associated with stomatitis.

    a. _____

    b. _____

    c. _____

    d. _____

    e. _____

2. Differentiate between primary and secondary stomatitis.

3. Match each of the following descriptions of primary stomatitis with the corresponding type.

Description

_____ a. Erythema, ulceration, and necrosis of gingival margins

_____ b. Uniformly sized vesicles on tongue, palate, and buccal mucosa

_____ c. Development at the site of an injury

_____ d. Shallow, painful ulcerations covered by a yellow-gray ulcer pseudomembrane and exterior erythematous ring

Type of Primary Stomatitis

1. Aphthous stomatitis
2. Herpetic stomatitis
3. Vincent's stomatitis
4. Traumatic stomatitis

True or False? Write T for true or F for false in the blanks provided. If a statement is false, correct it to make it true.

_____ 4. Lichen planus is an inflammatory mucocutaneous disease involving both the skin and the oral mucous membranes.

_____ 5. Nonsymmetric yellow lesions of various patterns appear on the tongue and buccal mucosa in the client with lichen planus.

_____ 6. Oral lichen planus may be associated with hepatitis C infection.

_____ 7. In oral candidiasis, uniform white ulcerations appear on the tongue, palate, pharynx, and buccal mucosa.

_____ 8. Candidiasis is a bacterial infection resulting from an infection elsewhere in the body.

_____ 9. Candidiasis is very common among HIV-infected individuals.

10. Oral care for the client with stomatitis includes which of the following?
    a. Using a hard-bristled toothbrush to thoroughly clean the oral cavity
    b. Rinsing the mouth out with a commercial mouthwash
    c. Frequently rinsing the mouth with warm saline, hydrogen peroxide solution, or sodium bicarbonate solution
    d. Frequently rinsing the mouth with cold tap water and vinegar solution

11. Chlorhexidine, an oral rinse, can be beneficial in preventing infection. The nurse must inform the client that it may cause stinging and burning and that it also causes a discoloration of the teeth (which can be removed with abrasives). What color would this discoloration be?
    a. Pink
    b. Brown
    c. Blue
    d. Green

12. For clients with oral candidal infection, an antifungal agent such as nystatin oral suspension is prescribed. Explain how the nurse would instruct the client to take this solution the proper way.

13. Identify the client data (both subjective and objective) you would include for your nursing assessment of a client with stomatitis.

14. Identify four measures that may be used to prevent stomatitis.

    a. _____

    b. _____

    c. _____

    d. _____

15. Develop a teaching plan for clients who have stomatitis.

16. Match the following types of oral cavity tumors with their corresponding descriptions.

Description

_____ a. Painless, raised purple nodule or plaque on the hard palate

_____ b. Red, raised, eroded areas on the lips, tongue, buccal mucosa, and oropharynx

_____ c. Thickened, white, firmly attached patches in the oral mucosa, lips, or tongue

_____ d. Raised scab, primarily on the lips; lesion evolves to an ulcer with a raised pearly border

_____ e. Red, velvety lesion on the tongue, palate, floor of the mouth, or mandibular mucosa

Type of Oral Cavity Tumors
1. Leukoplakia
2. Erythroplakia
3. Squamous cell carcinoma
4. Basal cell carcinoma
5. Kaposi's sarcoma

17. Identify at least five common causes and risk factors of malignant oral tumors.

    a. _____

    b. _____

    c. _____

    d. _____

    e. _____

18. List the client data (both subjective and objective) that you would include in your nursing assessment of the client with oral cavity tumors.

19. Identify common nursing diagnoses and interventions for clients with oral cancer.

20. Briefly describe seven preoperative teaching instructions that the nurse would provide to the client about to undergo a large surgical resection for oral cancer.

21. Briefly define a glossectomy.

22. List in priority order the steps in postoperative care for clients undergoing surgery for oral cancer by listing the relevant nursing diagnoses.

23. What intervention, using sterile technique, must be frequently used to maintain a patent airway in the client after extensive excision or resection (from oral cancer surgery)?

24. To protect the operative area (after oral cancer surgery), the nurse would elevate the head of the bed to at least _____ degrees to assist in decreasing edema by gravity.

25. Clients who have undergone surgery for oral carcinomas often describe their pain as _____ or _____.

26. The initial postoperative pain medication given to clients who have had surgery for oral carcinomas is usually _____.

27. Identify three assessments the nurse would make when a client resumes oral liquids after oral surgery.

    a. _____

    b. _____

    c. _____

28. Develop a teaching plan for community-based care of clients with oral cancer.

29. Identify four expected outcomes, based on the evaluation of care, for the client with a tumor of the oral cavity.

    a. _____

    b. _____

    c. _____

    d. _____

30. Identify three common disorders of the salivary glands.

    a. _____

    b. _____

    c. _____

31. Identify three common causes of acute sialadenitis.

    a. _____

    b. _____

    c. _____

32. Describe five nursing interventions the nurse would include in an attempt to help treat the underlying cause and increase the flow of saliva in the client with acute sialadenitis.

    a. _____

    b. _____

    c. _____

    d. _____

    e. _____

33. Briefly describe xerostomia.

34. What outcome may be the result of facial nerve involvement with tumors of the salivary glands?

35. Identify the relevant data the nurse would collect while performing an assessment of the client's facial nerve.

    a. _____

    b. _____

    c. _____

    d. _____

    e. _____

    f. _____

    g. _____

36. Briefly define parotidectomy.

Interventions for Clients with Esophageal Problems

LEARNING OUTCOMES

1. Explain the pathophysiology of gastroesophageal reflux disease (GERD).
2. Assess the client who is experiencing GERD.
3. Plan the nursing care for clients with GERD.
4. Identify medications that are used for GERD and nursing implications for each classification.
5. Develop a postoperative teaching plan for the client having a hiatal hernia repair.
6. Identify the differences in the incidence of esophageal cancer among cultural groups.
7. Describe the risk factors for esophageal cancer.
8. Analyze assessment data to determine common nursing diagnoses for the client with esophageal cancer.
9. Discuss the priorities for postoperative care of the client undergoing surgery for esophageal cancer.
10. Plan community-based care for clients diagnosed with esophageal cancer.

LEARNING ACTIVITIES

1. Before completing the study guide exercises in this chapter, it is recommended that you review the following:
   - Anatomy and physiology of the gastrointestinal (GI) system
   - Anatomy and physiology of the esophagus
   - Assessment of the GI system
   - Care of nasogastric (NG) and nasointestinal tubes
   - Care of feeding tubes and preparation of tube-feeding formulas

2. Analyze assessment data to determine common nursing diagnoses for the client with esophageal cancer.

3. Discuss the priorities for postoperative care of the client undergoing surgery for esophageal cancer.

4. Plan community-based care for clients diagnosed with esophageal cancer.
   - Principles of total parenteral nutrition (TPN) and care of peripheral and central line catheter
   - Normal fluid and electrolyte values
   - Perioperative nursing management

- Postoperative nursing management
- Concepts of grief, loss, death, and dying
- Concepts of body image and self-esteem

5. Review the boldfaced terms and their definitions in Chapter 58 to enhance your understanding of the content.

STUDY/REVIEW QUESTIONS

Answers to the Study/Review Questions are provided on the companion Evolve Learning Resources Web site at http://evolve.elsevier.com/Iggy/.

1. How would the nurse describe esophageal reflux to the client?

2. Which physiologic factor contributes to gastroesophageal reflux disease (GERD)?
   a. Accelerated gastric emptying
   b. Irritation from refluxate
   c. Competent lower esophageal sphincter
   d. Increased esophageal clearance

3. Identify two anatomic factors that support the normal function of the lower esophageal sphincter (LES).

   a. _____

   b. _____

4. Briefly describe Barrett's epithelium.

5. The degree of esophageal inflammation is which of the following?
   a. Inversely related to the acid concentration of refluxed stomach contents
   b. Directly dependent on the number of reflux episodes of stomach contents
   c. Primarily determined by the duration of exposure to irritating material
   d. A result of increased peristaltic activity as irritants return to the stomach

6. Briefly describe the relationship between nighttime reflux and GERD.

7. Match each of the following GERD-associated conditions with the corresponding definition.

Definition

_____ a. Pain described as a substernal or retrosternal burning sensation that tends to move up and down the chest in a wavelike fashion

_____ b. Difficulty in swallowing

_____ c. Occurrence of warm fluid traveling up the throat with a sour or bitter taste

_____ d. Painful swallowing

_____ e. Reflex salivary hypersecretion in response to reflux

GERD-Associated Conditions
1. Dyspepsia
2. Regurgitation
3. Water brash
4. Dysphagia
5. Odynophagia

8. List the client data (subjective and objective) you would include when performing a nursing assessment of a client with GERD.

9. Briefly describe the Bernstein test.

10. In regard to dietary modifications, the nurse would counsel an adult client with GERD to do all of the following except:
    a. Eat four to six small meals a day.
    b. Avoid spicy and acidic foods.
    c. Avoid carbonated beverages.
    d. Include evening snacks, particularly 1 to 2 hours before going to bed.

11. The lifestyle adjustment a client may have to make to best control GERD would be which of the following?
    a. Sleep in the Trendelenburg position.
    b. Attain and maintain ideal body weight.
    c. Wear snug-fitting belts and waistbands.
    d. Engage in strenuous exercise such as weightlifting.

12. The physician has prescribed Maalox for a client with GERD. The nurse instructs him to take the antacid _____ hour(s) before and _____ hour(s) after each meal.

13. Histamine blockers such as famotidine (Pepcid), ranitidine (Zantac), and cimetidine (Tagamet) act by inhibiting _____.

14. Identify the primary action of metoclopramide.

15. Differentiate between sliding hernia and rolling hernia, two types of hiatal hernias.

16. List the client data (subjective and objective) you would include when performing a nursing assessment of the client with a hiatal hernia.

17. Briefly describe a fundoplication.

Read the following interventions for the client who has had a fundoplication procedure and decide whether each is true or false. Write T for true or F for false in the blanks provided. If a statement is false, correct it to make it true.

_____ 18. The nurse elevates the head of the client's bed 10 degrees to lower the diaphragm and facilitate lung expansion.

_____ 19. Incentive spirometry and deep breathing are routinely used after surgery to maintain patency of the airways.

_____ 20. Nasogastric drainage is initially dark brown with old blood but should become normal yellowish-green within the first 48 hours after surgery.

_____ 21. The nurse explains to the client that meals consumed will need to be much larger and less frequent than before.

_____ 22. The nurse teaches the client to avoid drinking carbonated beverages, eating gas-producing foods, chewing gum, and drinking with a straw.

_____ 23. The client is taught to inspect the healing incision daily. The nurse explains that if swelling, redness, tenderness, discharge, or fever occur, the client should not worry because these are all common responses to the procedure.

24. Briefly describe achalasia.

25. Identify four complications that can result from achalasia.

   a. _____

   b. _____

   c. _____

   d. _____

26. Following esophageal dilation of a client, the nurse does which of the following?

   a. Monitors the client for subcutaneous emphysema, hemoptysis, fever, and signs of perforation

   b. Encourages the client to consume a small meal immediately after the procedure

   c. Massages the client's shoulder when he or she complains of shoulder pain

   d. Teaches the client to swallow any oral secretions that accumulate

27. Which of the following statements about esophageal tumors is false?

   a. Esophageal tumors exhibit rapid local growth.

   b. Esophageal tumors can protrude into the esophageal lumen and cause thickening.

   c. Leiomyomas are malignant tumors and are almost always fatal.

   d. Most malignant esophageal tumors arise from the epithelium.

28. Identify six risk factors associated with esophageal cancer.

   a. _____

   b. _____

   c. _____

   d. _____

   e. _____

   f. _____

29. The greatest incidence of adenocarcinoma of the esophagus in the United States can be found in what demographic group?

30. The incidence of squamous cell cancer of the esophagus has greatly increased in the United States over the past several decades, particularly in what demographic group?

31. The incidence of esophageal cancer is extremely high in areas of the Transeki region of southern Africa, the Caspian Sea (around Russia and Iran), Japan, and the northwest area of what other country?

32. Identify the primary clinical manifestations in clients with esophageal cancer.

   a. Dysphagia and weight loss

   b. Sialorrhea and eructation

   c. Xerostomia and anorexia

   d. Weight gain and abdominal distention

33. Identify the relevant assessment data (subjective and objective) the nurse would collect and analyze to determine appropriate nursing diagnoses for the client with esophageal cancer.

34. Identify the priority nursing diagnosis for clients with cancer of the esophagus.

35. Formulate additional nursing diagnoses based on your assessment in Question 33.

36. For the client with cancer of the esophagus, list the treatment options available that can assist in both disease management and nutrition management.

    a. _____

    b. _____

    c. _____

    d. _____

    e. _____

    f. _____

    g. _____

Read the following seven statements related to treatment options for esophageal cancer and decide whether each is true or false. Write T for true or F for false in the blanks provided. If a statement is false, correct it to make it true.

_____ 37. The nurse encourages the client to consume semisoft foods and thickened liquids because they are easier to swallow.

_____ 38. When performing swallowing therapy for a client, the nurse would assist the client in positioning the head in hyperextension and placing the food in the front of the mouth in preparation for swallowing.

_____ 39. For clients receiving radiation therapy, frequent gentle mouth care is important because the client is at risk for monilial esophagitis.

_____ 40. Immediately after photodynamic therapy, the client is instructed to sunbathe as often as possible.

_____ 41. Esophageal dilation provides permanent relief for dysphagia.

_____ 42. Chemotherapy appears to be more effective when given in combination with radiation.

_____ 43. Radical surgery represents the only definitive treatment for esophageal cancer and is the preferred treatment for clients in advanced disease stages.

44. Identify the preferred surgical procedure for the client with esophageal cancer.

45. The client who has had surgery for esophageal cancer requires meticulous postoperative care and is at risk for multiple serious complications. In prioritizing your nursing care for the client, care of what would be your highest priority?

46. Identify two postoperative pulmonary complications and give interventions for each.

47. List three interventions the nurse would institute with the client following extubation.

    a. _____

    b. _____

    c. _____

48. The nurse assesses the client for decreased breath sounds and shortness of breath at least every _____ to _____ hours.

49. The nurse keeps the client in a _____ or _____ position to support ventilation and prevent _____.

50. The nurse ensures patency of the water seal drainage system for chest tubes and monitors for changes in the _____ or _____ of the drainage.

51. For the client who has undergone lymph node dissection, the nurse monitors for signs and symptoms of _____.

52. Identify three conditions the nurse assesses for in the postoperative client.

    a. _____

    b. _____

    c. _____

53. Following esophageal surgery irrigation or repositioning, the NG tube is which of the following?
    a. An independent intervention
    b. A collaborative intervention
    c. An intervention that can be delegated
    d. Contraindicated for the first 72 hours

54. Develop a teaching plan for community-based care for clients diagnosed with esophageal cancer.

55. Briefly define diverticula.

56. Identify the two most common ways in which diagnosis of esophageal diverticula is made.

    a. _____

    b. _____

57. Identify the two major interventions for controlling symptoms related to diverticula.

    a. _____

    b. _____

58. Identify five sources of trauma to the esophagus.

   a. _____

   b. _____

   c. _____

   d. _____

   e. _____

59. The client with trauma to the esophagus is at risk for what conditions?

   a. _____

   b. _____

   c. _____

   d. _____

   e. _____

60. Nonsurgical management for the client with trauma to the esophagus may include which of the following?

   a. Total parental nutrition (TPN) and anti-fungal agents

   b. Broad-spectrum antibiotics and oral NSAIDs

   c. Opioid and non-opioid analgesics

   d. High-dose corticosteroids and vigorous oral hygiene.

Interventions for Clients with Stomach Disorders

LEARNING OUTCOMES

1. Compare etiologies and assessment findings of acute and chronic gastritis.
2. Describe the key components of collaborative management for clients with gastritis.
3. Compare and contrast assessment findings associated with gastric and duodenal ulcers.
4. Identify the most common medical complications that can result from peptic ulcer disease (PUD).
5. Analyze assessment data to determine common nursing diagnoses associated with PUD.
6. Discuss drug therapy for gastritis and PUD.
7. Develop a teaching plan related to drug therapy for clients experiencing PUD.
8. Prioritize interventions for clients with upper gastrointestinal (GI) bleeding.
9. Plan preoperative and postoperative care for the client undergoing gastric surgery.
10. Develop a community-based plan of care for clients who have undergone gastric surgery.
11. Evaluate outcomes for clients with PUD.
12. Explain Zollinger-Ellison syndrome and its associated clinical manifestations.
13. Analyze risk factors for gastric carcinoma, including cultural considerations.
14. Plan postoperative care for clients who have undergone surgery for gastric cancer.
15. Discuss the psychological and emotional concerns of clients with gastric cancer.

LEARNING ACTIVITIES

1. Before completing the study guide exercises in this chapter, it is recommended that you review the following:
   - Anatomy and physiology of the stomach
   - Assessment of the abdomen
   - Effect of the central and autonomic nervous systems on the stomach
   - Special diets (such as bland, liquid, and pureed) for clients with stomach disorders
   - Care of nasogastric tubes
   - Care of feeding tubes and preparation of tube-feeding formulas
   - Principles of total parenteral and central line catheters
   - Normal fluid and electrolyte values
   - Perioperative nursing management
   - Concepts of body image and self-esteem
   - Concepts of grief, loss, death, and dying

2. Explain Zollinger-Ellison syndrome and its associated clinical manifestations.

3. Analyze risk factors for gastric carcinoma, including cultural considerations.

4. Plan postoperative care for clients who have undergone surgery for gastric cancer.

5. Discuss the psychological and emotional concerns of clients with gastric cancer.

6. Review the boldfaced terms and their definitions in Chapter 59 to enhance your understanding of the content.

STUDY/REVIEW QUESTIONS

Answers to the Study/Review Questions are provided on the companion Evolve Learning Resources Web site at http://evolve.elsevier.com/Iggy/.

1. How would the nurse describe gastritis to the client and family?

2. Identify the function of the mucosal barrier.

3. Describe the early pathologic manifestation of gastritis.

4. Briefly differentiate between acute and chronic gastritis.

5. Match each of the following etiologic factors with the corresponding type of gastritis. *Answers may be used more than once.*

Etiologic Factor

_____ a. Long-term alcohol use

_____ b. NSAID use

_____ c. Ingestion of corrosive substances

_____ d. Pernicious anemia

_____ e. A client who is NPO

_____ f. History of smoking

_____ g. Physiologic stress

Type of Gastritis
1. Acute gastritis
2. Chronic gastritis

6. Compare and contrast acute and chronic gastritis:

	Acute Gastritis	Chronic Gastritis
Pain location		
Appetite		
Pain relief		
Nausea and vomiting		
Bleeding		
Cramping		

7. How would the nurse describe to the client the diagnostic test most commonly used to diagnose gastritis?

8. What are the two goals of management of gastritis?

   a. _____

   b. _____

9. Match the following commonly used drugs for the client with gastritis to their primary mode of action.

Drug Action

_____ a.   Antacids used as buffering agents

_____ b.   Prevention or treatment of pernicious anemia

_____ c.   Blocks gastric secretions

_____ d.   A mucosal barrier fortifier

Drugs Used to Treat Gastritis
1. H_2-receptor antagonists
2. Sucralfate
3. Maalox, Mylanta
4. Vitamin B_{12}

10. Collaborative management of gastritis includes which of the following?
    a. Instructing the client to take antacids with medications to reduce acidity
    b. Encouraging the client to engage in stress reduction techniques
    c. Instructing the client to take aspirin and ibuprofen to control pain
    d. Introducing new foods into the diet several at a time

11. Define peptic ulcer disease (PUD).

12. List the three types of ulcers and give their common locations.

    a. _____

    b. _____

    c. _____

13. Identify the four most common medical complications that can result from PUD.

    a. _____

    b. _____

    c. _____

    d. _____

14. Match each of the following assessment findings in the client with PUD to its corresponding complication. *Answers may be used more than once.*

Assessment Finding

_____ a.   Melena (occult blood in a tarry stool)

_____ b.   Tender, rigid, boardlike abdomen

_____ c.   Abdominal bloating, nausea, and vomiting

_____ d.   Despite treatment, recurrent pain and discomfort that interfere with activities of daily living

_____ e.   Hypokalemia

_____ f.   Sudden, sharp pain beginning at midepigastric region and spreading to entire abdomen

_____ g.   Vomiting of bright red blood

_____ h.   Metabolic alkalosis

_____ i.   Granular dark vomitus with a coffee-ground appearance

_____ j.   No longer responding to conservative management

_____ k.   Assumes a knee-chest position

Complications of PUD
1. Hemorrhage
2. Pyloric obstruction
3. Perforation
4. Intractable disease

15. Identify the data (subjective and objective) you would include when performing an assessment on the client with PUD.

16. Formulate common nursing diagnoses for the client with PUD.

17. What is the major diagnostic test for PUD?

18. Identify the four primary goals of drug therapy in the treatment of PUD.

    a. _____

    b. _____

    c. _____

    d. _____

Provide the appropriate teaching plan related to each of the following drug therapies used for the client experiencing PUD.

19. Antisecretory agents

20. H$_2$-receptor antagonists

21. Prostaglandin analogues

22. Antacids

23. Mucosal barrier fortifiers

24. What are the purposes of interventions to reduce bleeding in the client with PUD?

25. The nurse monitors the client for signs and symptoms indicating GI bleeding. Describe the assessment findings you would expect for the following clients.

    a. The client with mild bleeding (less than 500 mL)

    b. The client with blood loss exceeding 1 L/24 hr

26. What type of therapy may be required to replace blood loss?

27. Identify and prioritize the goals of therapeutic intervention for bleeding secondary to PUD.

    a. _____

    b. _____

28. Identify the four therapeutic, nonsurgical interventions used to control acute bleeding and prevent recurrent bleeding.

    a. _____

    b. _____

    c. _____

    d. _____

29. Briefly describe the three primary methods of endoscopic therapy that may be effective for an acute bleeding episode.

    a. _____

    b. _____

    c. _____

30. In planning preoperative care for the client with PUD, explain why the nurse inserts an NG tube and connects it to suction to remove secretions and empty the client's stomach.

31. Provide a rationale for why the NG tube would remain in place postoperatively for the client who undergoes gastric surgery.

32. Identify and describe the most commonly performed surgical procedures for the client with PUD.

Read the following three statements related to postoperative nursing care and decide whether each is true or false. Write T for true or F for false in the blanks provided. If a statement is false, correct it to make it true.

_____ 33. The nurse monitors the NG tube for patency and carefully secures the tube to prevent dislodgement.

_____ 34. The nurse routinely irrigates and repositions the NG tube after gastric surgery.

_____ 35. Acute gastric dilation is manifested by vertigo, sweating, and confusion.

36. Signs and symptoms of dumping syndrome include which of the following?
    a. Severe pain
    b. Bradycardia
    c. Profuse vomiting
    d. Vertigo

37. In teaching the client to manage dumping syndrome, which of the following instructions by the nurse would be appropriate?
    a. Consume a low-protein, high-fat, high-carbohydrate diet.
    b. Consume a high-protein, high-fat, low-carbohydrate diet.
    c. Increase liquid intake with meals.
    d. Increase the amount of food taken in at one meal.

38. Develop a community-based plan of care for clients who have undergone gastric surgery. Use a separate sheet of paper for your answer, if necessary.

39. Identify the expected outcomes for clients with PUD.

   a. _____

   b. _____

   c. _____

   d. _____

   e. _____

   f. _____

   g. _____

   h. _____

   i. _____

40. Briefly describe Zollinger-Ellison syndrome (ZES).

41. How would the nurse define steatorrhea to the client?

42. What is the goal of medical therapy for the client with ZES?

43. Briefly describe the methods of gastric carcinoma extension.

   a. _____

   b. _____

   c. _____

   d. _____

   e. _____

44. Identify 13 risk factors associated with the development of gastric carcinoma.

   a. _____

   b. _____

   c. _____

   d. _____

   e. _____

   f. _____

   g. _____

   h. _____

   i. _____

   j. _____

   k. _____

   l. _____

   m. _____

45. Which three cultural groups are two times as likely to develop gastric cancer as compared with whites?

   a. _____

   b. _____

   c. _____

46. What are the two most common symptoms in the client with early gastric carcinoma?

   a. _____

   b. _____

47. Which of the following statements about the management of gastric cancer is correct?
    a. Combination chemotherapy for advanced disease is less effective than single-agent therapy.
    b. The response to combination chemotherapy is unaffected by radiation therapy.
    c. Combining chemotherapy and radiation therapy after surgery has proven to be effective and is preferred.
    d. High-dose radiation therapy is the recommended adjuvant therapy to surgical treatment.

48. Which of the following statements about surgical interventions for gastric cancer is true?
    a. Surgery has the lowest cure rate for early gastric cancer.
    b. Neoplasm location in the stomach determines the type of surgical procedure.
    c. Palliative resection can help the cure rate for clients with advanced disease.
    d. The primary surgical procedure for the treatment of gastric cancer is gastroenterostomy.

49. List complications that the nurse will instruct the client may follow gastric surgery.

    a. _____

    b. _____

    c. _____

    d. _____

    e. _____

    f. _____

    g. _____

    h. _____

    i. _____

    j. _____

50. Which of the following statements about postoperative nursing care is false?
    a. Auscultate the lungs for adventitious sounds.
    b. Auscultate the abdomen for return of bowel sounds.
    c. Inspect the operative site every day for the presence of redness, swelling, or drainage.
    d. Ensure proper positioning of the client to prevent aspiration from reflux.

51. Anemia as well as vitamin B_{12} and folate deficiency can result after a gastrectomy. What interventions can help correct these deficiencies?

52. Briefly discuss the indications for placing a client on total parenteral nutrition (TPN) after gastric surgery.

53. Briefly describe the psychological and emotional concerns of clients with gastric cancer.

Interventions for Clients with Noninflammatory Intestinal Disorders

LEARNING OUTCOMES

1. Develop a teaching-learning plan for clients with irritable bowel syndrome (IBS).
2. Differentiate the most common types of hernias.
3. Develop a plan of care for a client undergoing a minimally invasive inguinal hernia repair.
4. Interpret assessment findings for clients with colorectal cancer (CRC).
5. Identify health promotion practices to prevent CRC.
6. Discuss the psychosocial aspects associated with CRC and related surgeries.
7. Explain the role of the nurse in managing the client with CRC.
8. Develop a perioperative plan of care for a client undergoing a colon resection and colostomy.
9. Construct a community-based teaching-learning plan for clients requiring colostomy care.
10. Identify community-based resources for clients with CRC.
11. Analyze the differences between small-bowel and large-bowel obstructions.
12. Explain the role of the nurse when caring for clients with nasogastric tubes.
13. Develop a plan of care for a client experiencing intestinal obstruction.
14. Prioritize nursing care for the client with abdominal trauma.
15. Develop a teaching-learning plan for clients having hemorrhoid surgical procedures.
16. Explain the pathophysiology of malabsorption syndrome.

LEARNING ACTIVITIES

1. Before completing the study guide exercises in this chapter, it is recommended that you review the following:
   - Anatomy and physiology of the small bowel and large intestine, including the rectum and anus
   - Assessment of the gastrointestinal (GI) system
   - Effect of the central and autonomic nervous systems on the gastrointestinal organs
   - Normal nutrition, including essential vitamins, minerals, and recommended food groups
   - Special diets (e.g., low protein, high carbohydrate, low fiber, liquid, and pureed) for clients with GI organ disorders
   - Care of nasogastric and nasointestinal tubes
   - Principles of total parenteral nutrition (TPN) and care of peripheral and central line catheters
   - Perioperative and postoperative nursing care

- Concepts of body image
- Concepts of grief, loss, death, and dying

2. Review the boldfaced terms and their definitions in Chapter 60 to enhance your understanding of the content.

STUDY/REVIEW QUESTIONS

Answers to the Study/Review Questions are provided on the companion Evolve Learning Resources Web site at http://evolve.elsevier.com/Iggy/.

1. Briefly describe the most commonly seen digestive disorder in clinical practice and give three characteristics of it.

2. Distinguish between IBS and a true colitis.

3. Identify three factors that may contribute to IBS.

   a. _____

   b. _____

   c. _____

4. IBS is commonly characterized by which of the following?
   a. Chronic constipation
   b. Chronic diarrhea
   c. Alternating diarrhea and constipation
   d. Normal bowel habits with flatulence

5. Which of the following statements about IBS is true?
   a. Individual lifestyle is relatively unaffected.
   b. Most clients can identify factors that precipitate exacerbations.
   c. IBS is estimated to occur in less than 5% of the population in the United States.
   d. IBS has not been associated with the use of analgesics.

6. Identify the assessment data (both subjective and objective) you would include relevant to the client with IBS.

Read the following five statements related to client education for IBS and decide whether each is true or false. Write T for true or F for false in the blanks provided. If a statement is false, correct it to make it true.

_____ 7. Information would be provided to the client regarding what constitutes normal bowel function and laxative abuse.

_____ 8. The client is advised to increase caffeine intake but limit alcohol use.

_____ 9. Fiber supplements are never recommended because they may cause more diarrhea.

_____ 10. The client is advised to limit fluid intake.

_____ 11. Bentyl and Pro-Banthine can help relieve abdominal cramping and intestinal spasm.

12. Which of the following statements indicates that the client with IBS understands his or her home maintenance regimen?
    a. "I enjoy having a glass or two of wine with my dinner."
    b. "I can continue to eat my cheese sandwiches."
    c. "When I feel the urge to have a bowel movement, I should wait an hour and then go."
    d. "I will enroll in a stress management workshop."

13. The nurse would be prepared to instruct the client what six causes of increased intra-abdominal pressure that can lead to a hernia?

    a. _____

    b. _____

    c. _____

    d. _____

    e. _____

    f. _____

14. Categorize each of the following descriptions with the type of hernia.

Description

_____ a. Contents of the sac can be replaced into the abdominal cavity

_____ b. Occurs when the canal enlarges, allowing peritoneum through

_____ c. Occurs in the region of the navel

_____ d. Hernia pushes downward at an angle in the inguinal canal

_____ e. Cannot be replaced back into the abdominal cavity

_____ f. Blood supply to the herniated bowel segment is cut off

_____ g. Occurring at the site of a prior surgical incision

Type of Hernia
1. Femoral
2. Incarcerated
3. Indirect
4. Reducible
5. Strangulated
6. Umbilical
7. Ventral

15. Which of the following statements about hernias is correct?
    a. Direct hernias are the most common type.
    b. Umbilical hernias are more common in the elderly.
    c. Indirect inguinal hernias occur most often in men.
    d. Incisional hernias are common in obese people.

16. List the client data (subjective and objective) you would include relevant to hernias for your nursing assessment.

17. Interventions for the client who uses a truss for a hernia include which of the following?
    a. Using a surgical binder to hold the truss in place
    b. Removing the truss only for bathing
    c. Applying the truss while sitting on the edge of the bed
    d. Applying powder to the skin under the truss daily

18. Identify and briefly describe the two common types of hernia repair.

    a. _____

    b. _____

19. Which activity should the nurse teach the client to avoid after surgery for a hernia repair?
    a. Ambulating
    b. Turning
    c. Coughing
    d. Deep breathing

20. Postoperative measures for the male client who has had an inguinal herniorrhaphy include which of the following?
    a. Applying a warm pack to the scrotum
    b. Elevating the scrotum on a pillow
    c. Encouraging use of a bedpan to void
    d. Decreasing fluid intake to decrease bladder emptying

21. Number the following steps describing the growth and spread of an intestinal tumor in sequential order.

    _____ a. Enlargement into the bowel lumen

    _____ b. Presence of a polyp in the bowel

    _____ c. Malignant cells found in the liver

    _____ d. Malignant cells line the bowel wall

    _____ e. Local invasion into layers of the bowel wall

    _____ f. Spread via the lymphatic system or circulatory system

22. Identify five sites where intestinal tumors can metastasize and indicate which is the most common.

    a. _____

    b. _____

    c. _____

    d. _____

    e. _____

23. Identify four risk factors that are involved in the development of colorectal cancer.

    a. _____

    b. _____

    c. _____

    d. _____

24. List the client data (subjective and objective) you would include in your assessment relevant to intestinal cancer.

Read the following statements related to diagnostic assessments and decide whether each is true or false. Write T for true or F for false in the blanks provided. If a statement is false, correct it to make it true.

_____ 25. Hemoglobin and hematocrit values are usually increased as a result of the intermittent bleeding associated with the tumor.

_____ 26. A negative test result for occult blood in the stool confirms bleeding in the GI tract.

_____ 27. Colonoscopy with biopsy is the definitive test for the diagnosis of colon cancer.

_____ 28. A liver scan is used to remove polyps.

29. Identify four psychosocial implications associated with colon cancer.

    a. _____

    b. _____

    c. _____

    d. _____

30. Briefly describe a hemicolectomy.

31. Briefly describe a colostomy.

32. Why would the nurse caring for a client who is about to undergo a hemicolectomy and colostomy consult an enterostomal therapist (ET)?

33. What training is required for one to be an ET?

34. Develop a perioperative plan of care for the client undergoing a colon resection and colostomy.

35. After colostomy surgery, the nurse does which of the following?
    a. Covers the stoma with a dry, sterile dressing
    b. Applies a pouch system as soon as possible
    c. Makes a hole in the pouch for gas to escape
    d. Watches for the colostomy to start functioning on day 1

36. The nurse immediately reports to the surgeon all but which of the following signs and symptoms related to a colostomy?
    a. Liquid stool immediately postoperatively
    b. Bleeding
    c. Signs of ischemia and necrosis
    d. Mucocutaneous separation

37. Which of the following should the client who has a perineal wound and cavity be instructed to report to the physician immediately?
    a. Serosanguineous drainage from the wound
    b. Sensations of having a bowel movement
    c. Constant perineal odor and pain
    d. Occasional perineal pain and itching

38. The client with a colostomy could safely include which of the following in the diet?
    a. Burritos
    b. Chicken noodle soup
    c. Cabbage
    d. Carbonated beverages

39. Identify and discuss community-based resources for the client with colon cancer.

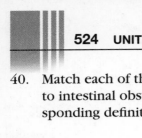

40. Match each of the following terms related to intestinal obstruction with the corresponding definition.

Definition

_____ a. Blockage of the bowel lumen resulting from internal or external factors

_____ b. Incomplete blockage of intestine

_____ c. Blockage of bowel lumen caused by decreased intestinal activity

_____ d. Total blockage of intestinal lumen

_____ e. Blockage with compromised blood flow

_____ f. Bands of scar tissue encircling intestine and constricting lumen

Term Related to Intestinal Obstruction
1. Adhesions
2. Complete obstruction
3. Mechanical obstruction
4. Nonmechanical obstruction
5. Partial obstruction
6. Strangulated obstruction

41. Identify five of the common causes of mechanical obstructions: two of the small intestine and three of the large bowel.

Small intestine:

a. _____

b. _____

Large bowel:

a. _____

b. _____

c. _____

42. Match the following metabolic disturbances with their levels of bowel obstruction.

Level of Bowel Obstruction

_____ a. High in the small intestine

_____ b. Below the duodenum but above the large bowel

_____ c. Below the terminal ileum

Metabolic Disturbance
1. Insignificant imbalance
2. Metabolic acidosis
3. Metabolic alkalosis

43. Describe assessment findings associated with mechanical and nonmechanical obstructions.

44. Nursing care of the client with a newly inserted nasointestinal tube includes which of the following?
   a. Anchoring the tube firmly to the client's cheek
   b. Irrigating with 30 mL of sterile saline as needed
   c. Changing the client's position every 2 hours
   d. Setting the tube to low continuous suction

45. Which of the following NG tubes would be connected to low intermittent suction?
   a. Salem sump
   b. Levin
   c. Anderson
   d. Carney

46. List three assessments the nurse would make for the client with an NG tube and indicate the frequency with which these assessments should be made.

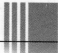

47. Describe the appropriate technique for measuring abdominal girth.

48. The client with an NG tube is assessed for what symptoms of abdominal distress?

49. Interventions for clients with Fluid Volume Deficit related to an intestinal obstruction include which of the following?
    a. Frequent mouth care with lemon glycerin swabs
    b. Ice chips to suck on before surgery
    c. A small glass of water
    d. Assessing for edema from third spacing

50. Which of the following observations of the client with an intestinal obstruction should the nurse report immediately?
    a. A urinary output of 1000 mL in an 8-hour period
    b. The client's request for something to drink
    c. Abdominal pain changing from colicky to constant discomfort
    d. The client who is changing positions frequently

51. Discharge instructions for the client who has had an intestinal obstruction caused by fecal impaction include which of the following?
    a. Encouragement to report abdominal distention, nausea or vomiting, and constipation
    b. Providing a written description of a low-fiber diet
    c. Reminding the client to limit activity
    d. Reminding the client to decrease fluid intake

52. Identify the two major categories of abdominal injury and identify examples of each.
    a. _____
    b. _____

53. Identify the three main issues health care providers focus on in the emergency phase of treatment for abdominal injury.
    a. _____
    b. _____
    c. _____

54. Identify the two priority nursing assessments for the client with abdominal injury.
    a. _____
    b. _____

55. To assess the abdomen for possible trauma, the nurse does which of the following?
    a. Exposes only the area from the xiphoid process to the symphysis pubis
    b. Immediately removes antishock trousers
    c. Palpates deeply over the abdominal wall for masses and areas of tenderness
    d. Inspects for symmetry, abrasions, lacerations, ecchymosis, and penetrating wounds

56. Ecchymosis following abdominal trauma may signify what?

57. Describe how the nurse would assess for Ballance's sign and identify its significance.
    a. Assessment

    b. Significance

58. Briefly discuss why the nurse would place at least two large-bore IV catheters in the client with abdominal trauma.

59. Briefly explain why serial hemoglobin and hematocrit levels are assessed for the client with abdominal injury.

60. If the client has an open abdominal wound or evisceration, the nurse would cover it with a _____ unless the physician orders otherwise.

61. Identify two reasons why the nurse would insert an NG tube in the client with abdominal trauma.

    a. _____

    b. _____

62. Explain why all clients who have suffered abdominal trauma are taught the signs and symptoms to report, regardless of whether they have had surgery or not.

63. Are the following statements about intestinal polyps true or false? *Write T for true or F for false in the blanks provided. If a statement is false, change it to make it true.*

    _____ a. Most polyps are malignant.

    _____ b. Polyps of certain tissue types are more likely to become malignant.

    _____ c. Most intestinal polyps are attached to the surface of the intestine.

    _____ d. Hyperplastic polyps are always malignant.

    _____ e. Villous adenomas tend to be benign.

    _____ f. Pedunculated polyps are stalklike.

    _____ g. Sessile polyps become elongated as peristalsis pulls them into the lumen of the intestine.

    _____ h. Familial polyposis is characterized by progressive development of colorectal adenomas.

    _____ i. Polyps frequently cause pain and rectal bleeding.

    _____ j. A polypectomy can be done during a colonoscopy.

64. Which of the following would be included in the nurse's care of the client who has had a colorectal polypectomy?
    a. Examining stools for blood or muco-purulent drainage on a weekly basis.
    b. Monitoring the client for abdominal distention and pain
    c. Reassuring the client that recurrence is unlikely
    d. Discouraging follow-up examinations

65. What are the two most common symptoms of hemorrhoids?

    a. _____

    b. _____

66. Which of the following interventions is contraindicated in the nonsurgical management of hemorrhoids?
    a. Diets low in fiber and fluids
    b. Witch hazel soaks for pain
    c. Warm sitz baths three or four times a day
    d. Cleansing the anal area with moistened cleaning tissues

67. Identify three potential postoperative complications that may occur after a hemorrhoidectomy.

    a. _____

    b. _____

    c. _____

68. Identify the types of disorders that may result in malabsorption, and provide an example of which nutrients are not absorbed in each disorder.

    a. _____

    b. _____

    c. _____

    d. _____

    e. _____

    f. _____

69. What is the classic symptom of malabsorption?

70. Identify six clinical manifestations relevant to malabsorption.

    a. _____

    b. _____

    c. _____

    d. _____

    e. _____

    f. _____

71. List two interventions that are the focus for most malabsorption syndromes.

    a. _____

    b. _____

72. Which of the following drugs would be used to treat tropical sprue?
    a. Bentyl
    b. Lomotil
    c. Steroids
    d. Bactrim

CASE STUDY: THE CLIENT WITH A BOWEL OBSTRUCTION

Answer Guidelines for the Case Study questions are provided on the companion Evolve Learning Resources Web site at http://evolve.elsevier.com/Iggy/.

You are working in the emergency department of the hospital when a 47-year-old man comes in complaining of acute upper to mid-abdominal, sporadic pain and cramping. Upon assessment you observe abdominal distention and high-pitched bowel sounds. The physician has ordered flat plate and upright abdominal x-rays that show distention of loops of intestine, with fluid and gas in the small intestine in conjunction with absence of gas in the colon. The physician has diagnosed a bowel obstruction.

1. Based on the findings, identify which type of bowel obstruction this client most likely has and why.

2. What other signs and symptoms would you observe for in this client?

3. Identify the most likely interventions for this client, based on his type of bowel obstruction.

4. It is found that the client has a small fecal impaction. Identify how fecal impaction usually resolves.

Interventions for Clients with Inflammatory Intestinal Disorders

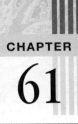

CHAPTER

61

LEARNING OUTCOMES

1. Differentiate common types of acute inflammatory bowel disease.
2. Prioritize nursing care for the client who has peritonitis.
3. Discuss the common causes of gastroenteritis.
4. Compare and contrast the pathophysiology and clinical manifestations of ulcerative colitis and Crohn's disease.
5. Analyze priority nursing diagnoses and collaborative problems for clients with chronic inflammatory bowel disease (IBD).
6. Explain the purpose of and nursing implications related to drug therapy for clients with IBD.
7. Formulate a postoperative plan of care for a client undergoing a colon resection/colectomy and colostomy or ileostomy.
8. Identify expected outcomes for clients with chronic IBD.
9. Explain the role of diet therapy in managing the client with diverticular disease.
10. Describe the comfort measures that the nurse can use for the client with an anal abscess, fissure, or fistula.
11. Discuss ways that helminthic infestation, parasitic infection, and food poisoning can be prevented.

LEARNING ACTIVITIES

1. Before completing the study guide exercises in this chapter, it is recommended that you review the following:
   - Anatomy and physiology of the small bowel, large intestine, rectum, and anus
   - Effect of the central and autonomic nervous systems on the gastrointestinal organs
   - Assessment of the gastrointestinal system
   - Normal nutrition, including essential vitamins, minerals, and recommended food groups as well as special diets (e.g., high protein, high carbohydrate, low fiber, liquid, bland, and pureed) for clients with gastrointestinal disorders
   - Perioperative nursing management
   - Principles of nasogastric (NG), total parenteral nutrition (TPN), and peripheral and central line catheters
   - Principles of infection control
   - Principles of enema administration

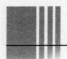

- Concepts of body image
- Concepts of grief, loss, death, and dying

2. Review the boldfaced terms and their definitions in Chapter 61 to enhance your understanding of the content.

STUDY/REVIEW QUESTIONS

Answers to the Study/Review Questions are provided on the companion Evolve Learning Resources Web site at http://evolve.elsevier.com/Iggy/.

1. Describe the function of the appendix.

2. Number the following events related to appendicitis in sequential order.
   - _____ a. Infection causes more swelling
   - _____ b. Gangrene from hypoxia or perforation
   - _____ c. Blood flow to the appendix is restricted
   - _____ d. Peritonitis
   - _____ e. Mucosa continues to secrete fluid
   - _____ f. Lumen of appendix becomes obstructed
   - _____ g. Further reduction of blood flow to the appendix
   - _____ h. Pressure within the lumen exceeds venous pressure
   - _____ i. Bacteria invade the wall of the appendix

3. Define fecalith and its relationship to obstruction of the appendix.

4. Which of the following statements about appendicitis is correct?
   a. The peak incidence is between the ages of 20 and 30 years.
   b. The peak incidence is between the ages of 15 and 25 years.
   c. Appendicitis affects more women than men.
   d. Appendicitis affects more women than men before the age of 25.

5. List the client data (both subjective and objective) you would include relevant to appendicitis for your nursing assessment.

6. Identify three complications of appendicitis that may result from the diagnosis of Altered Tissue Perfusion.

   a. _____

   b. _____

   c. _____

7. A 25-year-old carpenter has just been admitted to your unit with acute appendicitis. He began to experience periumbilical pain, fever of 100.2° F, and nausea and vomiting while working on a house. Currently his pain is constant and located to the right lower quadrant. He is requesting that you bring him a heating pad to relieve his pain. His WBC count is 15,000 with a "shift to the left." His appendectomy is scheduled for today. Use this information and the information presented in your textbook to develop rationales for the following interventions that have been selected for this client.
   a. Explain to client why you cannot give him the heating pad.

   b. Position client in a semi-Fowler's position.

c. Maintain client's NPO status.

d. Administer IV fluids as ordered.

e. Do not administer a laxative or enema.

8. Which of the following interventions regarding postoperative nursing care for a client who has had an appendectomy is correct?
   a. Administer IV antibiotics as needed.
   b. Encourage client to do abdominal exercises.
   c. Observe for and report any unusual bleeding immediately.
   d. Encourage client to get back to work the next day.

9. Describe primary peritonitis and secondary peritonitis.

10. The fluid shift that occurs in peritonitis may result in which of the following?
    a. Intracellular fluid moving into the peritoneal cavity
    b. A significant increase in circulatory volume
    c. Eventual renal failure and electrolyte imbalance
    d. Increased bowel motility caused by increased fluid volume

11. The respiratory problems that may accompany peritonitis are a result of which of the following?
    a. Associated pain interfering with ventilation
    b. Decreased pressure against the diaphragm
    c. Fluid shifts to the thoracic cavity
    d. Decreased oxygen demands related to the infectious process

12. List the client data (subjective and objective) you would include relevant to peritonitis for your nursing assessment.

13. Which of the following is an expected assessment finding in the client with generalized peritonitis?
    a. Soft, supple abdomen
    b. High urine output
    c. Low-grade fever
    d. Tachycardia

14. Which of the following would be included in nonsurgical management for the client with peritonitis?
    a. Monitoring of weekly weight and intake and output
    b. Insertion of an NG tube to decompress the stomach
    c. Ordering a breakfast tray because the client is hungry
    d. Administering NSAIDs for pain

15. Interventions following abdominal surgery for peritonitis include which of the following?
    a. Maintaining the client in a supine position
    b. Using clean technique for peritoneal irrigation
    c. Ambulating client on day 1
    d. Monitoring level of consciousness at least hourly initially after surgery

16. Briefly define gastroenteritis.

17. What are the two types of organisms responsible for gastroenteritis?

   a. _____

   b. _____

18. Identify three circumstances in which invading organisms can infect a person and result in gastroenteritis.

   a. _____

   b. _____

   c. _____

19. Identify the three organisms most commonly responsible for bacterial gastroenteritis.

   a. _____

   b. _____

   c. _____

20. Briefly describe the primary route of transmission for invading organisms causing gastroenteritis.

21. Identify four ways in which to avoid contamination and prevent the spread of gastroenteritis.

22. Briefly describe the pathophysiology of ulcerative colitis.

23. Identify the complications associated with ulcerative colitis.

   a. _____

   b. _____

   c. _____

   d. _____

   e. _____

   f. _____

   g. _____

   h. _____

24. Identify the client data (both subjective and objective) relevant to ulcerative colitis for your nursing assessment.

25. Before an invasive diagnostic workup, what are the client's stools examined for?

26. Nonsurgical management of ulcerative colitis includes which of the following?
   a. A high-fiber, high-roughage diet
   b. Antidiarrheal agents
   c. Regular exercise
   d. All clients being on NPO status

27. Identify and analyze priority nursing diagnoses and collaborative problems for the client with ulcerative colitis.

28. Match each of the following descriptions of common medications used for ulcerative colitis to the corresponding drug category. *Answers may be used more than once.*

Description

_____ a. As single agents, these drugs are not effective in the treatment of ulcerative colitis.

_____ b. Drugs are administered orally or rectally to reduce inflammation.

_____ c. Oral or IV therapy may be prescribed during exacerbations.

_____ d. Take with a full glass of water and with meals to prevent GI discomfort.

_____ e. These drugs can precipitate colonic dilation and toxic megacolon.

_____ f. The nurse observes for side effects, some of which may include thrombocytopenia, leukopenia, anemia, and renal failure.

_____ g. Long-term adverse effects of this drug can include hyperglycemia, osteoporosis, PUD, and increased risk for infection.

Drug Category
1. Salicylate compounds
2. Corticosteroids
3. Immunosuppressive drugs
4. Antidiarrheal drugs

29. A client who has had a total proctocolectomy with a traditional permanent ileostomy would most likely have the stoma placed where?

30. A client who has had a total colectomy with a continent ileostomy would have the pouch located where?

31. Explain how the client would drain the pouch with a Kock's ileostomy.

32. The nurse teaches the client with an ileostomy to include adequate amounts of _____ and _____ in the diet because the ileostomy promotes the loss of these.

33. Formulate a postoperative plan of care for the client with a colon resection/colectomy, colostomy, and ileostomy.

34. Identify the expected outcomes for the client with ulcerative colitis.

    a. _____

    b. _____

    c. _____

    d. _____

    e. _____

    f. _____

    g. _____

35. Briefly describe Crohn's disease.

36. Identify two common complications of Crohn's disease.

    a. _____

    b. _____

37. Discuss the implications that a fistula has for the client with Crohn's disease.

38. Which of the following differentiates Crohn's disease and ulcerative colitis?
    a. Stools may show evidence of blood.
    b. The etiology is unknown.
    c. Hemorrhage may occur.
    d. Severe malabsorption by the small intestine is more common.

39. Which of the following statements about Crohn's disease is correct?
    a. The peak incidence is in the 15- to 40-year age group.
    b. There is a decreased incidence of Crohn's disease in the Jewish population.
    c. The incidence is 20% greater in men than in women.
    d. No known familial link correlates with its incidence.

40. Identify the client data (both subjective and objective) relevant to Crohn's disease you would include for your nursing assessment.

41. Differentiate between Crohn's disease and ulcerative colitis by matching each of the following characteristics to its corresponding chronic disease. *Answers may be used more than once.*

Characteristic

_____ a. Slowly progressive

_____ b. Begins in the rectum and proceeds in a continuous manner to cecum

_____ c. Remissions and exacerbations

_____ d. Patchy involvement, all layers of the bowel

_____ e. Hemorrhage more common

_____ f. Unknown etiology

_____ g. Can have 10 to 20 liquid, bloody stools per day

_____ h. Terminal ileum, site most affected

Chronic Disease
1. Crohn's disease
2. Ulcerative colitis
3. Both Crohn's and ulcerative colitis

42. Sepsis can result from abscesses or fistulas that may be present with Crohn's disease. Identify the category of drugs that can mask the symptoms of infection, thus making it essential that the nurse monitor the client vigilantly for signs and symptoms of infection.

43. List four features of treatment of the client with a fistula.

    a. _____

    b. _____

    c. _____

    d. _____

44. Identify and analyze priority nursing diagnoses and collaborative problems for clients with Crohn's disease.

45. Identify the nursing diagnoses related to a serious life-threatening complication seen in Crohn's disease that does not normally occur in ulcerative colitis.

46. Develop a teaching plan for a client needing community-based care for a new ostomy.

47. Briefly describe diverticula.

48. Which of the following statements about diverticular disease is correct?
    a. Most diverticula occur in the descending colon.
    b. Diverticula are uncomfortable even when not inflamed.
    c. High-fiber diets contribute to diverticula occurrence.
    d. Diverticula form where intestinal wall muscles are weak.

49. Preventive measures for diverticular disease include which of the following?
    a. Excluding whole-grain breads from the diet
    b. Avoiding fresh apples, broccoli, and lettuce
    c. Taking bulk agents such as psyllium hydrophilic mucilloid
    d. Taking routine anticholinergics to reduce bowel spasm

50. Briefly explain why invasive radiographs or diagnostic tests are not done for the client with acute diverticulitis.

51. Identify the complications that would indicate that a client with diverticulitis will need surgery.

    a. _____

    b. _____

    c. _____

    d. _____

    e. _____

    f. _____

52. Which of the following types of stomas will the client with diverticulitis most likely have postoperatively?
    a. Ileostomy
    b. Kock's pouch
    c. Colostomy
    d. Cecostomy

53. All clients with diverticular disease require education regarding a diet high in what substance?

54. Develop a teaching plan explaining the role of diet therapy for the client with diverticular disease.

55. Match each of the following anorectal problems with the corresponding description.

Description

_____ a. Duct obstruction and infection

_____ b. Perianal laceration, superficial erosion

_____ c. Communicating tract

Anorectal Problem
1. Anal fissure
2. Anal fistula
3. Anorectal abscess

56. The nurse focuses on comfort measures that can be used for the client with anorectal problems. Identify four such measures for helping the client maintain comfort.

    a. _____

    b. _____

    c. _____

    d. _____

57. Describe the significance of warm sitz baths as an intervention in managing anorectal problems.

58. Identify the most common route of transmission of parasitic infection.

59. Briefly explain why other household members and sexual partners of the infected clients should also be examined for parasites.

60. Which type of food poisoning is the most life threatening and why?

61. Complete the following table by comparing and contrasting food poisoning and gastroenteritis.

Characteristic	Food Poisoning	Gastroenteritis
Communicability		
Incubation period		
Immunity status after recovery		
Diarrhea		
Nausea and vomiting		

62. Describe ways that parasitic infection, helminthic infestation, and food poisoning could be prevented.

CASE STUDY: THE CLIENT WITH DIVERTICULITIS

Answer Guidelines for the Case Study questions are provided on the companion Evolve Learning Resources Web site at http://evolve.elsevier.com/Iggy/.

An 18-year-old body-builder has just come into your office complaining of left lower quadrant abdominal pain, temperature of 100.8° F, constipation, and blood-streaked stool. On examination of the abdomen, you observe slight distention and tenderness on palpation, especially in the left lower quadrant. This client has an elevated white blood cell count and his stool for occult blood is positive. Diverticulitis is diagnosed.

1. Identify key findings noted in the examination and indicate the significance.

2. The client says, "Oh, I'll just go home and take a laxative or an enema and I'll be fine." Explain why these should be avoided.

3. Nonsurgical management has been selected for this client, and he may return home after receiving special instructions. Identify a key factor, based on your assessment, on which you would need to instruct him.

4. Provide this client with discharge instructions.

Interventions for Clients with Liver Problems

CHAPTER

62

LEARNING OUTCOMES

1. Describe the pathophysiology and complications associated with cirrhosis of the liver.
2. Interpret laboratory test findings commonly seen in clients with cirrhosis.
3. Analyze assessment data from clients with cirrhosis to determine priority nursing diagnoses and collaborative problems.
4. Formulate a collaborative plan of care for the client with severe late-stage cirrhosis.
5. Identify emergency interventions for the client with bleeding esophageal varices.
6. Evaluate care for clients with cirrhosis.
7. Develop a community-based teaching plan for the client with cirrhosis of the liver.
8. Compare and contrast the transmission of hepatitis A, B, and C viral infections.
9. Explain ways in which each type of hepatitis can be prevented.
10. Discuss the primary concerns about the increasing incidence of hepatitis C in the United States.
11. Identify treatment options for clients with cancer of the liver.
12. Describe the typical complications that result from liver transplantation.

LEARNING ACTIVITIES

1. Before completing the study guide exercises in this chapter, it is recommended that you review the following:
   - Anatomy and physiology of the liver
   - Normal F and E levels
   - Principles of infection control (universal, body substance precautions)
   - Principles of blood and blood product administration
   - Perioperative nursing management
   - Postoperative nursing management
   - Principles of TPN and care of peripheral and central line catheters
   - Special diets (such as low fat, low protein, high protein, high carbohydrate, and liquid) for clients with liver disorders
   - Concepts of body image and self-esteem
   - Concepts of grief, loss, death, and dying

2. Review the boldfaced terms and their definitions in Chapter 62 to enhance your understanding of the content.

STUDY/REVIEW QUESTIONS

Answers to the Study/Review Questions are provided on the companion Evolve Learning Resources Web site at http://evolve.elsevier.com/Iggy/.

1. Match each of the following descriptions with the corresponding type of liver cirrhosis. *Answers may be used more than once.*

Description

_____ a. Viral induced

_____ b. Vascular congestion

_____ c. Hobnailed capsule

_____ d. Associated with bile stasis

_____ e. Fatty infiltration of hepatocytes

_____ f. Chemical hepatotoxin-induced

_____ g. Alcohol-induced

_____ h. Liver anoxia

_____ i. Massive hepatocyte death

_____ j. Severe obstructive jaundice

_____ k. Increased hepatic volume

_____ l. Diffuse hepatic fibrosis

Type of Liver Cirrhosis
1. Laënnec's cirrhosis following alcoholic hepatitis
2. Postnecrotic cirrhosis
3. Biliary cirrhosis
4. Cardiac cirrhosis

2. Match each of the following descriptions of pathophysiology with the corresponding complication of liver cirrhosis.

Pathophysiology

_____ a. Bilirubin not excreted

_____ b. Vitamin K deficiency

_____ c. Backflow of blood to liver and spleen

_____ d. Impaired ammonia metabolism

_____ e. Plasma leaking into peritoneal cavity

_____ f. Kidneys unable to excrete solutes

_____ g. Thin-walled distended veins

Complication of Liver Cirrhosis
1. Portal hypertension
2. Ascites
3. Bleeding
4. Esophageal varices
5. Jaundice
6. Encephalopathy
7. Hepatorenal syndrome

3. Identify the most common form of cirrhosis in the United States and discuss how it can be prevented.

4. The cause of cirrhosis varies with the type. Identify the top cause of cirrhosis in the world.

5. List the client data (both subjective and objective) relevant to cirrhosis of the liver for your nursing assessment.

6. Analyze your assessment data and identify priority nursing diagnoses and collaborative problems for the client with cirrhosis.

7. Match each of the following abnormal laboratory findings in the cirrhotic client with the corresponding cause. *Answers may be used more than once.*

Abnormal Laboratory Finding

_____ a. Serum aspartate aminotransferase elevated

_____ b. Globulins elevated

_____ c. Total proteins decreased

_____ d. Ammonia increased

_____ e. Serum alanine aminotransferase elevated

_____ f. Prothrombin time prolonged

_____ g. Total serum bilirubin increased

_____ h. Albumin decreased

_____ i. Lactate dehydrogenase elevated

_____ j. Alkaline phosphatase elevated

Cause
1. Hepatocyte death
2. Biliary obstruction
3. Decreased liver synthesis
4. Increased immune response
5. Decreased conversion

8. A client with cirrhosis has been admitted to your unit with ascites. Use the information presented in your textbook as a basis for developing appropriate rationales for the following interventions that have been selected for this client.
   a. Placing her on a low-sodium diet

   b. Placing her on fluid restriction

   c. Adding vitamin supplements to her IV fluids

   d. Administering a diuretic

   e. Assessing intake and output

f. Weighing her daily

g. Measuring her abdominal girth

h. Monitoring electrolyte balance

i. Administering potassium supplements

j. Administering low-sodium antacid therapy

k. Elevating head of bed at least 30 degrees

9. Which of the following would indicate the need for the physician to perform a paracentesis?
   a. Client discomfort
   b. Decreased blood pressure
   c. Fetor hepaticus
   d. Respiratory distress

10. Briefly explain why the client with cirrhosis who has medically unmanageable ascites is a poor surgical risk for a shunting procedure.

11. Briefly explain the purpose of a peritoneovenous shunt.

12. Before surgery for a peritoneovenous shunt, what interventions would help the client achieve an optimal physical state?

13. An adult client has come to your emergency department with bleeding esophageal varices, and emergency interventions must be initiated to control rapid blood loss. Identify six methods the emergency team could institute to control the bleeding in this client.

    a. _____

    b. _____

    c. _____

    d. _____

    e. _____

    f. _____

14. Nursing responsibilities related to esophagogastric balloon tamponade include which of the following?
    a. Initially inflating each balloon according to the manufacturer's guidelines
    b. Attaching the esophageal and gastric drainage lumens to low continuous suction
    c. Ensuring that balloon pressures are kept at levels needed to control bleeding
    d. Repositioning the tube if it migrates upward and causes airway obstruction

15. Identify the types of intravenous products that the nurse may need to administer in cases of massive esophageal hemorrhage.

    a. _____

    b. _____

    c. _____

    d. _____

16. Vasopressin (Pitressin) therapy results in which of the following?
    a. Improved blood flow in the portal system
    b. Relaxation of vascular bed smooth muscle
    c. Effective long-term control of variceal bleeding
    d. Decreased blood flow to the abdominal organs

17. Identify the nonsurgical procedure that is considered a last-resort intervention for clients with portal hypertension and esophageal varices.

18. After shunting procedures, clients are susceptible to oliguria and often become hypovolemic. The nurse administers the ordered fluid volume and assesses the effects of the volume by monitoring for:

    a. _____

    b. _____

    c. _____

19. For the client with portal-systemic encephalopathy, identify what food group may be totally eliminated from the diet as the client's mental status deteriorates.

20. Which of the following drugs is usually prescribed for the client with portal-systemic encephalopathy to reduce serum ammonia levels?
    a. Levodopa (Dopar)
    b. Diazepam (Valium)
    c. Lactulose (Cephulac)
    d. Morphine sulfate

21. Formulate a collaborative plan of care for the client with severe late-stage cirrhosis.

22. Develop a community-based teaching plan for the client with cirrhosis of the liver.

23. Identify six expected outcomes based on the nursing diagnoses and collaborative problems for the client with cirrhosis of the liver.

   a. _____

   b. _____

   c. _____

   d. _____

   e. _____

   f. _____

24. Briefly describe hepatitis.

25. Number in chronologic order the following steps describing the pathologic changes that occur in hepatitis.

   _____ a. Intrahepatic jaundice results from edema of bile channels

   _____ b. Liver enlargement and congestion resulting from inflammatory cells, edema, and lymphocytes

   _____ c. Portal circulation impaired because of distorted lobular pattern

   _____ d. Eventual regeneration of liver cells

   _____ e. Widespread inflammation, necrosis, and hepatocellular regeneration

   _____ f. Exposure to causative agents occurs

   _____ g. Active phagocytosis and enzyme activity remove damaged cells

26. Identify the types of viral hepatitis.

   a. _____

   b. _____

   c. _____

   d. _____

   e. _____

27. Identify the type of viral hepatitis that is of most concern to health care workers.

28. Match each of the following descriptions with its corresponding type of hepatitis. *Answers may be used more than once.*

Description

_____ a.   Occurs only in the presence of hepatitis B virus

_____ b.   Rarely life threatening

_____ c.   Does not lead to chronic infection

_____ d.   Often goes unrecognized

_____ e.   Spread by contaminated water, shellfish

_____ f.   Transmitted from mother to fetus

_____ g.   Leading cause of cirrhosis worldwide

_____ h.   Concentrations of virus are found in semen and saliva

_____ i.   Approximately one half of liver transplantations in United States are for end-stage (of this virus)

_____ j.   Spread by sexual contact with multiple partners

_____ k.   Rarely transmitted sexually, although virus is present in blood

Type of Hepatitis
1. Hepatitis A
2. Hepatitis B
3. Hepatitis C
4. Delta hepatitis (hepatitis D)
5. Hepatitis E

29. Identify two ways in which hepatitis A, B, and C infection could be prevented.
    a.   Hepatitis A

    b.   Hepatitis B

    c.   Hepatitis C

30. Briefly explain the primary concerns about the increasing incidence of hepatitis C infection in the United States.

31. Match the following complications of viral hepatitis with their descriptions.

Description

_____ a.   Chronic active hepatitis

_____ b.   Chronic persistent hepatitis

_____ c.   Fulminant hepatitis

Complication of Viral Hepatitis
1. Nonprogressive liver damage
2. Progressive liver damage with necrosis, inflammation, and fibrosis
3. Severe and often fatal failure of liver cells to regenerate

32. Describe the development of jaundice in hepatitis.

33. Which of the following drugs is contraindicated for managing nausea in the client with viral hepatitis?
    a.   Trimethobenzamide hydrochloride (Tigan)
    b.   Prochlorperazine maleate (Compazine)
    c.   Dimenhydrinate (Dramamine)
    d.   Ranitidine (Zantac)

34. Instructions for the client with viral hepatitis would include all but which of the following?
    a. Avoid sharing bathroom towels with family members.
    b. Avoid alcohol, sedatives, and acetaminophen (Tylenol).
    c. Begin an exercise program at the local health spa.
    d. Eat small, frequent meals with a high-carbohydrate, low-fat content.

35. Categorize each of the following descriptions with the corresponding liver disorder. *Answers may be used more than once.*

Description

_____ a. Bacterial invasion

_____ b. Result of faulty metabolism

_____ c. Penetrating or blunt injury

_____ d. Sudden onset of symptoms

_____ e. Hemorrhagic shock

_____ f. Confirmed by liver biopsy

_____ g. Hepatomegaly

_____ h. Right shoulder pain

_____ i. Associated with chronic alcoholism

_____ j. Anorexia, weight loss

_____ k. Requires administration of multiple blood products

Liver Disorder
1. Fatty liver
2. Hepatic abscess
3. Liver trauma

36. The liver is a common site for metastasis from what cancer sources?

    a. _____

    b. _____

37. Identify the possible causes of liver cancer.

    a. _____

    b. _____

    c. _____

    d. _____

    e. _____

    f. _____

    g. _____

38. Identify five treatment options for clients with cancer of the liver.

    a. _____

    b. _____

    c. _____

    d. _____

    e. _____

39. Describe the type of client who would be a potential candidate for liver transplantation.

40. Describe the type of client who would not be considered a candidate for liver transplantation.

41. Donor livers are obtained primarily from what source?

42. Identify the complications that may result from liver transplantation.

    a. _____

    b. _____

    c. _____

    d. _____

    e. _____

    f. _____

    g. _____

    h. _____

    i. _____

43. When is organ rejection most likely to occur following liver transplantation?

44. Identify four clinical manifestations the nurse would observe for when assessing the client who may be experiencing acute rejection after liver transplantation.

    a. _____

    b. _____

    c. _____

    d. _____

45. Identify the drug therapy used to prevent organ rejection in the client who has had a liver transplantation.

    a. _____

    b. _____

    c. _____

    d. _____

CASE STUDY: THE CLIENT WITH CIRRHOSIS AND ESOPHAGEAL BLEEDING

Answer Guidelines for the Case Study questions are provided on the companion Evolve Learning Resources Web site at http://evolve.elsevier.com/Iggy/.

A recently retired locomotive engineer is looking forward to his retirement so that he and his wife "can finally enjoy" their lives together. He states he feels he has maintained sobriety quite well, but occasionally "sneaks a little drink now and then," and unfortunately his cirrhotic liver has never fully recovered from 25 years of fairly heavy drinking. Periodically, and through the years, he still has symptoms of residual effects. For the past several days he states he has been coughing on and off. His wife states that this morning he coughed up "bright red blood" and that is why she made him come to the hospital. As for now, he is not coughing or bleeding but has been admitted for observation. As you are doing your rounds, his wife comes out of his room hysterical; you enter his room and observe blood all over his gown and bed linens. He appears terrified.

1. What would you need to do immediately?

2. The physician enters the room to perform an esophagogastric balloon tamponade. Before the physician inserts the tube, (a) identify your priority nursing intervention and what measures you would take to ensure it. (b) What would your responsibility be in assisting the physician before insertion of the tube?

4. In preparing him for discharge, identify two essential health concerns for maintaining or improving your client's health after esophageal bleeding.

3. After insertion of the tube and placement has been verified, explain how you would assist the physician with securing the tube and applying traction.

Interventions for Clients with Problems of the Biliary System and Pancreas

LEARNING OUTCOMES

1. Identify the common causes of cholecystitis and cholelithiasis (gallbladder disease).
2. Interpret diagnostic test results associated with gallbladder disease.
3. Compare postoperative care of clients undergoing a traditional cholecystectomy with that of clients undergoing a laparoscopic cholecystectomy.
4. Develop a community-based teaching plan for clients with gallbladder disease, including care of a T-tube.
5. Compare and contrast the pathophysiology of acute and chronic pancreatitis.
6. Interpret common assessment findings associated with acute pancreatitis and those associated with chronic pancreatitis.
7. Prioritize nursing care for clients with acute pancreatitis and clients with chronic pancreatitis.
8. Explain the use and precautions associated with enzyme replacement for chronic pancreatitis.
9. Develop a postoperative plan of care for clients undergoing a Whipple procedure.
10. Construct a discharge plan for care of clients with pancreatic cancer in the community.
11. Discuss the psychosocial needs of the client with pancreatic cancer and associated nursing interventions.

LEARNING ACTIVITIES

1. Before completing the study guide exercises for this chapter, it is recommended that you review the following:
   - Anatomy and physiology of the gallbladder and pancreas
   - Special diets (such as low fat, low protein, high protein, high carbohydrate, and liquid) for clients with disorders of the gallbladder and pancreas
   - Principles of total parenteral nutrition (TPN) and care of peripheral and central line catheters
   - Principles of administration of blood and blood products
   - Perioperative nursing management
   - Postoperative nursing management
   - Normal F and E values
   - Care of nasogastric (NG) and nasointestinal tubes, care of feeding tubes, and preparation of tube-feeding formulas

- Concepts of body image and self-esteem
- Concepts of grief, loss, death, and dying

2. Review the boldfaced terms and their definitions in Chapter 63 to enhance your understanding of the content.

STUDY/REVIEW QUESTIONS

Answers to the Study/Review Questions are provided on the companion Evolve Learning Resources Web site at http://evolve.elsevier.com/Iggy/.

1. Differentiate between acute and chronic cholecystitis.

2. Cholecystitis can be caused by the formation of gallbladder calculi. Identify other possible causes.

   a. _____

   b. _____

   c. _____

   d. _____

   e. _____

   f. _____

   g. _____

   h. _____

   i. _____

   j. _____

   k. _____

3. Obstructive jaundice can result in which of the following?
   a. Pruritus
   b. Pale urine in increased amounts
   c. Pink discoloration of sclera
   d. Dark tarry stools

4. Identify the common underlying factor that contributes to the etiology of acute cholecystitis.

5. A high incidence of biliary tract disease and cholecystitis is associated with which of the following?
   a. Leading an active lifestyle
   b. Having a familial tendency
   c. Being slightly underweight
   d. Having non–insulin-dependent diabetes

6. Identify the client data (both subjective and objective) relevant to biliary disorders for your nursing assessment.

7. Because there is no specific laboratory test for gallbladder disease, explain the course of action taken in determining a diagnosis for gallbladder disease.

8. What is the best diagnostic test for cholecystitis?

9. Which of the following medications is usually not given to clients for pain management in gallbladder disease?
   a. Morphine
   b. Lomine
   c. Bentyl
   d. Demerol

10. What is the usual surgical treatment for clients with cholecystitis?

11. Preoperatively for the client about to undergo a traditional cholecystectomy, the nurse reinforces teaching methods to prevent respiratory complications. What teaching demonstrations will be included?

12. List three possible sites of drainage following a cholecystectomy.

    a. _____

    b. _____

    c. _____

13. The client's T-tube can remain in place for how long?

14. Management of a T-tube in a client who has had gallbladder surgery includes which of the following?
    a. Routinely irrigating the tube with 30 mL of normal saline every shift
    b. Keeping the client in a supine position
    c. Giving synthetic bile salts as ordered
    d. Keeping the drainage system above the level of the gallbladder

15. After the removal of the gallbladder, the client's dietary intake of fat should be which of the following?
    a. Eliminated completely
    b. Adjusted according to individual tolerance
    c. Limited to less than 10% of the diet
    d. Increased to more than 50% of the diet

16. Contrast laparoscopic cholecystectomy with one done via laparotomy.

17. Postoperatively with laparoscopic procedures, some clients have a problem with "free air pain." What will the nurse teach the client about managing this phenomenon?

18. What is the rationale for administering anti-emetic medications early in the postoperative phase following a cholecystectomy?

19. After having a laparoscopic procedure done, most clients are able to resume usual activities after how long?

20. Identify the most common cause of inflammation in clients with cholelithiasis.

21. Match the following terms related to gall-bladder disorders with their definitions.

Definition

_____ a. Common bile duct stones

_____ b. Gallbladder stones

_____ c. Inflammation of bile ducts (involves infection)

_____ d. Inflammation of biliary tree

Term Associated with Gallbladder Disorders
1. Ascending cholangitis
2. Cholangitis
3. Choledocholithiasis
4. Cholelithiasis

22. Identify the substances that are normally found in gallstones.

a. _____

b. _____

c. _____

d. _____

e. _____

23. What examination permits radiographic visualization of the common bile duct, pancreas, pancreatic ducts, and biliary tree and permits the physician to pinpoint the nature of a biliary obstruction?

24. What is the rationale for giving antispasmodics for pain relief to the client with biliary colic?

25. Match the following procedures with their definitions.

Definition

_____ a. Powerful shock waves shatter gall-stones

_____ b. Incision into common bile duct for stone removal

_____ c. Removal of gallbladder

_____ d. Direct visualization of biliary tract

_____ e. Opening into the gallbladder

Procedure
1. Cholecystectomy
2. Cholecystotomy
3. Choledocholithotomy
4. Choledochoscopy
5. Extracorporeal shock wave lithotripsy

26. Develop a community-based teaching plan for clients with gallbladder disease, including care of a T-tube.

27. Identify and briefly describe the four major pathophysiologic processes that occur in acute pancreatitis.

a. _____

b. _____

c. _____

d. _____

28. Briefly define autodigestion.

29. Identify the theories that attempt to explain the triggering mechanisms leading to enzyme activation in acute pancreatitis.

    a. _____

    b. _____

    c. _____

    d. _____

30. Match the following complications of pancreatitis with their pathophysiologies.

Pathophysiology

_____ a. Disruption of alveolar-capillary membrane results in edema

_____ b. Release of glucagon and damaged islet cell

_____ c. Consumption of clotting factors and microthrombi formation

_____ d. Head of pancreas swells and restricts bile flow through common bile duct

_____ e. Seepage of digested proteins and lipids into mesentery

_____ f. Pancreatic exudate migrates via transdiaphragmatic coagulation lymphatics

Complication of Pancreatitis
1. Peritoneal irritation
2. Jaundice
3. Transient hyperglycemia
4. Pleural effusion
5. Adult respiratory distress syndrome (ARDS)
6. Disseminated intravascular coagulation (DIC)

31. Identify the two most common factors that cause injury to the pancreas.

    a. _____

    b. _____

32. List the client data (both subjective and objective) relevant to acute pancreatitis for your assessment.

33. Identify the two serum studies that are considered the "cardinal" diagnostic signs important in the diagnosis of pancreatitis.

    a. _____

    b. _____

True or False? Write T for true or F for false in the blanks provided. If a statement is false, correct it to make it true.

_____ 34. Abdominal pain is the prominent symptom of pancreatitis.

_____ 35. Anticholinergics are given to increase vagal stimulation, increase GI motility, and inhibit pancreatic enzyme and bicarbonate volume and concentration.

_____ 36. Pain management for acute pancreatitis should begin with rapid infusion of opioids by means of patient-controlled analgesia (PCA).

_____ 37. Helping the client to assume a cross-legged position may decrease the abdominal pain of pancreatitis.

_____ 38. Surgical intervention for acute pancreatitis is usually not indicated.

_____ 39. The client in the early stages of acute pancreatitis is usually maintained on NPO status.

_____ 40. If total parenteral nutrition (TPN) is used for nutritional support, the nurse assesses for glucose intolerance by monitoring for decreased blood glucose levels.

41. Prioritize nursing care needs for clients with acute pancreatitis.

42. Briefly describe chronic pancreatitis.

43. Differentiate between chronic calcifying pancreatitis and chronic obstructive pancreatitis.

44. Match each of the following complications of chronic pancreatitis with the related cause. _Answers may be used more than once._

Complication of Chronic Pancreatitis

_____ a. Steatorrhea

_____ b. Decrease in muscle mass

_____ c. Ketoacidosis

_____ d. Peripheral edema

_____ e. Hyperglycemia

Cause
1. Loss of endocrine function
2. Loss of exocrine function

45. What is the only definitive diagnostic test for chronic pancreatitis?

46. Identify the significant serum laboratory findings most commonly associated with chronic pancreatitis.

a. _____

b. _____

c. _____

d. _____

47. List the client data (both subjective and objective) relevant to chronic pancreatitis for your nursing assessment.

48. Discuss problems the nurse may encounter with pain management for the client with chronic pancreatitis.

Read the following seven statements related to chronic pancreatitis and decide whether each is true or false. Write T for true or F for false in the blanks provided. If a statement is false, correct it to make it true.

_____ 49. Pancreatic enzymes are essential dietary supplements.

_____ 50. Pancreatic enzymes are given on an empty stomach.

_____ 51. The nurse mixes the powdered form of pancreatic enzymes in milk.

_____ 52. Enzyme preparation should be mixed with foods containing protein.

_____ 53. After administration of the enzyme preparation, the nurse advises the client to wipe the lips with a dry napkin.

_____ 54. Glucose levels for the client should be checked daily, particularly for the client on TPN.

_____ 55. The health care provider may prescribe Zantac to increase gastric acid.

56. Discharge planning for the client with chronic pancreatitis includes which of the following?
    a. Renting a commode for bedside use
    b. Gradually tapering off the dosage of the pancreatic enzymes
    c. Asking a member of Alcoholics Anonymous to visit
    d. Encouraging the client to consume high-fat large meals

57. Prioritize nursing care needs for clients with chronic pancreatitis.

58. Identify the primary sources of tumors that metastasize to the pancreas.

    a. _____

    b. _____

    c. _____

    d. _____

    e. _____

59. Briefly explain why cancer of the pancreas has a poor prognosis.

60. Tumors in the head of the pancreas have which of the following characteristics?
    a. Are usually large and invade the entire organ
    b. Frequently cause jaundice and gallbladder distention
    c. Spread more extensively than tumors in the tail
    d. Are the least common of the pancreatic cancers

61. Which of the following is a common complication of pancreatic carcinoma?
    a. Seizures
    b. Pneumonia
    c. Thrombophlebitis
    d. Uncontrolled bleeding

62. Identify the test that is the most diagnostic for cancer of the pancreas.

63. The Whipple procedure is used to treat what condition?

64. What is the most common and most serious postoperative complication of the Whipple procedure?

65. A client had a Whipple procedure. Identify the rationales for the following postoperative nursing interventions.

   a.   Monitoring of wound drainage and drainage tubes

   b.   Maintaining patency of NG tube

   c.   Protecting the skin from wound drainage

   d.   Positioning in a semi-Fowler's position

   e.   Monitoring vital signs

   f.   Administering ordered IV fluids

   g.   Measuring hourly urinary output

   h.   Checking serum glucose levels

   i.   Monitoring the Swan-Ganz catheter

66. Develop a discharge plan for care of clients with end-stage pancreatic cancer in the community.

67. Describe the type of care measures that are planned for the client with pancreatic cancer who is discharged, and include the two major goals.

68. What is the most serious complication of pancreatitis and why is it so serious?

69. What is the task at hand for clients and family with end-stage pancreatic cancer and how can the nurse help?

70. The nurse might facilitate what kinds of closure work with the client and others?

71. How might the client deal with feelings of being left out or disenfranchised during the last days of illness?

72. Identify and explain psychosocial needs for the client with pancreatic cancer and associated nursing interventions.

73. Name and describe the most common neuroendocrine pancreatic tumor.

Interventions for Clients with Malnutrition and Obesity

LEARNING OUTCOMES

1. Interpret findings of a nutritional assessment.
2. Explain the potential consequences and complications associated with malnutrition.
3. Describe the risk factors for malnutrition, especially for older adults.
4. Discuss the role of laboratory testing in the diagnosis of malnutrition.
5. Analyze assessment data to determine common nursing diagnoses for the client with malnutrition.
6. Identify expected outcomes for clients who are malnourished.
7. Describe the nursing care of clients receiving total enteral nutrition (TEN).
8. Prioritize nursing care for clients receiving total parenteral nutrition (TPN).
9. Identify complications associated with TEN and TPN.
10. Explain the potential consequences and complications associated with obesity.
11. Discuss the multiple causes of obesity.
12. Identify the role of drug therapy in the management of obesity.
13. Develop a postoperative teaching plan for clients having bariatric surgery.

LEARNING ACTIVITIES

1. Before completing the study guide exercises for this chapter, it is recommended that you review the following:
   - Anatomy and physiology of the gastrointestinal system
   - Effect of the central and autonomic nervous systems on the gastrointestinal organs
   - Normal nutrition, including the essential vitamins, minerals, and foods in the recommended food groups
   - Care and management of NG tubes, feeding tubes, and preparation of tube-feeding formulas
   - Perioperative and postoperative nursing management
   - Principles of TPN, TEN, and care of peripheral and central line catheters
   - Normal fluid and electrolyte balance
   - Concepts of body image and self-esteem

2. Review the boldfaced terms and their definitions in Chapter 64 to enhance your understanding of the content.

STUDY/REVIEW QUESTIONS

Answers to the Study/Review Questions are provided on the companion Evolve Learning Resources Web site at http://evolve.elsevier.com/Iggy/.

1. Identify the four nutritional components the Recommended Dietary Allowance (RDA) has established as recommendations for a healthy population.

   a. _____

   b. _____

   c. _____

   d. _____

2. Recommended Dietary Allowance (RDA) is which of the following?
   a. Standard for determining malnutrition
   b. Guide for selecting daily food choices
   c. Standard for evaluation of nutritional problems
   d. Guide for estimating the adequacy of nutrient intake over time

3. Describe the lactovegetarian diet.

4. What vitamin is lacking in the diet of vegans that can contribute to the development of megaloblastic anemia?

5. In teaching the client about nutrition, what factors affecting nutrient requirements would be addressed?

   a. _____

   b. _____

   c. _____

6. What factors influence a person's nutrient intake?

   a. _____

   b. _____

   c. _____

   d. _____

   e. _____

   f. _____

7. In planning a nutritional status assessment, what components would the nurse include?

   a. _____

   b. _____

   c. _____

   d. _____

   e. _____

   f. _____

   g. _____

8. Briefly describe anthropometric measurements.

9. Identify three anthropometric measurements that the nurse can use to evaluate a client's nutritional status.

   a. _____

   b. _____

   c. _____

Read the following statements related to anthropometric measurements and decide whether each is true or false. Write T for true or F for false in the blanks provided. If a statement is false, correct it to make it true.

_____ 10. The nurse must obtain accurate measurements, because clients who report their own measurements tend to underestimate height and overestimate weight.

_____ 11. Clients should be measured and weighed while wearing minimal clothing and no shoes.

_____ 12. In determining height, the client should stand erect and look straight ahead, with the heels apart and the arms forward.

_____ 13. The nurse weighs all clients with an upright balance beam scale.

_____ 14. Height and weight are unaffected by any medical condition the client may have.

_____ 15. An involuntary weight loss of 10% at any time significantly affects nutritional status.

_____ 16. The body mass index is a measure of nutritional status that depends on frame size.

_____ 17. Skinfold measurements estimate body fat.

_____ 18. The midarm circumference can measure muscle mass only.

19. Energy balance refers to the relationship between what aspects of energy?

20. Protein-calorie malnutrition may present in three forms. Identify the three forms and give a brief description of each.

a. _____

b. _____

c. _____

21. Describe the progressive changes in a malnourished client.

22. Identify the complications associated with severe malnutrition.

a. _____

b. _____

c. _____

d. _____

e. _____

f. _____

g. _____

h. _____

i. _____

23. Identify the factors that may influence inadequate nutrient intake and give an example or rationale for each.

a. _____

b. _____

c. _____

d. _____

e. _____

f. _____

g. _____

h. _____

i. _____

j. _____

k. _____

l. _____

m. _____

n. _____

24. Describe how a client who was previously adequately nourished may develop acute protein-calorie malnutrition.

25. List the client data (both subjective and objective) relevant to malnutrition for your nursing assessment.

26. Older adults are particularly at risk for malnutrition. Identify six factors that have been associated with placing the older adult at risk for malnutrition.

a. _____

b. _____

c. _____

d. _____

e. _____

f. _____

27. Match the following laboratory test values with their indications of nutritional status.

Indication of Nutritional Status

_____ a. Indicates the body's protein status

_____ b. A sensitive indicator of protein deficiency

_____ c. Assesses immune function

_____ d. Value below 160 mg/dL could indicate malnutrition, sepsis, and anemia

_____ e. Iron deficiency anemia

_____ f. Total iron-binding capacity

Laboratory Test Value

1. Hemoglobin
2. Serum albumin
3. Serum transferrin
4. Thyroxine-binding prealbumin
5. Serum cholesterol
6. Total lymphocyte count

28. Identify the most common nursing diagnosis for the client with malnutrition.

29. Identify additional nursing diagnoses and collaborative problems based on your assessment.

30. Identify three expected outcomes for the client who is malnourished.

    a. _____

    b. _____

    c. _____

31. For the client who has difficulty chewing or is without teeth, the preferred diet would be which of the following?
    a. Clear liquid
    b. Full liquid
    c. Pureed food
    d. Regular food

32. Total enteral nutrition (TEN) would be contraindicated for which of the following clients?
    a. An older adult receiving chemotherapy
    b. A client who has had a stroke and has dysphagia
    c. A client who has had extensive jaw and mouth surgery
    d. A client who had intestinal obstruction that has progressed to diffuse peritonitis

33. Identify the type of feeding tube that is used primarily for clients requiring short-term enteral feedings.

34. Briefly describe a gastrostomy.

35. Match each of the following types of feeding tubes with the corresponding description.

Description

_____ a. Small amounts are continually infused over a specified time

_____ b. Infusion is stopped for a specified time

_____ c. Intermittent feeding of a specified amount at specified times

Types of Feeding Tubes
1. Bolus feeding tube
2. Continuous feeding tube
3. Cycle feeding tube

36. What is the most common problem associated with feeding tubes?

37. Identify the most accurate method of confirming the placement of a feeding tube.

38. Describe the risk that clients receiving enteral therapy have with respect to fluid.

39. In clients with inadequate renal and cardiac function who are receiving enteral nutrition, identify the major complication associated with increased osmolarity.

40. If the nurse delivers hyperosmolar enteral preparations too quickly, what might be a consequence?

41. Identify the two most common electrolyte imbalances associated with enteral nutrition.

    a. _____

    b. _____

The following descriptions relate to parenteral nutrition. If the phrase refers to partial parenteral nutrition, write PPN in the blank provided; if the phrase refers to total parenteral nutrition, write TPN in the blank provided.

_____ 42. Used when nutritional support is needed less than 2 weeks

_____ 43. Delivered through a cannula in a large distal vein of the arm

_____ 44. Delivered through access to central veins, usually the subclavian or internal jugular

_____ 45. Client should be able to tolerate large fluid volumes

_____ 46. Given when the client requires intensive nutritional support for an extended time

_____ 47. Solutions contain higher concentrations of dextrose and proteins

_____ 48. The two common solutions used are lipid emulsions and amino acid dextrose

49. Clients receiving PPN or TPN are at increased risk for fluid imbalance. Identify the underlying factor that contributes to this risk.

50. Describe interventions the nurse will use to monitor for complications of fluid imbalances for the client who is receiving parenteral nutrition.

51. Identify the three most common electrolyte imbalances associated with parenteral nutrition.

a. _____

b. _____

c. _____

52. Match the following terms related to obesity with their definitions.

Definition

_____ a. Weight that negatively affects health status

_____ b. Excessive amount of body fat

_____ c. Increase in body weight for height as compared to a standard

Term

1. Obesity
2. Overweight
3. Morbid obesity

53. Identify the complications of obesity that can improve with weight loss.

a. _____

b. _____

c. _____

d. _____

e. _____

f. _____

g. _____

h. _____

i. _____

54. Identify the five major causes of obesity and provide an example for each.

a. _____

b. _____

c. _____

d. _____

e. _____

55. With respect to race and gender, which groups have the highest incidence of obesity?

56. Identify five medical conditions the overweight female could be at risk for developing.

    a. _____

    b. _____

    c. _____

    d. _____

    e. _____

57. Identify expected outcomes for the client with obesity.

    a. _____

    b. _____

    c. _____

58. Which of the following diets promotes safe weight loss?
    a. Nutritionally balanced diet
    b. Liquid formula diet
    c. The grapefruit diet
    d. Short-term fasting

59. Anorectic drugs used for obesity work through what mechanism of action?

60. How does Orlistat bring about weight loss?

61. Identify the major side effects of drugs used to treat obesity.

    a. _____

    b. _____

    c. _____

    d. _____

    e. _____

    f. _____

62. Identify surgical procedures that may be performed to reduce food intake of an obese client; provide a brief description of each.

    a. _____

    b. _____

    c. _____

    d. _____

63. What is the rationale for not repositioning the NGT in a client who has had a gastroplasty?

64. What are the two indications that the client who has undergone an intestinal bypass is ready to have the NGT removed?

65. What is the most important focus for client education in obesity?

66. Formulate additional postoperative teaching for clients having a gastroplasty or intestinal bypass.

Assessment of the Endocrine System

LEARNING OUTCOMES

1. Describe the relationship between hormones and receptor sites.
2. Explain negative feedback as a control mechanism for hormone secretion.
3. Discuss the structure and function of the hypothalamus.
4. Discuss the structure and function of the anterior and posterior pituitary glands.
5. Discuss the structure and function of the adrenal glands.
6. Discuss the structure and function of the thyroid and parathyroid glands.
7. Discuss the structure and function of the pancreas.
8. Describe changes in the endocrine system associated with aging.
9. Identify laboratory tests that aid in determining endocrine function and dysfunction.

LEARNING ACTIVITIES

1. Before completing the study guide exercises for this chapter, it is recommended that you review the following:
   - Anatomy and physiology of the endocrine system
   - Hormones and their functions
   - Normal growth and development and the effects of the endocrine system on the aging process
   - Assessment of the endocrine system
   - Diagnostic laboratory tests for endocrine disorders
   - Gordon's functional health patterns

2. Review the boldfaced terms and their definitions in Chapter 65 to enhance your understanding of the content.

STUDY/REVIEW QUESTIONS

Answers to the Study/Review Questions are provided on the companion Evolve Learning Resources Web site at http://evolve.elsevier.com/Iggy/.

1. Identify the six glands that make up the endocrine system.

   a. _____

   b. _____

   c. _____

   d. _____

   e. _____

   f. _____

2. The substances that all these glands secrete are called _____.

3. Explain the meaning of a "ductless" gland.

4. Briefly describe neuroendocrine regulation.

5. Match each hormone with the corresponding gland. *Answers can be used more than once.*

Hormone

_____ a.   Somatostatin

_____ b.   Thyrocalcitonin (calcitonin)

_____ c.   Cortisol

_____ d.   Epinephrine and norepinephrine

_____ e.   Corticotropin-releasing hormone (CRH)

_____ f.   Growth hormone

_____ g.   Glucagon

_____ h.   Parathyroid hormone (PTH)

_____ i.   Aldosterone

_____ j.   Triiodothyronine (T_3)

_____ k.   Estrogen

_____ l.   Insulin

_____ m.   Testosterone

_____ n.   Antidiuretic hormone (ADH)

_____ o.   Oxytocin

_____ p.   Thyroxin (T_4)

_____ q.   Thyroid-stimulating hormone (TSH)

_____ r.   Adrenocorticotropic hormone (ACTH)

Gland

1. Anterior pituitary
2. Posterior pituitary
3. Adrenal cortex
4. Adrenal medulla
5. Thyroid gland
6. Alpha cells—Islets of Langerhans
7. Beta cells—Islets of Langerhans
8. Delta cells—Islets of Langerhans
9. Parathyroid
10. Ovaries
11. Testes
12. Hypothalamus

6. Hormones work on a negative feedback mechanism. Briefly explain how that works in the body.

7. The target tissue for ADH is which organ?

8. Read the following statements related to hormones and the endocrine system and decide whether each is true or false. If the statement is true, write T in the blank provided. If it is false, correct the statement to make it true.

_____ a. Usually, low concentration of hormone is all that is needed to have an effect on the body.

_____ b. When hormones are secreted, the duration of effect is long.

_____ c. Hormones must be bound to a plasma protein in order to be connected with a receptor site.

_____ d. All hormones are stored in significant amounts so that response can be immediate.

_____ e. All hormones must be able to attach themselves to a receptor site in order to be used by the body.

_____ f. Most hormones are "recycled" after use through reuptake by the secreting gland.

_____ g. Homeostasis involves the endocrine system working together with the nervous system for good hormone function.

_____ h. Tropic hormones have another endocrine gland as their target tissue.

_____ i. There are specific normal levels of each of the hormones.

_____ j. More than one hormone can be stimulated before the target tissue is affected.

_____ k. Only the hypothalamus has releasing and inhibiting factors that affect specific hormone production.

9. Which hormone is directly suppressed when circulating levels of cortisol are above normal?
    a. Corticotropin-releasing hormone (CRH)
    b. Antidiuretic hormone (ADH)
    c. Adrenocorticotropic hormone (ACTH)
    d. Growth hormone–releasing hormone (GH-RH)

10. The release of epinephrine into the bloodstream is an example of which of the following endocrine processes?
    a. "Lock and key" manner
    b. Neuroendocrine regulation
    c. Positive feedback mechanism
    d. Stimulus-response theory

11. The hypothalamus has a major role in regulating the endocrine function because it:
    a. Has only very specific endocrine functions
    b. Has two distinct lobes that function independently
    c. Is the connection with the central nervous system
    d. Produces hormones that affect fluid and electrolyte balance

12. Identify the hormones that would be secreted for each of the following endocrine glands.

Endocrine Glands	Principal Hormones Secreted
a. Hypothalamus	
b. Anterior pituitary	
c. Posterior pituitary	
d. Thyroid	
e. Parathyroid	
f. Adrenal cortex	
g. Pancreas	
h. Ovaries	
i. Testes	

13. Which of the following statements is correct about the pituitary gland?
    a. The main role of the posterior pituitary is to secrete tropic hormones.
    b. The posterior pituitary gland stores hormones produced by the hypothalamus.
    c. The anterior pituitary is connected to the thalamus gland.
    d. The anterior pituitary releases stored hormones produced by the hypothalamus.

14. The anterior pituitary gland secretes tropic hormones in response to which of the following hormones from the hypothalamus?
    a. Releasing hormones
    b. Target tissue hormones
    c. Growth hormones
    d. Demand hormones

15. Which of the following statements about pituitary hormones is correct?
    a. The adrenocorticotropic hormone (ACTH) acts on the adrenal medulla.
    b. Follicle-stimulating hormone stimulates sperm production in men.
    c. Growth hormone promotes protein catabolism.
    d. Vasopressin decreases systolic blood pressure.

16. Which of the following statements about the gonads is correct?
    a. Ovaries and testes develop from the same embryonic tissue.
    b. The function of the hormones begins at birth in low, undetectable levels.
    c. The placenta secretes testosterone for the development of male external genitalia.
    d. External genitalia maturation is stimulated by gonadotropins in late adolescence.

17. Which of the following statements about the adrenal glands is correct?
    a. The cortex secretes androgens in men and women.
    b. Catecholamines are secreted from the cortex.
    c. Glucocorticoids are secreted by the medulla.
    d. The medulla secretes hormones essential for life.

18. Which of the following is the major function of the hormones produced by the adrenal cortex?
    a. "Fight or flight" response
    b. Control of glucose, sodium, and water
    c. Regulation of cell growth
    d. Calcium regulation, stress regulation

19. True or False? If the following statements regarding the hormone cortisol secreted by the adrenal cortex are true, write T in the blank provided. If it is false, write F and change the statement to make it correct.

_____ a.   It affects only carbohydrate metabolism.

_____ b.   It is needed for other physiologic processes, such as secretion of insulin, to occur.

_____ c.   It is regulated by ACTH from the posterior pituitary and CRH.

_____ d.   Peaks occur late in the day, with lowest points 12 hours after each peak.

20. Stress causes an increase in the production of cortisol from the adrenal cortex. This may cause an increase in susceptibility to what problem, and why?

21. Identify assessment findings a nurse would monitor in response to catecholamines released by the adrenal medulla.

22. True or False? If the following statements about the thyroid gland and its hormones are true, write T in the blank provided. If they are false, write F and change the statements to make them correct.

_____ a.   The gland is located posteriorly in the neck directly below the cricoid cartilage.

_____ b.   Thyroid hormone production depends on sufficient iodine and potassium intake.

_____ c.   The gland has four distinct lobes joined by a thin isthmus.

_____ d.   Oxygen consumption decreases in response to thyroid hormones.

23. Which of the following is the hormone that responds to a low serum calcium by increasing bone resorption?
    a.   Parathyroid hormone
    b.   Thyroxine (T_4)
    c.   Triiodothyronine (T_3)
    d.   Calcitonin

24. Which of the following is the hormone that responds to elevated serum calcium by decreasing bone resorption?
    a.   Parathyroid hormone
    b.   Thyroxine (T_4)
    c.   Triiodothyronine (T_3)
    d.   Calcitonin

25. Which of the following statements is correct regarding T_3 and T_4 hormones? *Check all that are correct.*

    _____ a.   The basal metabolic rate is affected.

    _____ b.   Hypothalamus is stimulated by cold and stress to secrete thyrotropin-releasing hormone (TRH).

    _____ c.   These hormones need intake of protein and iodine for production.

    _____ d.   Circulating hormone in the blood directly affects the production of TSH.

26. Identify the target organs of parathyroid hormone in the regulation of calcium and phosphorus.

    a. _____

    b. _____

    c. _____

27. Which of following statements about the pancreas is correct?
    a.   Endocrine functions of the pancreas include secretion of digestive enzymes.
    b.   Exocrine functions of the pancreas include secretion of glucagon and insulin.
    c.   The islets of Langerhans are the only source of somatostatin secretion.
    d.   Somatostatin inhibits pancreatic secretion of glucagon and insulin.

28. Which of the following statements is correct about glucagon secretion?
    a.   It is stimulated by an increase in blood glucose levels.
    b.   It is stimulated by a decrease in amino acid levels.
    c.   It exerts its primary effect on the pancreas.
    d.   It acts to increase blood glucose levels.

29. Which of the following statements about insulin secretion is correct?
    a.   Insulin levels drop sharply following the ingestion of a meal.
    b.   Insulin is stimulated primarily by fat ingestion.
    c.   Basal levels are secreted continuously.
    d.   Insulin promotes glycogenolysis and gluconeogenesis.

30. In addition to the pancreas that secretes insulin, which of the following secretes hormones that affect protein, carbohydrate, and fat metabolism?
    a.   Posterior pituitary
    b.   Thyroid gland
    c.   Ovaries
    d.   Parathyroid

31. The bloodstream delivers glucose to the cells for energy production. Which of the following hormones control the cells' use of glucose?
    a. T_4
    b.   Growth hormone
    c.   Adrenal steroids
    d.   Insulin

32. Which of the following diseases involves a disorder of the islets of Langerhans?
    a.   Diabetes insipidus
    b.   Diabetes mellitus
    c.   Addison's disease
    d.   Cushing's disease

33. Identify the subjective data a nurse would obtain when performing an assessment of the endocrine system.

34. Identify the objective data a nurse would obtain when performing an assessment of the endocrine system

35. Which of the following statements is true about age-related changes in older adults and the endocrine system?
    a. All hormone levels are elevated.
    b. Thyroid hormone levels decrease.
    c. Adrenal glands enlarge.
    d. The thyroid gland enlarges.

36. For each of the following structures, identify a physiologic change associated with aging and name the cause of each change.
    a. Gonad
    b. Pancreas
    c. Posterior pituitary gland
    d. Thyroid

37. An older adult complains of a lack of energy and not being able to do the usual daily activities without several naps. These symptoms could indicate which of the following problems that is often seen in the older client?
    a. Hypothyroidism
    b. Hyperparathyroidism
    c. Overproduction of cortisol
    d. Underproduction of glucagon

38. A nurse is performing a physical assessment of the endocrine system. Which of the following glands can be palpated?
    a. Pancreas
    b. Thyroid
    c. Adrenal glands
    d. Parathyroids

39. Which of the following statements is correct about performing a physical assessment of the thyroid gland?
    a. The thyroid gland is easily palpated in all clients.
    b. The client is instructed to swallow to aid palpation.
    c. The anterior approach is preferred for thyroid palpation.
    d. The thumbs are used to palpate the thyroid lobes.

40. A client is to have a suppression/stimulation test completed. Briefly explain the purpose of this test.

41. Which of the following nursing interventions is most appropriate when collecting a 24-hour urine specimen for endocrine studies?
    a. Placing each voided specimen in a separate collection container
    b. Checking whether any preservatives are needed in the collection container
    c. Starting the collection with the first voided urine
    d. Weighing the client before beginning the collection

42. Which of the following instructions should be included in teaching a client about urine collection for endocrine studies? *Check all answers that are correct*.

    _____ a. Fast before starting the urine collection.

    _____ b. Measure the urine in mL rather than ounces.

    _____ c. Empty the bladder completely then start timing.

    _____ d. Time the test for exactly 24 hours.

    _____ e. Notify the laboratory of all medications the client is taking.

    _____ f. Empty the bladder at the end of the time period and keep that specimen.

43. Identify the types of radiographic tests that may be used for an endocrine assessment.

    a. _____

    b. _____

    c. _____

    d. _____

    e. _____

44. A client is suspected of having a pituitary tumor. Which radiographic test would aid in determining this diagnosis?
    a. Skull x-rays
    b. CT/MRI
    c. Angiography
    d. Ultrasound

45. After the ultrasound of the thyroid gland, which of the following diagnostic tests would determine the need for surgical intervention?
    a. CT scan
    b. MRI
    c. Angiography
    d. Needle biopsy

46. For each of the following Gordon's functional health patterns, identify one or more assessment findings that may indicate an actual or potential endocrine problem.
    a. Nutritional-metabolic pattern

    b. Elimination pattern

    c. Sleep-rest pattern

    d. Sexuality-reproduction pattern

    e. Activity-exercise pattern

47. The nursing diagnosis Risk for Falls related to the effect of pathologic fractures as a result of bone demineralization is pertinent to which of the following endocrine problems?
    a. Underproduction of parathyroid hormone
    b. Overproduction of parathyroid hormone
    c. Underproduction of thyroid hormone
    d. Overproduction of thyroid hormone

48. Calcium metabolism is regulated by the parathyroid hormone. Which of the following vitamins is directly involved in this metabolic process?
    a. Vitamin K
    b. Vitamin C
    c. Vitamin B complex
    d. Vitamin D

49. For thyroid hormones to be produced, a client needs to have sufficient intake of which type of food?
    a. Protein and iodine
    b. Protein and carbohydrates
    c. Calcium and protein
    d. Calcium and iodine

50. On physical assessment of a client with possible excess of adrenocortical hormones, the nurse notices reddish-purple "stretch marks" on the breasts and abdomen. The nurse would document these findings as which of the following?
    a. Vitiligo
    b. Hirsutism
    c. Striae
    d. Depigmentation

51. When performing a nursing assessment of the endocrine system, which of the following is a key piece of subjective data?
    a. Age at onset of menstruation
    b. Intake of daily supplemental vitamins
    c. Energy level and fatigue
    d. Lifestyle changes

52. Which of the following regulate aldosterone secretion? *Check all that apply.*

    _____ a. Renin-angiotensin system

    _____ b. Serum osmolarity

    _____ c. Serum potassium ion concentration

    _____ d. Serum calcium levels

    _____ e. Adrenocorticotropin hormone (ACTH)

53. Which hormones are involved in the "fight-or-flight" response to stress?
    a. Thyroid hormones
    b. Catecholamines
    c. Cortisol
    d. Insulin

54. Which cells of the parathyroid gland have endocrine function?

55. After palpation of a client's thyroid gland, the nurse notes that it is enlarged. Which of the following is the next step in assessment?
    a. Order an ultrasound to delineate the enlargement.
    b. Inspect the thyroid gland for symmetry.
    c. Auscultate the area of enlargement for bruits.
    d. Percuss the area of enlargement for dullness.

Interventions for Clients with Pituitary and Adrenal Gland Problems

LEARNING OUTCOMES

1. Compare the common clinical manifestations associated with pituitary hypofunction and pituitary hyperfunction.

2. Interpret clinical changes and laboratory data to determine the effectiveness of therapy for pituitary hypofunction.

3. Identify the teaching priorities for the client taking hormone replacement therapy for pituitary hypofunction.

4. Prioritize nursing care for the client immediately after a transsphenoidal hypophysectomy.

5. Interpret clinical changes and laboratory data to determine the effectiveness of therapy for pituitary hyperfunction.

6. Compare the problems associated with oversecretion and undersecretion of antidiuretic hormone on blood and urine volumes and blood and urine osmolarities.

7. Describe the mechanisms of action, side effects, and nursing implications for pharmacologic management of diabetes insipidus.

8. Interpret clinical changes and laboratory data to determine the effectiveness of interventions for diabetes insipidus.

9. Develop a community-based teaching plan for the client with diabetes insipidus.

10. Interpret clinical changes and laboratory data to determine the effectiveness of interventions for SIADH.

11. Develop a community-based teaching plan for the client with SIADH.

12. Compare the clinical manifestations of Cushing's syndrome and Addison's disease.

13. Interpret clinical changes and laboratory data to determine the effectiveness of interventions for Cushing's syndrome.

14. Develop a community-based teaching plan for the client with Cushing's syndrome or disease.

15. Describe the mechanisms of action, side effects, and nursing implications for pharmacologic management of adrenal insufficiency.

16. Interpret clinical changes and laboratory data to determine the effectiveness of therapy for adrenal insufficiency.

17. Develop a community-based teaching plan for the client with adrenal insufficiency.

18. Prioritize nursing interventions for the client experiencing acute adrenal insufficiency.

LEARNING ACTIVITIES

1. Before completing the study guide exercises in this chapter, it is recommended that you review the following:
   - Anatomy and physiology of the hypothalamus, pituitary gland, and adrenal glands
   - Functions of hormones of the pituitary gland and the adrenal glands
   - Normal growth and development and the effects of the pituitary and adrenal gland hormones on these processes
   - Normal laboratory values for serum and urine potassium and sodium levels and for urine specific gravity
   - Principles of fluid and electrolyte balance and acid-base balance
   - Concepts of human sexuality
   - Perioperative nursing care
   - Assessment of the endocrine system

2. Review the boldfaced terms and their definitions in Chapter 66 to enhance your understanding of the content.

STUDY/REVIEW QUESTIONS

Answers to the Study/Review Questions are provided on the companion Evolve Learning Resources Web site at http://evolve.elsevier.com/Iggy/.

1. Differentiate primary and secondary pituitary dysfunction and the end results that occur.
   a. Primary

   b. Secondary

   c. End results

2. Identify the most common and least common pituitary tumors:

   Most common: _____

   Least common: _____

3. Identify the six hormones that are produced and secreted by the anterior pituitary gland.

   a. _____

   b. _____

   c. _____

   d. _____

   e. _____

   f. _____

4. A malfunctioning posterior pituitary gland can result in which of the following disorders? *Choose all that apply.*
   a. Hypothyroidism
   b. Altered sexual function
   c. Diabetes insipidus
   d. Growth retardation
   e. Syndrome of inappropriate antidiuretic hormone (SIADH)

5. A malfunctioning anterior pituitary gland can result in which of the following disorders? *Choose all that apply.*
   a. Pituitary hypofunction
   b. Pituitary hyperfunction
   c. Diabetes insipidus
   d. Hypothyroidism

6. The assessment findings of a male client with anterior pituitary tumor include complaints of changes in secondary sex characteristics, such as episodes of impotence and decreased libido. The nurse explains to the client that these findings are a result of overproduction of which hormone? Identify a nursing diagnosis for this client.
   a. Gonadotropins inhibiting prolactin (PRL)
   b. Thyroid hormone inhibiting prolactin (PRL)
   c. Prolactin (PRL) inhibiting secretion of gonadotropins
   d. Steroids inhibiting production of sex hormones

   Nursing diagnosis: _____

7. A client with prolactin-secreting tumor would more than likely be treated with which of the following medications?
   a. Dopamine agonists
   b. Vasopressin
   c. Steroids
   d. Growth hormone

8. Interventions for the drug bromocriptine mesylate (Parlodel) include which of the following?
   a. Advising the client to get up slowly from a lying position
   b. Instructing the client to take medication on an empty stomach
   c. Taking daily for purposes of raising GH levels to reduce symptom of acromegaly
   d. Teaching the client to begin with a maintenance level dose

9. Clients diagnosed with an anterior pituitary tumor can have symptoms of acromegaly or gigantism. These symptoms are a result of overproduction of which hormone?
   a. ACTH
   b. Prolactin
   c. Gonatropins
   d. Growth hormone (GH)

10. Upon performing an assessment of an adult client with new-onset acromegaly, the nurse would expect to find which of the following?
    a. Extremely long arms and legs
    b. Thickened, oily facial skin
    c. Changes in menses with infertility
    d. Rough, extremely dry skin

11. Describe characteristic findings for acromegaly and gigantism. Identify a nursing diagnosis for these clients.

12. When analyzing laboratory values, the nurse would expect to find which of the following as a direct result of overproduction of growth hormone, and why?
    a. Hyperglycemia
    b. Hyperphosphatemia
    c. Hypocalcemia
    d. Hypercalcemia

13. Describe the type of pain a client may have with excessively high growth hormone levels.

14. Describe assessment findings a nurse could expect with deficient growth hormone from a hypofunctioning pituitary. Identify a nursing diagnosis related to these findings.

15. Deficiencies of what two hormones are the most life threatening? Explain.

16. Which of the following statements about the etiology of hypopituitarism is correct?
    a. Secondary dysfunction can result from radiation treatment to the pituitary gland.
    b. Primary dysfunction can result from infection or a brain tumor.
    c. Infarction following systemic shock results in secondary hypopituitarism.
    d. Severe malnutrition and body fat depletion can depress pituitary gland function.

17. Which of the following statements about hormone replacement therapy for hypopituitarism is correct?
    a. Once manifestations of hypofunction are corrected, treatment is no longer needed.
    b. The most effective route of androgen replacement is the oral route.
    c. Testosterone replacement therapy is contraindicated in men with prostate cancer.
    d. Clomiphene citrate (Clomid) is used to suppress ovulation in women.

18. Female clients receiving hormone replacement therapy should be instructed to do which of the following?
    a. Report any recurrence of symptoms, such as decreased libido, between injections.
    b. Monitor blood pressure at least weekly for potential hypotension.
    c. Treat leg pain, especially in the calves, with gentle muscle stretching.
    d. Take measures to reduce risk for hypertension and thrombosis.

19. The client who is suspected of having abnormal pituitary function has a circulating GH level of 9 ng/mL 1 hour after receiving 100 g of oral glucose. What is your interpretation of this finding?
    a. The client has anterior pituitary hypofunction.
    b. The client has posterior pituitary hypofunction.
    c. The client has anterior pituitary hyperfunction.
    d. The client has posterior pituitary hyperfunction.

20. Identify at least one preoperative teaching point regarding each of the following topics for a client going for a transsphenoidal hypophysectomy.
    a. Body image changes

    b. Nasal dressing and packing

    c. Preventive measures

    d. Bacteria cultures

    e. Postoperative hospital routines

    f. Hormone replacement

21. Following a hypophysectomy, the client would more than likely need instruction on hormone replacement for which of the following hormones? *Check all that apply*.

    _____ a.   Cortisol

    _____ b.   Thyroid

    _____ c.   Gonadal

    _____ d.   Vasopressin

22. Following a hypophysectomy, home care monitoring by the nurse would include assessing for which of the following? *Check all that apply*.

    _____ a.   Hypoglycemia

    _____ b.   Bowel habits

    _____ c.   Possible leakage of CSF

    _____ d.   24-hour intake of fluids and urine output

    _____ e.   24-hour diet recall

    _____ f.   Activity level

23. Postoperative care for the client who has had a transsphenoidal hypophysectomy includes which of the following?
    a. Encouraging coughing and deep breathing to decrease pulmonary complications
    b. Testing nasal drainage for glucose to determine whether it contains cerebrospinal fluid (CSF)
    c. Keeping the bed flat to decrease central CSF leakage
    d. Assisting the client with brushing of teeth to reduce risk of infection

24. While assessing a client's dressing after a transsphenoidal hypophysectomy, the nurse notes a light yellow color at the edge of the clear drainage on the dressing. What, if any, is the significance of this drainage?

25. A client with a hypophysectomy can post-operatively experience transient diabetes insipidus. Which manifestation alerts the nurse to this problem?
    a. Output much greater than intake
    b. A change in mental status indicating confusion
    c. Laboratory results indicating hyponatremia
    d. Nonpitting edema

26. The action of antidiuretic hormone (ADH) influences normal kidney function by stimulating which of the following?
    a. Glomerulus to control the filtration rate
    b. Proximal nephron tubules to reabsorb water
    c. Distal nephron tubules and collecting ducts to reabsorb water
    d. Constriction of glomerular capillaries to prevent loss of protein in urine

27. What is the term for the disorder that results from a deficiency of vasopressin (antidiuretic hormone ADH) from the posterior pituitary gland?
    a. Syndrome of inappropriate antidiuretic hormone (SIADH)
    b. Diabetes insipidus
    c. Cushing's syndrome
    d. Addison's disease

28. Read the following statements related to diabetes insipidus (ADH deficiency) and decide whether each is true or false. If the statement is true, write T in the blank provided. If it is false, write F and correct the statement to make it true.

    _____ a.   Because the fluid lost is isotonic, the client's plasma osmolality remains normal.

    _____ b.   The primary indication of diabetes insipidus is the client's decreased urinary output and thirst.

_____ c. The primary complications of diabetes insipidus are hypovolemia and shock.

_____ d. A diagnostic test of diabetes insipidus is urine specific gravity greater than 1.005.

_____ e. Urine output of greater than 4 L/24 hr is the first diagnostic indication of diabetes insipidus.

29. Clients with permanent diabetes insipidus must be instructed to:
    a. Continue vasopressin therapy until symptoms disappear.
    b. Monitor for recurrence of polydipsia and polyuria.
    c. Monitor and record their weight twice a week.
    d. Check urine-specific gravity three times a week.

30. A client uses desmopressin acetate metered dose spray as a replacement hormone for ADH. Which of the following is an indication for another dose? *Check all that apply.*

    _____ a. Excessive urination
    _____ b. Specific gravity of 1.003
    _____ c. Dark concentrated urine
    _____ d. Edema in the legs

31. A client is undergoing a dehydration test for diabetes insipidus. Which of the following statements are true regarding this test? *Check all that apply.*
    _____ a. Teach the client that fluid restriction must be maintained for accurate results.
    _____ b. Administer a normal water load followed by infusion of hypertonic saline.
    _____ c. Measure urine output, specific gravity, and osmolality hourly.
    _____ d. Five units of aqueous vasopressin are given for this test.

32. Which of the following oral medications is *not* used to treat mild diabetes insipidus, and why? Identify at least one nursing intervention for each of the correct answers.
    a. Chlorpropamide (Diabinese)
    b. Indomethacin (Indocin)
    c. Lithium (Eskalith)
    d. Lypressin (Diapid)

33. Upon taking a history, which of the following clients would be associated with the development of SIADH?
    a. A 27-year-old client on high-dose steroids
    b. A 47-year-old hospitalized adult client with acute renal failure
    c. A 58-year-old with metastatic lung or breast cancer
    d. An older adult with history of a stroke within the last year

34. Briefly compare diabetes insipidus (DI) with the syndrome of inappropriate antidiuretic hormone (SIADH).

35. Which of the following statements about the pathophysiology of SIADH is correct?
    a. ADH secretion is inhibited in the presence of low plasma osmolality.
    b. Water retention results in dilutional hyponatremia and expanded extracellular fluid (ECF) volume.
    c. The glomerulus is unable to increase its filtration rate to reduce the excess plasma volume.
    d. Renin and aldosterone are released and help to decrease the loss of urinary sodium.

36. Which of the following statements about the etiology and incidence of SIADH is correct?
    a. Malignant cells act on the posterior pituitary gland to decrease ADH release.
    b. Demeclocycline may be used to treat SIADH.
    c. Ectopic ADH production can result from benign gastrointestinal polyps.
    d. SIADH that results from vasopressin overdose in DI is irreversible.

37. The effect of increased ADH in the blood results in which of the following effects on the kidney?
    a. Urine concentration tends to decrease.
    b. Glomerular filtration tends to decrease.
    c. Tubular reabsorption of water increases.
    d. Tubular reabsorption of sodium increases.

38. In SIADH, as a result of water retention from excess ADH, which of the following laboratory values would the nurse expect to find? *Check all that apply.*

    _____ a. Increased urine osmolality (increased sodium in urine)

    _____ b. Elevated serum sodium level

    _____ c. Increased specific gravity (concentrated urine)

    _____ d. Decreased serum osmolarity

    _____ e. Decreased urine specific gravity

39. Which of the following is a priority nursing intervention of a client with SIADH?
    a. Restrict fluid intake.
    b. Monitor the neurologic status at least every 2 hours.
    c. Offer ice chips frequently to ease discomfort of dry mouth.
    d. Monitor urine tests for decreased sodium levels and low specific gravity.

40. Which of the following is the type of intravenous fluids that a nurse uses to treat a client with SIADH, and why?
    a. D_5 1/2 NS
    b. D_5W
    c. 3% NS
    d. NS

41. In addition to intravenous fluids, the client is on a fluid restriction as low as 500 to 600 mL/24 hr. Indicate the serum and urine results that would demonstrate effectiveness of this treatment. *Choose increases or decreases for each of the following.*
    a. Urine specific gravity results (increases or decreases)
    b. Serum sodium results (increases or decreases)
    c. Urine output (increases or decreases)

42. Which of the following statements is correct about pheochromocytoma?
    a. It is most often malignant.
    b. It is a catecholamine-producing tumor.
    c. It is found only in the adrenal medulla.
    d. It is manifested by hypotension.

43. A client in the emergency department is diagnosed with possible pheochromocytoma. What is a priority nursing intervention for this client?
    a. Monitor the client's intake and output and the specific gravity.
    b. Monitor blood pressure for severe hypertension.
    c. Monitor blood pressure for severe hypotension.
    d. Administer medication to increase cardiac output.

44. The nurse would expect to perform which of the following diagnostic tests for pheochromocytoma?
    a. 24-hour urine collection for sodium, potassium, and glucose
    b. Catecholamine stimulation test
    c. Administration of beta-adrenergic blocking agent and monitor results
    d. 24-hour urine collection for vanillylmandelic acid (VMA)

45. Interventions for the client with pheochromocytoma include which of the following?
    a. Assisting the client to sit in a chair for blood pressure monitoring
    b. Instructing the client not to smoke or drink coffee
    c. Encouraging the client to maintain an active exercse schedule including activity such as running
    d. Encouraging one glass of red wine nightly to promote rest

46. Which one of these interventions is contraindicated for the client with pheochromocytoma, and why?
    a. Monitoring blood pressure
    b. Palpating the abdomen
    c. Collecting 24-hour urine specimens
    d. Instructing the client to limit activity

47. Which of the following diuretics is ordered by the physician to treat hyperaldosteronism, and why?
    a. Furosemide (Lasix)
    b. Ethacrynic acid (Edecrin)
    c. Bumetanide (Bumex)
    d. Spironolactone (Aldactone)

48. Which of the following statements about hyperaldosteronism is correct?
    a. Painful "charley horses" are common from hyperkalemia.
    b. It occurs more often in men than in women.
    c. It is a common cause of hypertension in the population.
    d. Hypokalemia and hypertension are the main issues.

49. Identify two types of tests and the findings that are diagnostic for clients suspected of having hyperaldosteronism.

    a. _____

    b. _____

50. When diagnosed with Cushing's syndrome, the manifestations are most likely related to an excess production of which of the following hormones?
    a. Insulin from the pancreas
    b. ADH from posterior pituitary gland
    c. Prolactin from anterior pituitary gland
    d. Cortisol from the adrenal cortex

51. What is the most common cause of endogenous hypercortisolism, or Cushing's syndrome?
    a. Pituitary hypoplasia
    b. Insufficient ACTH production
    c. Adrenocortical hormone deficiency
    d. Hyperplasia of the adrenal cortex

52. Which of the following are physical findings of Cushing's syndrome? *Choose all that apply.*
    a. A "moon-faced" appearance
    b. Decreased amount of body hair
    c. Barrel chest
    d. Truncal obesity
    e. Coarse facial features
    f. Thin, easily damaged skin
    g. Excessive sweating
    h. Extremity muscle wasting

53. When assessing the client with Cushing's syndrome, the nurse would expect to find which of the following?
    a. Signs of dehydration
    b. Facial flushing
    c. Hypertension
    d. Muscle hypertrophy

54. Explain the reason that samples of plasma cortisol levels should always be taken at the same time each day.

55. A client suspected of a diagnosis of Cushing's syndrome is scheduled for a 3-day, low dose dexamethasone suppression test. What does a nurse include in client education for this test?

56. The positive urine tests for Cushing's syndrome would show _____ _____.

57. A nurse selects "Risk for Injury related to effects of demineralization of bone" as a nursing diagnosis for a client with Cushing's disease. Identify the nursing interventions for this client.

58. A female client with Cushing's syndrome expresses concern to the nurse about the changes in her general appearance. The nurse determines a nursing diagnosis of Disturbed Body Image. Which of the following is the desired outcome for this client?
    a. To verbalize an understanding that treatment will reverse many of the problems
    b. To ventilate about the frustration of these lifelong physical changes
    c. To verbalize ways to cope with the changes such as joining a support group or changing style of dress
    d. To achieve a personal desired level of sexual functioning

59. Match each of the following drugs with the corresponding clinical use for hypercortisolism.

Medication

_____ a. Mitotane (Lysodren)

_____ b. Aminoglutethimide (Cytadren)

_____ c. Cyproheptadine (Periactin)

Clinical Use
1. Adrenal cytotoxic agent used for inoperable adrenal tumors
2. Interferes with ACTH production
3. Adrenal enzyme inhibitor that decreases cortisol production

60. Indicate the two surgical procedures for adrenocortical hypersecretion.

    a. _____

    b. _____

61. A client is scheduled for bilateral adrenalectomy. Before surgery, steroids are to be given. Identify the name of the medication and the reason why this medication is administered.

    Name of medication: _____
    a. To promote glycogen storage by the liver for body energy reserves
    b. To compensate for sudden lack of adrenal hormones following surgery
    c. To increase the body's inflammatory response to promote scar formation
    d. To enhance urinary excretion of salt and water following surgery

62. What is the rationale for using strict aseptic technique for a client about to undergo adrenalectomy?

63. Discharge teaching about medications for the client following bilateral adrenalectomy includes emphasizing that:
    a. The dosage of steroid replacement medications will be consistent throughout the client's lifetime.
    b. The steroid medications should be taken in the evening so as not to interfere with sleep.
    c. The client should take the medication on an empty stomach.
    d. The client should learn how to give himself an intramuscular injection of hydrocortisone.

64. Describe how you would explain the significance of wearing a medical alert tag to a client who has had a bilateral adrenalectomy.

65. Which of the following statements is correct regarding a client with hyperaldosteronism following a successful unilateral adrenalectomy?
    a. The low-sodium diet must be continued postoperatively.
    b. Glucocorticoid replacement therapy is temporary.
    c. Spironolactone (Aldactone) must be taken for life.
    d. Additional measures are needed to control hypertension.

66. Identify the three reasons for the decreased production of adrenocortical steroids.

    a. _____

    b. _____

    c. _____

67. Which of the following clients is at risk for developing secondary adrenal insufficiency, and why?
    a. A client who suddenly stops taking high-dose steroid therapy
    b. A client who tapers the dosages of steroid therapy
    c. A client who is deficient in ADH
    d. A client with an adrenal tumor causing excessive secretion of ACTH

68. An ACTH stimulation test is the most definitive test for which disorder?
    a. Adrenal insufficiency
    b. Cushing's syndrome
    c. Pheochromocytoma
    d. Acromegaly

69. Briefly discuss Addisonian crisis.

70. A client in the emergency department complaining of lethargy, muscle weakness, nausea, vomiting, and weight loss over the past weeks is diagnosed with Addisonian crisis (acute adrenal insufficiency). The nurse would expect to administer which of the following?
    a. Beta blocker to control the hypertension and dysrhythmias
    b. Solu-Cortef IV along with IM injections of hydrocortisone
    c. IV fluids of D_5 NS with KCl added for dehydration
    d. Spironolactone (Aldactone) to promote diuresis

71. The nurse would determine that the administration of hydrocortisone for Addisonian crisis was effective when which of the following assessments is made?
    a. Increased urine output
    b. No signs of pitting edema
    c. Weight gain
    d. Lethargy improving; client alert and oriented

72. Complete the chart by comparing the clinical findings in adrenal insufficiency with those in Cushing's syndrome. Indicate by + for increased or − for decreased.

Clinical Finding	Adrenal Insufficiency	Cushing's Syndrome
a. Serum sodium level		
b. Serum potassium level		
c. ECF volume		
d. Blood pressure		
e. Serum glucose level		
f. Cortisol level		

73. Preventive measures for adrenocortical insufficiency include which of the following?
    a. Maintaining diuretic therapy
    b. Instructing the client on salt restriction
    c. Reducing high-dose glucocorticoid therapy quickly
    d. Reducing high-dose glucocorticoid doses gradually

74. The client on prolonged cortisone therapy should be instructed to observe for and report signs of which of the following?
    a. Anuria and hypoglycemia
    b. Weight gain and moon face
    c. Anorexia and muscle twitches
    d. Hypotension and fluid loss

75. Complete this chart comparing endocrine disorders. Use a separate sheet of paper if necessary.

| Categories | Pituitary Disorder | | Adrenal Disorder | |
	Excess	Deficit	Excess	Deficit
Common abnormal diagnostic laboratory test values				
Common abnormal radiologic tests				
Common clinical manifestations				
Common therapeutic drug regimen				
Diet therapy				

CASE STUDY: THE CLIENT WITH DIABETES INSIPIDUS

Answer Guidelines for the Case Study questions are provided on the companion Evolve Learning Resources Web site at http://evolve.elsevier.com/Iggy/.

A 22-year-old man has been admitted to the emergency department after his girlfriend found him lying in the floor of their apartment. He had fallen off a ladder 2 days ago but "seemed fine," according to the girlfriend, even though he had hit his head slightly when he fell. He never lost consciousness. He has a few abrasions on his arms, face, and legs, and is drowsy but arousable. His girlfriend states that yesterday he started "going to the bathroom nonstop" and he drank "everything in sight" because he was so thirsty. A magnetic resonance imaging (MRI) scan reveals a small intracerebral hemorrhage, and he is admitted to the intensive care unit with the diagnosis of head trauma and diabetes insipidus (DI).

1. What physical and laboratory findings led to the diagnosis of diabetes insipidus?

2. The physician is considering whether this client is a candidate for the fluid deprivation and hypertonic saline tests to confirm the diagnosis of DI. How is this determined?

3. Identify potential nursing diagnoses for this client based on the above data.

4. Identify nursing measures that would assist the client to maintain an adequate fluid balance. State the rationale for these measures.

5. The physician initially orders aqueous vasopressin (Pitressin) 10 units IM every 3 to 4 hours as indicated. How does the nurse determine when to give the medication?

6. The client recovers sufficiently to be dismissed to home care. He is to continue the vasopressin via nasal spray. Develop a teaching-learning plan for the client for self-administration of the vasopressin.

Interventions for Clients with Problems of the Thyroid and Parathyroid Glands

LEARNING OUTCOMES

1. Compare the common clinical manifestations of hyperthyroidism with those of hypothyroidism.

2. Explain the pathophysiology of Graves' disease.

3. Describe the mechanisms of action, side effects, and nursing implications for pharmacologic management of hyperthyroidism.

4. Interpret clinical changes and laboratory data to determine the effectiveness of interventions for hyperthyroidism.

5. Prioritize nursing care for the client during the first 24 hours following a total thyroidectomy.

6. Explain the pathophysiology of Hashimoto's thyroiditis.

7. Identify teaching priorities for the client taking thyroid hormone replacement therapy.

8. Interpret clinical changes and laboratory data to determine the effectiveness of interventions for hypothyroidism.

9. Compare the clinical manifestations of hyperparathyroidism with those of hypoparathyroidism.

10. Prioritize nursing care for the client during the first 24 hours following a parathyroidectomy.

11. Interpret clinical changes and laboratory data to determine the effectiveness of interventions for parathyroid problems.

LEARNING ACTIVITIES

1. Before completing the study guide exercises in this chapter, it is recommended that you review the following:
   - Anatomy and physiology of the thyroid and parathyroid glands
   - Functions of the hormones of the thyroid and parathyroid glands
   - Normal growth and development and the effects of aging on the thyroid and parathyroid glands
   - Sympathetic nervous system
   - Normal laboratory values for serum and urine sodium, calcium, and phosphorus
   - Principles of fluid and electrolyte balance and acid-base balance
   - Perioperative nursing care
   - Principles of airway management
   - Concepts of body image and self-esteem

- Concepts of fatigue
- Assessment of the endocrine system

2. Review the boldfaced terms and their definitions in Chapter 67 to enhance your understanding of the content.

STUDY/REVIEW QUESTIONS

Answers to the Study/Review Questions are provided on the companion Evolve Learning Resources Web site at http://evolve.elsevier.com/Iggy/.

1. When performing a physical examination of the thyroid gland, precautions are taken in performing the correct technique because palpation can result in which of the following?
   a. Damage to the esophagus, causing gastric reflux
   b. An obstruction of the carotid arteries causing a stroke
   c. Pressure on the trachea and laryngeal nerve causing hoarseness
   d. An exacerbation of symptoms by releasing additional thyroid hormone

2. Thyroid hormones affect the basal metabolic rate. Briefly describe the effect of excessive and inadequate thyroid hormone production on the basal metabolic rate and the resulting thyroid disorder.

3. Differentiate the general assessment findings by matching them with the corresponding type of thyroid deficiency. *Answers may be used more than once.*

Assessment Finding

_____ a. Weight loss with increased appetite

_____ b. Constipation

_____ c. Increased heart rate, palpitations

_____ d. Photophobia

_____ e. Manic behavior

_____ f. Decreased libido

_____ g. Dyspnea with or without exertion

_____ h. Insomnia

_____ i. Cold intolerance

_____ j. Increased stools

_____ k. Corneal ulcers

_____ l. Fatigue, increased sleeping

_____ m. Irritability

_____ n. Impaired memory

_____ o. Fine, soft, silky body hair

_____ p. Facial puffiness

_____ q. Increased libido

_____ r. Heat intolerance, warm skin

_____ s. Weight gain

_____ t. Dry, coarse, brittle hair

_____ u. Diaphoresis

_____ v. Tremors

Thyroid Deficiency
1. Hyperthyroidism
2. Hypothyroidism

4. Which of the following is the hallmark assessment finding signifying hyperthyroidism?
   a. Weight loss
   b. Increased libido
   c. Heat intolerance
   d. Diarrhea

5. Which of the following is a main assessment finding signifying hypothyroidism?
   a. Irritability
   b. Cold intolerance
   c. Constipation
   d. Fatigue

6. What is one of the first signals of hyperthyroidism that is often noticed by a client?
   a. Eyelid or globe lag
   b. Vision changes or tiring of the eyes
   c. Protruding eyes
   d. Photophobia

7. Which of the following laboratory results is consistent with hyperthyroidism?
   a. Decreased serum triiodothyronine (T_3) and thyroxine (T_4) levels
   b. Elevated serum thyrotropin-releasing hormone (TRH) level
   c. Decreased radioactive iodine uptake
   d. Increased serum T_3 and T_4

8. The laboratory results for a 53-year-old client indicate a low T_3 level and elevated TSH. What do these results indicate?
   a. Hyperthyroidism
   b. Hypothyroidism
   c. Malfunctioning pituitary gland
   d. Normal laboratory values for this age

9. The clinical manifestation resulting from an increase in thyroid hormone production is known as which of the following?
   a. Thyrotoxicosis
   b. Euthyroid function
   c. Graves' disease
   d. Hypermetabolism

10. What is the most common cause of hyperthyroidism?
    a. Radiation to thyroid
    b. Graves' disease
    c. Thyroid cancer
    d. Thyroiditis

11. Upon examination of a client with a goiter, the nurse notes that the mass is not visible with the neck in the normal position, but the goiter can be palpated and moves up when the client swallows. What grade would this goiter be classified as?
    a. Grade 0
    b. Grade 1
    c. Grade 2
    d. Grade 3

12. Describe each of the following assessment findings that are associated with hyperthyroidism and Graves' disease.
    a. Exophthalmos

    b. Pretibial myxedema

    c. Eyelid retraction (eyelid lag)

    d. Globe (eyeball) lag

13. Graves' disease and Hashimoto's disease are autoimmune disorders of the thyroid. Briefly describe the cause and pathophysiology of each disease.

14. Read the following statements regarding hypothyroidism and hyperthyroidism. If the statement is true, write T in the blank provided. If it is false, write F and correct the statement to make it true.

_____ a.   Exophthalmos only occurs in hyperthyroidism resulting from Graves' disease.

_____ b.   Graves' disease is hereditary.

_____ c.   A decreased metabolic rate results in TSH binding to thyroid cells, causing an enlarged thyroid.

_____ d.   Hypothyroidism can occur anytime throughout the life span.

_____ e.   Hypothyroidism and hyperthyroidism occur more frequently in women than men.

_____ f.   Simple goiter associated with hypothyroidism is usually due to insufficient iodine intake.

_____ g.   Hashimoto's disease is a type of hypothyroidism.

_____ h.   The effect of antithyroid medication can be delayed due to storage and release of large amounts of thyroid hormone.

_____ i.   Hypothyroidism causes elevated systolic pressure, wide pulse pressure, tachycardia, and dysrhythmias.

_____ j.   Thyroid storm following surgical intervention for hyperthyroidism is rare because of pretreatment with medications.

_____ k.   Euthyroid is defined as near-normal thyroid function.

_____ l.   Radiation precautions are required with treatment of ^{131}I for hyperthyroidism.

_____ m.   Nonsurgical treatment is the preferred treatment for hyperthyroidism.

15. A client has been diagnosed with having a thyroid goiter. Briefly define thyroid goiter and how it differs from thyroid nodule.

16. Laboratory findings of elevated T_3 and T_4, decreased TSH, and high thyrotropin receptor antibody titer indicate which of the following?
    a.   A multinodular goiter
    b.   Hyperthyroidism related to overmedication
    c.   A pituitary tumor suppressing TSH
    d.   Graves' disease

17. A client with hypothyroidism asks the physician about possible causes of this disorder. Briefly explain possible causes of decreased synthesis of thyroid hormones.

18.   A client who has been diagnosed with hypothyroidism has problems with constipation and dry, rough skin. What interventions can the nurse teach the client to perform in order to help relieve these problems?

19.   After a visit to the physician's office, a client is diagnosed with general thyroid enlargement and elevated thyroid hormone level. This would be an indication of which of the following?
    a.   Hyperthyroidism and goiter
    b.   Hypothyroidism and goiter
    c.   Nodules on the parathyroid gland
    d.   Thyroid or parathyroid cancer

20.   Which of the following conditions is a life-threatening emergency and serious complication of untreated or poorly treated hypothyroidism?
    a.   An endemic goiter
    b.   Myxedema coma
    c.   A toxic multinodular goiter
    d.   Thyroiditis

21.   A client with exophthalmos from hyperthyroidism complains of dry eyes, especially in the morning. The nurse teaches the client to perform which of the following interventions to help correct this problem?
    a.   Wear sunglasses at all times when outside in the bright sun.
    b.   Use cool compresses to the eye four times a day.
    c.   Tape the eyes closed with nonallergenic tape.
    d.   There is nothing that can be done to relieve this problem.

22.   A client was admitted to the hospital from the emergency department with a diagnosis of thyroid storm (crisis). Define thyroid storm. What triggers it? What clinical manifestations would a nurse expect to find on assessment?

23.   A client has the following assessment findings: elevated TSH level, low T_3 and T_4 level, difficulty with memory, lethargy, and muscle stiffness. These are clinical manifestations of which of the following?
    a.   Hypothyroidism
    b.   Hyperthyroidism
    c.   Hypoparathyroidism
    d.   Hyperparathyroidism

24.   With correction of hypothyroidism with thyroid hormone, the client can expect improvement in mental awareness within how long?
    a.   A few days
    b.   2 weeks
    c.   1 month
    d.   3 months

25.   Briefly describe interventions a nurse would perform for a client with a diagnosis of thyroid storm.

26. Management of the client with hyperthyroidism focuses on which of the following? *Check all that apply*.

_____ a. Blocking the effects of excessive thyroid secretion

_____ b. Treating the signs and symptoms the client experiences

_____ c. Establishing euthyroid function

_____ d. Preventing spread of the disease

27. Match each of the following characteristics with the corresponding intervention for hyperthyroidism. *Answers may be used more than once. Choose all answers that apply to each characteristic.*

Characteristic

_____ a. Discontinued if sore throat, fever, headache, or skin eruptions occur

_____ b. Use includes preoperative treatment to obtain euthyroid

_____ c. Action decreases the production of thyroid hormone

_____ d. Works to control symptoms related to sympathetic nervous system of tachycardia, palpations, anxiety, and diaphoresis

_____ e. Requires lifelong thyroid replacement

_____ f. Limited use due to side effects

_____ g. Taken with food

_____ h. Monitor for hypothyroidism over time

_____ i. Contraindicated in pregnancy; crosses placenta barrier

_____ j. Administered around the clock

_____ k. May require antithyroid medication for up to 8 weeks past treatment

_____ l. Acts to decrease blood flow to reduce hormone production with results in 2 to 6 weeks

_____ m. Works by damaging thyroid gland

_____ n. Removal of all of the thyroid gland

_____ o. Instruct client to avoid crowds and sick people due to reduced immune response

_____ p. Treatment for thyroid cancer

Intervention for Hyperthyroidism
1. Antithyroid drug Tapazole
2. Antithyroid drug PTU
3. Iodine preparations
4. Lithium carbonate
5. Beta-blocking agents (Inderal)
6. Radioactive iodine (^{131}I)
7. Subtotal thyroidectomy
8. Total thyroidectomy
9. Dexamethasone

28. Preoperative instructions for clients having thyroid surgery would include which of the following? *Check all that apply. Make changes to the incorrect answers to make them correct.*

_____ a. Teach postoperative restrictions such as no cough and deep breathing exercises to prevent strain on the suture line.

_____ b. Teach moving and turning technique of manually supporting the head and avoiding neck extension to minimize strain on the suture line.

_____ c. Inform the client that hoarseness for a few days after surgery is usually the result of a breathing tube (endotracheal tube) used during surgery but will be monitored with respiration and weakness of voice.

_____ d. Humidification of air maybe helpful to promote expectoration of secretions. Suctioning may also be used.

_____ e.   Clarify any questions regarding placement of incision, complications, and postoperative care.

_____ f.   Supine position and lying flat will be maintained postoperatively to avoid strain on suture line.

_____ g.   Teach the client to report immediately any respiratory difficulty, tingling around lips or fingers, or muscular twitching.

_____ h.   A drain may be present in the incision. All drainage and dressings will be monitored closely for 24 hours.

29.   A nurse is preparing to receive a client on the postoperative unit following thyroid surgery. Explain the purpose of each of the following items that should be available for this client. What assessment findings would indicate immediate notification of the physician and potential use of these items?
a.   Tracheostomy equipment
b.   Calcium gluconate or calcium chloride for IV administration
c.   Oxygen and suction equipment

30.   Following a thyroidectomy, a client complains of tingling around the mouth and muscle twitching. These assessment findings indicate to the nurse which of the following complications?
a.   Hemorrhage
b.   Respiratory distress
c.   Thyroid storm
d.   Hypocalcemia, parathyroid gland injury

31.   Postoperatively, the nurse monitors the client for the complication of laryngeal nerve damage. Identify assessment findings that may indicate this problem. What can you tell the client about these findings?

32.   Identify the three common nursing diagnoses for a client with hypothyroidism. Also, briefly describe both the rationale for your selection and the related nursing interventions.

33.   Describe the monitoring and teaching nursing interventions related to a client receiving thyroid hormone replacement therapy.

34.   Following hospitalization for myxedema, a client is prescribed thyroid replacement medication. Which of the following statements would demonstrate the client's correct understanding of this therapy?
a.   "I will be taking this medication until my symptoms are completely resolved."
b.   "I will be taking thyroid medication for the rest of my life."
c.   "Now that I am feeling better, no changes in my medication will be necessary."
d.   "I am taking this medication to prevent symptoms of an 'overactive thyroid gland.'"

35. Match each characteristic with the corresponding thyroid disorder. *Answers may be used more than once.*

Characteristic

_____ a. Defined as inflammation of the thyroid gland

_____ b. "Chronic thyroiditis"

_____ c. Common in age range 30s to 50s

_____ d. Caused by viral infection of thyroid gland after an upper respiratory infection

_____ e. Bacterial infection of thyroid gland

_____ f. Subtotal thyroidectomy is a form of treatment

_____ g. Treated with antibiotics

_____ h. Treated with thyroid replacement hormone

_____ i. Diagnosed by circulating antithyroid antibodies and needle biopsy

Thyroid Disorder
1. Thyroiditis
2. Hashimoto's disease
3. Acute thyroiditis
4. Subacute thyroiditis

36. Serum calcium levels are maintained by which of the following two hormones? *Select two answers.*

_____ a. Cortisol

_____ b. Calcitonin

_____ c. ADH

_____ d. PTH

37. Briefly explain how parathyroid hormone (PTH) and calcitonin maintain the serum calcium levels.

38. Match each hormone with the corresponding effect on the serum calcium levels.

Hormone

_____ a. Parathyroid hormone production

_____ b. Calcitonin production

Effect
1. Raises levels
2. Lowers levels

39. Bone changes in the older adult are often seen with endocrine dysfunction and increased secretion of which of the following?
   a. Parathyroid hormone
   b. Calcitonin
   c. Insulin
   d. Testosterone

40. In addition to regulation of calcium levels, parathyroid hormone and calcitonin regulate the circulating blood levels of which of the following?
   a. Potassium
   b. Sodium
   c. Phosphate
   d. Chloride

41. Briefly explain how the parathyroid hormone maintains phosphate balance.

42. A client has a positive Trousseau's or Chvostek's sign resulting from hypoparathyroidism. This assessment finding indicates which of the following?
   a. Hypercalcemia
   b. Hypocalcemia
   c. Hyperphosphatemia
   d. Hypophosphatemia

43. Which food should the client with hypo-
    parathyroidism avoid?
    a.   Canned vegetables
    b.   Fresh fruit
    c.   Red meat
    d.   Milk

44. A client in the emergency department who
    had continuous spasm of the muscles was
    diagnosed with hypoparathyroidism. The
    muscle spasms are a clinical manifestation
    of which of the following?
    a.   Nerve damage
    b.   Seizures
    c.   Tetany
    d.   Decreased potassium

45. Match the following causes with the para-
    thyroid disorder. *Answers may be used
    more than once.*

Cause

_____ a.   Chronic renal disease

_____ b.   Vitamin D deficiency

_____ c.   Removal of the thyroid gland

_____ d.   Neck trauma

_____ e.   Carcinoma of the lung, kidney, or GI
           tract producing PTH-like substance

_____ f.   Parathyroidectomy

Parathyroid Disorder
1.   Hypoparathyroidism
2.   Hyperparathyroidism

46. When interpreting laboratory values, what would the nurse expect to find in relation to hypopara-
    thyroidism and hyperparathyroidism? Indicate an increase (+) or decrease (–) in the adult normal
    range for the following laboratory tests.

Laboratory Test	Hyperparathyroidism (+/-)	Hypoparathyroidism (+/-)
a. Serum calcium		
b. Serum phosphate		
c. Serum parathyroid hormone (PTH)		

47. Which of the following is the most common
    initial treatment a client with hyperparathy-
    roidism and high levels of serum calcium
    will receive?
    a.   Force fluids (IV or PO) and administer
         Lasix
    b.   Calcitonin
    c.   Oral phosphates
    d.   Mithramycin

48. Postoperative nursing care for parathyroid-
    ectomy is similar to that of thyroid surgery
    with emphasis on monitoring and providing
    emergency intervention for which of the
    following?
    a.   Hypercalcemia
    b.   Hypocalcemia
    c.   Intake and output
    d.   Vitamin D deficiency

49. Identify the signs and symptoms of hypocalcemia.

50. Identify four medications that are frequently used to treat hypoparathyroidism.

    a. _____

    b. _____

    c. _____

    d. _____

51. Discharge planning for a client who has chronic hypoparathyroidism should include which of the following? *Choose all that apply.*

    _____ a. Reinforcing that the prescribed medications must be taken for the client's entire life

    _____ b. Teaching client to eat foods low in vitamin D and high in phosphorus

    _____ c. Teaching client to eat foods high in calcium but low in phosphorus

    _____ d. After several weeks, medications can be discontinued

    _____ e. Teaching that kidney stones are no longer a risk to the client

52. In older adults, assessment findings of fatigue, altered thought processes, dry skin, and constipation are often mistaken for signs of aging rather than assessment findings for which endocrine disorder?
    a. Hyperthyroidism
    b. Hypothyroidism
    c. Hyperparathyroidism
    d. Hypoparathyroidism

53. Which of the following conditions may precipitate myxedema coma? *Choose all that apply.*

    _____ a. Rapid withdrawal of thyroid medication

    _____ b. Vitamin D deficiency

    _____ c. Untreated hypothyroidism

    _____ d. Surgery

    _____ e. Excessive exposure to iodine

54. Complete the following chart comparing endocrine disorders. Use a separate sheet of paper if necessary.

Categories	Thyroid Disorder		Parathyroid Disorder	
	Excess	**Deficit**	**Excess**	**Deficit**
Common abnormal diagnostic laboratory test values				
Common abnormal radiologic tests				
Common clinical manifestations				
Common therapeutic drug regimen				
Diet therapy				

55. Complete the following chart comparing endocrine emergencies. Use a separate sheet of paper if necessary.

Categories	Myxedema	Thyroid storm
Events that precipitate the crisis		
Common abnormal lab and other diagnostic tests		
Priority emergency interventions		

Interventions for Clients with Diabetes Mellitus

CHAPTER

68

LEARNING OUTCOMES

1. Compare the age of onset, clinical manifestations, and pathologic mechanisms of type 1 and type 2 diabetes mellitus.

2. Identify clients at risk for type 2 diabetes mellitus.

3. Explain the effects of insulin on carbohydrate, protein, and fat metabolism.

4. Evaluate laboratory data to determine whether the client is using the prescribed dietary, medication, and exercise interventions for diabetes.

5. Explain the effect of aerobic exercise on blood glucose levels.

6. Describe the significance of ketone bodies in the urine of a diabetic client.

7. Discuss the dietary requirements of clients taking Humalog insulin before meals.

8. Identify eating habits and patterns that place the diabetic client at increased risk for hypoglycemia and hyperglycemia.

9. Compare the mechanisms of action of the sulfonylureas, meglitinide analogues, biguanides, alpha glucosidase inhibitors, and thiazolidinediones as antidiabetic agents.

10. Explain the effect of hypertension on the development of diabetic nephropathy and diabetic retinopathy.

11. Identify clients at risk for hypoglycemia.

12. Prioritize nursing interventions for the client with mild to moderate hypoglycemia and moderate to severe hypoglycemia.

13. Identify clients at risk for diabetic ketoacidosis (DKA).

14. Prioritize nursing interventions for clients with DKA.

15. Identify clients at risk for hyperglycemic-hyperosmolar nonketotic syndrome (HHNS).

16. Prioritize nursing interventions for clients with HHNS.

17. Use laboratory data and clinical manifestations to determine the effectiveness of the interventions for DKA and HHNS.

18. Describe the steps required for subcutaneous insulin administration.

19. Describe the correct technique to use when mixing different types of insulin in the same syringe.

20. Compare the clinical manifestations of hyperglycemia and hypoglycemia.

21. Perform foot assessment and foot care for the client with diabetes.

LEARNING ACTIVITIES

1. Before completing the study guide exercises for this chapter, it is recommended that you review the following:
    *   Anatomy and physiology of the pancreas and kidneys
    *   Function of insulin in the body
    *   Normal laboratory values for serum and urine glucose, osmolarity, and electrolytes
    *   Principles of fluid and electrolyte balance and acid-base balance
    *   Subcutaneous injections
    *   Assessment of the endocrine system

2. Review the boldfaced terms and their definitions in Chapter 68 to enhance your understanding of the content.

STUDY/REVIEW QUESTIONS

Answers to the Study/Review Questions are provided on the companion Evolve Learning Resources Web site at http://evolve.elsevier.com/Iggy/.

1. Briefly describe diabetes mellitus.

2. Define type 1 diabetes, type 2 diabetes, and gestational diabetes.

3. Which of the following statements is correct about insulin?
    a. It is secreted by alpha cells in the islets of Langerhans.
    b. It is a catabolic hormone that builds up glucagon reserves.
    c. It is necessary for glucose transport across cell membranes.
    d. It is stored in muscles and converted to fat for storage.

4. Why is glucose vital to the body's cells?
    a. It is used to build cell membranes.
    b. It is used by cells to produce energy.
    c. It affects the process of protein metabolism.
    d. It provides nutrients for genetic material.

5. Identify the counter-regulatory hormones released during episodes of hypoglycemia. Which one is considered the main counter-regulatory hormone?

    a. _____

    b. _____

    c. _____

    d. _____

    e. _____

Match the following terms with their correct definitions. For each term, briefly describe the pathophysiology that causes these classic symptoms.

Definition
a. Frequent urination
b. Frequent fluid intake
c. Frequent eating

Term

_____ 6. Polydipsia

_____ 7. Polyphagia

_____ 8. Polyuria

9. Which of the following individuals is at greatest risk for developing type 2 diabetes mellitus?
   a. A 25-year-old African-American woman
   b. A 36-year-old African-American man
   c. A 56-year-old Hispanic woman
   d. A 40-year-old Hispanic man

10. Which of the following four laboratory findings is most diagnostic of diabetes mellitus?
    a. Fasting blood glucose = 80 mg/dL
    b. 2-hour postprandial blood glucose = 110 mg/dL
    c. 1-hour glucose tolerance blood glucose = 110 mg/dL
    d. 2-hour glucose tolerance blood glucose = 210 mg/dL

11. Compare and contrast type 1 and type 2 diabetes mellitus. Underline similarities and highlight differences.

12. Untreated hyperglycemia results in which of the following?
    a. Respiratory acidosis
    b. Metabolic alkalosis
    c. Respiratory alkalosis
    d. Metabolic acidosis

13. What is the respiratory pattern of the client with untreated hyperglycemia?
    a. Rapid and shallow (tachypneic)
    b. Deep and labored (Cheyne-Stokes respiration)
    c. Rapid and deep (Kussmaul respiration)
    d. Shallow and labored (Biot respiration)

14. Which of the following electrolytes is most affected by hyperglycemia?
    a. Sodium
    b. Chloride
    c. Potassium
    d. Magnesium

15. Identify the three emergencies for clients with diabetes mellitus and their causes.

    a. _____

    b. _____

    c. _____

16. In determining whether a client is hypoglycemic, the nurse would look for which characteristics in addition to checking the blood glucose? *Check all that apply.*

       _____ a.   Nausea

       _____ b.   Hunger

       _____ c.   Irritability

       _____ d.   Rapid pulse

       _____ e.   Profuse perspiration

       _____ f.   Rapid deep respirations

17. The differences between diabetic ketoacidosis (DKA) and hyperglycemic-hyperosmolar-nonketotic syndrome (HHNS) include which of the following? *Check all that apply.*

       _____ a.   Level of hyperglycemia

       _____ b.   Amount of ketones produced

       _____ c.   Potassium levels

       _____ d.   Amount of volume depletion

18. A client is admitted with a blood glucose level of 900 mg/dL. Intravenous fluids and insulin are administered. Two hours after treatment is initiated, the blood glucose level is 400 mg/dL. Which of the following complications is the client most at risk for developing?
    a.   Hypoglycemia
    b.   Pulmonary embolus
    c.   Renal shutdown
    d.   Pulmonary edema

19. What type of insulin is used in the emergency treatment of DKA and HHNS?
    a.   NPH
    b.   Lente
    c.   Regular
    d.   Protamine zinc

20. Early treatment of DKA and HHNS includes intravenous administration of which of the following?
    a.   Glucagon
    b.   Potassium
    c.   Bicarbonate
    d.   Normal saline

21. Glucagon is used primarily to treat the client with which of the following?
    a.   DKA
    b.   Idiosyncratic reaction to insulin
    c.   Severe hypoglycemia
    d.   HHNS

22. Glucagon is given in a dextrose solution because dextrose does what?
    a.   Promotes more storage of glucose in the liver
    b.   Stimulates the pancreas to produce more insulin
    c.   Increases blood sugar levels at a controlled rate
    d.   Inhibits glycogenesis, gluconeogenesis, and lipolysis

23. When glucagon is administered, it:
    a.   Competes for insulin at the receptor sites
    b.   Frees glucose from hepatic stores of glycogen
    c.   Supplies glycogen directly to the vital tissues
    d.   Provides a glucose substitute for rapid replacement

Match each of the following etiologic factors with the corresponding type of diabetes mellitus. Answers may be used more than once.

Type of Diabetes Mellitus
a.   Type 1
b.   Type 2
c.   Gestational

Etiologic Factor

_____ 24. Aging process

_____ 25. Autoimmune process

_____ 26. Islet cell antibodies

_____ 27. Obesity

_____ 28. Heredity

_____ 29. Pregnancy

_____ 30. Viral infection

_____ 31. Decreased physical activity

32. Preventive measures for diabetes mellitus include which of the following?
    a. Controlling hypertension
    b. Prenatal care beginning the third trimester of pregnancy
    c. Working in a low-stress environment
    d. Maintaining ideal body weight

33. A diabetic client is scheduled to have a blood glucose test the next morning. Which of the following should the nurse tell the client to do before coming in for the test?
    a. Eat the usual diet but have nothing after midnight.
    b. Take the usual oral hypoglycemic tablet in the morning.
    c. Eat a clear liquid breakfast in the morning.
    d. Follow the usual diet and medication regimen.

34. The frequency with which a client should monitor capillary blood glucose levels depends on levels of which of the following?
    a. Urine glucose
    b. Serum ketones
    c. Serum glucose
    d. Urine ketones

35. Briefly discuss the significance of the presence of protein in the urine without renal symptoms.

36. If protein is present in the urine, what other tests should be performed?

37. Discuss the usefulness of monitoring urine glucose levels to manage diabetes mellitus.

Match each of the following oral antidiabetic medications with the corresponding nursing intervention.

Nursing Intervention
a. Give drug just before meals.
b. Hold drug for 48 hours if having x-ray with IV contrast dye (renal).
c. Hypoglycemic episodes are more likely to occur because of its long duration of action.
d. Give drug with first bite of each main meal.

Medication
_____ 38. Chlorpropamide (Diabinese)
_____ 39. Metformin (Glucophage)
_____ 40. Miglitol (Glyset)
_____ 41. Nateglinide (Starlix)

42. Identify the two most common side effects of administering oral antidiabetic agents.

    a. _____

    b. _____

43. When giving oral antidiabetic agents, the nurse should demonstrate caution with clients who are known to have what four types of body system problems?

    a. _____

    b. _____

    c. _____

    d. _____

44. Which of the following statements is correct about insulin?
    a. Exogenous insulin is necessary for management of all cases of type 2 diabetes.
    b. Insulin's effectiveness depends on the individual client's absorption of the drug.
    c. Insulin doses should be regulated according to self-monitoring urine glucose levels.
    d. Insulin administered in multiple doses per day decreases the flexibility of a client's lifestyle.

45. Which of the following statements is correct about insulin administration?
    a. Insulin may be given orally, intravenously, or subcutaneously.
    b. Insulin injections should be spaced no closer than one-half inch apart.
    c. Rotating injection sites improves absorption and prevents lipohypertrophy.
    d. In a mixed-dose protocol, the longer-acting insulin should be withdrawn first.

46. A diabetic is on a mixed-dose insulin protocol of 8 units regular insulin and 12 units NPH insulin at 7 AM. At 10:30 AM, the client reports feeling uneasy, shaky, and complains of a headache. Which is the probable explanation for this?
    a. The NPH insulin's action is peaking, and there is an insufficient blood glucose level.
    b. The regular insulin's action is peaking, and there is an insufficient blood glucose level.
    c. The client consumed too many calories at breakfast and now has an elevated blood glucose level.
    d. The symptoms are unrelated to the insulin administered in the early morning or diet taken in at lunchtime.

47. A client has orders for 40 units of insulin zinc suspension (Lente insulin) and 10 units of regular insulin every morning. Explain how these drugs should be prepared for administration. What should the client be told about these actions and the side effects of these medications?

48. Describe two problems with blood glucose levels that may occur during the night if a client is on insulin therapy.

49. The client who is to use an external insulin pump should be told that:
    a. Self-monitoring of blood glucose levels can be done only twice a day.
    b. The insulin supply must be replaced every 2 to 4 weeks.
    c. The pump's battery should be checked on a regular weekly schedule.
    d. The needle site must be changed every 1 to 3 days.

50. A 47-year-old client with a history of type 2 diabetes mellitus and emphysema who reports smoking three packs of cigarettes per day is admitted to the hospital with a diagnosis of acute pneumonia. The client is placed on his regular oral antidiabetic agents, sliding scale insulin, and antibiotic medications. On day 2 of hospitalization, the doctor orders prednisone therapy. What would the nurse expect the blood glucose to do?
    a. Decrease
    b. Stay the same
    c. Increase
    d. Return to normal

51. Identify the laboratory test that is the best indicator of the client's average blood glucose level and/or compliance to the diabetes mellitus regimen over the last 3 months.
    a. Postprandial test
    b. Oral glucose tolerance test (OGTT)
    c. Casual blood glucose test
    d. Glycosylated hemoglobin (HbA1c)

52. What is the earliest clinical sign of nephropathy?
    a. Proteinuria
    b. Ketonuria
    c. Glucosuria
    d. Microalbuminuria

53. The client's blood glucose level obtained from a fingerstick blood glucose monitor reads 20 mg/dL. Determine the next three priority nursing interventions.

   a. _____

   b. _____

   c. _____

54. A diabetic client has just returned from surgery with stable blood glucose levels between 120 and 180 mg/dL. Identify the appropriate IV solution to promote adequate hydration and stable blood glucose levels.
   a. D$_5$ 1/2 NS at 125 mL/hr
   b. D$_5$W at 125 mL/hr
   c. 0.45 % NSS at 100 mL/hr
   d. 0.9% NSS at 100 mL/hr

55. A client with type 2 diabetes mellitus, usually controlled with a sulfonylurea, develops a urinary tract infection. Due to the stress of the infection, she must be treated with insulin. She should be instructed that:
   a. The sulfonylurea must be discontinued and insulin taken until the infection clears.
   b. Insulin will now be necessary to control the client's diabetes for life.
   c. The sulfonylurea dose must be reduced until the infection clears.
   d. The insulin is necessary to supplement the sulfonylurea until the infection clears.

Match each of the following diabetic complications with the corresponding pathophysiology. Answers may be used more than once.

Pathophysiology
a. Nephropathy
b. Neuropathy
c. Retinopathy

Complication

_____ 56. Neovascularization

_____ 57. End-stage renal disease

_____ 58. Muscle weakness

_____ 59. Proteinuria

_____ 60. Hemorrhage into the eye

_____ 61. Pain or numbness

_____ 62. Hard exudates on fundus

_____ 63. Permanent blindness

64. Which of the following statements about sensory alterations in clients with diabetes is true? *Check all that apply and correct statements that are not true.*

   _____ a. Healing of foot wounds is reduced because of impaired sensation.

   _____ b. Sensory neuropathy, ischemia, and infection are the leading causes of foot disease among diabetics.

   _____ c. Very few clients with diabetic foot ulcers have peripheral sensory neuropathy.

   _____ d. Loss of pain, pressure, and temperature sensation in the foot increases the risk for injury.

65. According to the Diabetes Control and Complication Trial (DCCT) study of type 1 diabetes mellitus clients, intensive therapy with good glucose control resulted in what types of health benefits?

66. Match the definition with the foot condition described.

Definition

_____ a. Hyperextended toes, causing increased pressure on the ball of the foot.

_____ b. Deformity where the foot is warm, swollen, painful, and walking causes the arch to collapse, giving the foot a "rocker bottom" shape.

_____ c. Turning of the great toe

Foot Condition
1. Hallux valgus
2. Claw toe deformity
3. Charcot foot

67. Identify the factors that should be considered when developing an individualized meal plan for the diabetic client.

a. _____

b. _____

c. _____

d. _____

68. Which of the following is a basic principle of meal planning for the client with type 1 diabetes?
   a. Five small meals per day plus a bedtime snack
   b. Taking extra insulin when planning to eat sweet foods
   c. High-protein, low-carbohydrate, and low-fiber foods
   d. Considering the effects and peak action times of the client's insulin

69. Identify the food groups in the exchange system of diabetic meal planning.

a. _____

b. _____

c. _____

70. Which of the following statements about dietary concepts for the diabetic client is correct?
   a. Alcoholic beverage consumption is unrestricted.
   b. Carbohydrate counting is emphasized when adjusting dietary intake of nutrients.
   c. Sweeteners should be avoided because of the side effects.
   d. Both soluble and insoluble fiber foods should be limited.

71. The recommended protocol for type 2 diabetic clients who must lose weight is to do which of the following?
   a. Participate in aerobic program twice a week for 20 minutes each session.
   b. Slowly increase insulin dosage until mild hypoglycemia occurs.
   c. Reduce calorie intake moderately and increase exercise.
   d. Reduce daily calorie intake to 1000 calories and monitor urine for ketones.

72. What is the recommended calorie reduction for the diabetic client who must lose weight?
   a. 500 calories/week
   b. 1500 calories/week
   c. 2500 calories/week
   d. 3500 calories/week

73. The diabetic client who swims for exercise should be taught to administer insulin in which area of the body?
   a. Abdomen
   b. Thighs
   c. Arms
   d. Hips

74. Discuss the purpose of having a supply of simple sugar available for the diabetic client when he or she is exercising.

75. Diabetic foot care includes which of the following?
    a. Using rubbing alcohol to toughen the skin on the soles of the feet
    b. Wearing open-toed shoes or sandals in warm weather to prevent perspiration
    c. Applying moisturizing cream to the feet after bathing, but not between the toes
    d. Using cold water for bathing feet to prevent inadvertent thermal injury

76. A 25-year-old female client with type 1 diabetes tells the nurse, "I have two kidneys and I'm still young. I expect to be around for a long time, so why should I worry about my blood sugar?" Which of the following is the nurse's best reply?
    a. "You have little to worry about as long as your kidneys keep making urine."
    b. "You should discuss this with your physician because you are being unrealistic."
    c. "You would be correct if your diabetes could be managed with insulin."
    d. "Keeping your blood sugars under control now can help to prevent damage to both kidneys."

77. Self-monitoring of blood glucose levels is most important in which of the following clients? *Check all that apply.*
    _____ a. Clients with multiple daily insulin injections
    _____ b. Clients with mild type 2 diabetes
    _____ c. Clients with hypoglycemic unawareness
    _____ d. Clients using a portable infusion device for insulin administration

78. Which of the following statements about sexual intercourse for diabetic clients is correct?
    a. The incidence of sexual dysfunction is lower in men than women.
    b. Retrograde ejaculation does not interfere with male fertility.
    c. Impotence is associated with diabetes mellitus in male clients.
    d. Sexual dysfunction in female clients includes inability to achieve pregnancy.

79. Identify at least four psychosocial nursing diagnoses that may be found in a client with diabetes.
    a. _____
    b. _____
    c. _____
    d. _____

80. An insulin-dependent diabetic client is planning to travel by air and asks the nurse about preparations for the trip. The nurse should tell the client to do which of the following?
    a. Pack insulin and syringes in a labeled, crushproof kit in the checked luggage.
    b. Carry all necessary diabetes supplies in a clearly identified pack aboard the plane.
    c. Ask the flight attendant to put the insulin in the galley refrigerator once on the plane.
    d. Take only minimal supplies and get the prescription filled at his or her destination.

81. Which of the following statements reflects that the diabetic client understands the principles of self-care?
    a. "I don't like the idea of sticking myself so often to measure my sugar."
    b. "I plan to measure the sugar in my urine at least four times a day."
    c. "I plan to get my spouse to exercise with me to keep me company."
    d. "If I get a cold, I can take my regular cough medication until I feel better."

82. After a 2-hour glucose challenge, impaired glucose tolerance is present when the values are between _____ and _____ mg/dL.

83. A 50-year-old client was seen in the emergency department for complaints of nausea, vomiting, and dehydration. When admitted to the hospital, the fasting blood glucose was over 500 mg/dL. A blood gas showed a pH of 7.38. He was diagnosed with diabetes and treated with insulin and fluids. What does this situation tell you about this client?
    a. His diabetes is temporary.
    b. He will only require insulin when he is stressed or ill. His diabetes is temporary.
    c. His pancreas is producing enough insulin to prevent ketoacidosis.
    d. His pancreas is not producing enough insulin to prevent ketoacidosis.

84. A client with type 2 diabetes often has which of the following laboratory values?
    a. Elevated thyroid studies
    b. Elevated triglycerides
    c. Ketones in the urine
    d. Low hemoglobin

85. A newly diagnosed client with diabetes is being seen for instruction regarding insulin administration. Identify points of emphasis in teaching this client.

86. A client with type 1 diabetes takes two shots a day of mixed NPH and regular insulin. The client takes one shot in the morning and one in the evening. What instruction would you give this client regarding a meal regimen?

87. A client with type 1 diabetes notifies the physician of flu-like symptoms with nausea. What do you tell this client about sick day rules?

88. Hypovolemic shock can be a complication of diabetic ketoacidosis or hyperglycemic-hyperosmolar nonketotic syndrome (HHNS). Describe the key cause of hypovolemic shock in these clients.

89. What are the signs and symptoms of hypoglycemia?

90. A client with type 1 diabetes is taking a mixture of NPH and regular insulin at home. He is now NPO after midnight and scheduled for surgery the next day.
    A. On the day of surgery, what action would the nurse take regarding the morning dose of insulin?
       1. Administer the dose that is routinely prescribed at home since he has type 1 diabetes and needs the insulin.
       2. Administer half the dose because the client is NPO.
       3. Hold the insulin with all the other medications because the client is NPO and there is no need for insulin.
       4. Contact the physician for a physician's order regarding the insulin.
       5. Administer just the NPH because it is the long-acting insulin and should have good coverage for the day.
       6. Administer just the regular insulin because he will be going to surgery.
    B. Which of the above actions would the nurse take if the client has type 2 diabetes?

91. A client with diabetes has signs and symptoms of hypoglycemia. The client is alert and oriented with a blood glucose of 56.
    A. The nurse would administer which of the following?
       1. A glass of orange juice with two packets of sugar and continue to monitor the client
       2. A glass of orange or other type of juice and continue to monitor the client
       3. A complex carbohydrate and continue to monitor the client
       4. D50 IV push and give the client something to eat
    B. Which of the above actions would the nurse take if the client was not alert and oriented or unable to take PO fluids?

92. The client has been receiving insulin in the abdomen for three days. On day 4, where should the nurse give the insulin injection?
    a. In the deltoid
    b. In the thigh
    c. In the abdomen, near the navel
    d. In the abdomen, but in an area different from yesterday's injection
    e. Site rotation is only necessary for multiple injections within the same day.

93. Place the following injection sites in order of speed of absorption, with 1 having the fastest absorption and 4 having the slowest absorption.

    _____ a. Buttocks

    _____ b. Abdomen

    _____ c. Deltoid

    _____ d. Thigh

94. Match the insulin characteristics with the type of insulin. *Answers may be used more than once.*

Insulin Characteristic

_____ a. This type of insulin is used in most regimens for basal insulin coverage.

_____ b. A long-acting insulin analogue that is given once daily at bedtime for basal insulin coverage.

_____ c. When mixing insulins, this type is always drawn up first.

_____ d. This type of insulin should be given 30 minutes before meals.

_____ e. This type of insulin should not be diluted or mixed with any other insulin or solution.

Type of Insulin
1. Insulin glargine (Lantus)
2. Regular insulin
3. NPH insulin

95. Compare the conditions using the chart below. Use a separate sheet of paper for your answers if necessary.

	Hypoglycemia	Hyperglycemia	Diabetic ketoacidosis	Hyperglycemic-hyperosmolar nonketotic syndrome
Events that precipitate the crisis				
Common abnormal laboratory and other diagnostic tests				
Priority emergency interventions				

CASE STUDY: THE CLIENT WITH DIABETES MELLITUS

Answer Guidelines for the Case Study questions are provided on the companion Evolve Learning Resources Web site at http://evolve.elsevier.com/Iggy/.

Your client is a 48-year-old woman who is admitted to the emergency department, and she is unconscious. She has a known history of type 1 diabetes mellitus. Her daughter accompanies her and tells the staff that her mother has had the "flu" and has been unable to eat or drink very much. The daughter is uncertain whether her mother has taken her insulin in the past 24 hours. The client's vitals signs are temperature 101.8° F; pulse 120, weak and irregular; respiration, 22, deep and fruity odor; and blood pressure, 80/42. Blood specimens and arterial blood gases are drawn and an intravenous infusion begun.

1. Based on this client's history, give the probable changes in laboratory results for serum glucose, serum osmolarity, serum acetone, BUN, arterial pH, and arterial P_{CO_2}. What medical emergency do these data indicate?

2. What type of intravenous solutions should the nurse be prepared to administer to this client? What drugs should the nurse be prepared to give? Explain your answers.

3. The client is placed on continuous cardiac monitoring. What is the rationale for this intervention?

4. During the first 24 hours, what complications should the nurse monitor for in this client? Why?

5. The client eventually becomes normoglycemic, regains consciousness, and begins a 1500-calorie diabetic diet. Develop a teaching-learning plan for her about this diet.

6. Before this emergency, this client had been monitoring urine glucose and ketones for self-care and insulin administration. Her physician prescribes blood glucose monitoring instead of urine testing. What is the rationale for this change?

7. Which aspect of diabetic self-care should the nurse discuss with this client before her discharge?

8. The client is to be discharged on a mixed-dose regimen for insulin. She is to receive 10 units regular insulin and 18 units NPH insulin before breakfast and another 5 units regular insulin and 12 units NPH at dinner time. Develop a teaching-learning plan for these medications.

9. Considering the client's insulin protocol, the client should keep in mind what principles about the actions of the insulins she is taking?

10. What should the nurse discuss with this client about diabetes, insulin, and illness? What can this client do to prevent future emergency episodes? Consider "Instructions for Sick Day" rules.

Assessment of the Skin, Hair, and Nails

LEARNING OUTCOMES

1. Compare the structures and function of the dermis with those of the epidermis.
2. Describe the integumentary changes associated with aging.
3. Use proper terminology to describe different skin lesions.
4. Describe techniques to assess skin changes in clients with dark skin.
5. Distinguish between normal variations and abnormal skin manifestations with regard to skin color, texture, warmth, and moisture.
6. Explain the role of melanocytes in determining skin color.
7. Describe the ABCD method of assessing skin lesions for cancer.
8. Prioritize educational needs for the client undergoing an excisional biopsy for a skin lesion.

LEARNING ACTIVITIES

1. Before completing the study guide exercises for this chapter, it is recommended that you review the following:
   - Anatomy and physiology of the skin and its appendages
   - The ABCD method of assessing skin lesions
   - The effects of sun and ultraviolet exposure on the skin
   - Principles of fluid and electrolyte balance
   - Principles of infection control
   - Concepts of body image and self-esteem

2. Review the boldfaced terms and their definitions in Chapter 69 to enhance your understanding of the content.

STUDY/REVIEW QUESTIONS

Answers to the Study/Review Questions are provided on the companion Evolve Learning Resources Web site at http://evolve.elsevier.com/Iggy/.

1. Match each of the following properties with the appropriate layer of skin.

Property

_____ a. Contains elastin
_____ b. Serves as insulator
_____ c. Contains no cells
_____ d. Collagen is main component
_____ e. Does not have a separate blood supply
_____ f. Provides padding
_____ g. Innermost layer of skin
_____ h. Rich in sensory nerves
_____ i. Synthesis of vitamin D
_____ j. Melanin production

Layer of Skin

1. Fat
2. Dermis
3. Epidermis

2. Which of the following is a clinical example of a secondary lesion?
   a. Cysts
   b. Acne
   c. Psoriasis
   d. Hives

3. What is the most significant factor leading to the degeneration of the skin components?
   a. Systemic disease
   b. Genetic background
   c. Sun exposure
   d. Hormonal changes

4. In regulating body temperature, evaporative water loss can be as much as which of the following?
   a. 600 mL/day
   b. 900 mL/day
   c. 2 L/day
   d. 10 to 12 L/day

5. Which of the following statements are true about integumentary changes in older adults? *Check all that apply.*

   _____ a. Decreased thickness in the epidermal layer results in increased skin transparency and fragility replacement.

   _____ b. Thinning of the fat layer decreases the susceptibility to hypothermia.

   _____ c. Increased blood flow to the nail bed increases longitudinal nail ridges.

   _____ d. Decreased number of Langerhans cells increases cutaneous inflammatory response.

   _____ e. Decreased eccrine and apocrine gland activity increases susceptibility to dry skin.

6. Correct the statements in Question 5 that were not true.

7. Identify two characteristics for each of the following lesions, and cite one example for each lesion.
   a. Nodules:

   b. Papules:

   c. Wheals:

8. Match the terminology with the corresponding definitions.

Term

_____ a.   Serpiginous

_____ b.   Circinate

_____ c.   Diffuse

_____ d.   Coalesced

_____ e.   Annular

Definition
1. Lesions merging with each other
2. Widespread
3. Ringlike with raised borders around flat, clear centers of normal skin
4. Having wavy borders
5. Circular

9. Pallor in dark-skinned clients may be detected by which of the following?
    a.   Ash-gray color of mucous membranes
    b.   Reddish pink color of the skin
    c.   Whitish color of the skin
    d.   Bluish tinge of the nail beds

10. In dark-skinned clients, a color change of the _____ is the best indicator of jaundice.
    a.   Conjunctiva
    b.   Palms of the hands
    c.   Soles of the feet
    d.   Oral mucous membranes

11. Match each alteration in color listed below to the underlying cause or condition.

Underlying Cause or Condition

_____ a.   Pregnancy (melasma), Addison's disease

_____ b.   Bleeding from vessels into tissue

_____ c.   Liver disorders, chronic renal failure, or increased hemolysis of red blood cells

_____ d.   Vasoconstriction, sudden emotional upset

_____ e.   Fever, cellulitis

Alteration in Color
1. Blue
2. Yellow-orange
3. Red (erythema)
4. Brown
5. White (pallor)

12. Describe the ABCD method of assessing skin lesions for cancer.

13. Complete the following table regarding vascular skin lesions:

Lesion	Location	Description	Significance, or is it normal?
Port wine stain			
Telangiectasia			
Cherry angioma			
Spider angioma			

14. Explain the difference between primary and secondary skin lesions, and give examples of each.

15. Explain the difference between petechiae and ecchymoses.

16. Name the skin lesion described in each scenario:

    a. A man notices linear cracks in the soles of his feet while taking a shower.

    b. After spending a day outside in the sun, a child notices small, flat lesions on her nose, cheeks, and lower arms.

    c. A woman discovers a 3-cm round, elevated lesion that is filled with clear fluid on her thumb after spending the day raking leaves.

    d. While examining a female client, the nurse notices scattered lesions across the client's back. These lesions vary in size, but are less than 1 cm in diameter, and are small, firm, and elevated.

    e. After pulling weeds along a field fence, a teenage boy notices that he has elevated, irregularly shaped swollen lesions on his arms and hands.

17. To differentiate between color changes in the nail bed related to vascular supply and those from pigment disposition, the nurse should do which of the following?

    a. Examine the nail plate under a Wood's light.
    b. Assess for thickness.
    c. Blanch the nail bed.
    d. Evaluate for lesions.

18. Identify the probable causes for each skin manifestation identified below.

    a. Increased body hair growth on the face in a female client

    b. Drumstick appearance of nail shape

    c. Decreased skin turgor

    d. "Heaped up" appearance on a older adult's toenail

19. Your adult client is scheduled for an excisional biopsy and is very apprehensive about pain. Describe what the nurse should do to reassure this client.

20. Which test would be performed to determine whether the client has a fungal infection of the skin?

    a. Shave biopsy
    b. Punch biopsy
    c. Wood's light examination
    d. KOH test

Interventions for Clients with Skin Problems

LEARNING OUTCOMES

1. Prioritize nursing care for a client with dry skin.
2. Compare wound healing by first, second, and third intention.
3. Identify clients at risk for pressure ulcer development.
4. Plan an individualized strategy for pressure ulcer prevention for a specific client at increased risk.
5. Differentiate the clinical manifestations for stage I through stage IV pressure ulcers.
6. Prioritize the nursing interventions for a client with a stage III pressure ulcer.
7. Evaluate the effectiveness of interventions for pressure ulcer management.
8. Compare the clinical manifestations and modes of transmission for bacterial, viral, and fungal skin infections.
9. Prioritize nursing care and educational needs for clients who have parasitic skin infections.
10. Describe the mechanisms of action, side effects, and nursing implications for pharmacologic management of psoriasis.
11. Explain the rationale for ultraviolet therapy for psoriasis.
12. Develop a community-based teaching plan for the client with psoriasis.
13. Identify interventions for prevention of skin cancer.
14. Describe the clinical manifestations of melanoma.

LEARNING ACTIVITIES

1. Before completing the study guide exercises for this chapter, it is recommended that you review the following:
   - Anatomy and physiology of the skin and its appendages
   - Principles of fluid and electrolyte balance
   - Principles of infection control
   - Concepts of body image and self-esteem
   - Pain management
   - Principles of wound healing and wound care
   - Principles of general nutrition

2. Review the boldfaced terms and their definitions in Chapter 70 to enhance your understanding of the content.

STUDY/REVIEW QUESTIONS

Answers to the Study/Review Questions are provided on the companion Evolve Learning Resources Web site at http://evolve.elsevier.com/Iggy/.

1. Which of the following is the most common symptom of pruritus?
   a. Blisters
   b. Itching
   c. Flaking
   d. Tenderness

2. Which of the following statements regarding pruritus are true? *Check all that apply.*

   _____ a. It can be associated with a systemic disease rather than skin disease.

   _____ b. It is worse at night.

   _____ c. It is better to rub an itchy area rather than to scratch it.

   _____ d. It is an objective assessment finding.

3. How or when should creams or lotions be applied to facilitate rehydration of the skin?
   a. Within 2 to 3 minutes after bathing
   b. With vigorous and circular motions
   c. To completely dry skin
   d. After the first sign of flakiness appears

4. Which of the following statements about xerosis are true? *Check all that apply.*

   _____ a. It is worse in dry climates.

   _____ b. Wind, cold, and sunlight contribute to the problem.

   _____ c. Frequent bathing with deodorant soap and hot water relieve the problem.

   _____ d. Using a dehumidifier during humid days decreases the risk of getting xerosis.

   _____ e. Avoiding caffeine and alcohol ingestion is helpful in preventing this condition.

5. Management of urticaria includes which of the following? *Check all that apply.*

   _____ a. Avoiding overexertion and warm environments

   _____ b. Using antihistamines as the drug of choice

   _____ c. Restricting alcohol consumption

   _____ d. Avoiding scratching and touching the lesions

6. A client is complaining about painful sunburn. Describe what treatment information the nurse would share.

7. In wound healing, which of the following statements describes healing by second intention?
   a. There is minimal tissue destruction with no open areas or dead spaces.
   b. The wound is closed surgically after it was open for several days.
   c. The chronic wound is allowed to heal from the inside out.
   d. The wound is surgically made and has minimal tissue reaction.

8. Identify the two factors that affect the degree to which epithelialization and contraction can restore wound integrity.

   a. _____

   b. _____

9. How long does partial-thickness wound healing by epithelialization take?
   a. 24 hours
   b. 2 to 3 days
   c. 5 to 7 days
   d. 12 to 14 days

10. Which of the following are true about a full-thickness wound? *Check all that apply.*

_____ a. Requires necrotic tissue to be removed for healing to occur

_____ b. Results in unstable epithelial surface

_____ c. Heals by primary intention

_____ d. Heals by granulation

11. Identify three reasons why older adults are at risk for pressure ulcers.

a. _____

b. _____

c. _____

Questions 12 and 13 refer to the following client.

An 89-year-old nursing home client is now bed-ridden and has been losing weight steadily. The dietitian is working with her family to improve her diet and encourage her eating. She has been identified as high risk for development of a pressure ulcer.

12. What interventions can prevent her from getting a pressure ulcer?

13. It was noted that this client has developed a pressure ulcer from friction of the sheets. It is described as an intact blister on her left heel that is 6 cm long and 5 cm wide with no signs of cellulitis. This is a stage _____ pressure ulcer.

14. What two nutritional factors are important for intact skin and wound healing?

a. _____

b. _____

15. Complete the following statements.
   a. A _____ dressing material is beneficial when the wound is relatively free of drainage.
   b. To prevent maceration with a draining wound, a _____ dressing is used.

16. Which of the following are necessary for a successful skin graft? *Check all that apply.*

_____ a. The graft area must have an adequate blood supply

_____ b. The graft area must be free of infection.

_____ c. The graft area must be completely immobilized.

_____ d. The graft area must be irrigated frequently.

17. Which of the following statements is true about herpes zoster (shingles)?
   a. It is manifested by pain, itching, and tenderness.
   b. It usually causes a larger, single lesion.
   c. It is usually painless.
   d. It lasts 1 to 2 days.

18. Match each tinea infection with the corresponding location.

Location		Infection	
_____ a.	Feet	1.	Tinea capitis
_____ b.	Hands	2.	Tinea manus
_____ c.	Groin (jock itch)	3.	Tinea barbae
_____ d.	Scalp	4.	Tinea pedis
_____ e.	Beard	5.	Tinea corporis
_____ f.	Smooth skin surfaces	6.	Tinea cruris

19. Which of the following is typical of pediculosis capitis?
    a. It is treated with chemical agents.
    b. It is more common in men than in women.
    c. It is seen in adults.
    d. Its course is self-limiting.

20. A client who complains of intense itching at night may have which of the following?
    a. Tinea corporis
    b. Scabies
    c. Furuncles
    d. Contact dermatitis

21. Determine the type of skin infection based on each description of the clinical manifestations.
    a. Cracks and fissures at the corners of the mouth; creamy white plaques on oral mucous membranes

    b. Fever, redness, warmth, lymphadenopathy

    c. Group of blisters on anterior trunk, painful, itching

22. Psoriasis is an inflammatory dermatosis that:
    a. Can be cured with proper management of systemic drugs and topical agents.
    b. Is a scaling disorder with underlying dermal inflammation.
    c. Slows the rate of shedding at the outermost stratum corneum.
    d. Is infected with *Staphylococcus aureus*.

23. Which of the following are the characteristic lesions of psoriasis?
    a. Plaques surmounted by silvery-white scales
    b. Circular areas of redness
    c. Multiple blisters with a yellowish crust
    d. Patches of tender raised areas limited to extremities

24. Treatment for psoriasis can include which of the following? *Check all that apply.*
    _____ a. UV light therapy
    _____ b. Calcipotriene (Dovonex) topical cream
    _____ c. Topical methotrexate
    _____ d. Oral ciprofloxacin

25. Which of the following are examples of benign tumors? *Check all that apply.*
    _____ a. Cysts
    _____ b. Nevus
    _____ c. Hemangioma
    _____ d. Actinic keratoses
    _____ e. Keloids

26. Match the skin disorder with the description.

Description

    _____ a. Most common cause: ultraviolet exposure; metastasis is rare
    _____ b. Invades locally and is potentially metastatic; arises from epidermis
    _____ c. Pigmented skin cancer that is highly metastatic
    _____ d. Premalignant lesions of the cells of the epidermis

Skin Disorder
1. Melanoma
2. Basal cell carcinoma
3. Actinic keratosis
4. Squamous cell carcinoma

27. Identify four ways to prevent skin cancer.

    a. _____
    b. _____
    c. _____
    d. _____

28. You have a 25-year-old client who has recently had a rhinoplasty as part of reconstruction after cancer treatment. He is swallowing repeatedly and belching. What is this an indication of?

29. Which of the following statements about isotretinoin (Accutane) are true? *Check all that apply.*

    _____ a. It may cause dry, chapped lips.

    _____ b. It is the first choice for acne treatment.

    _____ c. Strict birth control measures are necessary.

    _____ d. Liver function studies should be monitored while on this therapy.

    _____ e. It is used for superficial lesions.

30. Nursing care for a client with toxic epidermal necrolysis (TEN) should include which of the following? *Check all that apply.*

    _____ a. Assessment of input and output

    _____ b. Monitoring fluid and electrolyte balance

    _____ c. Monitoring for hyperthermia

    _____ d. Managing inflammation with steroid creams

31. Which of the following describes how rewarming frostbite tissue is done?
    a. Slowly to avoid more damage
    b. In a water bath at 90° F to 107° F
    c. With warm water compresses of normal saline applied directly to the area
    d. After the blisters are punctured to facilitate healing

32. Match the disorders with their description. *Answers may be used more than once.*

Description

_____ a. A rash caused by toxic injury to the skin as a result of contact with an irritant substance

_____ b. A chronic, contagious, systemic mycobacterial infection of the peripheral nervous system with skin involvement

_____ c. A drug-induced skin reaction that may include a mix of vesicles, erosions, and crusts

_____ d. Painless lesions and eschar that form regardless of treatment used

_____ e. Ingrown toenail

_____ f. A rare, acute drug reaction of the skin that gradually heals in 2 to 3 weeks with widespread peeling of the epidermis

_____ g. Purple, flat-topped, itchy papules over the wrists and inner surfaces of the forearms

_____ h. Also known as leprosy

_____ i. Comedone lesions

Disorder
1. Toxic epidermal necrolysis
2. Stevens-Johnson syndrome
3. Contact dermatitis
4. Lichen planus
5. Hansen's disease
6. Acne
7. Unguis incarnatus
8. Cutaneous anthrax

33. Explain the following statement: "A wound that is exposed is always contaminated but is not always infected."

34. A mother calls the pediatric clinic for help because her toddler is miserable with a severe case of chicken pox. Which type of bath would be most appropriate to help relieve the toddler's discomfort?
    a.   Antibacterial bath
    b.   Emollient bath
    c.   Tar bath with Polytar formula
    d.   Aveeno colloidal oatmeal bath

35. A client has a stage III pressure ulcer over the left trochanter area that has a thick exudate. The wound bed is visible and beefy red, and the edges are surrounded with swollen, pink tissue. The exudate has an odor. Which dressing is appropriate for this wound? *Check all that apply.*

    _____   a.   Transparent dressing

    _____   b.   Alginate dressing

    _____   c.   Continuous dry gauze dressing

    _____   d.   Wet to damp gauze dressing

CASE STUDY: MALIGNANT MELANOMA

Answer Guidelines for the Case Study questions are provided on the companion Evolve Learning Resources Web site at http://evolve.elsevier.com/Iggy/.

A 44-year-old Caucasian woman is admitted for local wide excision of a large mole on her upper thigh that has been diagnosed as malignant melanoma. Her past history is negative for serious illness. She was hospitalized for the birth of her three children. She admits to being an "avid sun worshipper" and is noted to have very dark brown skin and some premature aging in the facial skin.

1. Considering the possible etiology of melanoma, what effect does the exposure to sunlight have on this form of cancer?

2. During her preoperative instructions, the client asks why she is going to have a 4-inch circle of skin and tissue removed to get rid of a "mole." What information should the nurse consider before responding to her question?

The client has a wide excision of the melanoma, and the surgical site is closed with a split-thickness skin graft from the opposite thigh. Following surgery, the wound is dressed with a bulky dressing, and the donor site is covered with a pressure dressing. When assessing the dressings, the client asks the nurse to "peek" at the surgical site so that she can see where the mole had been.

3. How should the nurse respond?

4. On the following morning, the client complains that the donor site "hurts worse than the cancer site." What should the nurse say and what interventions are appropriate?

On the third day after surgery, the bulky dressing is removed. The wound appears wet with cloudy fluid oozing from it, and the skin graft is unattached to the wound. The surrounding tissues are red and swollen.

5. What is the likely cause of these features in the graft site?

Interventions for Clients with Burns

LEARNING OUTCOMES

1. Identify burn clients at risk for inhalation injury.
2. Compare the clinical manifestations of superficial, partial-thickness, and full-thickness burn injuries.
3. Explain the expected clinical manifestations of neural and hormonal compensation during the emergent phase of burn injury.
4. Calculate the total body surface area (TBSA) involved in a burn injury.
5. Identify clients at risk for problems of oxygenation.
6. Prioritize nursing care for the client during the emergent phase of burn injury.
7. Use laboratory data and clinical manifestations to determine the effectiveness of fluid resuscitation during the emergent phase of burn injury.
8. Use the Parkland formula to establish the correct rate and timing of fluid replacement.
9. Describe methods to prevent infection from autocontamination and cross-contamination in clients with burn injuries.
10. Prioritize nursing care for the client during the acute phase of burn injury.
11. Explain the alteration of nutritional needs for the burn client during the acute phase of burn injury.
12. Evaluate wound healing in the client during the acute phase of burn injury.
13. Compare pain management strategies for clients in the emergent and acute phases of burn injury.
14. Describe the characteristics of infected burn wounds.
15. Explain the positioning and range-of-motion interventions for the prevention of mobility problems in the client with burns.
16. Prioritize nursing care for the client during the rehabilitation phase of burn injury.
17. Discuss the potential psychosocial problems associated with burn injury.
18. Develop a community-based teaching plan for the client recovering from a burn injury.
19. Identify populations at risk for burn injury and discuss preventive measures.

LEARNING ACTIVITIES

1. Before completing the study guide exercises for this chapter, it is recommended that you review the following:
   - Anatomy and physiology of the skin and its appendages
   - Principles of fluid and electrolyte balance
   - Principles of acid-base balance
   - Principles of infection control
   - Concepts of body image and self-esteem
   - Pain management
   - Principles of wound healing and wound care
   - Perioperative care
   - Principles of general nutrition
   - Procedure for application of topical medications
   - Concepts of human sexuality
   - Concepts of loss, grief, death, and dying
   - The principles of airway management

2. Review the boldfaced terms and their definitions in Chapter 71 to enhance your understanding of the content.

STUDY/REVIEW QUESTIONS

Answers to the Study/Review Questions are provided on the companion Evolve Learning Resources Web site at http://evolve.elsevier.com/Iggy/.

1. Tissue destruction caused by a burn injury causes local and systemic problems. Identify six of these potential problems.

   a. _____

   b. _____

   c. _____

   d. _____

   e. _____

   f. _____

2. Match each of the following terms with the corresponding definitions.

Term

_____ a. Dermal appendages

_____ b. Anesthetic

_____ c. Avascular

_____ d. Eschar

_____ e. Desquamation

_____ f. Fasciotomy

_____ g. Viable

_____ h. Hyperkalemia

_____ i. Hyponatremia

_____ j. Hemoconcentration

_____ k. Catabolism

Definition

1. Decreased sodium levels
2. Peeling of dead skin
3. Living
4. Sweat and oil glands, and hair follicles
5. Burn crust
6. Elevated potassium levels
7. Without a blood supply
8. Incision through the eschar and fascia
9. Does not transmit sensation
10. Fat and protein breakdown
11. Elevated blood osmolarity, hemoglobin, and hematocrit

3. When a burn injury occurs, the skin can regenerate as long as which of the following occurs?
   a. The epidermis layer is present.
   b. Nerve tissue is intact.
   c. Parts of the dermis layer remain.
   d. There is no infection present.

4. Which of the following statements are true? *Check all that apply*.

_____ a. The depth of dermal appendages is equal across body areas.

_____ b. Full-thickness burn is identified by the total destruction of the dermis.

_____ c. Full-thickness burn results in loss of excretory ability.

_____ d. All burn injuries are painful.

_____ e. The skin can tolerate temperatures of 158° F.

_____ f. The magnitude of the injury is based on the depth and extent of the total body surface burn.

_____ g. Blood transfusions are critical in the first 24 hours for all burns.

5. Complete the following table on the classification by burn thickness.

Classification	Color	Healing Time	Examples
Superficial			
Partial thickness, superficial			
Deep partial thickness			
Full thickness			
Deep full thickness			

6. Partial thickness wounds can convert to full thickness when which of the following occurs?
   a. Scar formation is large.
   b. Tissue damage increases with ischemia.
   c. Blisters are present.
   d. Skin integrity is impaired.

7. Which of the following describes full-thickness wound healing? *Check all that apply*.

_____ a. Healing occurs by wound contraction.

_____ b. Eschar must be removed.

_____ c. Large blisters are protective and left undisturbed.

_____ d. Skin grafting may be necessary.

8. Which of the following describes third spacing or capillary leak syndrome in a client with severe burns?
   a. Usually happens in the first 36 to 48 hours
   b. Is a leak of plasma fluids into the interstitial space
   c. Is present even in unburned tissues
   d. Can usually be prevented

9. As a result of third spacing, during the acute phase, which of the following electrolyte imbalances may occur? *Check all that apply.*
   _____ a. Hyperkalemia
   _____ b. Hypokalemia
   _____ c. Hypernatremia
   _____ d. Hyponatremia
   _____ e. Hypokalemia
   _____ f. Hypercalcemia

10. Because of the fluid shifts in burns, which of the following regarding cardiac output is correct?
    a. It is not affected.
    b. It may be depressed up to 36 hours after the burn.
    c. It is improved with fluid restriction.
    d. It responds to diuretics.

11. What is the major source of respiratory problems related to burn injury?

12. Which of the following is a serious gastrointestinal problem that can occur with a major burn?
    a. Increased motility
    b. Increased flow of blood to the area
    c. Decreased secretion of catecholamines
    d. Paralytic ileus

13. The hypermetabolic state with a significant burn causes which of the following? *Check all that apply.*
    _____ a. Fat breakdown and the rapid use of glucose and calories
    _____ b. A decrease in the secretion of catecholamines
    _____ c. An increase in caloric needs
    _____ d. An increase in core temperature

14. Which of the following statements about fluid remobilization are true? *Check all that apply.*
    _____ a. Anemia may be present.
    _____ b. Metabolic alkalosis may occur.
    _____ c. Hyponatremia may develop.
    _____ d. Hyperkalemia may develop.

15. Tissue injury is a threat to homeostasis. What are the two compensatory responses?
    a. _____
    b. _____

16. Identify the sources of burn injuries.
    a. _____
    b. _____
    c. _____
    d. _____
    e. _____
    f. _____

17. Local tissue resistance to electricity varies in different parts of the body. Which of the following has the *most* resistance?
    a. Skin epidermis
    b. Tendons and muscle
    c. Fatty tissue
    d. Nerve tissue and blood vessels

18. Identify the age-related changes that increase morbidity and mortality in the older adult.

19. Identify information that should be included in a history.

20. A client who has been rescued from a burning house has been treated with oxygen. His breath sounds previously included wheezing, but after 30 minutes, the wheezing has stopped. What action, if any, should the nurse take at this time?

21. Which of following laboratory results would be expected during the emergent period? *Check all that apply.*

    _____ a. Potassium level of 3.2 mEq/L

    _____ b. Glucose level of 180 mg/dL

    _____ c. Hematocrit of 49%/dL

    _____ d. pH of 7.20

22. Which of the following statements are true about carbon monoxide poisoning? *Check all that apply.*

    _____ a. It causes "cherry-red" color in burn clients.

    _____ b. The partial pressure of oxygen (Pao_2) dissolved in the arterial blood is reduced.

    _____ c. Carbon monoxide binds to the hemoglobin molecule 250 times more tightly then oxygen.

    _____ d. It has a high mortality rate.

23. What should a nurse assess relevant to the cardiovascular system for the client with severe burns? *Check all that apply.*

    _____ a. Presence and strength of peripheral and central pulses

    _____ b. Capillary refill

    _____ c. Presence of edema

    _____ d. Noninvasive blood pressure

24. Which of the following is the best way to assess renal function in a client with severe burns?
    a. Measuring urine output and comparing this value with fluid intake
    b. Weighing the client
    c. Noting the amount of edema
    d. Measuring abdominal girth

25. Why it is important to be accurate when evaluating the size of the burn injury?

26. For an African-American client with a burn injury, an additional blood test may be appropriate. Which test is it and why?

27. Hypovolemic shock occurs in burned clients as a result of which of the following?
    a. Erratic lymphatic drainage
    b. Altered osmotic pressure in vessels
    c. Albumin trapped in the interstitial spaces
    d. A marked increase in capillary permeability

A 70-kg woman with 50% TBSA burn arrived at 11 AM and was burned at 9 AM, according to her family. Answer the following four questions relating to this client.

28. Using the Parkland (Baxter) formula, calculate the fluids needed for the first 8 hours after injury.

29. What time does the first 8-hour period end?

30. How much fluid is required for the 24 hours?

31. Hourly urine output is adjusted to _____ mL/kg.

32. Which of the following statements are true about escharotomies and fasciotomies? *Check all that apply.*
    _____ a. They are frequently done under general anesthesia.
    _____ b. No anesthesia is required.
    _____ c. Sedation and analgesia are commonly given to reduce anxiety.
    _____ d. They are often done at the bedside.

33. Airway maintenance for a client with a burn injury and respiratory involvement includes which of the following?
    a. Monitoring for signs and symptoms of upper airway edema during fluid resuscitation
    b. Inserting a nasopharyngeal or oropharyngeal airway when the client's airway is completely obstructed
    c. Securing loose dressing with a rib binder instead of tape
    d. Weighing the client three times a week for fluid overload

34. When does fluid remobilization occur?
    a. Within the first 4 hours after the burns were sustained
    b. After the scar tissue is formed and fluids are no longer being lost
    c. After 36 hours, when the fluid is reabsorbed from the interstitial tissue
    d. Immediately after the burns occur

35. Which of the following statements is true about pain associated with burn injuries?
    a. The pain is both chronic and acute.
    b. The preferred route of administration of narcotics in the emergent state is intravenous.
    c. Massaging nonburn areas may reduce pain.
    d. Maintain a cool room temperature to reduce discomfort from the burn injuries.

36. Which of the following statements about the acute phase of the burn injury is true? *Check all that apply.*
    _____ a. It begins at 24 hours after the injury and lasts until the wound closure is complete.
    _____ b. During this time, the client is at a high risk for infection.
    _____ c. Caloric requirements are decreased during this phase.
    _____ d. Pneumonia is a potential complication during this phase.

37. Which of the following applies to the debridement procedure? *Check all that apply.*

    _____ a. Remove eschar and other cellular debris from the wound.

    _____ b. Nonviable tissue is removed during hydrotherapy.

    _____ c. Sterile saline is used during debridement.

    _____ d. Small blisters are usually opened.

    _____ e. Includes both mechanical and enzymatic actions.

38. What is a biologic dressing called that uses skin from a cadaver provided from a skin bank?
    a. Heterograft
    b. Xenograft
    c. Allograft
    d. Autograft

39. What type of wound is created in the typical donor site?
    a. Stage 1
    b. Partial thickness
    c. Full thickness
    d. Stage 4

40. Drug therapy to reduce the risk of wound infection in the burn client includes which of the following? *Check all that apply.*

    _____ a. Tetanus toxoid given IM prophylactically once early in the hospitalization

    _____ b. Silver nitrate solution covered by dry dressings applied every 4 hours

    _____ c. Silver sulfadiazine (Sulfadine) on full-thickness injuries every 4 hours

    _____ d. Broad-spectrum antibiotics given intravenously

41. Early detection of wound infection is important. The wound should be examined for which six signs of infection?

    a. _____

    b. _____

    c. _____

    d. _____

    e. _____

    f. _____

42. Nutritional requirements for a client with a relatively large burn area can exceed which of the following?
    a. 1500 kcal/day
    b. 2000 kcal/day
    c. 3000 kcal/day
    d. 5000 kcal/day

43. After a dressing is applied to a client's ankle, the ankle is placed in which of the following positions?
    a. Dorsiflexion
    b. Adduction
    c. External rotation
    d. Hyperextension

44. The client with severe burns progresses through typical stages and exhibits which of the following feelings? *Check all that apply.*

    _____ a. Denial

    _____ b. Regression

    _____ c. Anger

    _____ d. Suicidal tendencies

45. Which of the following interventions best promotes a positive image in a burn client?
    a. The physician discusses future scar revision with the client.
    b. The dietitian helps the client select choices from the menus.
    c. The spouse plays cards with the client.
    d. The nurse applies the pressure garment upon discharge.

46. A 28-year-old male client sustained second-and third-degree burns on his legs (30%) when his clothing caught fire while he was burning leaves. He was hosed down by his friend and has arrived at the burn center in severe discomfort. Identify the priority nursing diagnosis for this client at this time.
    a. Acute Pain related to damaged or exposed nerve endings
    b. Deficient Fluid Volume related to electrolyte imbalance
    c. Risk for Pulmonary Edema
    d. Disturbed Body Image related to the appearance of legs

47. After his stay at the center, this client is discharged but has some minimal wound areas remaining open. Describe what kinds of needs should be addressed before he is discharged.

48. A client's burn wound has developed an infection with methicillin-resistant *Staphylococcus aureus* organism (MRSA). Is this an example of autocontamination or cross-contamination? Explain your answer.

49. Which of the following clients has the highest risk for a fatal burn injury?
    a. A 4-year-old child
    b. A 32-year-old man
    c. A 45-year-old woman
    d. A 77-year-old man

50. Complete the puzzle by answering the questions below.

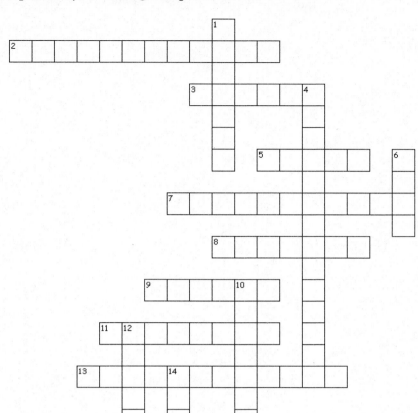

Across

2. A client has noticed that the skin is peeling off 3 days after a severe sunburn. What is this called?

3. Also known as "burn crust."

5. The nurse monitors for this severe complication of a full-thickness burn by watching for tachycardia, decreased blood pressure, decreased peripheral pulses, and other signs of decreased cardiac output.

7. After spending the day at the beach, a teenage girl has a severe sunburn. This is an example of a _____-thickness burn.

8. _____-thickness burn involves the entire epidermis and varying parts of the dermis.

9. To assess whether a superficial partial-thickness wound is present, the nurse notes that the wound is red, moist, and _____ when pressure is applied.

11. A client is admitted to a burn trauma unit after suffering a severe electrical shock. He is in the _____ phase of burn injury.

13. The client in Question 11 has severe edema. This is due to a fluid shift, known as _____ _____ (two words).

Down

1. A client who was admitted with a severe burn after spilling hot liquid on his legs will be receiving a heterograft. The most common heterograft, which is compatible with human skin, is made from _____.

4. After 48 hours, the client in Question 11 begins to produce large amounts of urine. This is known as fluid _____.

6. A client is admitted after a house fire with severe burns across her body. The burns have destroyed the entire epidermis and dermis layers. This is known as a _____-thickness wound.

10. A camper spills bacon grease on his foot while cooking breakfast. This type of burn is a ____ burn.

12. An elderly man tips over a tea kettle with boiling water and burns the skin of his abdomen and thighs. This type of heat injury is a _____ burn, or a scald.

14. A client suffers burns on her arms after the sleeves of her robe catch fire while she is cooking breakfast. This type of burn injury is known as a _____ heat injury.

Assessment of the Renal/Urinary System

LEARNING OUTCOMES

1. Compare and contrast kidney function with functions of the ureters, bladder, and urethra.
2. Describe the roles of the afferent and efferent arterioles in glomerular filtration.
3. Explain the influence of antidiuretic hormone and aldosterone on urine formation and composition.
4. Describe age-related changes in the renal/urinary system.
5. Use laboratory data to distinguish between dehydration and renal impairment.
6. Describe how to obtain a sterile urine specimen from a client with a Foley catheter.
7. Identify teaching priorities for a client who needs to obtain a 24-hour urine specimen.
8. Identify teaching priorities for a client who needs to obtain a "clean-catch" urine specimen.
9. Describe the correct techniques to use in physically assessing the renal system.
10. Prioritize nursing care for the client during the first 24 hours following intravenous (IV) urography.

LEARNING ACTIVITIES

1. Before completing the study guide exercises in this chapter, it is recommended that you review the following:
   - Anatomy and physiology of the renal system
   - Process of excretion
   - Procedures for obtaining urine specimens

2. Review the boldfaced terms and their definitions in Chapter 72 to enhance your understanding of the content.

STUDY/REVIEW QUESTIONS

Answers to the Study/Review Questions are provided on the companion Evolve Learning Resources Web site at http://evolve.elsevier.com/Iggy/.

1. Identify the six ways the kidneys contribute to health.

   a. _____

   b. _____

   c. _____

   d. _____

   e. _____

   f. _____

2. Identify the parts of the renal system.

3. Define the retroperitoneal space where the kidney is located.

4. An ultrasound of the kidney that reveals a larger or smaller kidney is indicative of which possible problem?
   a. Hypertension
   b. Kidney stones
   c. Renal carcinoma
   d. Chronic renal disease

5. The outer surface of the kidney is the renal capsule that covers the kidney, except at which of the following?
   a. Renal artery
   b. Hilum
   c. Ureters
   d. Veins

6. Which of the following are functional renal tissue in the kidneys?
   a. Cortex and medulla
   b. Medulla and calyces
   c. Calyces and calipers
   d. Capsule and calyces

7. Which of the following describes the path of urine flow?
   a. Papilla to the calyx, merging to form the renal pelvis and become the ureter
   b. Papilla to the calyx to the renal pelvis and into the ureter
   c. Calyx to the papilla to the renal pelvis and into the ureter
   d. Calyx to the papilla, merging to form the renal pelvis and become the ureter

8. Construct a diagram and trace the blood supply to the kidney.

9. What percentage of the cardiac output do the kidneys receive?

10. Glomerular filtration does not occur when systolic blood pressure is which of the following?
    a. Less than 70 mm Hg
    b. Less than 50 mm Hg
    c. Greater than 120 mm Hg
    d. Greater than 200 mm Hg

11. Urine is removed from the blood by which structure?
    a. Medulla
    b. Nephron
    c. Calyx
    d. Capsule

12. The glomerulus is a series of specialized capillary loops that filter the blood to make urine; the excess blood exits which of the following structures?
    a. Afferent arterioles
    b. Peritubular capillaries
    c. Efferent arterioles
    d. Vas recta

13. The hormone renin regulates which of the following?
    a. Blood flow to the brain
    b. Glomerular filtration rate (GFR)
    c. Arterial blood pressure
    d. Cardiac rate and rhythm

14. Changes in blood volume and pressure are sensed by what structure, and what response to these changes occurs?

15. When the body's blood pressure or sodium level is low, renin does which of the following?
    a. Converts angiotensinogen to angiotensin I
    b. Converts aldosterone to angiotensinogen
    c. Converts angiotensin I to angiotensin II
    d. Converts angiotensin II to angiotensin III

16. The kidneys have both regulatory and hormonal functions. Identify which process each of the following involves. *Use R for regulatory and H for hormonal.*

    _____ a. Controls fluid
    _____ b. Vitamin D activation
    _____ c. Blood pressure
    _____ d. Acid-base balance
    _____ e. Controls electrolytes
    _____ f. Controls RBC formation

17. Identify the part of the kidney in which the filtrate is made.
    a. Proximal convoluted tubule
    b. Distal convoluted tubule
    c. Glomerular capillary wall
    d. Loop of Henle

18. Why are albumin and red blood cells usually absent from the urine of a healthy adult?
    a. They are too large to be filtered from the blood by the glomerular capillaries.
    b. These negatively charged substances adhere firmly to the positively charged walls of the renal tubules.
    c. They are moved by active transport through the tubular walls and returned back to systemic circulation.
    d. These substances bind to calcium, forming complex compounds called "casts."

19. What is the response of the glomerulus to conditions that dilate the afferent arteriole and simultaneously constrict the efferent arteriole?
    a. Decreased filtration pressure; increased urine output
    b. Decreased filtration pressure; decreased urine output
    c. Increased filtration pressure; increased urine output
    d. Increased filtration pressure; decreased urine output

20. During water reabsorption, the membrane of the distal convoluted tubule is more permeable to water due to the influence of which hormones?
    a. Renin
    b. Cortisol
    c. Calcitonin
    d. Antidiuretic hormone (ADH)

21. What is the primary function of the proximal convoluted tubule (PCT)?
    a. Secretion of angiotensinogen
    b. Excretion of erythropoietin
    c. Reabsorption of water and electrolytes
    d. Excretion of glucose, urea, and acids

22. The calcium level is controlled by which of the following?
    a. Calcitonin
    b. Renin
    c. Angiotensin
    d. Secretin

23. When does glucose appear in the urine?

24. During the selective tubular reabsorption process, which solute is not returned to the blood?

25. Which structures or tissues can change the composition of urine?
    a. Renal parenchyma
    b. Convoluted tubules
    c. Calyces
    d. Ureters

26. Identify the hormonal functions of kidneys.

27. Describe the effects of the release of renin.

28. In what way do prostaglandins affect kidney function?
    a. Antagonize erythropoietin
    b. Maintain renal vascular integrity
    c. Promote water and sodium excretion
    d. Conserve water while excreting waste products

29. How does bradykinin affect kidney function?
    a. Enhances renal excretion of potassium
    b. Maintains renal blood flow
    c. Decreases urine output
    d. Decreases urine pH

30. Why do clients with renal disease become anemic?

31. How does the kidney contribute to the absorption of calcium in the body?

32. Using the text and Figure 72-9, draw and label the structures of the urinary system from the kidneys on a separate sheet of paper.

33. Identify the three areas where the ureters narrow.

34. What is the normal length of each ureter in the healthy adult?
    a. 12 to 18 cm
    b. 12 to 18 inches
    c. 3 to 6 cm
    d. 3 to 6 inches

35. List and describe the layers of the ureters.

36. Urine is moved through the ureter by which of the following functions?
    a. Peristalsis
    b. Gravity
    c. Pelvic pressure
    d. Backflow

37. At which area of the bladder does the urethra connect?
    a. Ureterovesical junction
    b. Pubic symphysis
    c. Detrusor
    d. Trigone

38. Which events promote continence?
    a. Detrusor muscle relaxation; internal urethral sphincter relaxation
    b. Detrusor muscle relaxation; internal urethral sphincter constriction
    c. Detrusor muscle constriction; internal urethral sphincter relaxation
    d. Detrusor muscle constriction; internal urethral sphincter constriction

39. Which events allow micturition?
    a. Detrusor muscle relaxation; internal urethral sphincter relaxation
    b. Detrusor muscle relaxation; internal urethral sphincter constriction
    c. Detrusor muscle constriction; internal urethral sphincter relaxation
    d. Detrusor muscle constriction; internal urethral sphincter constriction

40. Identify the renal changes and effects seen with aging.

41. Impairment in the thirst mechanism of older adults increases the incidence of which of the following?
    a. Dehydration
    b. Hypocalcemia
    c. Hypokalemia
    d. Hyponatremia

42. Sodium retention problems are more prominent in which culture?
    a. Caucasian-Americans
    b. African-Americans
    c. Asian-Americans
    d. Native-Americans

43. (1) For women, changes in the bladder result in which of the following?
    a. Incontinence
    b. Hematuria
    c. Retention
    d. Dysuria

    (2) But for men, changes in the bladder are related to which of the following?
    a. Prolapsed bladder
    b. Enlarged prostate
    c. Dehydration
    d. Rectocele

44. What is one primary indicator of kidney disease?
    a. Hypernatremia
    b. Hypertension
    c. Dehydration
    d. Hypokalemia

45. (1) ESRD has an increased incidence in which culture?
    a. Caucasian-Americans
    b. African-Americans
    c. Asian-Americans
    d. Native-Americans

    (2) The above cultural differences are due to a high incidence of which of the following?
    a. Hypertension
    b. Bowel disease
    c. Liver disease
    d. Diabetes mellitus

46. Identify the areas the nurse should cover when taking a history of a client with renal disease.

47. The client states that she uses all of the following over-the-counter products on a regular basis. Which one should you explore further for potential impact on renal function?
    a. Peroxide-containing mouthwash
    b. Milk of magnesia laxative
    c. Vitamin C
    d. NSAIDs

48. Which urine characteristic listed on a urinalysis arouses your suspicion of a problem in the urinary tract?
    a. Cloudiness
    b. Straw color
    c. Ammonia odor
    d. One cast per high-powered field

49. List changes the nurse should ask about during an assessment for urologic problems.

50. List symptoms that a client with renal colic presents with.

51. The client presents with the following symptoms: anorexia, nausea, and vomiting, muscle cramping, and pruritus. What condition does this suggest to the nurse?

52. List areas where edema can be found in the client with a renal disorder.

53. What sound is heard by auscultation when a bruit is present in a renal artery?
    a. A quiet pulsating sound
    b. A swishing sound
    c. A faint wheezing
    d. No sound at all

54. Describe how to percuss the abdomen to determine whether the bladder is distended.

55. A report of dysuria by the client should lead the nurse to suspect which of the following?
    a. Urethral irritation
    b. Increased urine
    c. Less voiding
    d. Nocturia

56. Which of the following is an excellent indicator of kidney function?
    a. Urine osmolarity
    b. Serum creatinine
    c. Urine pH
    d. Color of urine

57. The serum creatinine level is closely monitored by the nurse and doctor because:
    a. The level does not change until 50% of renal function is lost.
    b. The level does not change until 25% of renal function is lost.
    c. The level changes suddenly.
    d. The level changes slowly.

58. The blood urea nitrogen (BUN) test measures which of the following?
    a. Renal excretion of nitrogen
    b. Glomerular filtration
    c. Creatinine clearance
    d. Urine output

59. In addition to kidney disease, what other condition may cause the BUN to rise above the normal range?
    a. Anemia
    b. Asthma
    c. Infection
    d. Malnutrition

60. In the client with dehydration, laboratory tests would show which of the following?
    a. BUN and creatinine ratio stay the same.
    b. BUN rises faster than creatinine level.
    c. Creatinine rises faster than BUN.
    d. BUN and creatine have a direct relationship.

61. Match each urine specimen finding with the corresponding characteristic.

Finding

_____ a. Color

_____ b. Odor

_____ c. Turbidity

_____ d. Specific gravity

_____ e. pH

_____ f. Glucose

_____ g. Ketone bodies

_____ h. Protein

_____ i. Microalbuminuria

_____ j. Sediment

_____ k. Cells

_____ l. Cast

_____ m. Crystals

_____ n. Bacteria

Characteristic
1. Less than 7 acidic, greater than 7 alkaline
2. Byproduct of fatty acid metabolism, not seen in urine
3. Only identified by microscopic examination for protein
4. Structure found around cell, bacteria, protein, and clumps
5. Urine is normally sterile; these multiply and grow
6. Urochrome pigment
7. 1.000 to 1.35
8. Not normally in the urine
9. Cells, casts, crystals, and bacteria
10. Various salts
11. Epithelial cells, RBC, WBC, tubular cells
12. Not seen in urine until blood sugar above 220 mg/dL
13. Clear urine
14. Faint ammonia

CASE STUDY: ASSESSMENT OF THE RENAL/URINARY SYSTEM

Answer Guidelines for the Case Study questions are provided on the companion Evolve Learning Resources Web site at http://evolve.elsevier.com/Iggy/.

A 74-year-old man is scheduled to have a series of urologic studies for diagnostic purposes. The physician orders the following: urinalysis, urine for culture and sensitivity, BUN, serum creatine, and 24-hour urine for creatinine clearance. The tests will be conducted on an outpatient basis.

1. Describe what the nurse should do to instruct the client in the collection of these laboratory specimens.

2. Which specimens should be collected first?

3. The client returns the collection container with a 24-hour urine specimen to the physician's office. As he gives it to the nurse, he comments, "I had a hard time remembering to save it all. Actually, I think I missed some when I forgot and used a bathroom at the shopping mall yesterday." What should the nurse do?

4. Further tests are ordered for the client, including a renal ultrasound and intravenous pyelography (IVP). These are scheduled at an outpatient radiology clinic. Design a teaching-learning plan for the client to prepare him for these studies.

5. Following the ultrasound and IVP, what assessments should be made for the client?

Interventions for Clients with Urinary Problems

LEARNING OUTCOMES

1. Describe the clinical manifestations of cystitis.
2. Develop a community-based teaching plan for a person at risk for cystitis.
3. Describe nursing interventions to prevent urinary tract infections among hospitalized clients.
4. Compare the pathophysiology and manifestations of stress incontinence, urge incontinence, overflow incontinence, mixed incontinence, and functional incontinence.
5. Describe the mechanisms of action, side effects, and nursing implications for the management of a urinary tract infection with sulfonamide and fluoroquinolone antibiotics.
6. Describe the techniques used to assess pelvic floor strength in the client who is experiencing some incontinence.
7. Explain the proper application of exercises to strengthen pelvic floor muscles.
8. Explain the drug therapy for different types of incontinence.
9. Develop a community-based teaching plan for the client who must perform intermittent self-catheterization for incontinence.
10. Prioritize nursing care for the client with renal colic.
11. Describe the manifestations of urinary obstruction.
12. Describe the common clinical manifestations of bladder cancer.
13. Develop a community-based teaching plan for continuing care of clients who have a urinary diversion for bladder cancer.

LEARNING ACTIVITIES

1. Before completing the study guide exercises in this chapter, review the following:
   - Anatomy and physiology of the renal and urinary tract systems
   - Process of excretion
   - Intake and output procedure

2. Review the boldfaced terms and their definitions in Chapter 73 to enhance your understanding of the content.

STUDY/REVIEW QUESTIONS

Answers to the Study/Review Questions are provided on the companion Evolve Learning Resources Web site at http:// evolve.elsevier.com/Iggy/.

1. Complete the following chart. Use Chapter 73 text, tables, and charts.

Diagnosis	Pathology and Symptoms	Treatment	Medications	Complications	Nursing Diagnosis
Urethritis					
Cystitis					
Prostatitis					
Urosepsis					
Urethral strictures					

2. List three areas of life that are affected by having urinary disorders and give an example of each.

   a. _____

   b. _____

   c. _____

3. Toward what goals are nursing interventions directed for the client with a urinary disorder?

   a. _____

   b. _____

   c. _____

4. To determine treatment for urinary tract infection, what two determinations must be made?

5. Asymptomatic bacteriuria is a condition that is which of the following?
   a. Cancer
   b. Benign
   c. Infectious
   d. Contagious

6. Inserting a catheter into the bladder will typically cause a urinary tract infection (UTI) in what percentage of clients?
   a. 25%
   b. 50%
   c. 75%
   d. 0%

7. List four conditions that can lead to a UTI related to *Candida*.

   a. _____

   b. _____

   c. _____

   d. _____

8. What is the recommended action for treatment of a UTI that is caused by a parasitic infection in the vagina?

9. Identify and give examples of three causes of noninfectious cystitis.

   a. _____

   b. _____

   c. _____

10. Which of the following characterizes interstitial cystitis, which is a chronic inflammation of the bladder?
    a. It results from food allergies.
    b. It has the same symptoms as UTI, only more intense.
    c. It affects men five times more often than women.
    d. It does not require treatment.

11. For women older than 80 years of age, the cause of UTI is most commonly due to which of the following?
    a. Variation in estrogen release
    b. Changes in the skin and mucous membranes
    c. Decreased fluid intake
    d. Inappropriate sexual behavior

12. A vesicoureteral reflex is diagnosed by a _____ _____.

13. A cystoscope can identify the following bladder problems:

    a. _____

    b. _____

    c. _____

    d. _____

    e. _____

14. Which of the following is the most common treatment for a fungal urinary tract infection?
    a. Sulfa drugs
    b. Cephalosporins
    c. Ketoconazole
    d. Quinolones

15. Daily fluid intake to prevent a bladder infection should include which of the following?
    a. 2 to 3 L of water
    b. 3 to 6 cans of soda pop
    c. 4 to 6 cups of coffee
    d. 3 to 4 glasses of orange juice

16. Instruction for clients with a UTI should include what points about medication?

17. What is the risk of pyelonephritis in pregnant women?

18. Treatment for a urethral stricture usually includes which of the following?
    a. Dilatation
    b. Antibiotic therapy
    c. Fluid restriction
    d. Radiation

19. List the most common types of urinary incontinence.

20. Identify which factors contribute to urinary incontinence in older adults.

21. Define cystocele.

22. What may be determined about the urinary tract from a digital rectal examination?

23. Identify five tests that can be done on the urinary tract before surgical interventions.

    a. _____

    b. _____

    c. _____

    d. _____

    e. _____

24. Your client has been performing Kegel exercises for 2 months. How will you and your client know whether the exercises are working?
    a. Incontinence is still present, but client states that it is less.
    b. Client is able to stop urinary stream.
    c. There are no complaints of urgency from the client.
    d. Client still needs clothing protection.

25. After a bladder suspension, a suprapubic catheter is typically maintained for how long?
    a. 24 hours postoperatively
    b. 48 hours postoperatively
    c. Until client is able to void on her own
    d. Until client is able to void and residual is less than 50 mL

26. Use your textbook, charts, and tables to complete the chart below on types of incontinence. Use a separate sheet of paper if necessary.

Diagnosis	Pathology and Symptoms	Treatment	Medications	Complications	Nursing Diagnosis
Stress incontinence					
Urge incontinence					
Overflow incontinence					
Functional incontinence					

27. As the nurse, your care plan for teaching the client with incontinence problems should include the following:

    a. _____

    b. _____

    c. _____

    d. _____

    e. _____

    f. _____

    g. _____

    h. _____

    i. _____

28. Define the following terms related to how stones are formed in the urinary system.

    a. Urolithiasis: _____

    _____

    b. Nephrolithiasis: _____

    _____

    c. Ureterolithiasis: _____

    _____

29. Which dietary changes should you suggest to your client who has stress incontinence?
    a. Limit fluid intake to no more than 2 L/day.
    b. Peel all fruit before consuming.
    c. Avoid alcohol and caffeine.
    d. Avoid smoked or salted foods.

30. How does vaginal cone therapy improve incontinence?
    a. By mechanically obstructing urine loss from the urethra
    b. By repositioning the bladder to reduce compression
    c. By increasing the normal flora of the perineum
    d. By strengthening pelvic floor muscles

31. Your client with urinary incontinence is prescribed to take oxybutynin (Ditropan). What precautions or instructions should you provide related to this therapy?
    a. Avoid aspirin or aspirin-containing products.
    b. Take this drug 1 hour before or 2 hours after a meal.
    c. Have a gynecologic examination with a Pap test performed every 3 months while on this medication.
    d. Change positions slowly, especially when moving from a lying to a standing position.

32. Identify at least three nursing diagnoses specific to the client who also has a diagnosis of urinary incontinence.

    a. _____

    b. _____

    c. _____

33. True or False? Write T for true or F for false. Indicate why the false statements are incorrect.

    _____ a. Habit training is not appropriate for a client who is confused or cognitively impaired.

    _____ b. Limiting fluid intake decreases the risk for incontinence.

    _____ c. Penile clamps can be used safely for functional incontinence in male clients.

    _____ d. Drug therapy has no role as an intervention for reflex urinary incontinence.

34. For which client is intermittent self-catheterization for incontinence inappropriate?
    a. A 90-year-old female client
    b. A male client with paraplegia
    c. A 65-year-old client who is confused
    d. A 70-year-old client who wears absorbent briefs

35. What is the priority nursing diagnosis for a client who has a renal calculus in the ureter?
    a. Risk for Renal Failure
    b. Fear of Recurrence
    c. Altered Elimination
    d. Acute Pain

36. Which clinical manifestation indicates to you that the management intervention for your client with a kidney stone is ineffective?
    a. The urine is blood-tinged.
    b. The pulse rate is 128 and thready.
    c. The pulse pressure is 40 mm Hg.
    d. The client refuses to take oral liquids.

37. The urine output of a client who has a kidney stone has decreased from 40 mL/hr to 5 mL/hr. What is your best action?
    a. Notify the physician.
    b. Credé the client's bladder.
    c. Test the urine for ketone bodies.
    d. Document the finding as the only action.

38. Indicate which intervention is most appropriate for each type of stone.

Type of Stone

_____ a. Calcium-containing stone

_____ b. Uric acid–containing stone

_____ c. Oxalate-containing stone

_____ d. Cystine-containing stone

Intervention
1. Captopril
2. Thiazide diuretic
3. Sodium bicarbonate
4. Pyridoxine

39. Which client is at greatest risk for the development of bladder cancer?
    a. A 60-year-old male client with chronic alcoholism
    b. A 25-year-old male client with type 1 diabetes mellitus
    c. A 60-year-old female client who smokes two packs of cigarettes per day and works in a paint factory
    d. A 25-year-old female client who has had three episodes of bacterial (*Escherichia coli*) cystitis in the past year

40. Explain how a Kock's pouch is different from an ileal conduit.

41. What treatment should you expect for a client who has superficial bladder cancer?
    a. Intravesical instillation of BCG
    b. Radiation to the bladder, ureters, and urethra
    c. No treatment is needed for this benign condition
    d. Complete cystostomy with cutaneous ureterostomy

42. With which type of urinary diversion will male clients need to learn to sit to urinate?
    a. Kock's pouch
    b. Ileal conduit
    c. Cutaneous ureterostomy
    d. Diversion into sigmoid colon

43. Which nursing diagnoses are appropriate for a client in the community who has a Kock's pouch after surgery for bladder cancer?

44. A client is returning to your unit from the postanesthesia care unit after surgery for bladder cancer resulting in a cutaneous ureterostomy. Where should you expect the stoma to be located?
    a. On the perineum
    b. At the beltline
    c. On the posterior flank
    d. In the midabdominal area

45. Which intervention should you expect for a client who has sustained a simple bladder contusion?
    a. Hemodialysis
    b. Insertion of a Foley catheter
    c. Placement of a suprapubic catheter
    d. Surgical creation of a temporary urinary diversion

Interventions for Clients with Renal Disorders

CHAPTER 74

LEARNING OUTCOMES

1. Prioritize nursing care for the client with polycystic kidney disease.
2. Describe the clinical manifestations of hydronephrosis.
3. Identify clients at risk for pyelonephritis.
4. Describe the mechanisms of action, side effects, and nursing implications for drug therapy for pyelonephritis.
5. Use laboratory data and clinical manifestations to determine the effectiveness of therapy for pyelonephritis.
6. Compare the pathophysiology and clinical manifestations of acute glomerular nephritis and nephrotic syndrome.
7. Explain the relationship between hypertension and renal disease.
8. Prioritize nursing care for the client during the first 24 hours after a nephrectomy.
9. Explain how diabetic nephropathy can affect glucose metabolism and control in the client with diabetes mellitus.
10. Develop a community-based teaching plan for the client who has had a nephrectomy for renal cell carcinoma.
11. Describe strategies to prevent renal trauma.

LEARNING ACTIVITIES

1. Before completing the study guide exercises in this chapter, it is recommended that you review the following:
   - Anatomy and physiology of the renal system
   - Normal renal laboratory values
   - Assessment of the renal and urinary system
   - Acid-base balance
   - Intake and output
   - Infusion therapy
   - Fluid and electrolytes

2. Review the boldfaced terms and their definitions in Chapter 74 to enhance your understanding of the content.

STUDY/REVIEW QUESTIONS

Answers to the Study/Review Questions are provided on the companion Evolve Learning Resources Web site at http://evolve.elsevier.com/Iggy/.

1. List and give examples of seven types of renal disorders, by cause or origin.

   a. _____

   b. _____

   c. _____

   d. _____

   e. _____

   f. _____

   g. _____

2. Polycystic kidney disease (PKD) is the most common:
   a. Inherited disease of African-Americans
   b. Inherited disease of whites
   c. Acquired disease of African-Americans
   d. Acquired disease of whites

3. Treatment of polycystic kidney disease (PKD) would include what interventions?

4. Describe the causes of pain for clients with PKD.

5. What are the causes of hypertension and renal ischemia in a client with PKD?

6. The effect on the renin-angiotensin system in the kidney in PKD results in which of the following?
   a. Increased blood pressure
   b. Decreased blood pressure
   c. Decreased renal flow
   d. Increased renal flow

7. What is the risk involved with other organs and tissues in the progression of PKD?

8. Clients with PKD often have other tissue involvement. List several of the complications that can be present.

9. Compare the risk of inheritance of PKD by gender.

10. Match each characteristic of clients with polycystic disease to the corresponding gene trait. *Answers may be used more than once.*

Characteristic

_____ a. About 40 years of age at onset of manifestations

_____ b. Death in childhood

_____ c. Affects 5% to 10% of nephrons early in life

_____ d. Cysts develop everywhere and get larger

_____ e. Present at birth

_____ f. Kidneys are like bunches of grapes

_____ g. Slow cystic rate

_____ h. Progressive renal failure

Gene Trait
1. Autosomal recessive
2. Autosomal dominant

11. A client presenting with PKD typically has what symptoms?

12. Sharp pain followed by blood in the urine in the client with PKD is usually caused by which of the following?
    a. Infection
    b. A ruptured cyst
    c. Increased kidney size
    d. A ruptured renal artery aneurysm

13. As PKD becomes more severe, symptoms from berry aneurysms can include which of the following?
    a. Severe headache
    b. Pruritus
    c. Edema
    d. Fatigue

14. Nocturia in clients with PKD is due to which of the following?
    a. Increased fluid intake in the evening
    b. Increased hypertension
    c. Decreased renal concentrating ability
    d. Detrusor irritability

15. List reasons that clients diagnosed with PKD may need a nursing diagnosis of Impaired Coping.

16. What are typical findings of a urinalysis in a client with PKD?

    a. _____

    b. _____

    c. _____

17. Which laboratory abnormalities in a client with PKD indicates disease progression?
    a. Hypercalcemia
    b. Hypokalemia
    c. Proteinuria
    d. Homocystinuria

18. Of the following diagnostic studies, which can show PKD with minimal risk?
    a. KUB
    b. Urography
    c. Renal sonography
    d. MRI with contrast

19. Which drug category should be avoided or used with caution in a client with PKD who is having pain?
    a. NSAIDs
    b. Meperidine
    c. Morphine sulfate
    d. Sulfa-containing antibiotics

20. Which pain management strategy should the nurse teach a client who has pain from progressive PKD?
    a. Take nothing by mouth.
    b. Increase the dose of aspirin.
    c. Assume a high Fowler's position.
    d. Apply dry heat to the abdomen or flank.

21. The client with PKD usually experiences constipation. What topic of instruction should the nurse provide?
    a. Stool softener and increased fluids.
    b. Decreased dietary fiber and laxatives.
    c. Laxatives and decreased fluids.
    d. Daily tap water enemas and fiber supplements.

22. The client with PKD has nocturia and should do which of the following?
    a. Drink 2 L of fluid daily.
    b. Restrict fluid in the evening.
    c. Only drink 1000 mL/24 hr.
    d. Take diuretics as ordered.

23. Which of the following is the best choice of medication to control hypertension in a client with PKD?
    a. ACE inhibitors
    b. Beta blockers
    c. Calcium channel blockers
    d. Potassium-sparing diuretics

24. Identify priority nursing care needs for clients with polycystic kidney disease.

25. After the nurse instructs a client with PKD on his home care, the client should know to contact the physician immediately when what happens?
    a. The urine is blood-tinged.
    b. Weight has increased by 3 pounds in 3 days.
    c. Two days have passed since the last bowel movement.
    d. Morning systolic blood pressure has decreased by 5 mm Hg.

26. Hydronephrosis, hydroureter, and urethral stricture have much in common because they are all forms of what?
    a. Stones
    b. Tumors
    c. Obstructions
    d. Congenital deformities

27. Which clinical manifestations in a client with an obstruction in the urinary system is associated specifically with a hydronephrosis?
    a. Flank asymmetry
    b. Chills and fever
    c. Urge incontinence
    d. Decreased urine volume

28. List three outcomes of a decrease in the glomerular filtration rate.

    a. _____

    b. _____

    c. _____

29. Indicate which of the factors or manifestations listed below are primarily:
    1. Associated with acute pyelonephritis
    2. Associated with chronic pyelonephritis
    3. Common to both acute and chronic pyelonephritis
    4. Common to neither acute nor chronic pyelonephritis

    _____ a. Obstruction with reflex

    _____ b. Abscess formation

    _____ c. Alcohol abuse

    _____ d. Active bacterial infection

    _____ e. Decreased urine specific gravity

    _____ f. CVA tenderness/pain

30. Which client is at greatest risk for the development of chronic pyelonephritis?
    a. An 80-year-old woman who takes diuretics for mild heart failure
    b. An 80-year-old man who drinks four cans of beer per day
    c. A 36-year-old woman with diabetes mellitus who is pregnant
    d. A 36-year-old man with diabetes insipidus

31. In acute pyelonephritis, acute inflammation is followed by which of the following?
    a. Tubular cell necrosis and abscess formation
    b. Abscesses in capsule, cortex, and medulla
    c. Fibrous cyst formation
    d. a then b then c

32. Describe vesicoureteral and intrarenal reflux.

33. Explain the differences between an ascending and a descending urinary tract infection.

34. The most common causes of pyelonephritis among people living in the community are which of the following gastrointestinal tract organisms?
    a. *Escherichia coli* and *Enterococcus faecalis*
    b. *Proteus mirabilis* and *Klebsiella* species
    c. *Pseudomonas aeruginosa* and *Klebsiella* species
    d. *Staphylococcus aureus*, *Salmonella* species, and *Candida* species

35. Screening a client for pyelonephritis testing would include what procedures?

36. Nonsurgical management of pyelonephritis could include what interventions?

37. What surgeries may be performed to preserve the kidney of a client with pyelonephritis?

38. Which of the following is the priority nursing diagnosis for a client with pyelonephritis?
    a. Deficient Knowledge
    b. Excess Fluid Volume
    c. Acute/Chronic Pain
    d. Activity Intolerance

39. Postoperative instruction for a client with pyelonephritis is important and will include all of the following except:
    a. Controlling the blood pressure
    b. Fluid restriction
    c. Protein restriction
    d. Ingesting at least 2 L of fluid per day

40. Which is the most important action for a client with pyelonephritis?
    a. Complete all antibiotic regimens.
    b. Report episodes of nocturia.
    c. Stop taking the antibiotic when pain is relieved.
    d. Notify physician of any over-the-counter drugs.

41. List three outcomes for a client with pyelonephritis.

    a. _____

    b. _____

    c. _____

42. List three places where renal abscess can occur.

    a. _____

    b. _____

    c. _____

43. List two ways renal abscess can be identified.

    a. _____

    b. _____

44. In addition to antibiotics, treatment for a renal abscess may include which of the following?
    a. Surgical incision or needle aspiration
    b. Hemodialysis
    c. Insertion of a suprapubic catheter
    d. Cystostomy

45. The treatment for renal tuberculosis includes which of the following?
    a. Immunosuppressive drugs
    b. Glucocorticoid drugs
    c. Antitubercular therapy
    d. Opioid analgesics

46. Acute glomerulonephritis has which of the following causes? *Choose all that apply.*
    a. Immunologic basis
    b. Underlying genetic basis
    c. Fungal infections
    d. Bacterial infections

47. Renal tissue changes in chronic glomerulonephritis are caused by which of the following? *Choose all that apply.*
    a. Hypertension
    b. Ischemia
    c. Fluid and electrolyte imbalance
    d. Trauma

48. Which health care problem reported to you by a client who has acute glomerular nephritis could be considered a causative factor for the disorder?
    a. Cystitis 6 months ago
    b. Strep throat 3 weeks ago
    c. Sprained ankle 6 days ago
    d. Mild hypertension diagnosed 1 year ago

49. The glomerular filtration rate (GFR) of a client who has acute pyelonephritis is 50 mL/minute. What is your interpretation of this finding?
    a. The GFR is normal; therapy is effective.
    b. The GFR is high; the client is at risk for dehydration.
    c. The GFR is low; the client is at risk for shock.
    d. The GFR is low; the client is at risk for fluid overload.

50. Upon physical assessment, the client with acute glomerulonephritis may tell the nurse:
    a. The urine has been smoky or cola-colored.
    b. The urine has been clear.
    c. That nocturia has been a problem.
    d. That diaphoresis has been present at night.

51. Which of the following diagnostic tests and results would you expect in acute glomerulonephritis? *Check all that apply.*

    _____ a. UA revealing hematuria

    _____ b. UA revealing proteinuria

    _____ c. Microscopic red blood cell casts

    _____ d. Normal urine sedimentation assay

    _____ e. 24-hour urine for creatinine clearance decreased

    _____ f. Serum nitrogen level decreased

    _____ g. Serum albumin levels decreased

    _____ h. Antistreptolysin-O titers increased

    _____ i. Type III cryoglobulin present

52. Which of the following statements is true regarding treatment of a client with late-stage chronic glomerulonephritis?
    a. The appropriate anti-infective medication is used for treatment.
    b. Dialysis or transplantation is needed.
    c. The client is treated with radiation.
    d. Immunosuppressive agents are used.

53. List four interventions to prevent complications from acute glomerulonephritis.

    a. _____

    b. _____

    c. _____

    d. _____

54. Which nursing intervention is appropriate for a client with acute glomerular nephritis?
    a. Restricting visitors to adults only
    b. Using a lift sheet to turn the client
    c. Inspecting the vascular access
    d. Measuring abdominal girth daily

55. Rapidly progressive glomerulonephritis is related to which of the following?
    a. Previous multisystem disease
    b. Tuberculosis
    c. Urinary tract infection
    d. Pyelonephritis

56. Which is most commonly associated with chronic glomerular nephritis?
    a. History of antibiotic allergy
    b. Intense flank pain
    c. Malnutrition and weight loss
    d. Mild edema and hypertension

57. Which manifestation is a hallmark for nephrotic syndrome rather than another type of kidney problem?
    a. Flank asymmetry
    b. Serum albumin 2.2 g/dL
    c. Serum sodium 148 mmol/L
    d. Serum cholesterol (total) 190 mg/dL

58. Immune alterations may produce which type of renal disorders?
    a. Tubercular
    b. Interstitial
    c. Degenerative
    d. Infectious

59. What is the underlying pathology of nephrosclerosis?
    a. Decreased renal blood flow, ischemia, renal fibrosis
    b. Renal hypertension, parenchymal ischemia, necrosis
    c. Abscess formation, inflammation, narrowing of the renal tubules
    d. Increased capillary permeability, cortical edema, urinary obstruction

60. Renovascular disease affects the renal arteries by stenosis or thrombosis and has which of the following characteristics?
    a. Sudden onset of hypertension after 50 years of age
    b. Associated with chronic cystitis
    c. Leads to renal calculus formation
    d. Most common in men

61. Treatment for renal artery stenosis includes all of the following except:
    a. Renal transplant
    b. Control hypertension
    c. Percutaneous transluminal balloon angioplasty
    d. Renal bypass surgery

62. What change in diabetic therapy may be needed for a client who has stage IV diabetic nephropathy?
    a. Fluid restriction
    b. Dietary protein restriction
    c. Decreased insulin dosages
    d. Increased dietary fat intake

63. In a client with diabetic nephropathy, changes in what organ correlate with damage to renal microvascular changes?
    a. Heart
    b. Retina
    c. Oral mucosa
    d. Feet

64. Explain how renal insufficiency affects insulin availability for clients with type 1 or type 2 diabetes mellitus.

65. Which of the following are symptoms of renal cell carcinoma? *Check all that apply.*

    _____ a. Urinary tract infection

    _____ b. Erythrocytosis

    _____ c. Hypercalcemia

    _____ d. Liver dysfunction

    _____ e. Decreased sedimentation rate

    _____ f. Elevated BUN

    _____ g. Hematuria

    _____ h. Hypertension

66. List three hormonal changes brought about by tumor cells in renal cell carcinoma and give outcomes of these changes.

67. A renal cell carcinoma that has metastasized to the lungs would be considered what stage?
    a. Stage I
    b. Stage II
    c. Stage III
    d. Stage IV

68. The client with renal cell carcinoma typically presents with which of the following?
    a. Flank pain, gross hematuria, palpable renal mass, and renal bruit
    b. Gross hematuria, hypertension (HTN), diabetes, and oliguria
    c. Dysuria, dehydration, and renal mass
    d. Nocturia and urinary retention

69. What is the best treatment for renal cancer?
    a. Chemotherapy
    b. Surgical removal
    c. Hormonal therapy
    d. Radiation therapy

70. A client who had a left radical nephrectomy for renal cell carcinoma returns to your unit and is concerned because he has severe pain on the right side. What should you tell this client?
    a. "The right kidney was repositioned to take over the function of both kidneys."
    b. "I'll call your doctor for an order to increase your pain medication."
    c. "The pain is likely to be from being positioned on your right side during surgery."
    d. "Would you like to talk with someone who had this surgery last year and now is fully recovered?"

71. What does a decrease in blood pressure in the postoperative nephrectomy client means?
    a. Hypertension has been corrected.
    b. Possible internal hemorrhage.
    c. The other kidney is failing.
    d. The client is responsive to medication.

72. Postoperative urine flow in the client following nephrectomy should be at least which of the following?
    a. 10 to 20 mL/hr
    b. 30 to 50 mL/hr
    c. 60 to 80 mL/hr
    d. Over 100 mL/hr

73. Analgesics for the client who has had a nephrectomy should be:
    a. Limited because they slow respiration
    b. An oral analgesic
    c. Given parenterally as needed for 3 to 5 days
    d. Given parenterally on a schedule

74. Of the levels of renal trauma, which one needs immediate repair?
    a. Major
    b. Minor
    c. Pedicle
    d. Palliative

75. For a client with pedicle injury, what is the best diagnostic test?
    a. Urinalysis
    b. Renal arteriography
    c. CT
    d. Intravenous urography

76. List five nursing diagnoses for the client with renal trauma.

    a. _____

    b. _____

    c. _____

    d. _____

    e. _____

Interventions for Clients with Acute and Chronic Renal Failure

LEARNING OUTCOMES

1. Compare the pathophysiology and causes of acute renal failure (ARF) with those of chronic renal failure (CRF).
2. Identify clients at risk for development of ARF.
3. Identify clients at risk for development of CRF.
4. Use laboratory data and clinical assessment to determine the effectiveness of therapy for renal failure.
5. Discuss interventions to prevent ARF.
6. Prioritize nursing care for the client with ARF.
7. Describe the mechanisms of action, side effects, and nursing implications for pharmacologic management of renal failure.
8. Compare the clinical manifestations of stage I, stage II, and stage III CRF.
9. Discuss the mechanisms of peritoneal dialysis (PD) and hemodialysis (HD) as renal replacement therapies.
10. Prioritize nursing care for the client with end-stage renal disease.
11. Prioritize teaching needs for the client using continuous ambulatory PD.
12. Develop a community-based teaching plan for the client with a permanent vascular access for long-term HD.
13. Compare the dietary modifications needed for the client undergoing HD with those for the client undergoing PD.
14. Plan prevention strategies for the complications of PD.
15. Discuss the criteria for kidney donation.
16. Prioritize nursing care for the client during the first 24 hours after kidney transplantation.
17. Develop a community-based teaching plan for the client who has received a kidney transplant.

LEARNING ACTIVITIES

1. Before completing the study guide exercises in this chapter, it is recommended that you review the following:
   • Anatomy and physiology of the renal system
   • Assessment of the renal and urinary systems

- Normal renal laboratory values
- Intake and output
- Fluid and electrolyte
- Infusion therapy
- Diuretics

2. Review the boldfaced terms and their definitions in Chapter 75 to enhance your understanding of the content.

STUDY/REVIEW QUESTIONS

Answers to the Study/Review Questions are provided on the companion Evolve Learning Resources Web site at http://evolve.elsevier.com/Iggy/.

1. What is the most common cause of renal failure?

2. Chronic renal function deteriorates the kidney slowly; significant failure is not seen until what percent of the nephrons are destroyed?
   a.   30% to 50%
   b.   50% to 60%
   c.   60% to 75%
   d.   90% to 95%

3. Acute renal failure may occur with only what percent of nephrons functioning?
   a.   30%
   b.   50%
   c.   75%
   d.   90%

4. How do acute renal failure and chronic renal failure compare with respect to effect on other body systems?

5. Compare and contrast the pathophysiology and causes of chronic renal failure and acute renal failure. Use the textbook and Tables 75-2, 75-6, and 75-7.

6. Identify clients at risk to develop acute renal failure (ARF).

7. Discuss intervention to prevent ARF.

8. Describe how the kidney uses an autoregulatory response to compensate for decreased renal blood flow.

9. Explain how injury to the tubular cells of the kidney can occur as a result of decreased renal blood flow.

10. Renal insufficiency is present when:
    a. The BUN and creatinine levels rise and remain constant.
    b. The BUN rises faster than creatinine level.
    c. The BUN is lower than creatinine level.
    d. Both BUN and creatine levels decrease.

11. Match each cause to the corresponding urologic change. *Answers may be used more than once.*

Cause

_____ a. Urethral cancer

_____ b. CHF

_____ c. Vasculitis

_____ d. Sepsis

_____ e. Exposure to nephrotoxins

_____ f. Renal calculi

_____ g. Atony of bladder

_____ h. Renal artery stenosis or thrombosis

_____ i. Shock

Urologic Change
1. Prerenal
2. Intrarenal
3. Postrenal

12. Which of the following drugs are nephrotoxic?
    a. Aspirin and NSAIDs
    b. Antibiotics and aspirin
    c. Antibiotics and NSAIDs
    d. Antihypertensives and antibiotics

13. List three interventions to reverse prerenal azotemia.

    a. _____

    b. _____

    c. _____

14. When the vascular volume is depleted, the nurse can expect the signs of which of the following?
    a. Decreased urine output, postural hypotension, and tachycardia
    b. Increased urine output, postural hypotension, and tachycardia
    c. Tachycardia, hypertension, and decreased urine output
    d. Tachycardia, hypertension, and increased urine output

15. Which of the following is an early sign of renal tubular damage?
    a. Elevated BUN
    b. Decreased urine specific gravity
    c. Increased serum electrolytes
    d. Oliguria

16. List three things the nurse should monitor when a client is taking a nephrotoxic drug.

    a. _____

    b. _____

    c. _____

17. List four things the nurse should note when taking a history of a client with prerenal failure.

    a. _____

    b. _____

    c. _____

    d. _____

18. The symptoms of a client with prerenal azotemia mimic those of a client with what other conditions?

19. Identify the symptoms of prerenal azotemia:

    a. _____

    b. _____

    c. _____

    d. _____

    e. _____

    f. _____

20. Identify the symptoms of intrarenal acute renal failure that are different from those of prerenal azotemia.

    a. _____

    b. _____

    c. _____

    d. _____

    e. _____

    f. _____

    g. _____

    h. _____

    i. _____

21. Identify two conditions a flat plate x-ray could reveal about the kidneys.

    a. _____

    b. _____

22. How can most renal obstructions be diagnosed?

23. Identify priorities for care of clients with acute renal failure.

24. For clients in prerenal azotemia, a fluid challenge is done to promote renal perfusion by which of the following?
    a. Administering normal saline 500 to 1000 mL infused over 1 hour
    b. Administering drugs to suppress aldosterone release
    c. Instilling warm, sterile normal saline into the bladder
    d. Discontinuing diuretic therapy

25. What drug may enhance renal perfusion or elevate blood pressure?

26. In the client with acute renal failure, what are calcium channel blockers used to do?
    a. Prevent buildup of calcium stones in the kidneys.
    b. Prevent buildup of vitamin D in the kidneys.
    c. Limit renal perfusion.
    d. Maintain cell integrity and improve GFR.

27. Clients in acute renal failure have a high rate of catabolism that is related to which of the following?
    a. Increased levels of catecholamines, cortisol, and glucagon
    b. Inability to excrete excess electrolytes
    c. Conversion of body fat into glucose
    d. Presence of retained nitrogenous wastes

28. What should be done when the client with acute renal failure is anorexic?
    a. Give normal saline to prevent dehydration.
    b. The dietitian will prescribe a calculated diet.
    c. TPN can be ordered if laboratory results are monitored.
    d. Fat emulsion can be added to TPN.

29. The goal of TPN is to:
    a. Preserve lean body mass
    b. Promote tubular reabsorption
    c. Create a negative nitrogen balance
    d. Prevent infection

30. Identify the indications for dialysis in the client with acute renal failure.

31. What is the rationale for having a double lumen catheter for hemodialysis?

32. List three advantages of using peritoneal dialysis instead of hemodialysis.

33. Identify three types of clients for whom continuous arteriovenous hemodialysis and filtration (CAVH) would be used.

    a. _____

    b. _____

    c. _____

34. Describe the rationale for the use of a pump in CAVH and list a risk of this pump.

35. Match each characteristic with the corresponding device. *Answers may be used more than once.*

Characteristic

_____ a. Requires placement of arterial and venous catheter

_____ b. Requires a double-lumen venous catheter

_____ c. Uses pump

_____ d. Arterial pressure of at least 60 mm Hg

_____ e. Removes water and electrolytes

_____ f. Risk of air embolus

_____ g. Uses dialysate to remove nitrogenous waste

Device
1. CAVH
2. CAVHD
3. CVVH

36. Prioritize teaching needs for the client using continuous ambulatory peritoneal dialysis (CAPD).

37. Identify each of the following terms and abbreviations:

ESRD

Uremia

Uremic syndrome

Azotemia

CRF

Hyposthenuria

Isosthenuria

Polyuria

GFR

HTN

38. Match each characteristic with the corresponding stage of renal failure. *Answers may be used more than once.*

Characteristic

_____ a. Excessive waste products

_____ b. Increased BUN and creatinine

_____ c. Dialysis

_____ d. Reduced function

_____ e. Nephrons compensation

_____ f. Hypertension (HTN)

_____ g. Stress of illness can compromise this stage fast

_____ h. Medical management very important

_____ i. Severe fluid overload

_____ j. Electrolyte and acid-base imbalances

_____ k. Renal osteodystrophy

Stage
1. Diminished renal reserve
2. Renal insufficiency
3. End-stage renal disease

39. The GFR functions can maintain kidney function until only 20% of the nephrons are left, and then nephrons:
a. Become edematous
b. Decrease water absorption
c. Increase water absorption
d. Begin to atrophy

40. As the client with end-stage renal disease experiences hyposthenuria, polyuria, and then isosthenuria, the nurse needs to be alert for which of the following?
a. The diuretic stage
b. Fluid volume overload
c. Dehydration
d. Alkalosis

41. Ideally, when should renal replacement therapy for a client who has chronic renal failure (CRF) begin?
a. Stage I
b. Stage II
c. Stage III
d. Stage IV

42. What are the most accurate ways to monitor kidney function?

43. Identify the cause of sodium depletion seen in early CRF.

44. Briefly describe the stages of renal failure.

45. Which of the following is a result of kidney failure?
    a. Excessive hydrogen ions cannot be excreted.
    b. Excessive hydrogen ions are counteracted by ammonia.
    c. Excessive hydrogen ions are balanced by excessive bicarbonate.
    d. Excessive hydrogen ions cause metabolic alkalosis.

46. With acid retention, respiratory compensation is manifested as which of the following?
    a. A Cheyne-Stokes respiratory pattern
    b. An increased depth of breathing
    c. Decreased respiratory rate and depth
    d. Increased arterial carbon dioxide levels

47. Describe the changes in the relationship between calcium and phosphorus in the client with renal failure.

48. A client in uremia will have all of the following except:
    a. Uremic halitosis or stomatitis
    b. Hiccups and anorexia
    c. Spider hemangiomas
    d. Nausea and vomiting

49. Identify the two most common causes of CRF.

    a. _____

    b. _____

50. Identify clients at risk for the development of CRF.

51. The nurse taking a history on a client with CRF needs to be aware of characteristic symptoms. Review Chart 75-7 and identify effects on each body system.

52. A client with CRF can use many nursing diagnoses as the condition changes daily. Identify the three diagnoses that apply until transplant or death.

    a. _____

    b. _____

    c. _____

53. How does dialysis affect the dietary needs of the client?

54. How do the protein needs of a client receiving hemodialysis compare to those of a client receiving peritoneal dialysis?

55. Identify assessments the nurse should instruct the CRF client to document at home.

56. What precautions to prevent infection would the nurse teach the client with CRF?

57. Identify drugs typically given to clients with CRF. Note important side effects or toxicities that can result from poor kidney function.

58. What are the expected outcomes of treating a client with CRF with recombinant erythropoietin?

59. What signs and symptoms does the nurse assess for in possible pulmonary edema?

60. List interventions appropriate for a client suffering from pulmonary edema.

61. Identify the medications commonly ordered for the client with pulmonary edema.

62. Hemodialysis is initiated immediately for what reasons?

63. What is the basis for calculating the duration of survival for a client on hemodialysis?

64. Compare and contrast dietary modifications needed for a client on hemodialysis with those for a client on peritoneal dialysis. Use Table 75-8.

65. Discuss mechanisms of peritoneal dialysis and hemodialysis as renal replacement therapies.

66. Prioritize teaching for a client using CAPD.

67. Briefly describe the process of dialysis.

68. Why is it unnecessary for the dialysate to be sterile to protect the client during dialysis?

69. List four important facts about heparin that the nurse must know about the client on hemodialysis.

70. Prioritize teaching needs with permanent vascular access device for long-term dialysis.

71. List four precautions for a client with AV fistula or AV graft.

a. _____

b. _____

c. _____

d. _____

72. Identify the complications that can occur regardless of type of access for renal replacement therapies.

a. _____

b. _____

c. _____

d. _____

e. _____

f. _____

73. What is the most common infectious agent in the client with a AV fistula or graft, and how is it usually introduced?

74. The client exhibits the following progressive symptoms: headache, nausea, and vomiting; decreased level of consciousness; seizures and coma. What syndrome do these suggest to the nurse?

75. How is the syndrome identified in Question 74 treated?

76. What practices have helped reduce the incidence of hepatitis and HIV in dialysis clients?

77. In peritoneal dialysis, what is the membrane through which the process occurs?

78. What is used to prevent fibrin clot formation in peritoneal dialysis?

79. Identify the types of peritoneal dialysis and note the difference of each.

80. How is peritonitis identified and diagnosed in the client receiving dialysis?

81. The client reports to the nurse about out-flow from the first peritoneal dialysis. What does the nurse instruct the client about this?

82. Identify the source of possible problems with the flow of dialysate in clients with peritoneal dialysis.

83. What do the following appearances indicate about the outflow of peritoneal dialysis dialysate?
    a. Red or pink

    b. Brown color

    c. Yellow color

    d. Cloudy

84. Identify the reasons a client may not qualify for transplantation.

85. Describe the qualifications for kidney donors.

86. Describe the necessity of matching organ size for adults and children who receive kidney transplants.

87. Before a kidney is determined a suitable donor for transplant, the client and kidney undergo what testing?

    a. _____

    b. _____

    c. _____

88. In order to increase graft survival, a kidney transplant recipient receives what two procedures before transplantation?

89. Identify two postoperative assessments the nurse will use to monitor the kidney recipient.

    a. _____

    b. _____

90. Prioritize nursing care for the client during the first 24 hours after kidney transplant.

91. Identify the possible complication indicated by oliguria.

92. Indicate types of rejections, how they are identified, how they are treated, and which is the most common.

93. What interventions may be implemented to save the transplant when acute tubular necrosis is present?

94. In a transplant client, a sudden decrease in urine at 2 to 3 days postoperative is a sign of which of the following?
    a. Rejection
    b. Thrombosis
    c. Stenosis
    d. Other complications

95. What places a kidney recipient at risk for fatal viral, fungal, bacterial, or protozoal infections?

96. Identify the drugs used for immunosuppression following a kidney transplant.

97. The nurse is responsible for teaching a client in-home care. Use Chart 75-12 to develop a teaching plan for the home care client on dialysis and after transplantation. Include the family.

98. Briefly describe the changing moods of the client on dialysis and how the nurse can provide psychosocial support.

99. Identify two sources of ongoing costs of care after transplantation.

    a. _____

    b. _____

CASE STUDY: CONTINUOUS AMBULATORY PERITONEAL DIALYSIS (CAPD)

Answer Guidelines for the Case Study questions are provided on the companion Evolve Learning Resources Web site at http://evolve.elsevier.com/Iggy/.

A 36-year-old woman is married and has two adopted children. She is diagnosed with polycystic kidney disease (PKD). She will soon have to go on dialysis or consent to a renal transplant.

1. Develop a teaching-learning plan for the client that explains hemodialysis, peritoneal dialysis, CAPD, and renal transplantation.

2. What additional data should the nurse collect to help the client make the best decision for herself?

3. Due to the long distance the client lives from the medical center, she elects to begin CAPD. Develop a plan of care for the client for this procedure.

4. Develop a teaching-learning plan for CAPD management.

Assessment of the Reproductive System

LEARNING OUTCOMES

1. Review the anatomy and physiology of the male and female reproductive systems.
2. Discuss the components of a health history for reproductive health problems using Gordon's Functional Health Patterns.
3. Explain the procedures for physical assessment of the male and female reproductive systems.
4. Describe the client preparation for common reproductive diagnostic tests.
5. Interpret common reproductive laboratory diagnostic test findings.
6. Develop a teaching plan for a client undergoing one of the endoscopic studies for reproductive health problems.
7. Explain the importance of selected reproductive screening tests in promoting and maintaining health (e.g., Pap test).

LEARNING ACTIVITIES

1. Before completing the study guide exercises for this chapter, it is recommended that you review the following:
   - Anatomy and physiology of the male and female reproductive systems
   - Effect of the endocrine system on genitoreproductive tissue
   - Concepts of human sexuality
   - Concepts of body image and self-esteem
   - Normal growth and development

2. Review the boldfaced terms and their definitions in Chapter 76 to enhance your understanding of the content.

STUDY/REVIEW QUESTIONS

Answers to the Study/Review Questions are provided on the companion Evolve Learning Resources Web site at http://evolve.elsevier.com/Iggy/.

1. A mother is very concerned that her 13-year-old son is not showing any physical signs of puberty but her daughter was fully developed and menstruating by the age of 13. The nurse's best response to the mother would be which of the following?
   a. "Your son will start his growth spurt by his 14th birthday, so I would not worry at this time."
   b. "Boys usually mature physically before girls, so your son needs to see your family doctor."
   c. "Girls usually mature physically about 2 years before boys, so I wouldn't be concerned at this time."
   d. "Boys and girls generally mature at about the same age, so you need to take your son to the doctor immediately."

2. Which order of the phases of the menstrual cycle is correct?
   a. Proliferative, secretory, sloughing, follicular
   b. Sloughing, proliferative, secretory, ischemic
   c. Follicular, proliferative, sloughing, secretory
   d. Proliferative, secretory, sloughing, ischemic

3. Your client, 13½ years of age, experienced menarche 4 months ago. Her mother is very concerned that her daughter has had very irregular menstrual cycles since then. Which of the following is the nurse's best response to the mother?
   a. Her daughter needs to see a doctor for a pelvic examination.
   b. Her daughter needs to have a pregnancy test done.
   c. Her daughter's irregularity will adjust itself within the next 2 years.
   d. Her daughter's irregularity is normal following the onset of menstruation.

4. The menstrual cycle is regulated by a feedback control system of interrelated cycles. What are these interrelated cycles?
   a. Mammary, ovarian, and uterine cycles
   b. Hypothalamic-pituitary, ovarian, and endometrial cycles
   c. Ovarian, pituitary, and gonadal cycles
   d. Hypothalamic-pituitary, mammary, and ovarian cycles

5. During a sex education class, the nurse is explaining the function of the female breasts to a group of seventh grade students. The nurse's best statement would be which of the following?
   a. The female breasts have only one function: serving as a source of sexual pleasure.
   b. The function of the female breasts is to provide nourishment for the mother's baby.
   c. The female breasts provide nourishment for the mother's baby and are a source of sexual sensation.
   d. The main function of the female breasts is to allow for passive transfer of antibodies to the baby after birth.

6. What is the normal pH of the vagina necessary to decrease the vagina's susceptibility to infection?
   a. 5.0
   b. 4.5
   c. 4.0
   d. 6.0

7. Which of the following is the inner layer of the uterus that allows for implantation of the fetus and that is shed during menses?
   a. Myometrium
   b. Parametrium
   c. Endometrium
   d. Peritoneum

8. Which of the following statements is true concerning artificial menopause?
   a. It is a pseudomenopause.
   b. Estrogen levels usually increase.
   c. It can be surgically corrected.
   d. It can be surgically induced.

9. What part of the internal reproductive system of the male aids in maturation of the sperm?
    a. Vas deferens
    b. Epididymis
    c. Seminal vesicles
    d. Ejaculatory glands

10. Identify three things that the fluid excreted by the prostate does in the male reproductive cycle.

    a. _____

    b. _____

    c. _____

11. Identify three factors that can have a direct negative effect on reproductive health in both men and women.

    a. _____

    b. _____

    c. _____

12. Identify the three most common symptoms presented in problems associated with the reproductive system.

    a. _____

    b. _____

    c. _____

13. Which of the following points would the nurse make to instruct a client about a pelvic exam?
    a. The client needs to douche before the examination to allow for better visualization of the cervix.
    b. The client needs to have a full bladder so it is easier to identify on palpation.
    c. The pelvic examination is indicated every 3 years if a client is sexually active.
    d. The pelvic examination can be used to assess for infection or menstrual irregularities.

14. Which of the following is a common occurrence in the client after a pelvic examination?
    a. Abdominal pain
    b. Orthostatic hypotension
    c. Bleeding for 1 to 2 hours
    d. Nausea or anorexia

15. Annual digital rectal examinations and prostate-specific antigen (PSA) blood tests are recommended for all men older than what age?
    a. 35 years of age
    b. 40 years of age
    c. 45 years of age
    d. 50 years of age

16. Which of the following statements is true concerning a genitourinary reproductive examination of a male?
    a. The left and right side of the scrotal sac should be symmetrical.
    b. The epididymis and inguinal hernias cannot be palpated by external examination.
    c. The prostate gland is examined by a digital rectal examination.
    d. Penile discharge can only be assessed by an internal examination.

17. Which test would best evaluate the presence of a tubal dysfunction?
    a. Hysterosalpingography
    b. Computed tomography
    c. Urologic studies
    d. Radioimmunoassay

18. Which of the following radiologic assessment tests does not require any specific client preparation?
    a. IVP
    b. KUB
    c. Barium enema
    d. Hysterosalpingography

19. Which of the following diagnostic procedures necessitates performing a small incision?
    a. Laparoscopy
    b. Hysteroscopy
    c. Colposcopy
    d. Cystoscopy

20. Which of the following biopsies would require the use of a local or general anesthesia?
    a. Cervical biopsy
    b. Excisional biopsy of the breast
    c. Needle aspiration of the prostate
    d. Endometrial biopsy

21. An adult client presents to the clinic for her annual physical examination. She tells the nurse practitioner that she has been performing breast self-examination as directed, but was wondering when to have her first mammogram. The nurse tells the client that a baseline mammogram needs to be performed at what age?
    a. 40 years of age
    b. 30 years of age
    c. Between 50 and 55 years of age
    d. Between 35 and 40 years of age

22. Your adult client is scheduled to have an endometrial biopsy. The nurse is responsible for teaching her about this test. The nurse will teach this client which of the following?
    a. Abdominal cramping will last 1 to 2 weeks.
    b. Vaginal discharge will be heavy at times but will last only 10 to 14 days.
    c. Sexual activity should be postponed until the vaginal discharge stops.
    d. General anesthesia will be used for the procedure.

23. A client's Pap smear results were reported as having epithelial cell abnormalities with no evidence of dysplasia. These results are indicative of what classification based on the Papanicolaou scale?
    a. Class I
    b. Class II
    c. Class III
    d. Class IV

24. Why does a bilateral vasectomy function as a male contraceptive?
    a. Sperm production is prohibited.
    b. Ejaculation is prevented.
    c. Penile erection is limited.
    d. Passage of sperm to the semen is prevented.

25. Which of the most common cancers in young adult males can be treated effectively if found early?
    a. Prostate
    b. Colon
    c. Penile
    d. Testicular

26. Match each diagnostic test with the corresponding definition.

Diagnostic Test

_____ a. Culture

_____ b. Radioimmunoassay method

_____ c. Serologic test

_____ d. VDRL

_____ e. Pap smear

_____ f. FTA-ABS

_____ g. Wet smear specimen

_____ h. ELISA

_____ i. PSA

_____ j. 24-hour urine sample

Description

1. Detects cancerous and precancerous cells of the cervix
2. Screens for prostate cancer
3. Detects the causative agent of syphilis
4. Detects levels of estrogen, progesterone, and testosterone
5. Test used to screen for syphilis
6. Involves the use of a spray on preparation and a glass slide
7. Determines the occurrence of ovulation by levels of hormones
8. Detects antigen-antibody reactions
9. Detects the presence of a chlamydial infection
10. Determines appropriate antibiotic therapy

27. Match each etiology with the resulting dysfunction.

Etiology

_____ a.　Low levels of body fat or poor nutrition

_____ b.　Infertility in women

_____ c.　Substance abuse

_____ d.　Low rubella titers in child-bearing women

_____ e.　Mumps in postpubertal males

_____ f.　Endocrine disorders

_____ g.　Chronic disorders of nervous, respiratory, or cardiovascular system

_____ h.　Medications such as MAOIs, antihypertensives, antihistamines, and opioids

_____ i.　PID, salpingitis

Dysfunction
1. Teratogenic effects
2. Vaginal dryness, increased yeast infections, impotence
3. Impaired fertility
4. Ovarian dysfunction
5. Decreased spermatogenesis, libido, or impotence
6. Increased risk of endometrial cancer
7. Pelvic scarring and adhesions or infertility
8. Altered sexual response
9. Orchitis, sterility

28. Describe six of the physical changes that occur in a woman's body during climacteric and include the etiology of the physical change.

29. Discuss the difference between the terms menopause and climacteric.

30. State at least five causes of reproductive system dysfunction common to both males and females.

a. _____

b. _____

c. _____

d. _____

e. _____

31. Identify the different areas to be included in a genitoreproductive nursing history.

a. _____

b. _____

c. _____

d. _____

e. _____

f. _____

32. State five nursing diagnoses most often associated with diagnostic assessment of the male or female reproductive system.

a. _____

b. _____

c. _____

d. _____

e. _____

Interventions for Clients with Breast Disorders

CHAPTER 77

LEARNING OUTCOMES

1. Compare assessment findings associated with benign breast lesions with those of malignant breast lesions.
2. Describe the three-pronged approach to early detection of breast masses: mammography, clinical breast examination (CBE), and breast self-examination (BSE).
3. Teach a client how to do BSE.
4. Explain the options available to a woman at high genetic risk for breast cancer.
5. Analyze assessment data to determine priority nursing diagnoses and collaborative problems for a woman with breast cancer.
6. Develop a plan of care for a client with breast cancer.
7. Discuss the psychosocial aspects related to having breast cancer and undergoing surgery for breast cancer.
8. Formulate a community-based teaching plan for clients undergoing surgery for breast cancer.
9. Explain what options are available to a client considering breast reconstruction.

LEARNING ACTIVITIES

1. Before completing the study guide exercises for this chapter, it is recommended that you review the following:
   - Anatomy and physiology of male and female breast
   - Effect of the endocrine system on breast tissue
   - Concepts of human sexuality
   - Concepts of body image and self-esteem
   - Normal growth and development of breast tissue
   - Concepts of grief, loss, death, and dying

2. Review the boldfaced terms and their definitions in Chapter 77 to enhance your understanding of the content.

STUDY/REVIEW QUESTIONS

Answers to the Study/Review Questions are provided on the companion Evolve Learning Resources Web site at http://evolve.elsevier.com/Iggy/.

1. The nurse is teaching a 24-year-old client about breast self-examination (BSE). The nurse tells her that BSE needs to be performed how often?
   a. The day before her menstrual flow is due
   b. On the third day after her menstrual flow starts
   c. When ovulation occurs
   d. 1 week after her menstrual flow starts

2. Your young female adult client is suspected of having breast cancer. Based on the nurse's knowledge of types and frequencies of breast cancer, which of the following types is this client most likely to be diagnosed as having?
   a. Adenocystic
   b. Infiltrating ductal carcinoma
   c. Invasive lobular
   d. In situ breast

3. Cancer surveillance in high-risk women involves BSE, clinical breast examination (CBE), and mammography. Cancer surveillance is used to detect cancer in its early stages and is referred to as which of the following?
   a. Primary prevention
   b. Secondary prevention
   c. Tertiary prevention
   d. Prophylactic prevention

4. A female client has returned from surgery for breast reconstruction. She has a Jackson-Pratt drain in place that is patent and draining serosanguineous fluid. The nurse notices that at 8:00 AM the drainage container is full. It was last emptied at 6:00 AM. The total drainage for the last 2 hours is measured at 145 mL. Which of the following would be the priority nursing intervention?
   a. Notify the physician of the amount and type of drainage over the last 2 hours.
   b. Empty the drain every 2 hours so the suction will be more effective.
   c. Chart the type and amount of drainage.
   d. Report to the charge nurse that the night nurse really did not empty the drainage container.

5. Which of the following statements is true concerning fibrocystic breast disease?
   a. Seventy percent of women will have fibrocystic changes sometime during their lives.
   b. A diet of low salt, no caffeine, and the addition of vitamins C, E, and B is recommended.
   c. Fibrocystic disease occurs in several stages, which are characterized by painless, fluid-filled cysts.
   d. Danazol is the drug of choice for treating all types of fibrocystic disease.

6. Current research has identified several risk factors for the development of breast cancer. According to the latest studies, which of the following women has the greatest risk of developing breast cancer?
   a. A physician, age 56, who had her first child at 38
   b. A ballet dancer, age 20, who has a 5-year-old son
   c. A radiation tech, age 24, who had her menarche at age 13
   d. A postmenopausal woman, age 52, who had breast reduction surgery at age 26

7. A modified radical mastectomy involves the removal of which of the following?
   a. The involved breast and all of the axillary lymph nodes and chest muscles on the affected side
   b. The breast tumor, all surrounding breast tissue, and axillary lymph nodes on the affected side
   c. Only the breast tumor itself
   d. The entire breast only on the affected side

8. A client had a partial mastectomy yesterday. The nurse writes on the nursing care plan: "Risk for Anxiety related to removal of breast tissue." The nurse's priority intervention is which of the following?
   a. Use distraction until the client is better and able to think more clearly.
   b. Encourage the client to have a positive attitude so she will heal faster.
   c. Ensure that the client takes her pain medicine every 4 to 6 hours as ordered.
   d. Encourage the client to discuss her fears and ask questions about her concerns.

9. When teaching an ambulatory surgery client about discharge instructions following a partial mastectomy regarding care of the arm on the affected side, the nurse tells the client which of the following?
   a. Start arm exercises as soon as the drains are removed from the incision.
   b. Keep the arm elevated so that the elbow is above the shoulder and the wrist is above the elbow.
   c. Blood pressures cannot be taken in the arm on the affected side for the first 6 months postoperatively.
   d. Push-ups and arm circles are the exercises of choice for a full recovery.

10. A female client has been told that her breast tumor is 3 cm, nonfixed, with axillary metastasis. Based on this information, what stage of breast cancer is the most likely for this client?
    a. Stage I
    b. Stage II
    c. Stage III
    d. Stage IV

11. Which of the following factors will result in the least favorable prognosis for the above client?
    a. Estrogen receptor–positive status of the cancer cells
    b. Accelerated growth rate of the cancer cells
    c. Well-differentiated tumor
    d. Low alteration of DNA content

12. Which of the following factors will have the most influence on the client's choice for treatment of breast cancer?
    a. Her age at the time of diagnosis
    b. Overall health status of client
    c. Her personal choice and type of insurance
    d. Extent and location of metastasis of the breast mass

13. The priority preoperative nursing diagnosis for the client with breast cancer will most probably be which of the following?
    a. Deficient Knowledge
    b. Decisional Conflict
    c. Fear
    d. Anxiety

14. Why is the mammogram a more sensitive screening tool than some others presently available for early detection of breast cancer?
    a. It has a higher compliance rate than BSE because it is less painful.
    b. Radioimmunoassay to identify tumor markers is very expensive.
    c. It is able to reveal masses too small to be palpated manually.
    d. It is able to differentiate between fluid and solid masses.

15. The three-pronged approach to early detection of breast cancer is defined as which of the following?
    a. Breast self-examination, annual clinical breast examination, and ultrasound
    b. Clinical breast examination, mammogram, and ultrasound
    c. Mammogram, breast self-examination, and clinical breast examination
    d. Breast self-examination, mammogram, and ultrasound

16. Identify three breast changes the nurse would be most likely to see during the physical examination of a client with late-stage breast cancer.

    a. _____

    b. _____

    c. _____

17. The most common breast dysfunction found in the male breast is which of the following?
    a. Nipple discharge
    b. Nipple retraction
    c. Gynecomastia
    d. Disseminated breast cancer

18. A round, firm, nontender, mobile breast mass not attached to breast tissue or the chest wall is usually associated with which of the following?
    a. Fibroadenomas
    b. Fibrocystic disease
    c. Breast cysts
    d. Ductal ectasia

19. The treatment plan for the client with fibroadenoma will most likely include what interventions?

    a. _____

    b. _____

    c. _____

20. Identify places where breast cancer is most likely to metastasize.

    a. _____

    b. _____

    c. _____

    d. _____

21. Which of the following interventions would be the nurse's priority in the nursing care plan for a client after a modified radical mastectomy?
    a. Position the client on the affected side to aid with gravity flow of drainage from the incision site.
    b. Immobilize the arm on the affected side for the first 24 hours postoperatively.
    c. Assess the client for anxiety because it can impede the healing process.
    d. Teach the client signs and symptoms of infection and how to monitor for altered wound healing.

22. Which of the following organizations is a community resource available to women with breast cancer?
    a. Reach to Recovery
    b. Empty Arms
    c. Resolve
    d. Nami

23. A woman's acceptance of her postoperative appearance is most likely to be affected by which of the following?
    a. Preoperative teaching of expected appearance of the scar
    b. Ability to discuss her feeling and concerns
    c. Response of her partner and family to her postoperative appearance
    d. Ability to camouflage her postoperative appearance

24. The incidence of breast disease is most closely related to which of the following factors?
    a. Weight
    b. Age
    c. Ethnic background
    d. Socioeconomic status

25. What effect does prophylactic mastectomy have on the woman's risk for developing breast cancer?
    a. Increases
    b. Eliminates
    c. Decreases
    d. Doubles

26. What type of teaching increases the likelihood that a woman will be more compliant with the performance of regular monthly examinations?
    a. Learning from a pamphlet at home
    b. Learning at a clinic or office
    c. Practicing with a videotape
    d. Reading magazine articles

27. When do menopausal women need to perform BSEs?
    a. The first day of every other month
    b. One week after the last menstrual period
    c. The last day of each month
    d. Any day as long as the schedule is consistent

28. Fibroadenoma is the most common breast problem of women in what age range?
    a. 15 and 20 years old
    b. 20 and 30 years old
    c. 30 and 40 years old
    d. 40 and 50 years old.

29. Breast cancer has the highest death rate for women between what ages?
    a. 20 and 30 years
    b. 30 and 40 years
    c. 25 and 50 years
    d. 35 and 55 years

30. Which is the best synonym for the term "chemoprevention?"
    a. Chemotherapy
    b. Adjuvant treatment
    c. Prophylactic treatment
    d. Palliative treatment

31. Large-breasted women are at greater risk for which of the following?
    a. Fungal infections and backaches
    b. Difficulty nursing a baby
    c. Discharge from the nipples
    d. Fibrocystic disease

32. Ductal ectasia is associated with which symptoms?
    a. Nonpalpable mass and a serosanguineous nipple discharge
    b. Purulent nipple discharge and axillary pain
    c. Irregular palpable masses with enlarged axillary nodes
    d. Bilateral multicentric nodules and tenderness

33. Identify the most common procedure for breast reconstruction and distinguish it from other methods.

34. Compare and contrast a benign breast nodule to a malignant breast nodule on physical examination of the breast.

35. Identify five steps to assessing a breast mass.

    a. _____

    b. _____

    c. _____

    d. _____

    e. _____

36. Discuss four aspects of discharge home teaching in relation to physical care necessary for a positive postoperative course after a modified radical mastectomy.

37. Identify six instructions necessary for the nurse to teach a woman before having her demonstrate a breast self-examination.

CASE STUDY: FIBROCYSTIC BREAST DISEASE

Answer Guidelines for the Case Study questions are provided on the companion Evolve Learning Resources Web site at http://evolve.elsevier.com/Iggy/.

A 26-year-old woman reports during her annual gynecologic examination that she has been feeling fullness and soreness before her menstrual period and that she has felt some "marbles" in her breast. She is using contraceptive gel for prevention of pregnancy. The nurse palpates numerous nodules in both breasts and tells the client that this is most likely fibrocystic change in the breast tissue.

1. What will the nurse tell the patient about diagnostic testing that will be done?

2. What kinds of treatments might the nurse instruct the patient about after the diagnosis of fibrocystic breast disease (FBD) is confirmed?

3. What teaching will the nurse do to prepare the client to care for her symptoms?

Interventions for Clients with Gynecologic Problems

LEARNING OUTCOMES

1. Compare the pathophysiology, manifestations, and treatments of common menstrual cycle disorders.
2. Discuss common assessment findings associated with menopause.
3. Describe the mechanisms of action, side effects, and nursing implications for pharmacologic management of endometriosis.
4. Develop a teaching plan for a client with a vaginal inflammation or infection.
5. Prioritize care after surgery for the client undergoing an anterior or posterior repair.
6. Analyze assessment data for clients with leiomyomas to determine nursing diagnoses and collaborative problems.
7. Formulate a plan of care for a client undergoing a hysterectomy.
8. Identify the risk factors for gynecologic cancers.
9. Discuss the psychosocial issues associated with gynecologic cancers.
10. Explain the purpose of radiation and chemotherapy for clients with gynecologic cancers.
11. Develop a community-based plan of care for clients with gynecologic cancers.

LEARNING ACTIVITIES

1. Before completing the study guide exercises for this chapter, it is recommended that you review the following:
   - Anatomy and physiology of the female reproductive system
   - Effect of the endocrine system on the female reproductive system
   - Concepts of human sexuality
   - Concepts of body image and self-esteem.
   - Normal growth and development
   - Concepts of grief, loss, death, and dying
   - Perineal care
   - Sitz baths
   - Enema administration
   - Care of the patient undergoing chemotherapy and radiation therapy
   - The principles of perioperative nursing management
   - Assessment of the reproductive system

2. Review the boldfaced terms and their definitions in Chapter 78 to enhance your understanding of the content.

STUDY/REVIEW QUESTIONS

Answers to the Study/Review Questions are provided on the companion Evolve Learning Resources Web site at http://evolve.elsevier.com/Iggy/.

1. One current treatment of primary dysmenorrhea with a therapeutic intervention of medication includes the use of which of the following?
   a. MAOIs
   b. Beta blockers
   c. NSAIDs
   d. Prostaglandin stimulators

2. Which of the following women is at greatest risk for having premenstrual syndrome?
   a. 26-year-old with her first child
   b. 35-year-old with no children
   c. 32-year-old whose father died 6 months ago
   d. A 34-year-old mother of four with a recent postpartum tubal ligation

3. A 36-year-old woman has been having hot flashes, crying spells, and mood swings. Her physician wants to put her on hormone replacement therapy for her perimenopausal symptoms. The nurse realizes that this client's age means that she is experiencing which of the following?
   a. Early-onset menopause
   b. Late-onset menarche
   c. Normal menopause
   d. Signs of ovarian cancer

4. Hormone replacement therapy increases the menopausal client's risk of which of the following?
   a. Breast cancer
   b. Heart attack
   c. Deep vein thrombosis
   d. Osteoporosis

5. A client is diagnosed with vaginitis as the cause of her vaginal itching and discharge. The nurse is aware that a common cause of vaginitis is which of the following?
   a. Taking antibiotics
   b. Swimming in lakes
   c. Wiping front to back
   d. Inappropriate clothing

6. Which of the following is a treatment choice for vulvitis, which is caused by a nonpathologic condition?
   a. Vaginal creams
   b. Analgesics
   c. Sitz baths
   d. Antibiotics

7. Which of the following is the antigenic organism involved in toxic shock syndrome?
   a. *Escherichia coli*
   b. *Staphylococcus aureus*
   c. *Haemophilus influenzae*
   d. Beta-hemolytic *Streptococcus*

8. A nurse is teaching a group of teenagers about risk factors and toxic shock syndrome. The nurse will teach the class that women who use tampons are at an increased risk for toxic shock syndrome due to what characteristics of the product?

9. Which of the following symptoms would the nurse expect to observe in a woman with toxic shock syndrome?
   a. Hypertension and rash
   b. Sore throat and swollen lymph nodes
   c. Rash and chills
   d. Headache and constipation

10. The most common complaint reported of women with uterine leiomyomas (fibroids) is which of the following?
    a. Vaginal pressure and fullness
    b. Abnormal bleeding
    c. Intermittent pain
    d. Urinary dysfunction

11. What are three risk factors associated with cancer of the cervix?

    a. _____

    b. _____

    c. _____

12. Bartholin's cysts are commonly treated by which procedures?

13. A woman recovering from repair of a cystocele should be taught which of the following?
    a. To perform perineal floor exercises
    b. To take sitz baths three times a day
    c. To perform povidone-iodine douches every other day
    d. To take bedrest for the first 6 weeks

14. Which of the following is a priority nursing diagnosis commonly seen preoperatively as well as postoperatively in a woman with leiomyomas?
    a. Risk for Infection
    b. Acute Pain
    c. Risk for Altered Tissue Perfusion
    d. Anxiety

15. What is the treatment of choice for a symptomatic postmenopausal woman with recurring uterine leiomyomas?
    a. Myomectomy
    b. Hysterectomy
    c. Hormone replacement therapy
    d. Anteroposterior repair

16. Discharge teaching for the woman after having a total abdominal hysterectomy includes which of the following?
    a. Sexual activity may be resumed usually in 2 to 3 weeks if the incision has healed.
    b. Pain will decrease in about 2 to 3 days but may last for up to 6 weeks.
    c. Daily exercise such as walking is encouraged after the first 6 weeks.
    d. Wound care includes showering but no baths.

17. A client reports bleeding between her menstrual periods. What is this type of bleeding called?
    a. Dysmenorrhea
    b. Menorrhagia
    c. Metrorrhagia
    d. Polyrrhea

18. A client suffering from postmenopausal vaginal dryness can use which of the following to decrease sexual discomfort related to intercourse?
    a. Motrin
    b. Water-soluble gel
    c. Petroleum jelly
    d. Cream spermicide

19. Which is the most common symptom found to occur in women diagnosed as having endometrial cancer?
    a. Pelvic pain
    b. Nausea and anorexia
    c. Dysfunctional uterine bleeding
    d. Vaginal discharge

20. The nurse is giving instructions to a woman who is going to have intracavity radiation therapy (IRT). The nurse's postprocedure instructions should include which of the following?
    a. Bedrest with bathroom privileges only
    b. Maintain Trendelenburg position
    c. No visitors for 2 weeks
    d. Provision of a low-residue diet

21. A woman with complaints of abdominal pain and swelling, along with gastrointestinal disturbances, is generally diagnosed with which type of reproductive cancer?
    a. Endometrial
    b. Cervical
    c. Ovarian
    d. Vaginal

22. Amenorrhea can be the result of several physiologic and pathologic etiologies. Which of the following etiologies is characteristic of a pathologic state that causes unusual hair growth in addition to the amenorrhea?
    a. Anorexia nervosa
    b. Pregnancy with lactation
    c. Menopausal climacteria
    d. Polycystic ovarian disease

23. Which of the following physiologic factors is thought to be the etiologic cause of dysmenorrhea?
    a. Increased production of gonadotropin-releasing hormone
    b. Increased production of prostaglandins
    c. Decreased production of progesterone
    d. Decreased production of estradiol

24. Which of the following is the major reason for the onset of menopause and resulting atrophy of the vulvar organs?
    a. Decrease in levels of follicle-stimulating hormone
    b. Increase in levels of prostaglandin
    c. Decrease in levels of estrogen
    d. Increase in levels of luteinizing hormone

25. Which of the following is the most common and most serious cause of postmenopausal bleeding?
    a. Endometrial hyperplasia
    b. Increased production of gonadotropin-releasing hormone
    c. Atrophic vaginitis
    d. Toxic shock syndrome

26. Which of the following best describes endometriosis?
    a. Precursor to endometrial cancer
    b. Endometrial tissue implantation outside the uterus
    c. Progresses rapidly
    d. Exacerbates during pregnancy

27. Which of the following is the primary treatment for dysfunctional uterine bleeding in perimenopausal women?
    a. Hysterectomy
    b. Hormone replacement
    c. Radiation
    d. Chemotherapy

28. What type of cysts occur in young menstruating women and grow with hormonal influence?
    a. Corpus luteum cysts
    b. Follicular cysts
    c. Bartholin's cysts
    d. Theca-lutein cysts

29. Which of the following is treatment for ovarian cancer?
    a. Chemotherapy
    b. Hormone replacement
    c. Total hysterectomy and oophorectomy
    d. Radiation

30. Which of the following is the rarest of all gynecologic cancers?
    a. Vaginal
    b. Vulvar
    c. Fallopian
    d. Clitoral

31. What is the most common psychological complication following hysterectomy?
    a. Euphoria
    b. Depression
    c. Anger
    d. Increased libido

32. CIN (cervical intraepithelial neoplasia) is often treated with which of the following?
    a. Laser therapy
    b. Dilation and curettage
    c. Cryotherapy
    d. Radiation

33. Match each of the following terms to the corresponding definition.

Term

_____ a.   Uterine prolapse

_____ b.   Polycystic ovary

_____ c.   Cystocele

_____ d.   Ovarian fibroma

_____ e.   Urethrovaginal

_____ f.   Dermoid cyst

_____ g.   Fibroid

_____ h.   Rectocele

_____ i.   Theca-lutein cyst

_____ j.   Polyp

_____ k.   Chocolate cyst

_____ l.   Bartholin's cyst

Description
1. Area of endometriosis inside of an ovary
2. Protrusion of the bladder through the vaginal wall
3. Results in leakage of urine into the vagina
4. Ovarian cyst associated with a molar pregnancy
5. Protrusion of the rectum through the vaginal wall
6. Most common ovarian cyst of childhood
7. A common disorder of the vulva
8. Weakened pelvic floor muscles and a full feeling in the vagina
9. Ovarian cyst which causes endometrial hyperplasia
10. Most common benign tumor; can be very large and often occurs in postmenopausal women
11. Most common slow-growing pelvic tumor
12. Most common benign neoplastic growth of the cervix

34. Discuss primary dysmenorrhea, including its etiology and how it differs from secondary dysmenorrhea.

35. State four complementary and alternative treatment therapies for primary dysmenorrhea.

a. _____

b. _____

c. _____

d. _____

36. Identify eight major symptoms associated with premenstrual syndrome.

a. _____

b. _____

c. _____

d. _____

e. _____

f. _____

g. _____

h. _____

37. Compare primary amenorrhea to secondary amenorrhea. Include the etiology and fertility prognosis for both disorders.

38. Identify the most common methods of treating cancer of the reproductive organs.

a. _____

b. _____

c. _____

d. _____

e. _____

39. Postoperative nursing diagnoses for cancers of the reproductive tract are similar. Identify eight of these priority nursing diagnoses and collaborative problems.

a. _____

b. _____

c. _____

d. _____

e. _____

f. _____

g. _____

h. _____

CASE STUDY: ENDOMETRIOSIS

Answer Guidelines for the Case Study questions are provided on the companion Evolve Learning Resources Web site at http://evolve.elsevier.com/Iggy/.

A 28-year-old woman comes to the gynecologist's office with complaints of persistent lower abdominal pain, which peaks just before menstrual flow, and she has difficulty getting pregnant. She is very frustrated and wants to know "what's wrong" with her.

1. What will the nurse focus on during the history-taking?

2. What will the nurse tell the client about usual testing procedures for endometriosis?

3. What interventions will the nurse describe to the client as usual treatment for endometriosis?

4. What are the goals of nursing management of the client with endometriosis?

Interventions for Male Clients with Reproductive Problems

LEARNING OUTCOMES

1. Describe common physical assessment findings for the client with benign prostatic hyperplasia (BPH).
2. Describe the mechanisms of action, side effects, and nursing implications for pharmacologic management of BPH.
3. Discuss options for surgical management of the client with BPH.
4. Develop a postoperative plan of care for a client undergoing a transurethral resection of the prostate (TURP).
5. Identify the procedures for prostate cancer screening.
6. Explain the role of hormonal therapy in treating prostate cancer.
7. Develop a community-based plan of care for a client with prostate cancer.
8. Describe the options for treating erectile dysfunction.
9. Describe the mechanisms of action, side effects, and nursing implications for pharmacologic management of erectile dysfunction.
10. Discuss cultural considerations related to male reproductive problems.
11. Analyze assessment data to determine priority nursing diagnoses and collaborative problems for a man with testicular cancer.
12. Develop a plan of care for a client with testicular cancer.
13. Formulate a community-based teaching plan for continuing care of clients with testicular cancer.
14. Compare hydrocele, spermatocele, and varicocele.
15. Compare the four types of prostatitis.
16. Discuss issues related to sexuality and body image for a man experiencing male reproductive health problems.

LEARNING ACTIVITIES

1. Before completing the study guide exercises for this chapter, it is recommended that you review the following:
   - Anatomy and physiology of the male reproductive system
   - Effect of the endocrine system on the male reproductive tissue
   - Concepts of human sexuality

- Concepts of body image and self-esteem
- Normal growth and development
- Concepts of grief, loss, death, and dying
- Perineal care
- Sitz baths
- Enema administration
- Care of the patient undergoing chemotherapy and radiation therapy
- Principles of perioperative nursing management
- Assessment of the reproductive system

2. Review the boldfaced terms and their definitions in Chapter 79 to enhance your understanding of the content.

STUDY/REVIEW QUESTIONS

Answers to the Study/Review Questions are provided on the companion Evolve Learning Resources Web site at http://evolve.elsevier.com/Iggy/.

1. Identify three symptoms that would help in differentiating BPH, an obstructive dysfunction, from infection, a nonobstructive dysfunction.

   a. _____

   b. _____

   c. _____

2. Which of the following factors contribute to the development of prostate cancer?
   a. Family history, age younger than 40, and sexually transmitted diseases (STDs)
   b. Advancing age, family history, and history of STDs
   c. History of STDs, chicken pox, and decreasing testosterone levels
   d. Advancing age, diet, and history of cytomegalovirus infections

3. Prostate-specific antigen (PSA) is a glycoprotein produced solely by the prostate. After treatment for prostate cancer, an elevated PSA level can be used to indicate which of the following?
   a. Recurrence of the prostate cancer
   b. Responsiveness to cancer therapy
   c. Presence of a malignancy elsewhere in the body
   d. a and b

4. Which is the most common site for the metastasis of prostate cancer?
   a. Bone
   b. Lungs
   c. Liver
   d. Stomach

5. Clients with metastasis of their prostate cancer to the bone usually have an elevated level of which of the following?
   a. Alpha fetoprotein
   b. BUN
   c. Serum alkaline phosphatase
   d. Serum creatinine

6. What is the term for inflammation of the testicles associated with the occurrence of mumps in the postpubertal male?
   a. Prostatitis
   b. Epididymitis
   c. Orchitis
   d. Urethrits

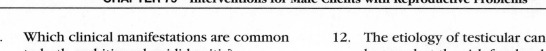

7. Which clinical manifestations are common to both orchitis and epididymitis?
    a. Scrotal pain and hematuria
    b. Scrotal pain and edema
    c. Scrotal edema and dysuria
    d. Scrotal edema and impotence

8. Your adult male client had a prostatectomy earlier this morning. He has a Foley catheter with a continuous bladder irrigation. Which of the following descriptions would the nurse expect to fit his urinary drainage?
    a. Light pink with small clots
    b. Bright red with small clots
    c. Dark burgundy with no clots
    d. Absent for the first 24 hours

9. Erectile dysfunction is commonly treated using all of the following except:
    a. Oral therapies
    b. Prostheses
    c. Vacuum devices
    d. Anticholinergics

10. Newly married at age 28, your male client has been performing testicular self-examinations since he was 16. He presents today because of a change in the size of his right testicle. Which of the following statements given to him by the nurse is correct information?
    a. Testicular cancer is always bilateral.
    b. Testicular cancer occurs most often in African-American men older than 25 years of age.
    c. An elevated alpha-fetoprotein level is used as a tumor marker for testicular cancer.
    d. An elevated alpha-fetoprotein level indicates metastatic disease of the testicular cancer.

11. Identify symptoms that the nurse would expect a client diagnosed with prostatitis to report.

12. The etiology of testicular cancer is still unknown, but the risk for developing a testicular tumor is reported to be higher in males with a history of which of the following?
    a. Hypospadias
    b. Recurrent urinary tract infections (UTIs)
    c. Cryptorchidism
    d. Orchitis

13. During the first 24 hours after prostatectomy, the nursing care plan would include the priority assessment for which of the following?
    a. Hemorrhage
    b. Risk for infection
    c. Risk for pneumonia
    d. Altered level of consciousness

14. An adult male client had surgery for his benign prostatic hyperplasia. He cannot remember the type of surgery but tells you he has no incision. As a nurse, you know that this client likely had which of the following procedures?
    a. Suprapubic prostatectomy
    b. Perineal prostatectomy
    c. Retropubic prostatectomy
    d. Transurethral resection

15. Which of the following nursing interventions can the nurse recommend to a client diagnosed with prostatitis?
    a. Take a stool softener to prevent straining.
    b. Take pain medications to prevent pain as needed.
    c. Use comfort measures such as sitz baths to provide pain relief.
    d. Use bladder antispasmodics to relieve bladder pain.

16. Benign prostatic hyperplasia is thought to result primarily from what conditions?

17. What approach is the most common type of closed procedure used for a prostatectomy?

18. What type of cancer is the most common malignancy in men 15 to 35 years of age?

19. How is a differential diagnosis made between organic erectile dysfunction and functional erectile dysfunction?

20. What is the primary complication resulting from a perineal prostatectomy?

21. The client with an indwelling catheter complains of the constant urge to void. What will the nurse tell him in teaching about this?

22. What is ordered to control painful bladder spasms after a prostatectomy?

23. How long after a prostatectomy can sexual activity usually resume?

24. Match each of the following terms with the corresponding fact.

Term

_____ a.   Spermatocele

_____ b.   Orchidopexy

_____ c.   Hydrocele

_____ d.   Phimosis

_____ e.   Varicocele

_____ f.   Cryptorchidism

_____ g.   Penectomy

_____ h.   Circumcision

_____ i.   Testicular torsion

_____ j.   Scrotal support

_____ k.   Priapism

_____ l.   Prostatitis

Fact

1. Results from a disorder in the lymphatic drainage of the scrotum, causing a mass around the testis

2. Uncontrolled penile erection without sexual desire, which is very painful

3. Surgical implantation of the testicle into the scrotal sac

4. Increased risk of suicide after this procedure

5. Inflammation can result from a viral or bacterial infection, STD, or a psychosexual problem

6. If not done at birth, requires strict personal hygiene to clean the prepuce

7. Very painful; a medical emergency

8. Palpation reveals a "wormlike" mass

9. Usually requires no intervention unless the client reports discomfort

10. Promotes drainage and comfort after surgery

11. Corrected by circumcision

12. Surgery for this condition may reduce the risk of testicular cancer

25. Prostate cancer is diagnosed by a combination of which two tests?

a.   _____

b.   _____

26. State five approaches for the medical treatment of prostate cancer.

a.   _____

b.   _____

c.   _____

d.   _____

e.   _____

27. Identify six common causes of organic erectile dysfunction.

    a. _____

    b. _____

    c. _____

    d. _____

    e. _____

    f. _____

28. Identify four common causes of priapism.

    a. _____

    b. _____

    c. _____

    d. _____

29. State three nursing diagnoses associated with male reproductive dysfunctions.

    a. _____

    b. _____

    c. _____

30. State four effects of benign prostatic hypertrophy on urinary elimination.

    a. _____

    b. _____

    c. _____

    d. _____

CASE STUDY: URINARY RETENTION SECONDARY TO PROSTATE ENLARGEMENT

Answer Guidelines for the Case Study questions are provided on the companion Evolve Learning Resources Web site at http://evolve.elsevier.com/Iggy/.

A 73-year-old man comes to the ambulatory urgent care center with complaints of burning on urination, urgency, dribbling of urine, and a feeling of bladder fullness. He states that he has noticed a gradual change in his urinary pattern over the past few months but attributes it to "old age." He adds that he would not have come in at all except that he noticed some burning when he urinated today. He also says his back has been hurting, but he attributes that to yard work and gardening.

1. When interviewing this client, what questions should be asked?

2. What areas should be the focus of the nursing assessment?

3. What laboratory tests and/or procedures can be expected for this client?

Interventions for Clients with Sexually Transmitted Diseases

CHAPTER

80

LEARNING OUTCOMES

1. Explain how sexually transmitted diseases (STDs) can be prevented.
2. Compare the stages of syphilis.
3. Prioritize nursing care for the client with syphilis at each stage.
4. Identify the role of drug therapy in managing clients with genital herpes (GH).
5. Discuss the psychosocial effects of having an STD.
6. Develop a community-based teaching plan for clients diagnosed with gonorrhea.
7. Describe the assessment findings that are typical in clients with *Chlamydia trachomatis* infection.
8. Analyze assessment data to determine common nursing diagnoses for women with pelvic inflammatory disease (PID).
9. Formulate a collaborative plan of care for a client with PID.
10. Describe the mechanisms of action, side effects, and nursing implications for drug therapy of PID.
11. Develop a community-based teaching plan for clients with PID.
12. Evaluate care for a client with PID.
13. Identify common causes of vaginal infections.

LEARNING ACTIVITIES

1. Before completing the study guide exercises for this chapter, it is recommended that you review the following:
   - Anatomy and physiology of the male and female reproductive system
   - Concepts of human sexuality
   - Perineal care
   - Principles of perioperative nursing management
   - Principles of infection transmission
   - Concepts of body image and self-esteem
   - Assessment of the reproductive system

2. Review the boldfaced terms and their definitions in Chapter 80 to enhance your understanding of the content.

STUDY/REVIEW QUESTIONS

Answers to the Study/Review Questions are provided on the companion Evolve Learning Resources Web site at http://evolve.elsevier.com/Iggy/.

1. List three complications associated with sexually transmitted diseases (STDs).

   a. _____

   b. _____

   c. _____

2. Syphilis is a disease with several stages. A client with central nervous system involvement, including hearing loss, would be diagnosed with what stage of syphilis?
   a. Primary
   b. Secondary
   c. Late tertiary
   d. Latent early

3. Which of the following is the medication of choice for treating any stage of syphilis?
   a. Penicillin-G
   b. Glucocorticoids
   c. Amoxicillin
   d. Tetracycline

4. What would be included in a nursing assessment of the client with symptoms of an STD?

5. What is the screening test for syphilis?
   a. ELISA serum test
   b. VDRL serum test
   c. FTA antibody test
   d. MHA assay test

6. A client has had genital herpes–HSV-2 for several years. She is at the clinic for her annual Papanicolaou smear and asks about long-term problems. The nurse's best response is based on the knowledge that HSV-2 infection is associated with which of the following?
   a. Pelvic inflammatory disease
   b. Vaginitis
   c. Cervical cancer
   d. Fetal infection

7. After being hospitalized for genital herpes, a female client is repeating discharge instructions to the nurse. The nurse knows that further teaching is necessary when she states:
   a. "I can be contagious even when I do not have any lesions."
   b. "If I get pregnant I need to tell my nurse midwife that I have genital herpes."
   c. "After taking all of my acyclovir, I will not have genital herpes anymore."
   d. "I need to have an annual Pap smear because of my increased risk for cervical cancer."

8. Which of the following is the medication of choice in the treatment of lymphogranuloma venereum?
   a. Doxycycline
   b. Penicillin-G
   c. Gentamicin
   d. Acyclovir

9. Identify the medications of choice used in the treatment of chancroid.

10. Many STDs involve genital lesions at the site of inoculation. A definitive diagnosis for granuloma inguinale is made from a cytologic smear from the ulcer and reveals the presence of which of the following?
    a. Koplik spots
    b. Barr bodies
    c. Janeway lesions
    d. Donovan bodies

11. Which of the following statements concerning sexually transmitted genital warts is true?
    a. Biopsy is not necessary for diagnosis because the lesion has a characteristic fern appearance.
    b. Treatment for genital warts must be on an inpatient basis and involves surgical removal of the lesions.
    c. The client must keep the genital area clean and dry and observe for secondary infections.
    d. Repeated treatments are not necessary once the external lesions are healed.

12. Complications of gonorrhea develop more often in women than in men because:
    a. Treatment for the disease can leave women infertile.
    b. The disease is asymptomatic in the early stages.
    c. Estrogen leaves the woman more resistant to antibiotic therapy.
    d. The disease is not curable in women.

13. How long is the usual incubation period for gonorrhea?
    a. 3 to 10 days
    b. 10 to 14 days
    c. 2 to 3 weeks
    d. 2 to 3 months

14. Identify three symptoms of gonorrhea.

    a. _____

    b. _____

    c. _____

15. Which is not a clinical manifestation of a chlamydial infection in men?
    a. Dysuria with voiding
    b. Urethritis
    c. Frequency of urination
    d. Thick green discharge

16. When obtaining a complete obstetric-gynecologic history, the nurse must also take a sexual history from the client. The nurse's most therapeutic approach to elicit information would be which of the following?
    a. Use a checklist to ask "yes" and "no" questions.
    b. Ask the client if there is anything she needs to tell you about her sexual history.
    c. Ask directly if the client has ever had an STD.
    d. Ask open-ended questions.

17. For the nurse to be an effective clinician when working with clients concerning sexuality, STDs, or other sexual concerns, the nurse must first do which of the following?
    a. Take a course on sexual relations and counseling.
    b. Know all about his or her client's concerns, problems, or needs.
    c. Be aware of his or her own sexual values, attitudes, and sexuality.
    d. Set up a meeting with the client's sexual partner.

18. A female client has an appointment today with her gynecologist physician because of a troublesome vaginal discharge. The discharge is diagnosed as trichomoniasis, and the client is given oral medication to treat the infection. The nurse will teach this client which of the following about the medication and her vaginal infection?
    a. Trichomonas vaginalis is self-limiting, but the medicine is needed to treat the vaginal itching.
    b. The client's sexual partner must be treated with the medication if the infection is to be resolved.
    c. The medication should be applied liberally to the external genitalia once a day.
    d. The vaginal infection can cause infertility in childbearing women.

19. An adult woman has been admitted to the gynecology floor with a diagnosis of pelvic inflammatory disease (PID). The nurse carefully assesses this client for complications because women with PID are at an increased risk for which of the following?
    a. Ovarian rupture
    b. Appendicitis
    c. Infertility
    d. STDs

20. What is the number one causative agent associated with PID?
    a. *Neisseria gonorrhoeae*
    b. *Escherichia coli*
    c. *Streptococcus* species
    d. *Chlamydia* species

21. What is the most common chief complaint that leads a client with PID to seek medical health care?
    a. Vaginal itching
    b. Lower abdominal pain
    c. Malaise with fever
    d. Abnormal menstrual flow

22. The activity orders for the client with PID are for bedrest with bathroom privileges. What position is best for her while on bedrest?
    a. Prone position
    b. Supine position
    c. Side-lying position
    d. Semi-Fowler's position

23. The client with PID is discharged home on oral antibiotics. The nurse should give her which of the following instructions regarding her monthly menstrual flow?
    a. "Use tampons only when your menstrual flow is heavy."
    b. "Follow your normal routine for using tampons unless the pain increases."
    c. "Use perineal pads until you are fully recovered."
    d. "Use tampons in the day and perineal pads at night."

24. When performing discharge teaching about the resumption of sexual relations to a client diagnosed with an STD, the nurse should teach the client which of the following?
    a. Sexual relations may be resumed, but she must douche within 24 hours after vaginal intercourse.
    b. Sexual relations are prohibited for 6 months.
    c. Sexual relations should be postponed until the treatment regimen is completed.
    d. Sexual relations are permitted unless there is an increase in abdominal pain.

25. What should the nurse tell the client with PID about the practice of vaginal douching?
    a. Increases a woman's risk for developing PID.
    b. Should be done daily during the course of the illness.
    c. Vinegar is the only safe solution to use.
    d. Use only disposable equipment.

26. Identify four reportable STDs.

    a. _____

    b. _____

    c. _____

    d. _____

27. Identify six indications for hospitalization of the client with PID.

    a. _____

    b. _____

    c. _____

    d. _____

    e. _____

    f. _____

28. Standards of care and treatment for STDs are developed by which organization?
    a. Family Planning
    b. American National Red Cross
    c. Centers for Disease Control and Prevention
    d. Food and Drug Administration

29. Identify eight categories of people at risk for HIV/AIDS.

    a. _____

    b. _____

    c. _____

    d. _____

    e. _____

    f. _____

    g. _____

    h. _____

30. Which statement about the treatment of genital herpes is correct?
    a. The infection is cured by medication.
    b. The goal of medication is to reduce symptoms and discomfort.
    c. Topical therapy is more effective than oral medications.
    d. Mild recurrent outbreaks respond well to antiviral therapy.

31. Match each of the following STDs with the corresponding definition.

Sexually Transmitted Disease

_____ a. Herpes simplex type 2

_____ b. Secondary syphilis

_____ c. Lymphogranuloma venereum

_____ d. Herpes genitalis

_____ e. Genital warts

_____ f. Primary syphilis

_____ g. Granuloma inguinale

_____ h. Gonorrhea

_____ i. Chancroid

_____ j. Chlamydia

_____ k. Hepatitis B

_____ l. Candida

Definition
1. Highly infectious state with the presence of a chancre
2. An infection limited to the vagina; very irritating, but has no long-term sequelae
3. The herpes virus responsible for the majority of genital and perianal lesions
4. Transmitted by direct sexual contact with mucosal surfaces and can be transmitted to the vaginally delivered neonate
5. Transient painless lesion that gives rise to secondary signs of infection as headache, malaise, or anorexia
6. Can lead to chronic disease state; vaccines are given as three injections over a period of 6 months
7. Most common sexually transmitted viral disease caused by the human papillomavirus (HPV)
8. Flu-like symptoms and a generalized rash
9. Nodules that ulcerate, grow together, and become a spreading ulcer, which can become mutilating
10. Most common STD in the United States
11. Genital lesions that are painful and bleed easily; known cofactor for HIV transmission
12. Initial infection that causes blisters, which rupture and cause painful lesions

32. State four methods for the transmission of organisms that cause STD.

    a. _____

    b. _____

    c. _____

    d. _____

33. Identify four reasons why women have more health problems associated with STDs than men.

34. Pregnant women are routinely screened for which STDs that can have devastating effects on the fetus or neonate?

    a. _____

    b. _____

    c. _____

    d. _____

35. Discuss four important facts about the treatment of gonorrheal infections the client needs to know before being released from treatment.

36. State four goals for the treatment of a client with genital herpes.

    a. _____

    b. _____

    c. _____

    d. _____

37. Describe six nursing responsibilities associated with the management of a client who is newly diagnosed with an STD.

Notes

Notes

Notes

Notes

Notes

Notes

Notes

Notes

Notes

Notes

Notes

Notes